NEONATAL AND INFANT EMERGENCIES

Caring for newborns and infants in the first year of life can be anxiety-provoking and challenging, especially for the emergency physician. This book was designed to address the most common complaints that an emergency provider may have to evaluate and treat. *Neonatal and Infant Emergencies* is divided into three sections for quick access to a variety of medical conditions. Section I covers the basics of neonate care in the emergency department and includes the general exam, airway management and sedation. Section II focuses on specific common complaints, such as failure to thrive, fever and seizures. Section III covers management of specific systems, including cardiology, dermatology and toxicology. The appendixes include handy pediatric formulas, immunization schedules and easy-to-use algorithms and tables. This book will serve as a practical resource for a wide range of health providers, from medical students, residents and Fellows to attending physicians.

Ghazala Q. Sharieff, MD, is Medical Director of the Rady Children's Hospital Emergency Care Center and Associate Clinical Professor, University of California, San Diego. She also serves as the Director of Pediatric Emergency Medicine for Palomar-Pomerado Health System and California Emergency Physicians.

Maureen McCollough, MD, is Associate Professor of Pediatrics and Emergency Medicine at the University of Southern California Keck School of Medicine and Director of the Pediatric Emergency Department, Department of Pediatrics. She is also Medical Director, Department of Emergency Medicine at Los Angeles County–USC Medical Center, Los Angeles, California.

Neonatal and Infant Emergencies

Edited by

GHAZALA Q. SHARIEFF

Rady Children's Hospital, San Diego, California

MAUREEN McCOLLOUGH

Los Angeles County–USC Medical Center

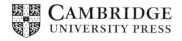

CAMBRIDGE
UNIVERSITY PRESS

CAMBRIDGE UNIVERSITY PRESS
Cambridge, New York, Melbourne, Madrid, Cape Town, Singapore, São Paulo, Delhi

Cambridge University Press
32 Avenue of the Americas, New York, NY 10013-2473, USA

www.cambridge.org
Information on this title: www.cambridge.org/9780521881135

First published 2009

Printed in the United States of America

A catalog record for this publication is available from the British Library.

Library of Congress Cataloging in Publication data

Neonatal and infant emergencies / edited by Ghazala Q. Sharieff, Maureen McCollough.
   p. ; cm.
Includes bibliographical references and index.
ISBN 978-0-521-88113-5 (hardback)
1. Neonatal emergencies – Handbooks, manuals, etc.   2. Pediatric emergencies – Handbooks,
manuals, etc.   I. Sharieff, Ghazala Q.   II. McCollough, Maureen, 1962–
[DNLM: 1. Emergencies.   2. Emergency Medical Services.   3. Infant, Newborn.   4. Infant.
WS 205 N438 2009]
RJ253.5.N42   2009
618.92′01–dc22   2008022709

ISBN   978-0-521-88113-5 hardback

To my husband, Javaid; my beautiful daughters, Mariyah and Aleena; and my friends and family who give me the inspiration and confidence to pursue dreams and transform them into reality – no matter how far out of reach they may seem.

Ghazala Q. Sharieff, MD

To my husband, Mike, and my daughters, Molly and Maggie . . . you are my life. To my parents, who inspired me to find a career that I would love . . . I hope that you are proud. To the providers of the world who care for children each and every day . . . this is for you.

Maureen McCollough, MD

CONTENTS

CONTRIBUTORS

Mohammed Al Mogbil, MD
Consultant
Pediatric Emergency Medicine
Department of Emergency Medicine
King Faisal Specialist Hospital and Research Center
Riyadh, Saudi Arabia

Joyce C. Arpilleda, MD, FAAP
Associate Clinical Professor, Department of Pediatrics
Associate Fellowship Program Director, Department of Emergency Medicine
University of California, San Diego
Attending Physician, Pediatric Emergency Department
Rady Children's Hospital
Children's Specialists of San Diego
San Diego, California

Adam Barouh, MD
Fellow
Pediatric Emergency Medicine
St. Christopher's Hospital for Children
Philadelphia, Pennsylvania

Michelle D. Blumstein, MD
Attending Physician
Pediatric Emergency Medicine
Division of Emergency Medicine
Miami Children's Hospital
Miami, Florida

Tonia J. Brousseau, DO
Attending Physician
Wolfson Children's Hospital
Jacksonville, Florida

James E. Colletti, MD, FAAP, FAAEM, FACEP
Assistant Professor
Department of Emergency Medicine

Mayo Clinic College of Medicine
Rochester, Minnesota

Stephanie J. Doniger, MD, FAAP, RDMS
Associate Director of Pediatric Emergency Ultrasound
Division of Emergency Medicine
Department of Surgery
Stanford University School of Medicine
Lucile Packard Children's Hospital
Palo Alto, California

Marla J. Friedman, DO
Attending Physician
Division of Emergency Medicine
Miami Children's Hospital
Miami, Florida

Stephen Gletsu, MD
Consultant
Department of Emergency Medicine
King Faisal Specialist Hospital and Research Center
Riyadh, Saudi Arabia

Jim R. Harley, MD
Emergency Medicine
Rady Children's Hospital
Emergency Medicine/Critical Care
Children's Specialists of San Diego
San Diego, California

Phyllis L. Hendry, MD, FAAP, FACEP
Associate Professor
Pediatric Emergency Medicine
University of Florida College of Medicine
Jacksonville, Florida

Martin I. Herman, MD, FAAP, FACEP
Professor of Pediatrics
Division of Emergency and Urgent Care Services
University of Tennessee Health Sciences Center
College of Medicine
Staff Physician
Emergency Department
Le Bonheur Children's Medical Center
Memphis, Tennessee

Paul Ishimine, MD
Associate Program Director
Pediatric Emergency Medicine
Rady Children's Hospital
San Diego, California

John T. Kanegaye, MD
Associate Clinical Professor
Department of Pediatrics
University of California, San Diego
Emergency Care Center
Rady Children's Hospital
San Diego, California

Kenneth T. Kwon, MD, RDMS, FACEP, FAAP
Associate Clinical Professor
Department of Emergency Medicine
University of California Irvine School of Medicine
Director
Pediatric Emergency Medicine
University of California Irvine Medical Center
Orange, California
Co-Director
Pediatric Emergency Services
Mission Regional Medical Center/Children's Hospital of Orange County at Mission
Mission Viejo, California

Audrey Le, MD
Fellow
University of Tennessee Health Sciences Center College of Medicine
Le Bonheur Children's Medical Center
Memphis, Tennessee

Jamie G. Lien, MD
Attending Physician
Rady Children's Hospital Emergency Care Center
San Diego, California

Merlin C. Lowe, Jr., MD, FAAP
Assistant Professor of Clinical Pediatrics
Department of Pediatrics
University of Arizona
Tucson, Arizona

Raemma P. Luck, MD, MBA, FAAP
Associate Professor
Department of Pediatrics and Emergency Medicine

Temple University School of Medicine
Director of Research
Deptartment of Emergency Medicine
St. Christopher's Hospital for Children
Philadelphia, Pennsylvania

Sharon E. Mace, MD, FACEP, FAAP
Professor of Medicine
Cleveland Clinic Lerner College of Medicine of Case Western Reserve University
Faculty, MetroHealth Medical Center Emergency Medicine Residency
Director, Pediatric Education/Quality Improvement
Director, Observation Unit
Cleveland Clinic
Cleveland, Ohio

P. Jamil Madati, MD
Assistant Clinical Professor
University of California San Diego School of Medicine
Division of Emergency Medicine
Children's Specialists San Diego
Rady Children's Hospital
San Diego, California

Christy A. Meade, MD
Pediatric Emergency Medicine
Rady Children's Hospital
San Diego, California

Maureen McCollough, MD
Associate Professor
Keck School of Medicine
University of Southern California
Medical Director
Department of Emergency Medicine
Los Angeles County–USC Medical Center
Los Angeles, California

Nadeem Qureshi, MD, FAAP, FCCM
Consultant, Pediatric Emergency Medicine
Chair, International Emergency Medicine Programe
King Faisal Specialist Hospital and Research Center
Riyadh, Saudi Arabia

Christiana R. Rajasingham, MD
Attending Physician
Emergency Care Center

Rady Children's Hospital
San Diego, California

Emily Rose, MD
Fellow
Pediatric Emergency Medicine
Loma Linda University
Loma Linda, California

Robert Sapien, MD
Professor, Emergency Medicine and Pediatrics
Chief, Division of Pediatric Emergency Medicine
Medical Director, EMS for Children
Department of Emergency Medicine
University of New Mexico Health Sciences Center
Albuquerque, New Mexico

Seema Shah, MD
Fellow
Pediatric Emergency Medicine
Rady Children's Hospital
San Diego, California

Ghazala Q. Sharieff, MD
Medical Director
Rady Children's Hospital Emergency Care Center
San Diego, California
Associate Clinical Professor
University of California, San Diego
San Diego, California

Virginia W. Tsai, MD
Fellow in Pediatric Emergency Medicine
Division of Emergency Medicine
Rady Children's Hospital
San Diego, California

Melissa A. Vitale, MD
Fellow
Pediatric Emergency Medicine
University of Pittsburgh School of Medicine
Children's Hospital of Pittsburgh
Pittsburgh, Pennsylvania

Dale P. Woolridge MD, PhD, FAAEM, FAAP, FACEP
Assistant Professor
Director, Pediatric Emergency Medicine

Director, Emergency Medicine/Pediatric Residency
Department of Emergency Medicine and Pediatrics
University of Arizona
Tucson, Arizona

Linton Yee, MD
Associate Professor, Department of Pediatrics
Division of Hospital and Emergency Medicine
Associate Professor, Department of Surgery
Division of Emergency Medicine
Director, Pediatric Emergency Medicine Education
Duke University School of Medicine
Durham, North Carolina

Noel S. Zuckerbraun, MD, MPH
Assistant Professor of Pediatrics
Department of Pediatrics
Division of Pediatric Emergency Medicine
University of Pittsburgh School of Medicine
Children's Hospital of Pittsburgh
Pittsburgh, Pennsylvania

PART I

NEONATAL AND INFANT CARE IN THE EMERGENCY DEPARTMENT – THE BASIC PRINCIPLES

1 Approach to the Newborn Examination

Merlin C. Lowe, Jr., and Dale P. Woolridge

INTRODUCTION

Newborns can be some of the most challenging patients evaluated in the emergency department (ED). It is important that health care providers understand the anatomical and physiological differences present in healthy newborns and very young infants. In addition, approximately one in five healthy newborns will have at least one congenital anomaly. As the number of congenital anomalies in an infant increases, the risk of major anomalies being present also increases.[1] A thorough, systematic approach to evaluating the newborn will help ensure that these anomalies, if present, are detected and that significant findings are not overlooked. It is important to recognize normal anomalies in order to prevent costly workups. It is also crucial for the practitioner not to miss an abnormal finding because he or she thinks that it is normal. Illness presentation in neonates can be subtle in that a direct history is not possible and the physical examination is often unreliable. The clinician must rely on vague symptoms, such as fussiness or eating less, and a comprehensive physical examination to detect illness.

A complete physical examination can be time-consuming. When time is limited, it is still important to have a concise yet thorough method for completing the examination. In the rapid examination, emphasis needs to be placed on the overall wellness of the infant, the heart, the lungs and the abdomen and any area identified as a potential problem area. A complete neurological examination is quite involved and may not be possible in the time available. The infant is observed for any signs of distress, including inconsolability and respiratory distress. The sleeping infant should be calm. While awake, the infant should be vigorous and interactive. Testing a few of the primitive reflexes generally can give a good sense of the baby's neurological condition. Monitor for symmetric facies and spontaneous limb movement. Any deficits need to be fully evaluated.

VITAL SIGNS

The general assessment also needs to include evaluation of the infant's vital signs. It is crucial to remember that the "normal" vital signs of an infant vary greatly depending on age. For example, a respiratory rate of 60 breaths per minute would be normal for a newborn but not for a 9 month old. Being unfamiliar with "normal" ranges for vital signs can lead to false views of the infant's overall well-being (Table 1.1. Vital signs also need to be correlated with other clinical indicators to better determine if the values are of concern (e.g., a heart rate of 150 beats per minute with poor perfusion is more concerning than a heart rate of 150 beats per minute with no signs of shock).

In neonates, fevers carry an increased association with serious bacterial infections, including osteomyelitis, sepsis, meningitis and urinary tract infections. The latter three are difficult to evaluate for during a physical examination. It is for this reason that infants younger than 28 days with a fever of 38°C (100.4°F) or higher are admitted to the hospital for a "rule out sepsis" evaluation. One should be aware that bundling an infant has often been attributed as the cause of a fever; however, it has been shown that bundling does not raise the core temperature and therefore should never be used as an excuse to avoid further evaluation.[2] One should also be alert for hypothermia in this age group as this can be an indicator of serious infection or other pathology. Hypothermia, fevers and temperature swings may be signals of not only infection but also of other problems such as hypoglycemia or hypo/hyperthyroidism.

The weight of a newborn infant should be considered another important vital sign. The body length and head

Table 1.1. Normal vital signs in the infant

Age	Heart rate[*]	Respiratory rate[†]	Systolic blood pressure
Newborn	90–180	40–60	60–90 mm Hg
1 mo	110–180	30–50	70–104 mm Hg
3 mo	110–180	30–45	70–104 mm Hg
6 mo	110–180	20–35	72–110 mm Hg

[*]Measured in beats per minute.
[†]Measured in breaths per minute.
Normal ranges for specified vital signs are listed. Ranges were obtained from *The Pediatric Emergency Medicine Resource*, revised 4th ed., 2006, Jones and Bartlett, p. 108.

circumference also may be crucial to consider, depending upon the chief complaint. These measurements, especially appropriate weight gain, can be early clues to potential problems or developing pathology. The average weight of a full-term newborn is 3.4 kg (7.5 lb). Parents often can recite the exact weight of their newborn at the time of the delivery. Newborns lose, on average, approximately 10% of their birth weight during the first few days after birth. This weight generally should be gained back by the end of the first 7 to 10 days. Average subsequent weight gain in the newborn period is 15 to 30 g (0.5–1 oz) per day. Standardized growth charts are available that can be used to determine appropriate weight for gestational age in premature infants. These growth charts are available for download from http://www.cdc.gov/growthcharts. Knowing the gestational age is important because a difference of 1 to 2 weeks can significantly change the average weight for a premature infant. By definition, an infant is the appropriate weight for gestational age if the weight is within 2 standard deviations (SD) of the mean. Several evaluation tools exist to help determine gestational age if it is unknown. These tools rely on the physical examination of the infant including neuromuscular development, skin findings such as creases, ear laxity, and breast/genital development.[3] When evaluating growth of infants, one should remember to correct the plotting on growth charts for gestational age. (e.g., a 6 month old who was born 32 weeks premature would be plotted on the 4-month-old line to account for the 8 weeks of prematurity.) This correction is continued until the infant reaches 2 years of age.

Babies who are large for gestational age (LGA) may have an underlying syndrome or may be large simply due to familial inheritance. If familial reasons are suspected, one can plot the parents' weight on growth charts to determine their percentiles. Parents in upper percentiles tend to have babies who are also in upper percentiles. Most commonly, LGA babies are born to diabetic mothers. (Infants of diabetic mothers have a variety of potential complications, including hypoglycemia, cardiac septal hypertrophy and meconium plug.)[4] Infants are particularly at risk for being LGA if the mother's blood sugar was poorly controlled during the last trimester.

Numerous syndromes can lead to LGA babies, including Soto, Beckwith-Wiedemann and Simpson-Golabi-Behmel syndrome. If a genetic syndrome is suspected, it is recommended that genetics consultation be obtained for further evaluation.

Similarly, small for gestational age (SGA) babies are at risk for congenital anomalies and complications; 20% of infants with serious congenital anomalies are SGA.[3] SGA infants should be monitored closely for development of hypoglycemia and temperature instability.

Both macrocephaly and microcephaly are associated with pathological findings. As an isolated finding, macrocephaly may be inherited from a parent. It shows an autosomal dominant inheritance pattern. Parental head circumference can be plotted to determine the percentiles using standard growth charts and plotting at the 18-year-old point.

Although macrocephaly may be inherited, most commonly it is associated with hydrocephalus.[5] Other physical findings that increase the suspicion of hydrocephalus include widening sutures or a bulging fontanel. A head circumference that is rapidly enlarging is very suspicious for hydrocephalus. Repeated examinations of the infant's skull over time allow for these changes to be noticed.

Microcephaly is more likely to be pathological and should be fully evaluated. Due to the open fontanel, a cranial ultrasound can provide significant information about underlying structures and spares the infant radiation that would be needed for a CT scan.

EVALUATION OF THE HEAD

The newborn skull is composed of a total of 22 bones: 8 encompass the brain and 14 form the facial skull. Most of these bones are not fused together at birth. This allows for significant molding to occur during the birth process. Resolution of molding typically occurs over the course of 3 to 5 days. This resolution can cause the head circumference

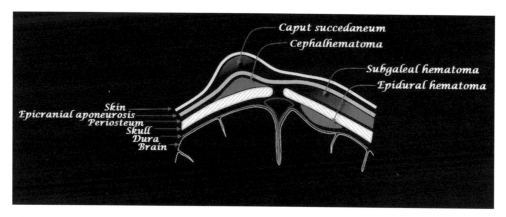

Figure 1.1. Caput succedaneum is the most common scalp injury due to birth trauma. Created by AMH Sheikh, Jan. 25, 2006. Used with permission.

to increase by as much as 1 cm and should not be mistaken for underlying hydrocephalus.[3]

Several other findings related to the birth process can present in the head as well. Caput succedaneum very commonly is seen; it is the most common scalp injury caused by birth trauma.[6] Caput succedaneum develops as a result of localized soft tissue edema. Vacuum extraction is particularly well known to cause it. The edema typically resolves within 48 hours (Figure 1.1). Caput succedaneum may cross suture lines, unlike a cephalhematoma. Cephalhematomas are blood collections that occur in the subperiosteal space. They occur in 1.5% to 2.5% of all deliveries. Vacuum and forceps extractions increase the incidence of a cephalhematoma to 9.8% to 14.8% and 4.1%, respectively.[6,7] Resolution of this bleed may take several days to weeks. Such a bleed also increases the risk of developing significant hyperbilirubinemia as the red blood cells break down.

Other important findings of the head examination include subgaleal bleeds, craniosynostosis and plagiocephaly, most commonly due to the infant repeatedly lying on the same side, with repeated pressure on one side of the head. One also should evaluate the fontanelles for their appropriate size and feel. A bulging fontanel is an indication of increased intracranial pressure. An overly large anterior fontanel may be associated with hypothyroidism. The anterior fontanel typically is closed by age 18 months. The posterior fontanel generally is closed within the first few months of life.[8]

The subgaleal space is a potential space that lies between the galeal aponeurosis and the periosteum. It can expand to allow significant amounts of blood into it. If this happens, the infant may require intensive resuscitation.

Mortality from a subgaleal bleed can reach 22%.[9] The skull will often take on a diffusely boggy feel when a subgaleal bleed is present.

In addition to evaluating for bleeds, the suture lines should be examined for pathology. Skull growth is driven by underlying brain growth. Infants have approximately 40% of their ultimate skull volume at birth. Brain growth rapidly occurs such that by age 3 years it has reached 80% of adult size.[10] Normally, the suture lines allow the skull bones to expand as the brain becomes larger. However, in cases of craniosynostosis (premature fusion of a suture line), skull growth is limited along the fused suture. As a result, skull growth continues perpendicular to that suture line causing significant plagiocephaly.

Craniosynostosis occurs with an incidence of 1 in 1700 to 2500 births with nonsyndromic cases and 1 in 25,000 births with syndromic cases.[11] Cases may involve a single suture line, termed *simple craniosynostosis*, or may be compounded, involving two or more sutures. The sagittal suture is most commonly involved, followed by the coronal, metopic and lambdoid sutures in decreasing incidence order.

Although it is the most uncommon, occurring in approximately 3 in 100,000 births, lambdoid suture synostosis can be confused with positional plagiocephaly.[10,11] Physical examination readily distinguishes between the two by evaluating ear position from above. In positional plagiocephaly, the skull is moved forward, causing the ear to be shifted forward on the affected side. In lambdoid synostosis, skull bone growth is restricted, causing the ear to remain posterior compared to the opposite side.

Craniosynostosis may be inherited, most commonly via an autosomal dominant pattern with varying degrees of penetrance and expressivity. Fibroblast growth factor receptor (FGFR) mutations have been implicated in several syndromes associated with craniosynostosis. As an example, three well-known syndromes, including craniosynostoses, Crouzon's disease and Apert's syndrome, are associated with mutations in the FGFR2 gene.[12]

Fontanel size can be easily evaluated in an infant by simple palpation of the skull. If molding is present, the fontanel may be somewhat obscured by overlapping skull bones; however, as molding resolves, the fontanel should take on its appropriate size. The fontanel size is determined by its surrounding bony structures, thus anything affecting fontanel growth will, in turn, affect its size. For example, skull bone growth is delayed in patients with congenital hypothyroidism, leading to an increased fontanel size. Fontanel size is determined as a measure of its greatest width and its greatest length. On day 1 of life, the average size of a full-term infant's anterior fontanel is 0.6 cm to 3.6 cm (0.2 – 1.4 inches).[13] Large fontanelles are also associated with Down syndrome, achondroplasia and increased intracranial pressure (due to the spreading of the skull bones).

EVALUATION OF THE EYES

The red reflexes of the eyes are easily evaluated using a direct ophthalmoscope. Eyes should be assessed for the presence of a red reflex as well as for any differences between the two eyes. *Leukocoria,* or a white reflex, may be present due to congenital cataracts (which may also present as black spots in the red reflex), retinal detachment, vitreous opacities or, the more commonly thought of, retinoblastoma. Findings of leukocoria warrant evaluation by an ophthalmologist to determine its cause. One should also remember that darker skinned babies often do not have a classic red reflex. Instead, the reflex is often more orange or lighter colored. The red reflex should not, however, be white. A *coloboma,* a hole or defect in one of the structures of the eye, such as eyelid, iris, lens, retina or optic disc, also can be searched for during the evaluation of the red reflex. Additionally, the papillary reflexes and strabismus can be seen during this evaluation.

Retinoblastoma has been shown to be associated with mutations or deletions of the q14 band of chromosome 13.[14] It is important to evaluate for as it presents with an incidence of 1 in 17,000 infants. Approximately 30% of cases will be bilateral.[15]

Congenital cataracts may present as black or white spots in the red reflex. They are present from birth but may not present until later in life. They occur in 0.44% of live births and may increase in size as the child ages; 23% of congenital cataracts are inherited (most often in an autosomal dominant pattern). When bilateral involvement occurs, there is an increased risk of an underlying metabolic or systemic disease including galactosemia, congenital infections (rubella, cytomegalovirus, herpes simplex virus and toxoplasma, in particular), Down syndrome and other trisomy syndromes and prematurity.[16]

A disconjugate gaze may be noticed during examination of the red reflexes. One can use the papillary light reflex to assess easily for this. A newborn may have eyes that are crossed or divergent. These findings will generally self-correct within 2 months.[17] Persistent disconjugate gaze may be an indicator of an underlying vision problem or other defect of one or both eyes. It is important to detect vision issues early to attempt to prevent permanent vision loss and amblyopia. Often, if one eye is weaker than the other, the stronger eye can be patched to encourage strengthening of the weaker eye. If patching is not performed while the child is young, the risk of permanent amblyopia increases.

The iris of newborns is typically grey or blue-grey at birth in lighter skinned infants and dark grey or brown in darker skinned infants.[16] Colobomas can affect the iris as well, often giving a keyhole appearance to the iris. The presence of colobomas should prompt a full evaluation of the child as they are commonly associated with other congenital syndromes.

Areas of stromal hyperplasia surrounded by areas of hypoplasia are referred to as *Brushfield spots.* They give a speckled appearance to the iris. They can be seen in normal infants; however, more commonly, they are seen in association with Down syndrome. Approximately 90% of Down syndrome infants will have Brushfield spots.[18]

Blue scleras often make the clinician suspicious of underlying osteogenesis imperfecta. A bluish coloring of the sclera also can be seen in other connective tissue disorders such as Ehlers-Danlos syndrome. Keep in mind that "normal" newborns also may have a bluish tint to their sclera due to the sclera being thinner at that age.[16]

Following birth, subconjunctival hemorrhages very commonly are seen. These can cause significant anxiety for the parent, although they are harmless to the infant. They are formed due to a ruptured blood vessel below the conjunctiva and will generally resorb within 1 to 2 weeks.

The examiner may also note nystagmus on examination. *Nystagmus* is repetitive, involuntary and rhythmic movement of the eyes in one direction. It may be horizontal, vertical or rotary in nature. This should be distinguished from opsoclonus, which is rapid, irregular and nonrhythmic movement that is associated with acute febrile episodes (especially when caused by Epstein-Barr, varicella, Coxsackie and West Nile viruses) or with conditions such as neuroblastoma (where it is seen in conjunction with myoclonus).[16,19]

Nystagmus may have several causes in neonates, both benign and pathological. It can be seen due to prematurity or with retinopathy of prematurity. It also may be seen in a condition known as *transient neonatal nystagmus,* which typically will develop before age 10 months, has a mean age of onset of 2.7 months and resolves spontaneously by 1 year of age. The cause of this condition is not yet known.[20]

Eye complaints are often what brings new parents into the ED with their newborn. Silver nitrate drops used in the delivery room cause a chemical conjunctivitis in 10% of newborns. Beginning in the first 24 hours, chemical conjunctivitis presents with bilateral mild conjunctival hyperemia and mild discharge that usually resolves within 48 hours. Gram stain will be negative and no intervention is necessary. Chlamydia, causing neonatal conjunctivitis, typically has an incubation period of 1 to 2 weeks but can occur earlier due to premature rupture of the membranes. The conjunctiva becomes hyperemic and edematous with the palpebral conjunctiva more involved. Usually, only one eye is affected. Otitis media or afebrile pneumonia also may be present. Chlamydia can lead to conjunctival scarring and micropannus formation. Diagnosis can be made by identifying the chlamydial antigen, identifying intracellular inclusions from the Giemsa stain, or isolating the organism by culture from the palpebral conjunctiva of the lower lid. Gram stain typically is not useful. Oral erythromycin (40–50 mg/kg/day) for 2 to 3 weeks will eliminate colonization of both the eyes and nose. Recent studies show that prophylaxis with erythromycin ointment at birth does not decrease the incidence of chlamydial conjunctivitis.[21]

Neisseria gonorrhea has a wide-ranging incubation period, from 1 to 31 days, but clinical symptoms usually occur within the first week. It typically presents as a bilateral purulent conjunctivitis, but conjunctival hyperemia, chemosis, eyelid edema and erythema also may be present. Gram stain will reveal gram-negative intracellular diplococci. Cultures on both blood and chocolate agar should be sent for examination. Infants with gonorrheal conjunctivitis also may have evidence of rhinitis, anorectal infection, arthritis or meningitis. If gonorrheal conjunctivitis is suspected or determined, then a complete septic workup is warranted, including a lumbar puncture. Treatment includes admission for intravenous (IV) ceftriaxone or cefotaxime and frequent irrigation of the eyes. Parents should be screened for gonorrhea.[21]

Other bacteria, such as *Staphylococcus aureus, Hemophilus, Streptococcus pneumoniae, Enterococcus, Corynebacterium, Lactobacillus* or *Bacteroides* can either cause conjunctivitis or be normal flora. In such cases of infection, the conjunctiva is typically red and edematous with some exudate. Diagnosis is made by both Gram stain and culture. Broad spectrum topical antibiotics are recommended. Untreated cases of conjunctivitis may lead to corneal ulceration, perforation, scarring or bacteremia.

Viral causes of conjunctivitis in neonates also are very common, with the most likely source being family members. Usually, these infections are self-limited. Topical antibiotics can be prescribed to avoid secondary infection and to treat a possible early bacterial infection due to self-inoculation from eye-rubbing. Washing hands and not sharing towels is also important to avoid spread. Herpes simplex, on occasion, may cause conjunctivitis in newborns. Usually appearing within the first 2 weeks of life, herpes conjunctivitis will show nonspecific lid edema, conjunctival injection and serosanguineous discharge. In newborns, microdendrites and geographic ulcers are more common than the typical dendrites seen in adults. Herpes becomes colonized in the newborn during the birth process; therefore, a history of herpes infection in the parents is important to obtain so the physician can initiate preventative measures. Herpes conjunctivitis can lead to more systemic infections with higher morbidity and mortality. Conjunctival scrapings may reveal multinucleated giant cells and intranuclear inclusions. A fluorescent antibody test and viral culture should be obtained. Herpes conjunctivitis in the newborn should be treated with IV acyclovir and topical 1% trifluiridine drops or 3% vidarabine ointment.[21]

Another common eye complaint in newborns that continues into infancy is a congenital nasolacrimal duct obstruction (dacryostenosis). Failure to canalize the valve of Hasner is the cause. Infants present with tearing and eyelid maceration. Congenital glaucoma can present not only with tearing but also with photophobia and a cloudy enlarged cornea. Treatment of dacryostenosis includes massaging of the lacrimal sac, prophylactic topical antibiotics and warm compresses. Most ductal obstruction spontaneously resolves by 12 months of age.

EVALUATION OF THE EARS

The ears should be examined for position in relation to the eyes as well as from a top-down perspective to look for posterior or anterior set ears. *Low set ears* (defined as ears with the top of the pinna below the middle of eye level) have been associated with numerous syndromes.

Preauricular skin tags or pitting is quite common. It was once stated that any preauricular pits or skin tags required an evaluation for renal anomalies; however, after further study, it is now expressed that no further workup is needed unless there is indication of other possible anomalies during the remainder of the examination. Familial preauricular pitting has been associated with hearing loss. These patients should have their hearing screened periodically.[3] More significant otic anomalies can be associated with genitourinary anomalies. A renal ultrasound is generally indicated in any such patient.

Lastly, visualization of the tympanic membrane is difficult in newborns due to tortuous canals. Amniotic fluid may remain behind the tympanic membrane for several days to a couple of weeks after birth.

EVALUATION OF THE NOSE, MOUTH AND PHARYNX

Newborns and very young infants are obligate nose breathers. When challenged by nasal congestion from an upper respiratory infection, many newborns are unable to compensate. The newborn's normal oral intake may decline. It is important to instruct the parents how to perform bulb suctioning of the nasal passages prior to feedings and sleep. Many normal variants can be found in the mouth. Epstein's pearls, Bohn nodules and natal teeth are commonly seen. Epstein's pearls and Bohn nodules have a white or yellow appearance, giving the look of a pearl. Epstein's pearls are located near the midpalatal raphe at the junction of the hard and soft palates. Bohn nodules are located on the alveolar ridges. Both represent remnants of embryonic development of the dental lamina. These findings will resolve spontaneously and do not cause any harm to the infant while present. *Natal teeth* are defined as teeth that erupt before 30 days of life. They are seen in approximately 1 in 3000 newborns. Generally, the mandibular incisors are involved.[22] These teeth lack any significant root system, thus they ultimately fall out. They need not be removed unless there is concern for aspiration of the tooth when it dislodges or if the tooth interferes with proper feeding.[23]

Cleft lip, cleft palate or a combination of the two represent the most common newborn head and neck anomaly; only clubfoot is more common overall. Of affected infants, 46% have a combination of cleft lip and palate, whereas 21% and 33% have an isolated cleft lip or palate, respectively. Most are quite obvious; however, a finger should be inserted into the mouth to palpate the palate as submucosal clefts can be difficult to identify without palpation. Infants with a cleft should be evaluated by a plastic surgeon because surgical correction of these anomalies generally produces excellent results. Delay in correction may cause unneeded difficulties in feeding and speech development.

Occasionally, parents or even inexperienced clinicians become concerned about a mass in the throat. Many times they are seeing the tip of the epiglottis that can extend upward into visual range in the newborn. The parents need to be reassured that this is normal in order to avoid unnecessary workup.

EVALUATION OF THE NECK

An infant with positional plagiocephaly should be evaluated for underlying congenital muscular torticollis (CMT), seen in 1 in 250 live births.[24] An infant with CMT presents with his or her head flexed and chin turned opposite the affected muscle. Approximately two-thirds of patients with CMT have a palpable mass in the affected muscle. When plagiocephaly is present, detection of CMT is important as uncorrected torticollis beyond 1 year of age tends to lead to persistent plagiocephaly.[25] Physical therapy generally is curative. Rarely, surgical intervention is needed. Recognition of this condition is important because plagiocephaly has an increased risk of becoming permanent if the torticollis is not corrected by age 1 year.[25]

Branchial cleft cysts, sinuses or other anomalies can present in the neck as well. The neck needs to be examined closely for any remnants of the branchial clefts or arches.

These may be found involving the pinna of the ear, the preauricular area or the lateral neck. Several syndromes are associated with branchial cleft anomalies, including Goldenhar syndrome and Pierre Robin syndrome.

Occasionally, a thyroglossal duct cyst that has become infected may present as a central neck cellulitis. Midline neck lesions should prompt examination for an underlying thyroglossal duct cyst.

EVALUATION OF THE CHEST AND LUNGS

When examining the chest, it is important to not become fixed on the lung sounds; the remainder of the chest should be evaluated for any possible anomalies as well. The clavicles should each be palpated for any feeling of crepitus or malalignment that may indicate a clavicle fracture. Clavicle fractures occur in 0.2% to 3.5% of births.[26] Fortunately, even severely angulated clavicle fractures will heal very well with no intervention. Parents should be instructed on the use of pain medications for their baby. Pain should subside quite quickly.

Newborns of both genders can develop breast enlargement and neonatal acne due to maternal hormones. These hormones also can cause vaginal bleeding in newborn girls. This triad has been termed *puberty of the newborn period*. Parental reassurance as to why this occurs is the only treatment that is needed. Occasionally, mastitis may develop in the newborn breast tissue. Any newborn diagnosed with mastitis should be admitted to the hospital for IV antibiotics. Choice of antibiotic should include methicillin-resistant *S. aureus* coverage as this organism appears to be increasing in frequency in the newborn period.[27] If an abscess is suspected, surgical consultation is mandatory. Much information can be gained about the respiratory status of a neonate by observing the chest while the infant is breathing. Chest movement should be symmetrical. Subcostal, suprasternal and intracostal retractions should be noted. So-called abdominal breathing can be a sign that the young infant is working harder to breathe. Nasal flaring and grunting also indicate respiratory distress. Fever and tachypnea may indicate an underlying pneumonia. Infants presenting with tachypnea, an increased oxygen requirement and lack of hypercapnia shortly after birth are likely to be experiencing transient tachypnea of the newborn (TTN). TTN is seen in approximately 0.3% to 0.5% of newborns and will resolve within 24 to 72 hours.[28] Infants with TTN-like symptoms that do not resolve within this time period should be reevaluated for a different cause of respiratory distress.

Periodic breathing is defined as periods of rapid breathing followed by short pauses. The pauses are not associated with mental status change, color change or limpness. Periodic breathing occurs in "normal" newborns. It can occur more often when newborns and young infants are tired or ill. Periodic breathing can be mistaken for apnea. *Apnea* is defined as a cessation of breathing that is either longer than 20 seconds or associated with cyanosis, mental status change or limpness. Any newborn diagnosed with apnea needs to be admitted to the hospital for a complete workup. Apnea can be caused by a variety of conditions, including sepsis, respiratory infections such as pertussis or respiratory syncytial virus (RSV), or apnea of prematurity.

EVALUATION OF THE CARDIOVASCULAR SYSTEM

Significant transitions occur within the cardiovascular system at the time of birth. Prior to birth, the infant is not using the lungs for ventilation, thus blood flow is generally shunted away from the lungs and back to the body. This occurs due to an elevated pulmonary blood pressure, a patent ductus arteriosus and a patent foramen ovale. At birth, the lungs need to become fully active and these bypass systems must adjust. As the lungs expand, the pulmonary pressures begin to drop. This transition lowers the right atrial pressure, allowing the foramen ovale to close. The ductus arteriosus typically will functionally close 10 to 15 hours after birth but may not fully fuse for up to 3 weeks.[29] Infants who require the ductus to be open to maintain systemic circulation, as in some individuals with congenital heart diseases, may not begin to close their ductus until days after birth. When this delayed closure finally occurs, the newborn typically will present with cyanosis or poor systemic cardiovascular perfusion (see Chapter 15). Pulmonary pressures typically continue to fall for 4 to 6 weeks after birth. Because of this, a newborn typically has a single S2 that becomes physiologically split as pressures fall. S1 is typically single and loudest near the apex of the heart. Additionally, near the apex, an S3 may be heard and is considered normal in infants. An S4 is not considered normal in neonates and should be evaluated further. Infants often have quite rapid heart rates that can make distinguishing heart sounds difficult. If in doubt, evaluation is prudent. Pulses should be palpated in all four extremities, noting their strength and regularity. Diminished pulses in the lower extremities may be an indication of coarctation of the aorta.

The newborn cardiac examination can reveal many murmurs that may or may not be considered innocent. Very commonly, a flow murmur can be heard. This murmur is a systolic ejection murmur and has a vibratory or musical sound to it. It is often heard best in the lower left sternal boarder area. This and other innocent murmurs are typically soft (I-II/VI in strength) and generally do not radiate.

A machinelike murmur that is heard just below the left clavicle is likely to be a patent ductus arteriosus (PDA) murmur. This murmur is often described as a continuous murmur that waxes and wanes in volume. As pulmonary pressures drop, a PDA murmur may become more prominent.

Murmurs that are harsh sounding are less likely to be physiologic. Holosystolic or diastolic murmurs are never innocent and should be evaluated. Most commonly, a holosystolic murmur is due to a ventricular septal defect (VSD). VSDs represent 15% to 20% of congenital cardiac defects.[30] The classic holosystolic murmur of the VSD may be absent at birth due to increased right-sided cardiac pressures preventing significant blood flow across the VSD. As pulmonary pressures decrease, blood flow increases and the murmur becomes apparent.

Many congenital syndromes are associated with predictable cardiac defects. When these defects are found, an underlying syndrome should be considered. As an example, 30% of patients with a complete atrioventricular septal defect (AVSD) have Down syndrome.[30]

If concern about the cardiovascular system exists, evaluation typically includes a chest x-ray, electrocardiogram (ECG) and echocardiogram. Just as vital signs vary with age, ECG standards vary as well. Tables of standard ECG values should be consulted when interpreting pediatric ECGs to ensure aberrations are not missed (see Chapter 15).

EVALUATION OF THE ABDOMEN

The assessment of the newborn abdomen includes the same components as with older children. The areas of the liver, spleen and kidneys are palpated.. The newborn liver edge frequently is located approximately 1 cm below the right costal margin. This extension is normal. At 1 week of age, a normal liver span is 4.5 to 5 cm.[31] Tables of normal liver spans for age exist and can be consulted, if needed. The liver edge is examined using the flats of the fingers as they are more sensitive to masses than the fingertips. Palpation should start in the left lower quadrant and move slowly to the right upper quadrant to avoid missing a dramatically enlarged liver.

The spleen should not be palpable, in general. It may become enlarged and palpable in several conditions that can present in the newborn. Any of the hemolyzing states, such as rhesus factor (Rh factor) or ABO incompatibility, or red cell defects, such as spherocytosis, can result in an enlarged liver. Typically, these are accompanied by prolonged or severe jaundice.

If the kidneys are enlarged, they are often easily palpable. (Note that it is often possible to palpate a normal kidney because infants have a compliable abdominal compartment.) Cystic or enlarged kidneys can be quite large at birth. If the kidneys are enlarged bilaterally, autosomal recessive polycystic kidney disease should be considered.[32]

The umbilical cord of a newborn should be inspected. A normal umbilical cord should have two arteries and one vein. Approximately 0.2% to 1% of newborns have a single umbilical artery. It has been shown that these infants have a three- and sixfold higher incidence, respectively, of severe renal anomalies and renal malformations compared with the general population.[33,34]

Often, parents complain of discharge or odor around the infant's healing umbilicus. Most often this is due to inadequate cleaning of the area. Parents should be instructed on good umbilical hygiene. Any nonhealing granulation tissue that remains after the cord falls off can be treated with silver nitrate application; it is important to avoid getting silver nitrate on the surrounding normal skin. Any redness surrounding the umbilical area should be considered the bacterial infection, omphalitis until proven otherwise. Etiology includes both gram-positive and gram-negative organisms such as *S. aureus*, group A Streptococcus, *Escherichia coli*, *Klebsiella pneumoniae* and *Proteus mirabilis*.

Newborns at higher risk for umbilical infection include those with premature rupture of membranes and those with umbilical catheterization. Other risk factors include patent urachus and immunodeficiency. Omphalitis is of concern as the infection may progress to fascial planes (necrotizing fasciitis), abdominal wall musculature (myonecrosis) and the umbilical and portal veins (phlebitis). Mortality rates are high, estimated at 7% to 15%. Admission to the hospital is mandatory. IV antibiotics such as oxacillin and gentamicin provide good gram-positive and gram-negative coverage. Recently, however, methicillin-resistant *S. aureus* has increased in frequency in the newborn period, thus better coverage may include vancomycin and gentamicin.[27] If more extensive infection is present, such as necrotizing fasciitis or myonecrosis, then anaerobic coverage should be added with metronidazole or clindamycin. If an abscess is present, then surgical consultation is also recommended.[35] The umbilical cord usually dries up and falls off within the first 2 weeks after birth. An umbilical cord that is still present after 4 weeks is of concern because it may indicate an immunodeficiency and should be investigated. A continuous or intermittent clear yellow discharge from the umbilicus also may be a sign of a patent urachus or urachal sinus. Crying, voiding, straining or lying in the prone position can increase the discharge. Evaluation of the fluid for urea or creatinine can prove the presence of urine. A patent urachus may be associated with a bladder obstruction due to posterior urethral valves. Ultrasound or a voiding cystourethrogram (VCUG) can be used to make the diagnosis. The patent tract may become inflamed with tenderness, swelling and a serosanguinous or purulent discharge. A patent ductus can be observed as some may spontaneously resolve in the first 2 months of life. Umbilical hernias also may be present at birth. These rarely produce incarceration of the bowel and most resolve by the age of 1 year. Parents should be discouraged from using home remedies such as the taping of a coin or abdominal binders on the newborn. If an umbilical hernia is still present when the infant is 1 year old, he or she can be referred to a pediatric surgeon for hernia repair. Infants with a congenital diaphragmatic hernia (CDH) may present with a scaphoid abdomen at birth. If CDH is suspected, the infant should be immediately intubated at birth to prevent introduction of air into the stomach, which may increase pressure on the lungs and mediastinum. Note that absence of a scaphoid abdomen does not rule out CDH. CDHs can, on occasion, present several weeks to months after birth, often when a significant lower respiratory tract infection such as RSV or pneumonia compromises the young infant. Rarely, an absence of the abdominal musculature may be seen. In combination with cryptorchidism and urinary tract anomalies, this condition is termed *prune belly syndrome* or the *Eagle-Barrett triad*. It occurs in 1 in 40,000 births; 95% of cases are found in males.[36]

EVALUATION OF THE GENITOURINARY TRACT

As this area is generally covered by the diaper, it may not get a proper evaluation; however, there are numerous genitourinary tract anomalies that are important to identify if present. Male infants should be evaluated for hypospadius or other urethral anomalies, inguinal hernias, varicoceles, hydroceles and undescended testes. The cremasteric reflex can be quite strong in infants. This reflex pulls the testes into the inguinal canal, which can give the impression of an undescended testis. In patients with a strong reflex, the testis can be brought fully into the scrotum. In approximately 3% to 4% of boys, the testis truly is not able to be brought fully into the scrotum at birth (termed *cryptorchidism*). By age 1 year, most testes have descended; only 0.3% remain undescended.[32] True undescended testes have a four- to tenfold higher risk of developing a malignancy (most commonly a seminoma) than do descended testes.[32] For this reason, the testis should be surgically brought down into the scrotum to allow for easy examination and earlier detection of masses.

Varicoceles and hydroceles can present with an enlarged scrotum. Varicoceles are often described as feeling like a "bag of worms" in the scrotum. They develop from a dilation of the pampiniform plexus and internal spermatic vein. They are more commonly seen on the left and when the infant is upright. Varicoceles should reduce easily with constant pressure while the infant is lying flat. If the varicoceles will not reduce or are found on the right, there should be suspicion of venous blockage. This may be indicative of an abdominal mass. Abdominal ultrasound is a fast, painless, noninvasive way to evaluate for this.[37]

Hydroceles can be distinguished easily from a varicocele or hernia by transillumination. A hydrocele is formed when the processus vaginalis fails to close fully but closes enough to prevent bowel herniation. Only fluid is allowed to enter the scrotum. This fluid easily transilluminates. Rarely, bowel also may transilluminate, giving the impression of a hydrocele, but palpation is likely to help distinguish the two. If necessary, ultrasound can be used to verify the diagnosis. Hydroceles resolve spontaneously by age 12 to 28 months in most cases.[38] Those that do not resolve can be surgically repaired. Inguinal hernias may present as a bulge in the scrotum, and bowel may be palpable. Inguinal hernias are found in 0.8% to 4.4% of boys. Approximately 60% are on the left, 30% are on the right and 10% are bilateral.[41] Inguinal hernias are found predominantly in boys but can occur in girls as well, with a male:female ratio of 6:1. If an inguinal hernia is present, it should be evaluated for incarceration. If the hernia is not reducible, surgical consultation should be obtained due to the risk of strangulation and bowel loss. Ambiguous genitalia can range from nearly female anatomy to nearly male anatomy in either boys or girls. The clinician should evaluate for micropenis or clitoromegaly and bifid scrotum or fusion of the labia. When ambiguous genitalia are recognized at birth, sex assignment should be postponed until further information can be obtained. Girls with ambiguous genitalia should be evaluated for congenital adrenal hyperplasia (CAH) with virilization. CAH occurs in 0.06 to 0.08 per 1000 live births. Of these, 90% are due to 21-hydroxylase deficiency.[39] Boys with ambiguous genitalia may fail to produce virilizing hormones, such as in 17 alpha-hydroxylase deficiency, or have end-organ resistance to these hormones, such as in androgen insensitivity.

EVALUATION OF THE EXTREMITIES

A thorough examination of all four extremities should be performed. Both hands and feet may be missing digits or have supranumary digits. Polydactyly is commonly a spontaneous occurrence; however, having a family history of polydactyly increases the chances of this anomaly tenfold. Polydactyly of the "pinky" side of the hand is quite common, occurring in 1 in 3000 infants.[40] Supranumary digits may range from skin tags to fully formed digits. Skin tags can be removed by tying a suture at the base, whereas more fully formed digits require surgical removal. The palms should be inspected for the presence of a single transverse palmar crease. Approximately 4% of the general population has a unilateral single transverse palmar crease and 1% has bilateral involvement. Single transverse palmar creases are seen in conjunction with several syndromes, with Down syndrome being the most well known.

The feet are not exempt from anomalies. Clubfoot, formally known as *talipes equinovarus,* is found in 1 in 1000 live births. Bilateral involvement is seen in 30% to 50%

of cases with a male:female ratio of 2:1.[40] Clubfoot is an intricate anomaly composed of four main abnormalities[41]:

1. The forefoot is inverted and adducted.
2. The heel and hindfoot are inverted.
3. Extension at the ankle and subtalar joint is limited.
4. The leg is internally rotated.

During examination, the foot cannot be brought back to midline. Clubfoot often is treated successfully by serial casting. If casting is unsuccessful, surgical correction is generally performed between 6 and 9 months.

EVALUATION OF THE NEUROLOGICAL SYSTEM

The complete neurological examination is quite involved. It is frequently not possible to perform the entire neurological examination due to time constraints. In these cases, a limited neurological examination can be performed that should include evaluation of tone, cranial nerves, sensation, strength and primitive reflexes (Table 1.2). If any deficits are detected, the complete neurological examination should be performed. Close observation can often show any abnormalities in most of these areas.

While observing the infant, note any asymmetries of the face. All extremities should move spontaneously and without difficulty. Observation of how the infant lies at rest can give insight into the underlying tone of the infant. Full-term infants typically keep their extremities flexed and pulled up into the body, whereas premature infants often lie with their extremities less flexed and resting on the bed due to their relative decreased tone. Strength can be assessed by watching the infant's ability to raise the head off the table while prone. The infant may not be able to maintain this elevation for long, nor will they necessarily be steady, but he or she should be able to raise the head off the table.[42] The cry of the infant should be strong and vigorous. Infants with various neurological problems produce weak or shrill, high-pitched cries.

As with adults, the cranial nerve examination in infants involves evaluation of all the nerves, often omitting cranial nerve one. Sensation evaluation is more difficult because the infant cannot tell the examiner if a specific sensation is felt. Consequently, the test is generally limited to light touch and pinprick because the infant likely will move the area examined in response to the stimulus.

When performing the neurological examination, the clinician is most likely to detect hypotonia. Hypotonia

Table 1.2. Common primitive reflexes

Rooting Reflex
Touch newborn on either cheek and baby turns toward stimulus.
Walking Reflex
Hold baby in vertical position. As feet touch ground, baby makes walking motion.
Tonic Neck (Fencing) Reflex
Rotate babies head leftward and the left arm stretches into extension and the right arm flexes up above head (opposite reaction if head is rotated rightward).
Moro Reflex (Startle Reflex)
Hold supine infant by arms a few inches above bed and gently release infant back to elicit startle. Baby throws arms out in extension and grimaces.
Hand-to-Mouth (Babkin) Reflex
Stroke newborn's cheek or put finger in baby's palm and baby will bring fist to mouth and suck a finger.
Swimmer's (Gallant) Response
Hold baby prone while supporting belly with hand. Stroke along one side of spine and baby flexes entire torso toward the stroked side.
Palmar
Stroke inner palm/sole and toes/fingers curl around ("grasp") examiner's finger.
Plantar
Stroke outer sole (Babinski) and toes spread with great toe dorsiflexion.
Doll's Eyes
Give one forefinger to each hand (baby grasps both) and pull baby to sitting position. Eyes open on coming to sitting (like a doll's eyes).
Protective Reflex
Soft cloth is placed over the baby's eyes and nose. Baby arches neck back, turns head side to side and brings both hands to face to swipe cloth away.
Crawling Reflex
Place newborn on abdomen and baby flexes legs under as if to crawl.

can be associated with many abnormalities. It can result from central or peripheral abnormalities. Central hypotonia can be seen in association with seizures, failure of eye fixation and failure to meet developmental milestones. Central hypotonia may be seen in syndromes such as Down syndrome and Prader-Willi syndrome and with other conditions such as hypoglycemia, hypothyroidism,

Table 1.3. Cranial nerve examination

CN II	Blink reflex: Shine a light in the infant's eye, the infant should blink.
CN III	Papillary reflex and eye movement
CN IV	Eye movement
CN V	Corneal light reflex: Touching the cornea produces a blink. Light touch/pinprick in the trigeminal areas
CN VI	Eye movement
CN VII	Blink reflex
CN VIII	Loud noises should evoke a blink.
CN IX	Swallow reflex
CN X	Swallow reflex
CN XI	Evaluation of the sternocleidomastoid muscle for fasiculations and movement
CN XII	Evaluation of the tongue for fasiculations and movement

hypoxic-ischemic encephalopathy and other metabolic/infectious disorders. As time goes on, central causes of hypotonia often slowly become more typical of "classic" central nervous system lesions with hypertonia and hyperreflexia.

Infants who present with severe hypotonia at birth, particularly following a difficult birth that may have included hyperextension of the neck, may have had a traumatic transection of the spinal cord. Severe respiratory failure may occur in these patients as well. In contrast to central hypotonia, peripheral hypotonia typically does not present with other central findings. The infant generally is able to respond to stimuli, although movement may be decreased due to diminished strength. Examples of peripheral hypotonia syndrome include neonatal botulism, spinal muscular atrophy and neonatal myasthenia gravis. Neonatal myasthenia gravis arises when the mother has myasthenia gravis. Maternal acetylcholine receptor antibodies cross the placenta and cause a myasthenic syndrome. Symptoms are very similar to those seen in adults, including hypotonia, diminished or absent Moro reflex, a weak suck and respiratory insufficiency. Symptoms may not be present immediately after birth and can develop up to 72 hours after delivery. As with symptoms, treatment of neonatal myasthenia gravis is similar to that for adults and includes the use of acetylcholinesterase inhibitors. As maternal antibodies are cleared from the infant, the symptoms resolve, generally around 12 weeks of age.

Spinal muscular atrophy type 1, also known as *Werdnig-Hoffmann* syndrome, results from degeneration of the anterior horn cells. This subsequently leads to weakness, decreased or absent reflexes and a weak suck. Sixty percent of these patients will present with hypotonia at birth. They continue to be alert and have facial reactions, setting it apart from hypotonia due to cerebral damage. Werdnig-Hoffmann syndrome typically presents between ages 0 to 6 months.[43]

During delivery, the brachial plexus is at risk for traumatic injury, particularly with breech deliveries or shoulder dystocia. The brachial plexus arises from spinal nerve roots C5 to T1. Part or all of the plexus may be injured, giving rise to various recognized palsies. Erb's palsy involves C5 and C6 with occasional involvement of C7. The lower part of the plexus, C8 and T1, give rise to Klumpke palsy. Erb palsy classically presents with the arm in a "waiter's tip" position. Klumpke palsy presents with full functionality of the upper arm with paralysis of the hand. Of all brachial plexus palsies, Klumpke palsy represents only 0.5% of cases.[3] Involvement of the total plexus yields a combination of the two palsies with resulting paralysis of the entire upper extremity. Erb and Klumpke palsies are typically transient, although permanent loss of function is possible with more severe damage to the nerve roots such as complete avulsions. Resolution generally occurs over the course of a few weeks or months.

EVALUATION OF THE SKIN

The skin examination in newborns can be challenging due to the vast array of possible skin findings. When there is doubt as to the diagnosis, specialist consultation should be requested. Often, however, visual diagnosis can be made easily by an experienced practitioner. Skin rashes result in numerous visits to the doctor's office for urgent care. Being able to diagnose common newborn skin findings and provide parental reassurance is important. Rashes and other skin conditions commonly seen in newborns and infants are reviewed in Chapter 16.

The vasomotor system in newborns is still fairly instable. Rapid changes in vasomotor tone can lead to several different skin findings including cutis marmorata, harlequin color changes and acrocyanosis. Cutis marmorata presents with a lacy, mottled look to the skin. It is brought about by changes in capillary blood flow. Cold exposure may induce its appearance. Its presence also may be a sign of sepsis. Unwrapping a bundled febrile young infant and finding mottled extremities should be concerning. Harlequin color changes are seen when the infant is turned on the side. When these occur there is generally a sharp color change at about the midpoint of the body. The upper portion becomes pale while the lower portion becomes red or bluish in color. Returning the baby to the supine position generally leads to rapid resolution of these color changes, but they may persist for up to 20 minutes.[44]

Acrocyanosis results in countless visits to the doctor due to concerns about low oxygen levels. The typical complaint is that the baby is turning blue. It is important to distinguish acrocyanosis from true central cyanosis, which may be indicative of a saturation problem. Acrocyanosis results from venous pooling of blood in the extremities, particularly in the hands and feet. This gives a bluish coloration to the areas. Cold temperatures may exacerbate the condition. As the child ages and vasomotor tone improves, this condition tends to resolve. Acrocyanosis should be distinguished from central cyanosis by examining the face, tongue and mucous membranes.

PITFALLS

- Failure to know the normal primitive reflexes in newborns
- Failure to routinely check for the red reflex
- Failure to undress the baby fully and examine the skin for lesions
- Failure to remove the diaper and check for hernias, undescended testes or other genital abnormalities.

REFERECES

1. Thilo E, Rosenberg AA. The newborn infant. In: Hay WW, Levin MJ, Sondheimer JM, et al., eds. *Current Diagnosis and Treatment.* New York, NY: Lange Medical Books/McGraw-Hill; 2007.
2. Grover G, Berkowitz CD, Lewis RJ, et al. The effects of bundling on infant temperature. *Pediatrics.* 1994;94(5):669–673.
3. Bland R. The newborn infant. In: Rudolph AM, Rudolph CD, et al, eds. *Rudolph's Pediatrics.* New York, NY: McGraw-Hill; 2007:55–222.

4. Macintosh M, Fleming KM, Bailey JA, et al. Perinatal mortality and congenital anomalies in babies of women with type 1 or type 2 diabetes in England, Wales, and Northern Ireland: population based study. *BMJ.* 2006;333(7560):157–158.

5. DeMyer W. Normal and abnormal development of the neuraxis. In: Rudolph AM, Rudolph CD, et al, eds. *Rudolph's Pediatrics.* New York, NY: McGraw-Hill;2003:2174.

6. Hillenbrand K. Birth trauma. In: Perkinswift JD, Newton DA, eds. *Pediatric Hospital Medicine.* Philadelphia, PA: Lippincott Williams & Wilkins; 2003:592–596.

7. Caughey A, Sanderber PL, Zlatnik MG. Forceps compared with vacuum: rates of neonatal and maternal morbidity. *Obstet Gynecol.* 2005;206(5, Part 1):908–912.

8. Introduction to clinically oriented anatomy. In: Moore K, Dalley AF, eds. *Clinically Oriented Anatomy.* Philadelphia, PA: Lippincott Williams & Wilkins; 1999:2–58.

9. Chadwick L, Pemberton PJ, Kurinczuk JJ. Neonatal subgaleal haematoma associated risk factors, complications and outcome. *J Paediatr Child Health.* 1996;32:228–232.

10. Kabbani H, Raghuveer T. Craniosynostosis. *Am Fam Physician.* 2004;69(12):2893–2896.

11. Carey J, Bamshad MJ. Clinical genetics and dysmorphology. In: Rudolph AM, Rudolph CD, et al, eds. *Rudolph's Pediatrics.* New York, NY: McGraw-Hill; 2003:713–786.

12. Wilkie AO, Slaney SF, Oldridge M, et al. Apert syndrome results from localized mutations of FGFR2 and is allelic with Crouzon syndrome. *Nat Genet.* 1995;9:165–172.

13. Popich G, Smith DW. Fontanels: range of normal size. *J Pediatr.* 1972;80:749–752.

14. Veeramachaneni V. Index of suspicion. *Pediatr Rev.* 2001;22(6):211–215.

15. Phillipi C, Christensen L, Samples J. Index of suspicion. *Pediatr Rev.* 2005;26(8):295–301.

16. Miller K, Apt L. The eyes. In: Rudolph AM, Rudolph CD, et al, eds. *Rudolph's Pediatrics.* New York, NY: McGraw-Hill; 2003:2351–2417.

17. Calhoun J. Consultation with the specialist: eye examination in infants and children. *Pediatr Rev.* 1997;18:28–31.

18. Izquierdo N, Townsend W. Down syndrome. [cited; Available from: http://www.emedicine.com.]

19. Hsieh D, Friederich R, Pelszynski MM. Index of suspicion. *Pediatr Rev.* 2006;27(8):307–313.

20. Lim S, Siatkowski RM. Pediatric neuro-ophthalmology. *Curr Opin Ophthalmol.* 2004;27(8):307–313.

21. Jatla KK, Zhao F. Neonatal conjunctivitis eMedicine from WebMD June 18, 2006.

22. Soames J, Southam JC. Other disorders of teeth: disorders of eruption and shedding of teeth. In: *Oral Pathology.* Oxford, United Kingdom: Oxford University Press; 2005.

23. Shusterman S. Pediatric dental update. *Pediatr Rev.* 1994;15(8):311–318.

24. Do T. Congenital muscular torticollis: current concepts and review of treatment. *Curr Opin Pediatr.* 2006;18(1):26–29.

25. Sponseller P. Bone, joint and muscle problems. In: McMillan JA, Feigin RD, DeAngelis C, et al, eds. *Oski's Pediatrics.* Philadelphia, PA: Lippincott Williams & Wilkins; 2006.

26. Kaplan B, Rabinerson D, Avrech OM, et al. Fracture of the clavicle in the newborn following normal labor and delivery. *Int J Gynaecol Obstet.* 1998;63(1):15–20.

27. Fortunov RM, Hulten KG, Hammerman WA, et al. Evaluation and treatment of community-acquired *Staphylococcus aureus* infections in term and late-preterm previously healthy neonates. *Pediatrics.* 2007;120:937–945.

28. Subramanian K, Bahri M. Transient tachypnea of the newborn. Nov. 21, 2006 [cited; Available from: http://www.emedicine.com].

29. Hoffman J. The circulatory system. In: Rudolph AM, Rudolph CD, et al, eds. *Rudolph's Pediatrics.* New York, NY: McGraw-Hill; 2003:1745–1904.

30. Bers M, Porter RS, Jones TV, et al. Congenital cardiovascular diseases. In: *The Merck Manual of Diagnosis and Therapy.* Whitehouse Station, NJ: Merck Research Laboratories; 2006.

31. Wolf AD, Levine JE. Hepatomegaly in neonates and children. *Pediatr Rev.* 2000;21(9):303–310.

32. Siegel N. Kidney and urinary tract. In: Rudolph AM, Rudolph CD, et al, eds. *Rudolph's Pediatrics.* New York, NY: McGraw-Hill; 2003:1629–1743.

33. Srinivasan R, Arora RS. Do well infants born with an isolated single umbilical artery need investigation? *Arch Dis Child.* 2005;90(1):100–101.

34. Bourke W, Clarke TA, Mathews TG, et al. Isolated single umbilical artery–the case for routine screening. *Arch Dis Child.* 1993;68(5):600–601.

35. Gallagher PG, Shah SS. Omphalitis eMedicine from Web MD August 18, 2006.

36. Available from: http://www.prunebelly.org/.

37. Pulsifer A. Pediatric genitourinary examination: a clinician's reference. *Urol Nurs.* 2005;25(3):163–168.

38. Nakayama D, Rowe MI. Inguinal hernia and the acute scrotum in infants and children. *Pediatr Rev.* 1989;11(3):87–93.

39. Goodman S. Endocrine alterations. In: Potts NL, ed. *Pediatric Nursing: Caring for Children and Their Families.* Clifton Park, NY: Thompson Delmar Learning; 2003.

40. Crawford A. Orthopedics. In: Rudolph AM, Rudolph CD, et al, eds. *Rudolph's Pediatrics.* New York, NY: McGraw-Hill; 2003:2419–2457.

41. Gore A, Spencer JP. The newborn foot. *Am Fam Physician.* 2004;69(4):865–872.

42. Mercuri E, Ricci D, Pane M, et al. The neurological examination of the newborn baby. *Early Hum Dev.* 2005;81:947–956.

43. Tsao B, Stojic AS, Armon C. Spinal Muscular Atrophy. Nov. 2, 2006 [cited; Available from: http://www.emedicine.com].

44. Morelli J, Burch JM. Skin. In: Levin M, Hay WW, Sondheimer JM, et al, eds. *Current Diagnosis and Treatment in Pediatrics.* New York, NY: Lange Medical Books/McGraw-Hill, 2007.

2   Premature Infants in the Emergency Department

Nadeem Qureshi, Stephen Gletsu and Mohammed Al Mogbil

INTRODUCTION

Premature infants are defined as those born before 37 weeks of gestational age (Table 2.1). They account for 10% of all births and typically weigh less than 2500 g (5 lb, 8 oz).[1] The infant mortality increases from 5 times normal at 37 weeks of gestational age to 45 times normal at 32 weeks of gestational age.[2] The majority of medical problems associated with prematurity occur in infants with birth weights of less than 1500 g (3 lb, 5 oz) and in those born before 32 weeks of gestational age. Recent advances in medical specialties have resulted in improved survival rates with a significant impact on the morbidity and mortality of these patients. This chapter outlines some of the complex medical problems experienced by these children, especially related to devices and their complications, which will bring them to the emergency department (ED).

GENERAL MANAGEMENT PRINCIPLES

Preterm infants may present to the ED with or without a technology-assisted device. At this point, the child's

Table 2.1. Terms related to prematurity

Premature Infant
An infant born at <37 weeks of estimated gestational age
Low Birth Weight
Birth weight <2500 g (5 lb, 8 oz)
Very Low Birth Weight
Birth weight <1500 g (3 lb, 5 oz)
Extremely Low Birth Weight
Birth weight <1000 g (2 lb, 3 oz)
Chronologic or Birth Age
Time since birth
Gestational Age
Estimated time since conception; postconceptional age
Corrected Age
Age corrected for prematurity

caregiver is a valuable source of information. The caregiver may provide information about the baseline status of the child, have medical summaries detailing the medical history, and carry spare necessary supplies such as gastrostomy tubes (GTs) or tracheostomy tubes. Therefore, it is invaluable to include caregivers in the medical decision-making process.

Premature infants or medically complex children (those with assisted devices) may have common pediatric illnesses that seem like more dangerous entities. For example, a child with a ventriculoperitoneal (VP) shunt may have gastroenteritis mimicking VP shunt malfunction. It is imperative not to overlook the presence of an indwelling device and to be familiar with any related complications such as infections and malfunctions that may occur. The following section addresses the common complications associated with different devices.

ASSESSMENT

ED physicians need to focus on the patient and not on the device. As usual, they start with airway, breathing and circulation (the ABCs). Premature infants with complex medical problems may be difficult to examine due to their physical disabilities.

At this point, key questions from the caregiver can aid in the evaluation and management of these chronically ill infants (Table 2.2).

Table 2.2. Device history

1. Why does the child need the device?
2. When was it placed?
3. When was it last changed?
4. What happens to the infant when this device malfunctions?

1. What are the child's symptoms today and how are they different from baseline?
2. What are the baseline developmental status, vital signs and weight?

APNEA OF PREMATURITY

Epidemiology

Apnea of prematurity (AOP) is defined as a sudden cessation of breathing that lasts for at least 20 seconds or that is accompanied by bradycardia or oxygen desaturation in an infant younger than 37 weeks gestational age. AOP is the most frequently encountered problem of respiratory control in the neonatal intensive care unit (NICU) and occurs in 85% of infants born at less than 34 weeks gestation.[3,4] AOP usually ceases by 37 weeks gestational age but may persist for several weeks beyond term, particularly in infants born before 28 weeks' gestation, and extreme episodes usually cease at approximately 43 weeks postconceptional age.[3]

Pathophysiology

Brainstem development and neural control of respiration are less mature in the preterm infant compared with the full-term infant. The physiologic maturity of various respiratory reflexes in late preterm infants of 34 to 37 weeks' gestation appears to lie on a continuum that extends from more immature infants to sometime beyond term.

The respiratory system in the newborn and especially the premature newborn is characterized by high chest wall compliance, and inward distortion of the anterior chest wall is commonly observed in preterm infants without respiratory disease. With maturation, chest wall compliance decreases, enhancing the mechanical stability of the respiratory system.

The airway of the newborn is more compliant than that of the adult, and the anatomic arrangement favors obstruction, particularly when the neck is flexed. In older infants and adults, laryngeal mechanoreceptor and chemoreceptor stimulation with the introduction of certain liquids results in cough and expiratory effort. In term and premature newborns in particular, this response can include apnea and bradycardia.

Finally, respiratory rate and tidal volume are regulated by feedback mechanisms that sense Pao_2 and $Paco_2$, triggering changes in minute ventilation to maintain normal concentrations of O_2, CO_2 and pH. In preterm infants, the intensity of this response is likely related to both gestational age and chronological age. Darnall et al. reported that the ventilatory response to hypercapnia is decreased in premature infants who have AOP compared with those who do not.[5]

Methylxanthine Therapy in Apnea of Prematurity

The methylxanthines (caffeine, theophylline and aminophylline) have been the mainstay of therapy for AOP for 3 decades and are believed to reduce the frequency of apnea and the need for mechanical ventilation during the first 7 days of life.[4] Caffeine is the preferred methylxanthine due to its wide therapeutic index.[6] Methylxanthines increase oxygen consumption in preterm infants and may diminish growth.[4] In addition, they are inhibitors of adenosine receptors, and adenosine has been shown to protect brain cells during hypoxia and ischemia.[4] It remains unclear whether methylxanthines have additional short- and long-term risks or benefits in preterm infants. A recent large multicenter randomized placebo-controlled trial of the use of parenteral caffeine citrate for the treatment of AOP in preterm, low birth weight infants[4] showed that those infants not treated with caffeine required respiratory support (supplemental oxygen alone, supplemental oxygen plus any positive airway pressure or positive airway pressure via endotracheal tube) for 1 week longer than those treated with caffeine. There was also a lower incidence of bronchopulmonary dysplasia in the caffeine treated group. No data are currently available regarding the long-term effects of caffeine from this study.

Apnea Monitoring in Premature Infants

Apnea monitors were first introduced in the mid-1960s for the management of AOP in hospital settings. Cardiorespiratory monitoring is now widely used in the care of infants with a variety of acute and chronic disorders.[3] The American Academy of Pediatrics proposed that apnea is the pathophysiologic precursor to sudden infant death syndrome (SIDS). This theory had never been proven despite extensive research. Despite the absence of evidence of efficacy, home cardiorespiratory monitoring continues to be a common practice in the United

States.[3] The Collaborative Home Infant Monitoring Evaluation (CHIME) monitored 1079 infants: infants with idiopathic apparent life-threatening events (ALTEs), siblings of infants who died of SIDS, preterm infants with clinically apparent apneic episodes, preterm infants without apneic episodes and healthy term infants.[3] This study showed that apnea and bradycardia occurred in all of these groups of infants. The only group with increased risk of clinically apparent apneic episodes compared with healthy term infants was the preterm infant group up to approximately 43 weeks gestational age. The mean age for SIDS occurrence is estimated to be 45.8 weeks gestational age for infants born at 24 to 28 weeks of gestational age compared to 52.3 weeks for term infants.[3] As this study shows, apnea appears to resolve at a postnatal age before which most SIDS deaths occur. There is no evidence that the presence of apnea and bradycardia identifies a group as at increased risk of SIDS, that home monitoring can provide warning in time for intervention or that intervention would be successful in preventing unexpected death.[3] Evidence does exist that preterm infants are at a greater risk of extreme apneic episodes than are term infants. This risk decreases with time and ceases at approximately 43 weeks gestational age.[3] There are no studies correlating long-term neurodevelopment outcome with these episodes.

The American Academy of Pediatrics Committee on Fetus and Newborn suggests that home cardiorespiratory monitoring after hospital discharge may be prescribed for some preterm infants and that monitoring usually may be discontinued after 43 weeks gestational age.[3]

Many types of monitors are available. Currently available monitors do not reliably detect obstructive apnea. Physicians are responsible for prescribing equipment with specific capabilities. Cardiac and respiratory activity must be monitored simultaneously, and monitors must be capable of event recording for downloading and retrospective review to allow for analysis of true versus false alarms.[3]

CEREBROSPINAL FLUID SHUNTS

Introduction

Cerebrospinal fluid (CSF) shunts are the mainstay therapy for hydrocephalus. CSF is produced in the lateral ventricles by the choroid plexus, at a rate of 0.5 mL/kg/hour. The CSF is diverted from the brain to another cavity in the body using these VP shunts. VP shunts can obstruct or

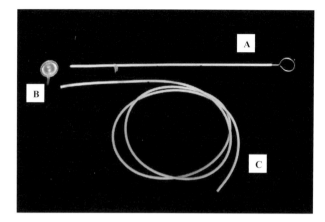

Figure 2.1. Components of a CSF shunt system. A, Ventricular catheter with stylet, B, Reservoir (palpable externally), C, Peritoneal catheter.

become infected (incidence of 2%-30%). The emergency management of premature children with CSF shunts focuses on diagnosing shunt obstruction and shunt infection. This section summarizes the clinical manifestations, diagnosis and treatment of shunt obstructions and infections.

Components

Most CSF shunts have three components: ventricular (proximal) shunt tubing, a reservoir system and peritoneal (distal) shunt tubing (Figures 2.1 and 2.2). The proximal (Silastic) shunt tubing has a fenestrated tip that is placed in the ventricle. The reservoir (bubble-shaped structure) is located directly over or slightly distal to the burr hole on the cranium. The distal shunt tubing is mostly positioned in the peritoneum, occasionally in the vascular system or pleural cavity.

Shunt Malfunction

Premature infants with mechanical shunt obstruction often present with vomiting, lethargy and irritability.[7]

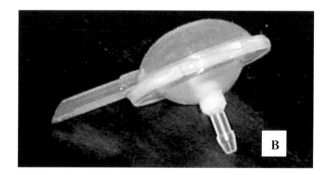

Figure 2.2. Close-up of reservoir.

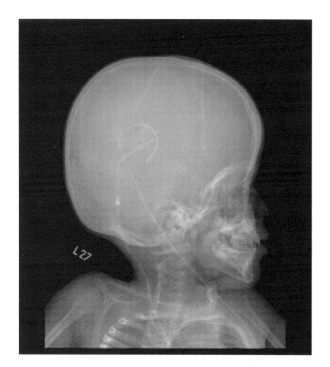
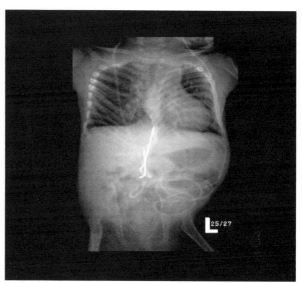

Figure 2.3. VP shunt series showing intact VP shunt system.

Altered mental status is the most common complaint. Parental history can provide crucial insights. The parents may say that the child "just isn't acting right," is less active than usual or showed similar symptoms during the last shunt obstruction episode. Sunsetting gaze, cranial nerve neurapraxia and vital sign changes (hypertension and bradycardia) may indicate increased intracranial pressure (ICP).

The ability to assess CSF shunt function at bedside by pumping shunt reservoir bubble and checking for refilling times upon release is a poor suboptimal test. Piatt[8] found that this maneuver had a positive predictive value of 21% and a negative predictive value of 78% in patients with definite shunt malfunction. This means that 22% of patients with shunt obstructions will have a normal pumping "test." Occasionally, frequent pumping of the shunt can cause entrapment of choroid plexus in the proximal shunt tubing and lead to proximal catheter obstruction.

A noncontrast computed tomography (CT) scan is often required to rule out shunt malfunction. Comparison with previous films is advantageous. A shunt series, which includes plain radiograph of the skull, chest and abdomen, assesses the components of the working system (Figures 2.3, 2.4 and 2.5). However, normal radiographic

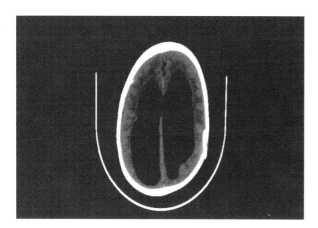

Figure 2.4. CT scans show enlarged ventricles compared to baseline CT exams.

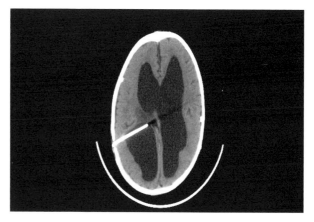

Figure 2.5. Post revision of the VP shunt, ventricular size starts to shrink.

studies should not supersede a strong clinical suspicion of a shunt malfunction based on symptoms and prior history.[9]

Shunt tapping is a useful diagnostic and therapeutic procedure. Although it is ideal to have a neurosurgeon perform this procedure, emergency physicians can tap a shunt with ease. A 23- or 25-gauge butterfly needle is inserted obliquely into the reservoir under sterile conditions. The butterfly tubing should be held perpendicular to the floor.[10] ICP can be estimated by noting the height of the CSF above the level of the tragus, measured in centimeters. Slow or absent flow suggests proximal shunt obstruction, whereas an ICP higher than 20 cm is indicative of distal shunt obstruction. CSF can be removed in 10 mL aliquots to reduce the ICP to normal levels of lower than 20 cm. Excessive or rapid removal of CSF may result in unwanted intracranial fluid shifts and subdural vessels disruption.[10,11]

In critically ill infants with suspected proximal shunt obstruction in whom a sudden rise in ICP is witnessed but rapid removal of CSF is difficult, intubation should be rapidly conducted. Followed by mild hyperventilation,[12] a dose of mannitol,[13] acetazolamide (Diamox) 30 mg/kg/day and dexamethasone (Decadron) 1.0 mg/kg/day may be useful until the shunt is replaced. The most effective use of hyperventilation is in acute situations to allow time for other, more definitive treatments to be put into action. Mannitol lowers ICP in 1 to 5 minutes, expands plasma volume and reduces blood viscosity, which increases cerebral blood flow and oxygen delivery to the brain.

Recently, hypertonic saline 3%[14] has been used to reduce ICP by creating an osmotic force to draw water from the brain parenchyma into the intravascular compartment. However, the use of 3% saline is still under investigation. Alternatively, lumen obstruction may be relieved by flushing a small amount of sterile water through the clogged tubing in an attempt to dislodge the obstruction. The only drawback to this is that a few more drops of water into the ventricles may in fact worsen the patient's condition. Burr hole puncture and fontanel tap are some other options for preoperative neurosurgical management of the unstable patient with a CSF shunt malfunction.[15]

Shunt Infection

CSF shunt-associated infections can take place in multiple anatomic locations along the track of the shunt, lumen of the shunt, the extra luminal ventricles, the cranial and distal surgical sites, and the peritoneal cavity. Therefore clinical manifestations of these infections are also variable. Most shunt infections occur within the first 6 months after shunt placement,[16–18] with approximately one half occurring within the first 2 weeks.

Etiology

The etiology of CSF shunt infections varies with the timing of the infection. Generally, infections occurring within the first 2 months of shunt placement are perioperative in nature and *Staphylococcus epidermidis* and *Staphylococcus aureus* are the most common organisms. Infections that occur more than 6 months after shunt placement are more likely due to gram-negative infections,[19] due to bowel erosion or pressure necrosis from the shunt apparatus.[19] Fungi are rare pathogens seen occasionally in premature infants.

Shunt infections can also include direct invasion. Necrosis or infection of the area around the reservoir can occur as a result of the constant pressure in infants or nonambulatory patients. Skin breakdown leading to visualization of the shunt mechanism is, by definition, a shunt infection and must be treated accordingly. Primary peritoneal infection may result in pseudocysts. These may be indolent in their presentation, and the shunt tap from the reservoir may not show evidence of infection. Shunt nephritis is a rare but serious complication of ventricular-atrial shunts, whereby renal deposition of antigen-antibody complexes leads to complement activation, which damages the renal tissue.

Clinical Presentations

Children with CSF shunt infections do not necessarily present with signs and symptoms of meningitis. Fever and irritability are the most common complaints in CSF shunt infections. Fever is not always present in patients with shunt infections and is uncommonly the only sign. Children with shunts infected by *S. epidermidis* may look particularly well, despite the presence of bacteria in their spinal fluid.[20] The symptoms of shunt infection overlap considerably with those of shunt malfunction, and, in fact, the infection can directly cause obstruction of the fenestrations in the catheters. Infection of the distal shunt mechanism may manifest as abdominal pain or vomiting.

Labs and Radiology

CSF Aspiration. The absolute leukocyte count is not always diagnostic and patients without infection can have a white blood cell count of up to 500/mm^3. Gram stain of CSF showing white blood cells with presumptive organism may be helpful in diagnosing shunt infection. Abdominal ultrasound or radiographs are helpful when looking for loculated CSF collection, pseudocyst or visceral perforation.

Treatment

The initial choice of empiric therapy in this era of methicillin-resistant *S. aureus* is vancomycin and cefotaxime. In one series, 17% of patients with shunt infection had normal CSF Gram stain, cell count and chemistries.[21] Therefore, maintain a broad spectrum coverage until sensitivities are confirmed before reducing the antibiotic coverage. For treatment of proximal CSF shunt infections, medical therapy alone has been found to have a relatively low success rate compared with a combined medical-surgical approach.[22] Potential surgical interventions include immediate shunt replacement or the insertion of an extraventricular drainage catheter followed by delayed shunt revision.[23,24]

Overdrainage

Occasionally, the CSF shunts can work "too well," resulting in low ICP. "Overshunting" is most common in infants who have had initial shunting before 6 months of age. Young infants may exhibit sunken fontanels, microcephaly or overriding parietal bones, and older children may exhibit intermittent symptoms of headache, nausea, vomiting and lethargy. In contrast to symptoms related to increased ICP, patients with intracranial hypotension are often worse when they are in the standing position or after they are awake for several hours.

CT scans may be unchanged from baseline or may reveal small ventricles (slit ventricles). Oral analgesics are usually effective in the management of these symptoms, although some cases need to be addressed surgically by altering the resistance of the valve.[11] If left unchecked, overdrainage can lead to shrinkage of brain tissue and concomitant subdural hematomas or effusions. Similarly, a decreased rate of head growth because of overdrainage can result in craniosynostosis in the infant.[11]

Other Complications

Seizures and Pseudocyst Formation

Patients with CSF shunts have an increased risk of seizures, caused by epileptogenic scars.[25] Intracranial hemorrhage or cyst increases the risk. Pseudocyst formation results from drainage of excess fluid into the peritoneum. These cysts may become infected.

CSF Shunt Leaks

Postoperatively, CSF leaks around the shunt tubing into the subgaleal space around the reservoir. Usually, it resolves spontaneously; therefore, there is no need to drain. In patients who are not postoperative, however, this indicates a shunt malfunction with CSF leaking through the path of least resistance.

Visceral Damage

Rarely, the distal portion of a CSF shunt apparatus can migrate, causing damage to viscera or acting as a fulcrum for intestinal volvulus.

Ventricular-Vascular Shunts

These shunts have been replaced by VP shunts. Major complications associated with ventricular-vascular shunts were an increased risk of bacteremia, deposition of bacteria in the renal system and antigen-antibody complex deposition causing complement activation and subsequently leading to shunt nephritis. Bacterial endocarditis, cardiac foreign body, atrial perforation, cardiac dysrhythmias and mural thrombus are rare but notable complications of ventricular-vascular shunts.

TRACHEOSTOMY TUBE

Use of tracheostomy tubes (TTs) to support respiratory function in different primary and secondary respiratory disorders is becoming increasingly common in children. TTs are subject to obstruction and infection. Infants with these airway devices may present to ED with respiratory distress. The size of the TT is usually listed on the rim of the tube, followed by a swivel device and followed by ventilator tubing (Figure 2.6).

TTs are made of polyvinyl chloride, a synthetic material with minimal tissue reactivity, and they are available from different manufacturers in different sizes. The most important characteristics are the inner and outer diameters of the TT, cuffed or uncuffed and length, so that an equivalent can be identified and it can be replaced, if needed.

The inner diameter is kept constant among manufacturers; however, the outer diameter and length are variable. Consequently, when replacing the TT, watch for

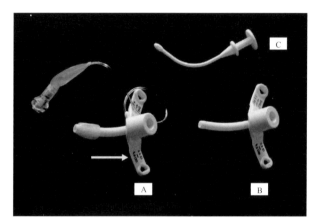

Figure 2.6. Tracheostomy tubes: cuffed (A), uncuffed (B) and obturator (C). *Arrow* indicates where the size is marked.

diameters. If you are having difficulty finding a replacement TT that has the same inner diameter, try using one size smaller.

Cuffed TTs are used in children; therefore, it is important to deflate the cuff before TT removal. Some patients with precarious airways may have TTs with inner cannulas, which provide a route for suctioning because the outer cannula keeps the airway patent.

Dislodgment or Obstruction

An infant with an artificial airway with respiratory distress is considered to have obstructed cannula or dislodgment until proven otherwise; therefore, an urgent TT change is mandated in this patient. Suctioning and supplemental oxygen may be helpful transiently. TT change is best accomplished by two people. One deflates the cuff and removes the tube. The other inserts the new TT. All the necessary equipment for airway management (endotracheal tube, lubricants, tapes and so on) should be readily available (Tables 2.3 and 2.4).

Table 2.4. Chest tube, nasogastric tube and urinary catheter sizes

	Neonate	6 mo	1-2 yrs	5yrs
Chest tube	12-18 Fr	14-20 Fr	14-24 Fr	20-32 Fr
Nasogastric tube	5-8 Fr	10 Fr	10-12 Fr	10-12 Fr
Urinary catheter	5-8 Fr (feeding tube)	10 Fr	10-12 Fr	12 F

Fr, French.

Infection

Patients with TTs usually are colonized with organisms in the trachea. Occasionally, these organisms become pathogenic and cause tracheitis and pneumonia. This scenario is usually difficult to diagnose. At this point, history of fever, malaise with worsening tachypnea, cough, retractions, increased supplemental oxygen requirements and changes in tracheal secretions' color and quantity provide indirect evidence of an acute infection. There is no reliable noninvasive test that can distinguish between colonization and active infection with 100% sensitivity and specificity. Treatment is oral or parenteral antibiotics, depending on the condition of the child.

ENTERAL FEEDING TUBES

Balanced nutrition is an important component for the growth of premature infants. Due to their limited energy reserve levels and poor physical growth, preterm infants have difficulty maintaining adequate oral feeding patterns. Enteral feeding tubes are routinely used to overcome this problem. A nasogastric tube (NGT) or GT is the preferred route (Figure 2.7A and B). NGTs are used when the duration of enteral feeding is expected to be less than 3

Table 2.3. Airway equipment by weight

Weight (g)	ET size (mm)	Suction catheter size (French)	Oral airway size	Laryngoscope straight blade no.
<1000	2.5	5	000	0
1000–1250	2.5, 3.0	5, 6	000	0
1250–2500	3.0	6	00	0, 1
2500–3000	3.0, 3.5	6, 8	0	1
>3000	3.0, 3.5, 4	8	0	1

ET size in mm = Gestational age in weeks/10
Total cm at gum line = 6 + weight of the infant in kilograms

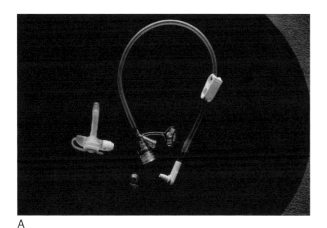 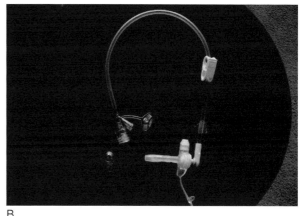

A   B

Figure 2.7. Mic-Key gastrostomy tube with attachment shown separately (A) and jointly (B).

months. GTs are used when long-term enteral feeding is anticipated (e.g., impaired swallowing due to brain damage, esophageal anomalies). GTs can be inserted via open technique or via percutaneous endoscopically.e. Percutaneous endoscopic gastrostomy is the most popular, safest method for placing gastrostomy tubes.[26]

Characteristics of Gastrostomy Tubes

Several different kinds of GTs are available. These are made of polyurethane or silicone. They vary in length, luminal diameter, number of ports and lumen. The most commonly used is the Mic-Key GT. This GT has a balloon located at the tip of the device, which is inflated after insertion and serves to anchor the tube tightly. To remove the tube, just deflate the balloon and remove the tube.

Complications of Gastrostomy Tubes

GT complications can be divided into device related or stoma associated.

Dislodgment

GT dislodgment is the most common complication. The size of the GT is marked on the rim. Parents may have a substitute GT available or know the size of the GT currently in place. Do not delay the replacement of the GT if it takes too long to confirm the size. To replace the GT, start by becoming familiar with the type of equipment present on the infant. First, carefully inspect the stoma for tears. Next, try to keep the stoma open. You can place a GT the same size as the current one; if the tube size is unknown,

then use a Foley catheter to keep the stoma stent open. Delay in placing the tube may result in constriction of the stoma and difficulty in replacing the same size tube. If the stoma constricts, use a smaller size Foley catheter and progressively dilate the opening with larger Foley catheters to reopen the partially constricted stoma.

Timing between dislodgment and initial placement of the GT is an important consideration. GT dislodgment within 1 month of placement is managed differently than tube that is more than 1 month old. If the dislodgment is less than 1 month old, the stoma is not well formed and the chance of false track insertion is high; therefore, the ED physician should seek the input of the service that initially placed the device. If the dislodgment is from a stable stoma ($\sim$>1 month old), then the GT should be replaced immediately with the same size GT. Once placed, confirm the position by aspiration and injection of 10 to 15 cc water to hear the borborygmi. If both test results are positive, no additional imaging studies are required.[27]

Obstruction

The second most common complication seen with GT is obstruction of the tube by solidified formula or a kink. Infusing fluids becomes difficult and a leak around the tube may also be present. Use of warm water to break the solidified food particles is most effective. Aspiration may be successful. Carbonated drinks may also be helpful. Do not attempt to push a stylet through the tube to overcome the obstruction because it may cause perforation (tube or visceral). Reposition the tube to relieve any kinks. If all of these maneuvers fail to relieve the obstruction, then the GT needs to be replaced.

Leak

Fluid leak around the GT is not an uncommon complaint. The leak may be due to stoma widening, a break in the GT apparatus, GT valve malfunction and balloon disruption.

Stoma widening may occur over time. This stretching of the stoma may lead to fluid leakage around the tube. The most important concerns regarding the fluid leak are pus, formula or gastric contents. Replacing the existing tube with a larger diameter tube or removing the tube briefly so as to allow stoma constriction can treat stoma widening.

A break in the GT apparatus, GT valve malfunction and balloon disruption will result in fluid leaks from the lumen itself. Replacing the GT should resolve these problems.

Gastric Irritation and Ulceration

A GT with an over-inflated balloon may result in local gastric irritation and ulceration. These infants may present to ED with signs of classical peptic ulcer disease: coffee ground drainage, dark stools and irritability. (See Chapter 18 for management of gastrointestinal bleeding.)

Gastric Outlet Obstruction

Too long of a tip on the gastric tube (Foley catheter tip) or migration of the GT tip can result in partial gastric outlet obstruction. The child may have sudden onset of emesis and appear uncomfortable. Radiographic assessment is required to locate the GT. The tube may need to be retracted to its original position or be changed to a smaller appropriate size.

Stomal Complications

Chemical/Allergic Dermatitis

Gastric secretions tend to irritate the stomal skin causing redness and irritation. Allergy to the GT itself may result in allergic rash around the stoma. Using adhesives, barrier creams and, occasionally, low-dose steroid cream and keeping the stoma dry will reduce these symptoms.

Granuloma

Granulomas are painless lesions around the peristomal area. These may occasionally become infected or bleed. Application of silver nitrate is the best therapy.

Cellulitis

At times, stoma dermatitis can progress to cellulitis. Erythema, induration swelling, occurs around the peristomal region. Staphylococci and streptococci are the most common organisms responsible for this. These infants require parenteral antibiotics.

Fungal skin infections are seen infrequently. Topical clotrimazole is adequate for these infections.

PITFALLS

- Failure to recognize that premature infants are at risk for significant morbidity, especially if the birth weight was less than 1500 g or if the gestational age was less than 32 weeks
- Failure to recognize that the respiratory system in the newborn, and especially the premature newborn, is characterized by high chest wall compliance
- Failure to recognize that premature infants with mechanical shunt obstruction often present with vomiting, lethargy and irritability. Altered mental status is the most common complaint. Parental history can provide crucial insights. The child "just isn't acting right," is less active than usual or similar symptoms were present during last shunt obstruction episode
- Failure to listen to the caregiver's concerns that the child is "not acting right"
- Failure to recognize that dislodgment of a GT that has been in place less than 1 month has a high incidence of false track insertion

REFERENCES

1. Berkowitz GS, Papiernik E. Epidemiology of preterm birth. *Epidemiol Rev.* 1993;15:414–443.
2. Wilcox AJ, Skjaerven R. Birth weight and perinatal mortality: the effect of gestational age. *Am J Public Health.* 1992;82:378–382.
3. American Academy of Pediatrics, Committee on Fetus and Newborn 2002–2003. Apnea, sudden infant death syndrome and home monitoring. *Pediatrics.* 2003;111(4):914–917.
4. Schmidt B, Roberts RS, Davis P, et al. Caffeine therapy for apnea of prematurity. *N Engl J Med.* 2006;354:2112–2121.
5. Darnall RA, Ariagno RL, Kinney HC. The late preterm infant and the control of breathing, sleep and brainstem development: a review. *Clin Perinatol.* 2006;33:883-914(4).
6. Wiswell TE, Tin W, Ohler K. Evidence-based use of adjunctive therapies to ventilation. *Clin Perinatol.* 2007;34(1).
7. Key CB, Rothrock SG, Falk JL. Cerebrospinal fluid shunt complications: an emergency medicine perspective. *Pediatr Emerg Care.* 1995;11:265–273.
8. Piatt JH. Physical examination of patients with cerebrospinal fluid shunts: is there useful information in pumping the shunt? *Pediatrics.* 1992;89:470–473.
9. Iskandar BJ, McLaughlin C, Mapstone TB, et al. Pitfalls in the diagnosis of ventricular shunt dysfunction: radiology reports and ventricular size. *Pediatrics.* 1998;101:1031–1036.
10. Grossman L. Section VII – Neurologic and Neurosurgical Procedures. Chapter 100 – Ventricular Shunt Evaluation And Aspiration. In: Eric R, Robert R. *Clinical Procedures*

in Emergency Medicine, 4th ed. Philadelphia, PA: Elsevier; 2004:901–908.

11. Walker M, Fried A, Petronio J. Diagnosis and treatment of the slit ventricle syndrome. *Neurosurg Clin N Am.* 1993;4:701–714.

12. Stocchetti N, Maas AI, Chieregato A, et al. Hyperventilation in head injury: a review. *Chest.* 2005;127:1812–1827.

13. Knapp JM. Hyperosmolar therapy in the treatment of severe head injury in children: mannitol and hypertonic saline. *AACN Clin Issues.* 2005;16:199–211.

14. Battison C, Andrews PJ, Graham C, et al. Randomized, controlled trial on the effect of a 20% mannitol solution and a 7.5% saline/6% dextran solution on increased intracranial pressure after brain injury. *Crit Care Med.* 2005;33:196–202.

15. Posner JC, Cronan K, Badaki O, Fein JA. Emergency care of the technology-assisted child. *Clinical Pediatric Emergency Medicine.* 2006;7(1):38–51.

16. Mancao M, Miller C, Cochrane B. Cerebrospinal fluid shunt infections in infants and children in Mobile, Alabama. *Acta Paediatr.* 1998;87:667–670.

17. Kontny U, Hofling B, Gutjahr P. CSF shunt infections in children. *Infection.* 1993;21:89–92.

18. Ronan A, Hogg GG, Klug GL. Cerebrospinal fluid shunt infections in children. *Pediatr Infect Dis J.* 1995;14:782–786.

19. Stamos JK, Kaufman BA, Yogev R. Ventriculoperitoneal shunt infections with gram-negative bacteria. *Neurosurgery.* 1993;33:858–862.

20. Madikians A, Conway EE. Cerebrospinal fluid shunt problems in pediatric patients. *Pediatr Ann.* 1997;26:613–620.

21. Ronan A, Hogg GG, Dlug GL. Cerebrospinal fluid shunt infections in children. *Pediatr Infect Dis.* 1995;14:782–786.

22. Morissette I, Gourdeau M, Francoeur J. CSF shunt infections: a fifteen-year experience with emphasis on management and outcome. *Can J Neurol Sci.* 1993;20:118–122.

23. Schreffler RT, Schreffler AJ, Wittler RR. Treatment of cerebrospinal fluid shunt infections: a decision analysis. *Pediatr Infect Dis J.* 2002;21:632–636.

24. Govender ST, Nathoo N, van Dellen JR. Evaluation of an antibiotic-impregnated shunt system for the treatment of hydrocephalus. *J Neurosurg.* 2003;99:831–839.

25. Johnson DL, Conry J, O'Donnell R. Epileptic seizure as a sign of cerebrospinal fluid shunt malfunction. *Pediatr Neurosurg.* 1996;24:223–227.

26. Gauderer MW. Percutaneous endoscopic gastrostomy. A 10 year experience with 220 children. *J Pediatr Surg.* 1991;26:288–294.

27. Graneto JW. Gastrostomy tube replacement. In: Christopher K. *Textbook of Pediatric Emergency Medicine Procedures.* Baltimore, MD: Williams & Wilkins; 1997:915–920.

Management of Pain and Sedation in the First Year of Life

P. Jamil Madati and Ghazala Q. Sharieff

INTRODUCTION

We have made significant strides in our knowledge of the ability of neonates to sense pain. Despite the recent growing body of evidence that repetitive painful procedures can lead to potentially harmful, both short-term and long-term, effects, there continues to be an insufficient use of appropriate analgesia or sedation for common painful procedures performed in both neonatal intensive care units (NICUs) and emergency departments (EDs).[1–3] The failure of this documented proof of neonatal pain to translate into appropriate bedside use of analgesia and sedation has been attributed to continued lack of awareness of neonatal pain and the developing neonatal nervous system, an inability of clinicians to appropriately assess neonatal pain and a pervading fear of adverse effects of prolonged or continuous analgesia administration.[4,5]

Neonates undergo numerous painful procedures, ranging from seemingly innocuous ones such as adhesive tape removal and heel sticks; to diagnostic procedures such as bladder catheterization and arterial, venous or lumbar punctures; to more invasive procedures such as chest tube placement, endotracheal intubation and circumcision. Existing studies have estimated that the average NICU patient receives anywhere from 2 to 14 painful procedures per day, with the smallest, most premature and potentially most vulnerable patients receiving a larger number of these procedures.[2,6] Repetitive painful stimuli has been linked to acute physiologic (increased heart rate, unstable blood pressure, increased intracranial pressure, desaturations) and hormonal (increased cortisol, epinephrine and norepinephrine, decreased insulin) changes.[5] Animal studies and, increasingly, human studies are beginning to show a link between inadequate analgesia leading to long-term harmful effects such as altered pain sensitivity

responses and behavioral, emotional and learning difficulties later in life.[7,8]

In order to prevent some of these potentially harmful short- and long-term effects that are caused by painful stimuli, the treating physician needs not only to be aware of the myriad of painful stimuli that neonates are exposed to but also to be knowledgeable of how to accurately assess whether or not a neonate is experiencing pain. Numerous studies and validated neonatal pain assessment scales exist in the literature. The majority take into account both physiologic (heart rate, desaturations, blood pressure), and behavioral (crying, facial expressions, sleeplessness) indicators into the overall assessment of the neonates' pain.

A table comparing these neonatal pain assessment tools can be reviewed in the 2006 American Academy of Pediatrics policy statement, "Prevention and Management of Pain in the Neonate: An Update."[7] All clinicians involved in the care of neonates need to be familiar with some of the common physiologic and behavioral signs a neonate exhibits in response to pain. This familiarity not only serves as a reminder to the clinician to administer appropriate analgesia and sedation but also allows the clinician to be able to reassess the adequacy of the analgesia or sedation given.

ANALGESIA

The International Association for the Study of Pain defined *pain* as "an unpleasant sensory and emotional experience associated with actual or potential tissue damage or described in terms of such damage."[9] This definition attempts to incorporate both the subjective nature of a patient's experience of pain as well as the more tangible and concrete anatomic and molecular disruption that occurs,

Table 3.1. Pain control combination therapies for common neonatal procedures[4]

Heel lance	1. Consider venipuncture 2. Sucrose pacifier 3. Kangaroo care/swaddling
Percutaneous venous and arterial catheter placement, venipunctue	1. Sucrose pacifier 2. Kangaroo care/swaddling 3. EMLA
Lumbar puncture	1. Sucrose pacifier 2. Lidocaine and prilocaine cream (EMLA) 3. Subcutaneous lidocaine infiltration
Subcutaneous or intramuscular injection	1. Use IV medication, if possible 2. Sucrose pacifier 3. Kangaroo care/swaddling 4. EMLA
Circumcision	1. Sucrose pacifier 2. EMLA 3. Dorsal penile nerve block, caudal nerve block, ring block 4. Acetaminophen for postoperative analgesia
Umbilical catheter insertion	1. Sucrose pacifier 2. Swaddling
Nasogastric or orogastric tube placement	1. Sucrose pacifier 2. Kangaroo care/swaddling
Catheterization for urinalysis	1. Sucrose pacifier 2. Swaddling

resulting in the neuroendocrine perception of pain. Analgesia is the inability to feel pain without the loss of consciousness.

Nonpharmacologic Pain Management

With the increase in knowledge and awareness that appropriate and adequate pain management in neonates leads to improved outcomes, there also has been an increase in the use of environmental and behavioral interventions that add to the overall well-being of a neonate in discomfort. These therapies are easy to implement and have little to no side effects. Although they might not provide complete analgesia when used alone, when used in conjunction with other pharmacologic analgesics they help shorten the period of discomfort of the neonate.

Environmental interventions include decreasing loud noises, dimming bright lights, limiting and clustering invasive procedures, swaddling, kangaroo care (skin to skin contact with mother). Breastfeeding and suckling pacifiers during or after procedures have been shown to decrease pain responses in neonates.[4,5,7] Having the patient use sucrose pacifiers or administering 0.1 to 2 mL of 24% to 50% sucrose orally 2 to 3 minutes before a painful procedure (doses <1 mL should be used in premature neonates [<32 weeks gestational age]) have been shown to significantly decrease neonatal pain scores during procedures. Sucrose administration is believed to release endogenous opioid neurotransmitters (β-endorphins), resulting in observed calming and analgesic effects. The duration of the calming effect is believed to be 2 to 3 minutes; therefore, the dose may be repeated as needed during the procedure. Use of sucrose for painful procedures is thought to be effective in newborns and infants younger than 6 months. The only theoretic, although not formally reported, risks of sucrose administration are hyperglycemia and necrotizing enterocolitis, the possibility of both of which are thought to increase with repeated administration.[5]

Table 3.1 lists recommended management strategies for common painful procedures in neonates.

Topical and Infiltrative Medications

Eutectic mixture of local anesthetics (EMLA): EMLA 5% cream, a mixture of lidocaine and prilocaine, has been shown to be effective in decreasing the pain of procedures such as circumcision, intravenous (IV) or intra-arterial

Table 3.2. Recommended acetaminophen dosing regimens

Acetaminophen	30 Weeks GA	34 Weeks GA	Term
PO Acetaminophen	10–15 mg/kg/dose Q12h Max: 25 mg/kg/day	10–15 mg/kg/dose Q8h Max: 45 mg/kg/day	10–15 mg/kg/dose Q6h Max: 60 mg/kg/day
PR Acetaminophen	15 mg/kg/dose Q12h	20 mg/kg/dose Q8h	20 mg/kg/dose Q6h
IV Propacetamol	20–25 mg/kg/dose Q6h	25–30 mg/kg/dose Q6h	20–30 mg/kg/dose Q4–6h

GA, gestational age.
Recommended doses obtained from results from studies by Anderson BJ, et al, and Allegaert K, et al.[13,14]

catheter insertion and lumbar puncture.[10,11] EMLA has not been shown to be effective for pain reduction from heel sticks.[12] Because EMLA is absorbed through the skin, it is not recommended for use in newborns younger than 36 weeks of gestational age or in preterm infants younger than 2 weeks of age due to the potential for systemic drug absorption.

EMLA is contraindicated in patients with glucose-6-phosphate dehydrogenase (G6PD) deficiency or congenital or idiopathic methemoglobinemia because these patients have an increased risk of developing methemoglobinemia due to the decreased amount of the nicotinamide adenine dinucleotide (NADH):cytochrome $b5$ reductase, the enzyme that reduces methemoglobin in the blood.[10] Patients who are taking phenobarbital, phenytoin, sulfonamides and acetaminophen who use EMLA are at risk for developing methemoglobinemia. The onset of action is 1 hour, with a duration of action of 45 to 60 hours after cream removal.[5] Due to concern about systemic absorption, repeat application is not recommended in neonates.

There are several other compounds and formulations for topical anesthetic use, many with proven efficacy in older children and adults. Medications such as lidocaine and tetracaine (Synera topical patch), 4% lidocaine cream (LMX4, ElaMax) and, more recently, lidocaine iontophoresis have been developed for use on intact skin. Unfortunately, these newer compounds have yet to be studied in neonates and infants. The use of agents such as tetracaine, adrenaline, and cocaine (TAC), which has now been replaced by lidocaine, epinephrine, and tetracaine (LET), on open wounds, also has not been studied in neonates precluding a recommendation for their routine use in this age group. Finally, there is no available literature regarding the safety or efficacy of vapocoolant sprays such as ethyl chloride on neonatal patients.

Infiltrative medications such as lidocaine and bupivicaine for local anesthesia or nerve blocks are also effective in newborns. Excessive doses of local anesthetics, however, may result in seizures and cardiac instability due to decreased metabolic clearance rates in children. The recommended dose of these agents is therefore lower in neonates. The maximum dose of lidocaine is 4 mg/kg without epinephrine and 5 mg/kg with epinephrine.[4] The maximum dose of bupivicaine is 2 mg/kg, regardless of the use of epinephrine.

Nonopioid Analgesics

Acetaminophen (*N*-acetyl-*p*-aminophenol, APAP), propacetamol/paracetamol: Recent studies in preterm and full-term neonates have concluded that acetaminophen is a safe analgesic and antipyretic medication in this age group. With the recent advent of propacetamol, the parenteral formulation of acetaminophen, there is now an additional option for pain management in postoperative patients. Although it has not been formally approved for use in neonates, there are numerous studies reporting its safety and efficacy. When infused, propacetamol is converted to paracetamol by plasma esterases in a ratio of 2:1 such that 1 g of propacetamol is converted into 0.5 g of paracetamol.[13–15] Prolonged use beyond 2 to 3 days is not recommended due to the increased risk of hepatotoxicity. See Table 3.2 for recommended dosing regimens.

Nonsteroidal anti-inflammatory drugs (NSAIDs): There are few studies that explore the use of nonselective cyclooxygenase inhibitors such as acetylsalicylic acid (ASA), ibuprofen and ketorolac for analgesia in neonates. Their anti-inflammatory, antipyretic and analgesic effects are well known but their safety is not established in neonates. These agents work by stopping prostaglandin synthesis by inhibiting the function of the cyclooxygenase enzyme. Prostaglandins are essential for protecting

Table 3.3. Opiate dosing guidelines[5]

Opioid medication	Route	Dose	Onset/duration	Side effects
Morphine sulfate	IV	0.05–0.1 mg/kg	4–6 min/2–4 hrs	Respiratory depression, hypotension, urinary retention, miosis, decreased gastrointestinal motility
	CI	0.01–0.03 mg/kg/hr		
Fentanyl citrate	IV	0.5–3 μg/kg	2–3 min/30–60 min	Chest wall rigidity, respiratory depression, hypothermia, hypotension, seizures, ↑ risk of hypoxemia and apnea when fentanyl used in conjunction with midazolam
	CI	0.5–2 μg/kg/hr		

IV, intravenous.

the gastrointestinal tract, aggregating platelets and maintaining a normal kidney glomerular filtration rate. Use of NSAIDs risks the increased chance of gastrointestinal tract bleeding, intraventricular hemorrhage and renal failure.[16,17] Although some centers in Europe have reported ketorolac use for pain management with some success and minimal side effects,[18] NSAIDs are not routinely recommended for pain management in preterm or term neonates in the United States.

Opioid Analgesics

Opioids are perhaps the most widely used analgesic for the management of moderate to severe pain in neonates. Adverse effects are related to the dose, the combination with other agents and the rate at which the medication is given. Side effects include respiratory depression, hypotension, decreased bowel motility and convulsions. With prolonged use and continuous infusions there is an increased risk of chemical dependence and/or tolerance; therefore, care should be taken to wean patient gradually off opioids so as to avoid withdrawal symptoms. Chest wall rigidity may occur with rapid IV administration of fentanyl.[4]

Although morphine can be used in neonates, renal clearance is slower, resulting in accumulation of active metabolites. The average half-life of morphine in preterm infants is 9 hours versus 6.5 hours in term neonates. The half-life in older children is only 2 hours. The accumulation of metabolites may cause respiratory depression and seizures.[19,20] Meperidine should be avoided in neonates as accumulation of its metabolite normeperidine can lead to seizures. Infants who receive opioids should be placed on continuous cardiac monitoring and pulse oximetry; naloxone should be readily available as should personnel

trained in advanced airway management. See Table 3.3 for dosing guidelines.

SEDATION

Many of the procedures being performed on infants that require analgesia also require some degree of simultaneously administered sedation. Painful procedures such as endotracheal intubation and tube thoracostomy, as well as less painful or relatively painless procedures such as sedating intubated patients or obtaining radiological scans, all require some degree of sedation. The use of sedative medications allows the clinician to safely and effectively complete many of the uncomfortable procedures for which a neonate is unable to hold still.

Varying degrees of sedation exist, and the definitions vary slightly, depending on the medical society that endorsed them. The level of sedation selected depends not only on the individual patient but also on the length, invasiveness and duration of the procedure being performed.

Following is a list of the definitions of the different types of sedation as outlined by the American Academy of Pediatrics and American College of Emergency Physicians:

- *Minimal sedation:* A drug-induced state during which patients respond normally to verbal commands. Although cognitive function and coordination may be impaired, ventilatory and cardiovascular functions are unaffected.[21]
- *Moderate sedation:* A drug-induced depression of consciousness during which patients respond purposefully to verbal commands. With moderate sedation, no intervention is required to maintain a patent airway, and spontaneous ventilation is adequate. Cardiovascular function is usually maintained.[21]

- *Deep sedation:* A drug-induced state of depressed consciousness or unconsciousness from which the patient is not easily aroused but does respond purposefully after repeated verbal or painful stimulation. The ability to independently maintain ventilatory function may be impaired. Patients may require assistance in maintaining a patent airway, and spontaneous ventilation may be inadequate. Cardiovascular function is usually maintained. A state of deep sedation may be accompanied by a partial or complete loss of protective reflexes.[21]
- *Procedural sedation and analgesia (PSA):* A technique of administering sedatives or dissociative agents with or without analgesics to induce a state that allows the patient to tolerate unpleasant procedures while maintaining cardiorespiratory function. Procedural sedation and analgesia is intended to result in a depressed level of consciousness but one that allows the patient to maintain airway control independently and continuously. Specifically the drugs, doses and techniques used are not likely to produce a loss of protective airway reflexes.[22]

As in many of the analgesics just listed, there is a relative paucity of studies reporting the efficacy, pharmacokinetics, safety and side effects of sedatives used in neonates. Despite the relative lack of literature to support their use in neonates, analgesics are still widely used by clinicians based on their effectiveness in older children.

With any sedative, it is important to have the appropriate equipment readily available when administering sedatives or performing PSA. The popular mnemonic SOAPME has been used to remember this essential checklist of items necessary for sedations[21]:

Suction apparatus with catheter
Oxygen delivery system capable of delivering >90% oxygen (positive-pressure)
Airway equipment (oropharyngeal tubes, functioning laryngoscopes, endotracheal tubes, etc.)
Pharmacy, that is, the requisite drugs/medications to induce sedation as well as the appropriate reversal agents
Monitoring equipment for cardiorespiratory function and oxygen saturation
Equipment for a safe sedation (e.g., defibrillator)

In addition to having these items readily available, it is imperative that the clinician adhere to the assessment, monitoring and documentation guidelines for sedation as outlined by the specific policy at his or her institution.

Benzodiazepines

Benzodiazepines, particularly midazolam and lorazepam, have been used extensively in neonates and infants for sedation. In addition to providing sedation, these drugs also produce muscle relaxation and anxiolysis, as well as possessing amnestic and anticonvulsant properties. Reported side effects include respiratory depression, hypotension, dependence and tolerance. Unlike midazolam and lorazepam, diazepam is not recommended for use in neonates because they have limited ability to metabolize it. Because benzodiazepines use the same glucuronidation pathway as bilirubin, their use can potentially decrease the metabolism of bilirubin thereby causing hyperbilirubinemia, particularly in preterm infants. See Table 3.4 for dosing guidelines.

Barbiturates

Barbiturates also have been used in neonates and infants for their sedative as well as their anticonvulsant properties. Commonly used barbiturates for sedating intubated patients or neonates experiencing withdrawal from neonatal abstinence syndrome include phenobarbital, pentobarbital and thiopental. Barbiturates are primarily metabolized in the liver. Side effects include significant hypotension, respiratory depression, tolerance and dependence. See Table 3.4 for dosing guidelines.

Chloral Hydrate

Chloral hydrate is a hypnotic drug used to sedate children for painless procedures such as obtaining radiological studies or echocardiograms. The breakdown products of metabolism, trichloroethanol and trichloroacetic acid reportedly can exacerbate hyperbilirubinemia and have been found to be carcinogenic in rat models. These metabolites have half-lives longer than 72 hours and with repeated doses, these metabolites accumulate and can increase the risk of adverse effects. Side effects include central nervous system depression, supraventricular tachycardias, renal failure and pulmonary edema. Caution should be taken when using chloral hydrate in neonates. See Table 3.4 for dosing guidelines.

Table 3.4. Sedative dosing guidelines[5,16,23–29]

Medication	Route	Dose (mg/kg)	Onset/duration	Side effects
Benzodiazepines				
Midazolam	IV	0.05–0.15	2–3 min/30–60 min	Respiratory depression, hypotension,
	CI	0.01–0.06 per hr	4–6 min/6–12 hr	dependence, tolerance
Lorazepam	IV	0.02–0.05		
Barbiturates				
Pentobarbital	IV/IM/Rectal	2–6	3–5 min/1–2 hr	Respiratory depression, hypotension,
Thiopental	IV	2–5	10–20 sec/5–8 min	dependence, tolerance
Chloral hydrate	PO	25–50	15–30 min/1–2 hr	Cardiovascular/respiratory/CNS depression, hyperbilirubinemia, supraventricular tachycardias, renal failure and pulmonary edema
Ketamine	IV	0.5–2	1–2 min/60 min	Tachycardia, increased blood pressure, bronchodilation, apnea, hypoxia, laryngospasm
Etomidate	IV	0.1–0.3	<1 min/3–5 min	Limited data in neonates for sedation. Few side effects in children and adults, emesis, myoclonic jerks
Propofol	IV	0.5–3	<1 min/5–10 min	Hypotension, respiratory depression, pain at injection site
	CI	0.15–0.3/min		

CI, continuous infusion; CNS, central nervous system; IV, intravenous; PO, per os.

Ketamine

Ketamine is a dissociative anesthetic that has sedative, analgesic and amnestic properties. Use of procedural sedation and analgesia has been well studied in older children, but limited studies exist in the neonatal population. Side effects include tachycardia, increased blood pressure, bronchodilation, apnea, hypoxia and laryngospasm. There is an increased risk of these respiratory side effects in patients younger than 3 months of age. Early animal studies linked ketamine administration in rat pups with increased neuronal apoptosis.[5,16] The significance of these findings is still unclear. Further studies need to be performed before ketamine can be recommended as a first-line medication for sedation in neonates. See Table 3.4 for dosing guidelines.

Etomidate

Etomidate is an ultrashort-acting sedative-hypnotic with onset of action in children older than 10 years of age of less than 1 minute and duration of approximately 3 to 5 minutes; etomidate has minimal cardiorespiratory effects. Standard dose is 0.1 to 0.3 mg/kg IV. Although etomidate has been used to ease intubations in infants, there are no studies to date addressing its safety and efficacy for sedation in neonates.[23] See Table 3.4 for dosing guidelines.

Propofol

Propofol is another ultrashort-acting sedative hypnotic with wide use in the adult population. As with most of the other sedatives, there are limited studies in neonates delineating its pharmacokinetics and safety. Propofol's onset of action is approximately 30 seconds, with IV infusion and an effective duration of action of fewer than 5 to 10 minutes. Standard initial dose is 0.5 to 3 mg/kg, followed by either repeated boluses of 0.5 mg/kg every 2 to 5 minutes or a constant infusion at 125 to 300 μg/kg/min. Propofol can cause pain at the site of infusion, has potent respiratory depressant effects and can produce significant hypotension. Specific studies regarding routine use of propofol in neonates in the ED setting are lacking; however, a recent pharmacokinetic study of propofol reported that there is increased peripheral distribution volume, reduced metabolic clearance and prolonged elimination time.[24–26]

PITFALLS

- Failure to recognize that neonates not only have the neuroendocrine mechanisms in place to feel pain but also that increasing studies show that they may have increased sensitivity to pain.[30,31]
- Failure to recognize that many sedatives have no analgesic properties; therefore, the clinician should always use

an appropriate analgesic in conjunction with the sedative when performing painful procedures.

- Failure to adjust the doses of sedatives and analgesics in newborns. There are limited studies on the safety and efficacy of a significant number of sedatives and analgesics in neonates.

REFERENCES

1. MacLean S, Obispo J, Young KD. The gap between pediatric emergency department procedural pain management treatments available and actual practice. *Pediatr Emerg Care.* 2007;23(2):87–93.
2. Simons SHP, van Dijk M, Anand KJS, et al. Do we still hurt newborn babies? A prospective study of procedural pain and analgesia in neonates. *Arch Pediatr Adolesc Med.* 2003;157(11):1058–1064.
3. Porter FL, Wolf CM, Gold J, et al. Pain and pain management in newborn infants: a survey of physicians and nurses. *Pediatrics.* 1997;100(4):626–632.
4. Anand KJS and the International Evidence-Based Group for Neonatal Pain. Consensus Statement for the Prevention and Management of Pain in the Newborn. *Arch Pediatr Adolesc Med.* 2001;155(2):173–180.
5. Khurana S, Hall RW, Anand KJS. Treatment of pain and stress in the neonate: when and how. *Neoreviews.* 2005;6(2):e76–86.
6. Stevens B, McGrath P, Gibbins S, et al. Procedural pain in newborns at risk for neurologic impairment. *Pain.* 2003;105(1–2):27–35.
7. American Academy of Pediatrics Prevention and management of pain in the neonate: an update. *Pediatrics.* 2006;118(5):2231–2241.
8. Zempsky WT, Schechter NL. What's new in the management of pain in children? *Pediatr Rev.* 2003;24(10):337–348.
9. Part III: Pain terms, a current list with definitions and notes on usage. In: H Merskey, N Bogduk, eds. *Classification of Chronic Pain,* 2nd ed. IASP Task Force on Taxonomy. Seattle: IASP Press; 1994:209–214.
10. Taddio A, Ohlsson A, Einarson TR, et al. A systematic review of lidocaine-prilocaine cream (EMLA) in the treatment of acute pain in neonates. *Pediatrics.* 1998;101(2):e1.
11. Brady-Fryer B, Wiebe N, Lander JA. Pain relief for neonatal circumcision. *Cochrane Database Syst Rev.*19 July, 2004(4):CD004217.
12. Stevens B, Johnston C, Taddio A, et al. Management of pain from heel lance with lidocaine-prilocaine (EMLA) cream: is it safe and efficacious in preterm infants? *J Dev Behav Pediatr.* 1999;20(4):216–221.
13. Allegaert K, Anderson BJ, Naulaers G, et al. Intravenous paracetamol (propacetamol) pharmacokinetics in term and preterm neonates. *Eur J Clin Pharmacol.* 2004;60(3):191–197.
14. Anderson BJ, van Lingen RA, Hansen TG, et al. Acetaminophen developmental pharmacokinetics in premature neonates and infants: a pooled population analysis. *Anesthesiology.* 2002;96(6):1336–1345.
15. Bartocci M, Lundeberg S. Intravenous paracetamol: the Stockholm protocol for postoperative analgesia of term and preterm neonates. *Pediatr Anesth.* 2007;17(11):1120–1121.
16. Anand KJS, Hall RW. Pharmacological therapy for analgesia and sedation in the newborn. *Arch Dis Child.* Fetal Neonatal Edition. 2006;91(6):F448–453.
17. Allegaert K, Vanhole C, Hoon J, et al. Nonselective cyclo-oxygenase inhibitors and glomerular filtration rate in preterm neonates. *Pediatr Nephrol.* 2005;20(11):1557–1561.
18. Papacci P, De Francisci G, Iacobucci C, et al. Use of intravenous ketorolac in the neonate and premature babies. *Paediatr Anaesth.* 2004;14(6):487–492.
19. Sinno HPS, Anand KJS. Pain control: opioid dosing, population kinetics and side-effects. *Semin Fetal Neonatal Med.* 2006;11(4):260–267.
20. Berde CB, Sethna NF. Analgesics for the treatment of pain in children. *N Engl J Med.* 2002;347(14):1094–1103.
21. Cote CJ, Wilson S, the Work Group on Sedation. American Academy of Pediatrics. Guidelines for monitoring and management of pediatric patients during and after sedation for diagnostic and therapeutic procedures: an update. *Pediatrics.* 2006;118(6):2587–2602.
22. Godwin SA, Caro DA, Wolf SJ, et al. Clinical policy: procedural sedation and analgesia in the emergency department. *Ann Emerg Med.* 2005;45(2):177–196.
23. Guldner G, Schultz J, Sexton P, et al. Etomidate for rapid-sequence intubation in young children: hemodynamic effects and adverse events. *Acad Emerg Med.* 2003;10(2):134–139.
24. Allegaert K, Peeters MY, Verbesselt R, et al. Inter-individual variability in propofol pharmacokinetics in preterm and term neonates. *Br J Anaesth.* 2007;99(6):864–870.
25. Miner JR, Burton JH. Clinical practice advisory: emergency department procedural sedation with propofol. *Ann Emerg Med.* 2007;50(2):182–187.
26. Pershad J, Godambe SA. Propofol for procedural sedation in the pediatric emergency department. *J Emerg Med.* 2004;27(1):11–14.
27. Krauss B, Green SM. Sedation and analgesia for procedures in children. *N Engl J Med.* 2000;342(13):938945.
28. Wada DR, Bjorkman S, Ebling WF, et al. Computer simulation of the effects of alterations in blood flows and body composition on thiopental pharmacokinetics in humans. *Anesthesiology.* 1997; 87(4):884–899.
29. Allegaert K, Daniels H, Naulaers G, et al. Pharmacodynamics of chloral hydrate in former preterm infants. *Eur J Pediatr.* 2005;164(7):403–407.
30. Porter FL, Grunau RE, Anand KJ. Long-term effects of pain in infants. *J Dev Behav Pediatr.* 1999;20(4):253–261.
31. Porter FL, Wolf CM, Miller JP. Procedural pain in newborn infants: the influence of intensity and development. *Pediatrics.* 1999;104(1):e13.

4 Pediatric Airway Management

Ghazala Q. Sharieff and Maureen McCollough

INTRODUCTION

Resuscitation of an infant or child can be one of the most challenging and anxiety-producing experiences in the emergency department (ED). The ability to recognize and treat life-threatening conditions requires advance preparation and the ability to secure an airway. The most common cause of cardiac arrest in children is respiratory failure; therefore, early attention to respiratory status is imperative. This chapter discusses airway techniques, rapid sequence intubation drugs and management of the difficult pediatric airway.

ANATOMY

The pediatric airway differs from the adult airway in numerous ways (Table 4.1); therefore, some special techniques are helpful for intubation in children. Because the occiput is large in younger children, a towel roll should be placed beneath the patient's shoulders and not behind the head as in adults. The shoulder roll helps to place the child in a more neutral position.[1,2] A child's airway is very anterior, and it is imperative that the person who is performing the intubation is looking up at the airway. Correct positioning cannot be emphasized enough (Figure 4.1); if necessary, the provider performing the intubation should squat in order to visualize the airway. A straight blade is recommended for use in infants as it helps to lift the floppy, U-shaped epiglottis out of the way (Figure 4.2). In an infant who has a very small mouth, have an assistant pull the baby's cheek to the side. This allows passage of both the laryngoscope and endotracheal tube (ETT).

The most common reasons for intubation are listed in Table 4.2. Potential combinations of agents that might be used for rapid sequence intubation are listed in Table 4.3.

Table 4.1. Anatomical differences between adult and pediatric airways

Prominent occiput, which can cause airway obstruction (use 1-in. towel roll below shoulders)

Dependence upon nasopharynx patency (avoid nasal airways in patients <1 year of age due to larger adenoidal tissue, which can bleed)

Lots of secretions

Loose primary teeth

Relatively larger tongues can obstruct the airway (may need to use an oral or nasal airway)

Epiglottis is U-shaped and floppy (use a straight laryngoscope blade to lift the epiglottis directly)

Larynx is more anterior and cephalad

Cricoid area is smallest area of the airway

Small trachea diameter and distance between rings makes tracheostomy or cricothyrotomy more difficult

AHA recommends needle cricothyrotomy for difficult airways (see text, Needle Cricothyrotomy [Jet Ventilation])

Much shorter tracheal length (newborn, 4–5 cm; 18 month old, 7–8 cm) (ETTs easily dislodged; reassess position of tube frequently)

Large airways are narrower (leads to greater resistance)

Ribs are more horizontal at a very young age; dependent upon diaphragm to move (decompress stomach with NG tube to ventilate easier, rough guide is two times ETT size)

AHA, American Heart Association; ETT, endotracheal tube; NG, nasogastric.

PROCEDURES

Bag Valve Mask Ventilation

Correct mask sizing is vital to proper bag valve mask (BVM) ventilation. The mask should fit snugly from the bridge of the nose to the cleft of the chin. A mask that is too large can place pressure on the eyes and result in vagal bradycardia. A mask that is too small will not allow for adequate oxygenation and ventilation. The mask should be held using a *CE grip*, in which the thumb and index finger grip the mask and the third, fourth and fifth fingers

Infant   Small Child

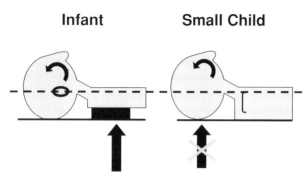

Figure 4.1. Optimal positioning of the neonate and child prior to intubation. Note that in the small child, a cushion may not be necessary for airway alignment.

are placed on the angle of the jaw. Avoid pushing on the soft tissue below the mandible as airway obstruction can occur.

The rate of bagged breaths per minute is best controlled by having the operator say "squeeze-release-release" while ventilating the patient. This will help to decrease the rapid rate of ventilation and the adverse effects that often occur in resuscitative events. The new American Heart Association Pediatric Life Support guidelines only recommend administering 8 to 10 breaths per minute in patients in full arrest once an advanced airway is placed.[3,4] If it is difficult to ventilate the patient, an oral or nasal airway can be used to facilitate BVM technique. Complications of BVM ventilation include gastric distention, pneumothorax, vomiting, aspiration and hypoxia.

Avoid stocking the ED with neonatal 250 cc bags as these bags are inadequate outside of the newborn period

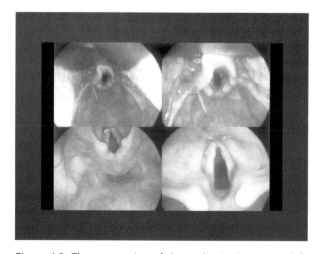

Figure 4.2. The progression of the pediatric airway: *top left*, infant; *top right*, toddler; *bottom left*, 8 year old; *bottom right*, teenager. (Courtesy of John Kanegaye, MD, Rady Children's Hospital, Emergency Care Center. San Diego, California.)

Table 4.2. Indications for airway management

Respiratory failure or impending respiratory failure:
  Respiratory rates < 12 or > 60 plus nonpurposeful or
  unresponsive to painful stimuli
Cardiopulmonary failure
Shock: Helps decrease the work of breathing
Emergency drug administration – lidocaine, epinephrine,
  atropine, Narcan (+ valium) – when no intravenous access
  in readily accessible
Neurological resuscitation: Pediatric GCS <8 or consider in
  anyone with GCS <12 and decreasing mental status;
  hyperventilate to Pco_2 of 30–35 mm Hg
Protection of the airway in patients without an intact gag
  reflex

GCS, Glasgow Coma Scale.

and can cause confusion in code situations. Appropriate bag sizing is as follows:

- 450 cc bag for infant or child younger than 5 years of age
- 750 cc or adult bag for older children

RAPID-SEQUENCE INTUBATION IN CHILDREN

Rapid sequence intubation enables the provider to secure the airway by decreasing the risk of aspiration and iatrogenic rise in intracranial pressure. In addition, it facilitates intubation in the agitated or seizing patient by rendering the patient completely unconscious. Preoxygenation is imperative prior to intubation attempts. An intubation timeline and drugs of choice are listed in Tables 4.4 through 4.6. In the case of a difficult airway in which paralysis of a breathing patient is not safe, an awake intubation may be attempted using a sedative agent alone.

Recommended ETT sizes for infants are listed in Table 4.7. With the advent of high volume, low pressure ETTs with cuffs, the dictum of using only uncuffed ETTs in

Table 4.3. Clinical scenarios

Clinical scenario	Induction agents
Isolated head injury	Propofol, thiopental, etomidate – no ketamine!
Status epilepticus	Thiopental, propofol, etomidate, midazolam
Asthma	Ketamine, etomidate – no thiopental!
Respiratory failure	Ketamine, etomidate, propofol

Courtesy of Al Sacchetti, MD.

Table 4.4. Pretreatment drugs (LOAD) for rapid sequence intubation

L   Lidocaine: An operating room–based study revealed that there was no effect on heart rate and blood pressure when using lidocaine pretreatment in children undergoing endotracheal intubation. However, as there is minimal risk of side effects and lidocaine can be potentially useful in older children, this agent is still used. It should be given 2 to 3 minutes prior to intubation in order to be effective.[8]

O   Opiates: Fentanyl 2–4 μg/kg can cause chest wall rigidity (no histamine release)

A   Atropine

D[†]   Defasciculating doses of paralytic agent

Drug	Dose (mg/kg)	Indication	Comments
Atropine	0.01–0.02mg/kg (minimum, 0.1mg)	Some advocate its use as prophylaxis against bradycardia with succinylcholine	Consider in children <5 years of age (20 kg) undergoing intubation[9]
Lidocaine	1.0–1.5	1. Elevated ICP* 2. Reactive airway disease	Mixed evidence of effectiveness

* ICP, intracranial pressure.

† There is no need to use a priming defasciculating dose of nondepolarizing paralytics in children <5 years of age as they do not have the muscle mass to fasciculate.

[8] Splinter WM. Intravenous lidocaine does not attenuate the hemodynamic response of children to laryngoscopy and tracheal intubation. *Can J Aneaesth.* 1990;37:440;443.

[9] Luten R. Approach to the pediatric airway. In: Walls R, Murphy M, Luten R, Schneider R, eds. *The Manual of Emergency Airway Management,* 2nd ed. Philadelphia, PA: Lippincott Williams & Wilkins; 2004.

Table 4.5. Commonly used paralytics for intubation in children

Drug	Dose (mg/kg)	Onset	Duration of action	Comments
Succinylcholine	1–2	<1 min	<10 minutes	Can cause bradycardia. Pretreat children <5 years of age with atropine. *Do not use in children with chronic muscular disorders.*
Rocuronium	1.0	<1 min	40–60 min	No change in potassium and does not cause malignant hyperthermia
Vecuronium	0.1 or 0.3	2–3 min or 60–90 sec	30–40 min or ≤100 min	Priming dose of 0.01 mg/kg may be given IV followed 2–3 sec later by induction agent and repeat vecuronium of 0.15 mg/kg.

Table 4.6. Induction agents

Drug	Dose (mg/kg)	Onset (sec)	Duration (min)	Blood pressure	ICP	Comments
Propofol	1–2	10–20	3–14	Decrease	Decrease	Antiepileptic effects. *Do not use in patients with soy or egg allergies.*
Etomidate	0.3	20–30	7–14	Neutral	May decrease	Adrenal suppression, myoclonic jerks,
Ketamine	IV: 1–2 IM: 4	15–60	IV: 10–15	Increase	Increase	Bronchial relaxation, myocardial depression
Thiopental	3.0–5.0	20–30	3–5	Decrease	Decrease	Antiepileptic effects, can cause bronchospasm
Midazolam	0.1–0.3	30–60	IV: 30	Decrease		Antiepileptic effects

ICP, intracranial pressure; IM, intramuscular; IV, intravenous.

Table 4.7. Endotracheal tube size

Newborn: 3.0 mm or, if large newborn, 3.5 mm
Infant: ≤6 months, 3.5–4.0 mm
Infant: 1 year, 4.0–4.5 mm

Table 4.8. Laryngoscope size and type

Age/weight	Size (type)
2.5 kg	0 (straight)
0–3 months	1.0 (straight)
3 months–3 years	1.5–2.0 (straight or curved) or 1.5 (Wisconsin)
3 years–12 years	2.0–4.0 (straight or curved)

children younger than 8 years of age is changing; therefore, it is possible to use a cuffed ETT in children. Currently, cuffed ETTs are not recommended in neonates.[5] A tube size smaller than that calculated when using an uncuffed ETT is typically recommended. Handy formulas for tube sizes are listed:

Uncuffed ETT:

$$4 + (\text{age in years}/4)$$

Cuffed ETT:

$$3 + (\text{age in years}/4)$$

Cuff inflation pressure should be kept at <20 cm H_2O. Nasotracheal intubations are more complicated in children than in adults for several reasons. The use of nasal airways generally is not recommended in children younger than 1 year of age as the small size of the nares makes passage of the tube difficult and large adenoids can be lacerated, resulting in profuse bleeding.

Incorrect ETT size can lead to the inability to ventilate if the tube is too small or airway trauma (e.g., subglottic edema) if the tube is too large. An easy way to estimate the depth of ETT placement is three times the ETT size (e.g., 4.0 mm ETT placed at the 12-cm mark at the lips) or 10 plus age in years at the lips. For premature infants, the following estimations are helpful:

Weight	Position at the lips
1 kg = →	7 cm
2 kg = →	8 cm
3 kg = →	9 cm
4 kg = →	10 cm

Approximate laryngoscope sizes are listed in Table 4.8. The Broselow Tape® also can assist with blade size; however, it is important to remember that the actual blade size needed will be determined not only by weight but also by body habitus and anatomic variation. In addition to having available an ETT one size smaller and one size larger than calculated, it is important to have a laryngoscope

available that is one size smaller and one size larger than anticipated.

Post-intubation assessment includes confirmation that the ETT is in correct position. Although direct visualization of the ETT passing through the cords is imperative, additional confirmation of tube placement should be performed. Listening first over the abdomen, and then over the axillae for breath sounds, is an excellent way to detect esophageal intubations. End-tidal capnometers and end-tidal CO_2 detectors are being used routinely as well. Pedi-Cap® by Nellcor should be used in infants weighing less than 15 kg. If the ETT is in the correct position, the color changes from purple to yellow on expiration when CO_2 passes across the filter paper. False positives can occur, however, if a large amount of air has been bagged into the stomach or if the patient has recently swallowed a carbonated beverage. CO_2 may not be detected in patients in full arrest or with poor perfusion.

Capnography may be used in patients in cardiopulmonary arrest to assess for the effectiveness of cardiac compressions. Although the Food and Drug Administration currently only approves the esophageal detector device in children weighing 20 kg or more, studies have shown it to be effective in infants heavier than 5 kg.[6,7]

Once ETT placement is confirmed, the tube should be secured. The ETT very easily becomes dislodged, particularly in young infants who have shorter tracheal lengths. In order to minimize ETT movement, place the patient in a cervical collar, even in the nontrauma setting. Place a nasogastric (NG) or orogastric (OG) tube as soon as possible. Any amount of gastric distention can make it difficult to ventilate and oxygenate a child. A rough rule of thumb for NG and OG tube size is that these tubes should be two times the ETT size. An OG tube should be used if there is concern about facial trauma due to the risk of intracranial passage of an NG tube. Complications of ETT placement include esophageal intubation, right mainstem intubation, dislodgement, obstruction, barotrauma, trauma to airway or subglottic stenosis.

Although the use of endotracheal medications is suboptimal, the ETT can be used to administer the following drugs (LEAN):

L Lidocaine
E Epinephrine
A Atropine
N Narcan (naloxone)

The ETT dosage of epinephrine is 10 times the IV or intraosseous (IO) dosage (0.1 mg/kg [0.1 cc/kg] of 1:1000 concentration). Lidocaine, atropine and Narcan typically are administered at two to three times the IV or IO dosage.

PROCEDURE FOR RAPID SEQUENCE INTUBATION

1. Time to intubation 5 minutes: Start preoxygenation
2. Time to intubation 3 minutes: Give any premedication (atropine, lidocaine)
3. Intubation time:
   - Push induction and paralytic agents
   - Apply cricoid pressure using the Sellick maneuver
   - BURP technique (*b*ackward, *u*pward and *r*ightward *p*ressure) (Can occlude the airway with too much pressure.)
4. Intubate after patient is fully relaxed
5. Immediately after intubation:
   - Check tube placement
   - Release cricoid pressure
   - Secure tube
   - Place NG tube

Initial Ventilator Settings

Initial ventilator settings typically are set by assessing the weight of the patient and the underlying etiology of respiratory distress. The following recommendations are for initial ventilatory management. Adjustments should be made according to blood gas measurements, end-tidal CO_2 and pulse oximetry monitors and patient status.

Children Weighing Less Than 10 kg

Use a pressure-limited system. The infant should be given sufficient O_2 to relieve cyanosis and maintain normal O_2 saturation (92%-96%) and/or normal Po_2 (60–90 mmHg).

Rate: Infant 20 to 60 breaths per minute (The ventilator should be cycled at the rate to produce a normal $Paco_2$ [35–45 mmHg].)

Fio_2: 100%

PEEP: 3 to 5 cm H_2O

PIP: 15 to 35 cm H_2O (The peak inspiratory pressure [PIP] should be sufficient to produce discernible chest wall movement.)

I:E ratio 1:2 (inspiratory time, 0.4–0.7 seconds; inspiratory:expiratory ratio, 1:2)

Children Weighing More Than 10 kg

Use a volume-limited system.

Initial volume 10 to 15 cc/kg (This is changing to smaller volumes of 6–8 cc/kg, particularly in asthmatic patients.)

Rate: Infant, 20 to 30 breaths per minute; child, 15 to 20 breaths per minute

Fio_2: 100%

PEEP: 3 to 5 cm H_2O

I:E ratio 1:2

THE DIFFICULT PEDIATRIC AIRWAY

The importance of having an immediate plan of action for patients who fail endotracheal intubation cannot be over-emphasized (Table 4.9).

FOREIGN BODY MANAGEMENT

One point to remember is that the tracheal rings in young children are quite pliable; therefore, an esophageal foreign

Table 4.9. Suggested essential equipment for pediatric airway management

Endotracheal tubes (uncuffed and cuffed)
Stylets
Face masks and self-inflating bags
Laryngoscope with varying blade sizes
Magill forceps
Nasal and oral airways
Suctioning equipment
Nasogastric and orogastric tubes
Laryngeal mask airways
Pediatric intubating stylets
Gum elastic bougie catheter
Transtracheal jet ventilation device for needle cricothyrotomy
Cricothyrotomy equipment for surgical airways

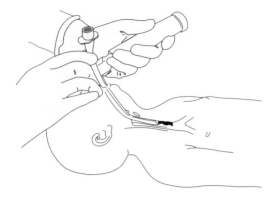

Figure 4.3. Diagram of how to push the foreign body further down the trachea and into a mainstem then pull back for oxygenation and ventilation

body can push from behind and cause airway compression.

If the patient has an active cough and is alert, there is no need for acute intervention. The patient should be kept in a comfortable position and arrangements should be made for the patient to be transported to the operating room for bronchoscopy. If the patient stops breathing effectively, however, then basic life support maneuvers should be initiated. First, a basic Heimlich maneuver may save this child. Abdominal thrusts are indicated in children older than 1 year, and a series of five back blows and five chest thrusts is recommended in infants.

If the Heimlich maneuver is not effective, then direct laryngoscopy should be performed; if a foreign body is visible, it should be removed using the Magill forceps. Be careful not to accidentally push the foreign body into the trachea with the tip of the laryngoscope blade. If no foreign body is visible, then an attempt can be made to intubate the patient with a stylet positioned in the ETT. Depending on the location of the foreign body, resistance may be met before the correct placement for the ETT is reached. When the ETT is in the correct position, and the patient is still unable to be ventilated, gentle pressure should be applied in an effort to push the foreign body lower in the tracheobronchial tree. The foreign body typically moves down the right mainstem bronchus, and at least oxygenation and ventilation of one lung may be achieved (Figure 4.3).

FAILED INTUBATION

In the event that endotracheal intubation is unsuccessful, there are several options for airway rescue. A pediatric intubating stylet is available and is used in the same manner as the Eschmann catheter or "gum bougie." The laryngeal mask airway (LMA) has the advantages of being easily

Table 4.10. Technique for placement of a laryngeal mask airway (LMA)

1. Check the cuff by inflating air. The LMA may be easier to insert if a small amount of air is left in the aperture, rather than collapsing it fully.
2. Lubricate the posterior surface of the LMA with K-Y Jelly.
3. Preoxygenate the patient and place the patient in the "sniffing" position.
4. Propofol is an ideal induction agent, but thiopental may be used.
5. While inserting the LMA, keep the cuff tip pressed against the posterior pharyngeal wall; this prevents the cuff from entering the valleculae or becoming caught against the epiglottis or arytenoids.
6. Face the aperture of the LMA forward, and use the index finger to guide the LMA into the hypopharynx until resistance is felt. Do not hold the jaw open during this step. An alternative technique is to use the thumb to guide the LMA into position
7. Inflate the cuff. There should be a smooth, oval swelling below the thyroid cartilage.
8. While inflating the cuff, let go of the LMA; it should automatically move forward out of the mouth.

placed without the need for laryngoscopy and showing little cardiac effect during the insertion process. Disadvantages include the lack of airway protection from vomiting or aspiration of gastric contents, the requirement that the patient be unconscious or sedated, and the fact that the LMA is not a definitive airway. There is now a pediatric LMA that will allow an ETT to pass through its lumen.

The technique for LMA replacement is listed in Table 4.10, and approximate LMA sizes are listed in Table 4.11. Complications of LMA placement include cough or bronchospasm, aspiration or regurgitation, airway trauma, lingual nerve palsy, vocal cord paralysis, hypoglossal nerve paralysis, hoarseness, stridor and pharyngeal or mouth ulcers.

Table 4.11. Laryngeal Mask Airway Sizing Recommendations for Children*

Size	Patient Weight
1	Neonates to 5 kg
1½	5–10 kg
2	10–20 kg
2½	20–30 kg
3	30–50 kg
4	50–70 kg
5	70–100 kg
6	>100 kg

* The sizes vary when using the pediatric LMA that allows intubation.

NEEDLE CRICOTHYROTOMY (JET VENTILATION)

Needle cricothyrotomy should be used when endotracheal intubation is not successful. It is most often indicated in children younger than 8 to 12 years of age in whom a surgical airway is technically difficult to perform. Most procedure texts discuss the use of a jet ventilator in order to ventilate through a needle cricothyrotomy; unfortunately, most EDs do not have access to a jet ventilator. This chapter describes various O_2 setups that can be used in any ED in order to ventilate using a needle cricothyrotomy without a jet ventilator attachment. The procedure for placing the needle is quite simple and is listed:

1. Identify cricothyroid membrane; prepare with povidone-iodine (Betadine), if possible.
2. Use a 12- to 14-gauge angiocatheter attached to a syringe to puncture the cricothyroid membrane. Direct the catheter at a 45-degree angle caudally (toward feet). Normal saline placed in the syringe will help to identify when air is aspirated.
3. Remove the needle from the angiocatheter.

Some experts advocate inserting another 14-gauge angiocatheter into the cricothyroid membrane in order to allow exhalation (be sure to occlude this second angiocatheter while squeezing the BVM bag and then unocclude it to allow exhalation). Using these methods, the child can be oxygenated, but ventilation (CO_2 exhalation) is limited. It is important to remember that needle cricothyrotomy is a temporizing measure and should be replaced as soon as possible with a definitive airway.

METHODS FOR VENTILATION (CHOOSE ONE)

1. Attach a 3-cc syringe barrel to the angiocatheter, then attach a 7.0 ETT adapter, then attach a BVM bag. Turn the wall O_2 up to 15 L and attempt to bag through the angiocatheter.
2. Attach a 3.0 ET tube adapter directly to the angiocatheter, then attach a BVM bag. Turn the wall O_2 up to 15 L and attempt to bag through the angiocatheter.
3. Attach a nasal cannula to the angiocatheter with one prong; use the other prong to regulate O_2 flow (1 second on, 4 seconds off).
4. Use the Cook Enk transtracheal ventilator kit.

Complication rates of needle cricothyrotomy range from 10% to 40% and include exsanguinating hematoma; perforation of the esophagus, posterior wall of the trachea or thyroid; infection; inadequate oxygenation (inadequate ventilation with a rise in CO_2 is inevitable – the goal is good oxygenation) and subcutaneous or mediastinal emphysema.

PITFALLS

- Failure to have available an ETT one size smaller and one size larger than calculated
- Failure to correctly position the child prior to attempting intubation
- Failure to oxygenate the patient prior to intubation attempts
- Failure to confirm ETT position
- Failure to rapidly place an NG or OG tube as soon as the ETT is secured

REFERENCES

1. Luten R. The pediatric patient. In: Walls R, Luten R, Murphy M, et al, eds. *Manual of Airway Management*. Philadelphia, PA: Lippincott Williams & Wilkins; 2000:143–152.
2. Luten R. The difficult airway in pediatrics. In: Walls R, Luten R, Murphy M, et al, eds. *Manual of Airway Management*. Philadelphia, PA: Lippincott Williams & Wilkins; 2000:112–118.
3. American Heart Association. Pediatric advanced life support and neonatal resuscitation guidelines. *Circulation*. 2005;112:167–195.
4. *Curr Emerg Cardiovasc Care*. 2005–2006;16(4):1–27.
5. Newth CJ, Rachman B, Patel N, Hammer J. The use of cuffed versus uncuffed endotracheal tubes in pediatric intensive care. *J Pediatr*. 2004;144:333–337.
6. Sharieff GQ, Rodarte A, Wilton N, et al. The self-inflating bulb as an esophageal detector device in children weighing more than twenty kilograms: a comparison of two techniques. *Ann Emerg Med*. 2003;41(5):623–629.
7. Sharieff GQ, Rodarte A, Wilton N, et al. The self-inflating bulb as an airway adjunct: is it reliable in children weighing less than 20 kilograms? *Acad Emerg Med*. 2003;10:303–308.
8. Splinter WM. Intravenous lidocaine does not attenuate the hemodynamic response of children to laryngoscopy and tracheal intubation. *Can J Aneaesth*. 1990;37:440–443.
9. Luten R. Approach to the pediatric airway. In: Walls R, Murphy M, Luten R, Schneider R, eds. *The Manual of Emergency Airway Management*, 2nd ed. Philadelphia, PA: Lippincott Williams & Wilkins; 2004: 143–152.

5 Pediatric Resuscitation: Basic and Advanced Life Support

Stephanie J. Doniger

INTRODUCTION

The majority of cardiac arrest in children results from a progression of shock and respiratory failure to cardiac arrest. The goal for resuscitation is to urgently reestablish substrate delivery to meet the metabolic demands of vital organs.[1] It is important to recognize that successfully applied techniques of basic and advanced cardiac life support (ACLS) are crucial to reduce neonatal and childhood mortality. Currently, there is no data about the incidence of pediatric resuscitations performed in the United States each year; however, it can be estimated by extrapolating data from childhood mortality rates (Figure 5.1A and B).

The 2005 American Heart Association (AHA) guidelines have further simplified resuscitation for pre-hospital as well as for advanced providers. For the lay rescuer, pediatric guidelines are applied to children 1 through 8 years of age, and adult ACLS guidelines applied to those patients older than 8 years of age. For the advanced provider, pediatric advanced life support (PALS) guidelines can be applied to children 1 year of age through the onset of puberty. Puberty is determined by the presence of secondary sexual characteristics, which usually occurs between 12 and 14 years of age.

Once it is recognized that a child needs resuscitation, it is important to approach the evaluation and management in a step-wise manner. First, the airway is assessed, then the breathing and finally the circulation. If there is an abnormality at any step of this airway, breathing and circulation (ABC) assessment, intervention must be initiated in order to stabilize the patient.[2] The goal of early, high quality cardiopulmonary resuscitation (CPR) and defibrillation is to improve overall survival from arrest. Only one third of cardiac arrest victims outside of hospital receive CPR prior to emergency medical services (EMS) arrival.[3] Those who actually receive CPR often do not receive effective CPR. When CPR is performed, suboptimal CPR is often performed with too few, too shallow (37%) and too weak chest compressions. Ventilations (61%) are often excessive, with too many interruptions in chest compressions.[4]

AIRWAY: BASIC LIFE SUPPORT

Evaluation for Airway Patency

The first priority in basic and advanced life support, is evaluating the airway. In order to assess upper airway patency, the provider should look, listen and feel whether there is adequate breathing. The provider should look for chest rise, listen for breath sounds and air movement and feel the movement of air at the nose and mouth. Clinical signs of an airway obstruction include breathing difficulty, inability to speak or breathe, poor air exchange, a silent cough and poor air exchange. It is crucial to determine whether the airway is maintainable by simple maneuvers or not maintainable, necessitating advanced interventions.[1]

Management: Opening the Airway

Simple measures to restore airway patency include positioning, suctioning and relieving a foreign body airway obstruction. Airway adjuncts such as oropharyngeal and nasopharyngeal airways may assist in opening the airway and facilitating in delivering oxygen by bag valve mask (BVM). More advanced interventions include endotracheal intubation (see Chapter 4).

The preferred method of opening the airway for the lay rescuer is the head tilt–chin lift maneuver for both

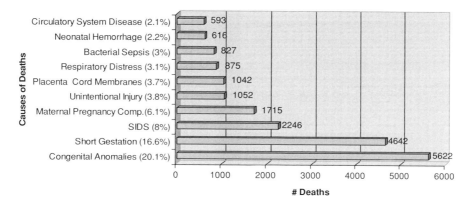

A

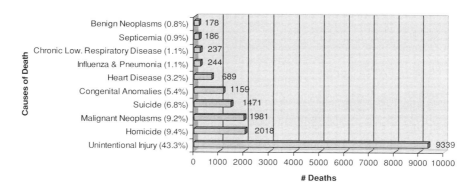

B

Figure 5.1. The top 10 causes of death in the United States in 2004, in children younger than 1 year of age (A), and in children 1 to 18 years of age (B). (Data source: Centers for Disease Control and Prevention/NCHS 2004 National Vital Statistics System, mortality.)

injured and noninjured victims. This method is also recommended for the health care provider in nontrauma settings. In trauma situations in which a cervical spine injury is suspected, a jaw thrust maneuver without a head tilt is recommended to open the airway and maintain manual stabilization of the head and neck. The jaw thrust is no longer recommended for lay rescuers because it is difficult to learn and perform, may be ineffective and may cause spinal movement.[5]

In situations of airway foreign bodies, action must be taken in those cases of severe airway obstruction. If the individual is unresponsive, it is recommended to activate EMS and perform CPR. Blind finger sweeps are not advised, and the jaw thrust maneuver is not recommended. This technique is difficult, especially for inexperienced providers. The preferred method of opening the airway for the lay rescuer is the head tilt-chin lift maneuver. The recommendation is to perform five back blows and five chest thrusts for infants, and to perform the Heimlich maneuver in older children.

Management: Respiratory Support

Rather than waiting for respiratory arrest, those who do not exhibit adequate breathing should receive rescue breaths. Try "a couple of times" to deliver two effective rescue breaths.[6] In those who are not breathing but who do have a pulse, only respirations should be delivered, without compressions. The health care provider should administer 12 to 20 breaths per minute (1 breath every 3–5 seconds) for infants and children and 10 to 12 breaths per minute (1 breath every 5–6 seconds) for adults. Rescue breaths should be given over 1 second, with enough volume to create visible chest rise. There are no indications stating specific tidal volumes as it is difficult to estimate tidal volumes delivered during rescue breaths. In fact, much less tidal volume is required during resuscitation than in normal healthy individuals. During CPR, there is 24% to 33% less blood flow to the lungs than during normal breathing. Therefore, fewer breaths with smaller volumes are needed for oxygenation and ventilation.[6]

The method of maintaining a proper airway depend on the skill level of the provider. For those untrained in advanced airway, one must focus on effective BVM technique.

AIRWAY: ADVANCED LIFE SUPPORT

Even for the advanced provider, adequate BVM technique is crucial in order to sustain a patient's airway. For those trained in endotracheal tube (ETT) placement, however, it is the preferred route of securing an airway. Because insertion of an advanced airway may cause a prolonged interruption in compressions, one must weigh the risks and benefits. The use of a cuffed ETT may be used in patients of all ages, except neonates. A cuffed ETT is especially useful for those with poor lung compliance, increased airway resistance or a large glottic air leak.[7] Attention must be paid to tube size, position and pressures. For children 1 to 10 years of age, the ETT size can be calculated by the following formulas[8]:

The size of a cuffed ETT is determined by:

$$\text{Diameter size (mm)} = (\text{age in years}/4) + 3$$

The size of an uncuffed ETT is determined by:

$$\text{Diameter size (mm)} = (\text{age in years}/4) + 4$$

Once placed, the ETT cuff pressure should be maintained at less than 20 cm H_2O.[9] When endotracheal intubation is not possible, a reasonable alternative is the placement of a laryngeal mask airway (LMA). However, the placement of LMAs is associated with a higher incidence of complications in children.[10]

Confirmation of tube placement should include clinical assessment and auscultation of breath sounds. In addition, it is recommended to measure exhaled CO_2 by a calorimetric detector or by capnography. However, their use is limited to those patients exhibiting a perfusing rhythm.[11] In those patients weighing more than 20 kg, one may

Table 5.1. Expected respiratory rates, according to age[1]

Age (years)	Breaths (per minute)
<1	30–60
1–3	24–40
4–5	22–34
6–12	18–30
13–18+	12–16

[1] From Ralston M, Hazinski M, Zaritsky A, et al. Pediatric assessment. *Pediatric Advanced Life Support, Provider Manual.* American Heart Association; 2006:1–32.

consider esophageal detector devices for confirmation of tube placement.[12] It is important to repeatedly verify ETT placement after the tube is inserted, during transport and after movement from one bed to another.

BREATHING: BASIC LIFE SUPPORT

Assessment of breathing includes an evaluation of the respiratory rate and effort, lung sounds and pulse oximetry. Normal respiratory rates depend on the age of the patient (Table 5.1). *Tachypnea* is defined as a rate that is more rapid than normal for age, whereas *bradypnea* is a rate that is slower than normal for age. *Apnea* is defined as a complete cessation of breathing for 20 seconds or more.

In regard to increased respiratory effort, a child may exhibit nasal flaring, retractions or accessory muscle use or irregular respirations. Further factors to assess are adequate and equal chest wall excursion and auscultation of air movement. Abnormal lung sounds include stridor, grunting, gurgling, wheezing and crackles.

BREATHING: ADVANCED LIFE SUPPORT

Once an advanced airway is in place, respirations should be administered simultaneously with chest compressions at a rate of 8 to 10 respirations per minute. Note that this rate is markedly lower than previous recommendations. Hyperventilation is not recommended as it actually can be harmful. Increased respiratory rates cause an increased intrathoracic pressure, thereby decreasing venous return and coronary perfusion pressure. This has been shown to decrease survival rates.[13]

AIRWAY AND BREATHING: NEONATES

In neonates, it is often necessary to provide positive pressure ventilation. This can be achieved with the use of a self-inflating bag, a flow-initiating bag or a T-piece device. The T-piece is a valved device that regulates pressure and limits flow.[14] The best indicator of successful ventilation is an increase in the heart rate.

Whenever positive pressure is indicated for resuscitation, supplemental oxygen is recommended. For those babies who are breathing but have central cyanosis, free-flow oxygen is indicated. The standard is to use 100% Fio_2; however, it is reasonable to begin with an oxygen concentration less than 100% or with room air. If there is no improvement after 90 seconds, oxygen should be administered. This updated recommendation reflects the possible adverse effects that high concentration oxygen has on the respiratory physiology and cerebral circulation of newborns.[15] Keeping in mind that oxygen deprivation and asphyxia cause further tissue damage, the goal is to provide adequate oxygenation, which is a balance between oxygen delivery and tissue demand.

In a vigorous infant, oropharyngeal and nasopharyngeal suctioning of meconium-stained amniotic fluid at the perineum is no longer recommended. A large multicenter trial showed that suctioning is ineffective in preventing meconium aspiration.[16] Those infants who are not vigorous warrant endotracheal suctioning immediately after birth.

CIRCULATION: BASIC LIFE SUPPORT

Evaluation

The assessment of cardiovascular function primarily includes heart rate, heart rhythm and blood pressure. Other indicators of adequate perfusion include peripheral and central pulses, capillary refill time and skin color and temperature. A delayed capillary refill time of greater than 2 seconds represents poor peripheral perfusion and may be a result of dehydration, shock or hypothermia. Advanced pediatric resuscitation includes the recognition and management of dysrhythmias, with the goal of restoring a perfusing heart rhythm.

Heart rate varies according to the child's age, and normal encompasses a wide range (Table 5.2). Typically, the rate is much slower in a sleeping or athletic child. *Tachycardia* is a heart rate faster than expected for a child's age, whereas *bradycardia* is slower than normal.

Similarly, blood pressures vary according to age (Table 5.3). *Hypotension* is defined as below the 5th percentile of

Table 5.2. Expected heart rates, according to age[1]

Age	Rate (mean) (beats per minute)
0–3 mo	80–205 (140)
3 mo–2 yrs	75–190 (130)
2–10 yrs	60–140 (80)
>10 yrs	50–100 (75)

[1]From Ralston M, Hazinski M, Zaritsky A, et al. Pediatric assessment. *Pediatric Advanced Life Support, Provider Manual.* American Heart Association; 2006:1–32.

expected blood pressures for age. Hypotension represents a state of shock, due to hemorrhage, sepsis or cardiac failure.

Management

The management recommendations for cardiovascular function include obtaining intravenous (IV) access and performing cardiac compressions.

IV or intraosseous (IO) routes are preferred for vascular access and for the administration of all drugs. Using an ETT to administer drugs is not recommended as drug delivery is unpredictable. In addition to lower drug concentrations in the blood, some drugs can cause detrimental β-adrenergic effects.[17] However, if vascular access is unavailable, lipophilic drugs may be administered at higher doses through the ETT. These drugs include

Table 5.3. Expected systolic and diastolic blood pressures* according to age[1]

Age	Systolic blood Pressure (mm Hg)	Diastolic blood Pressure (mm Hg)
0 day	60–76	30–45
1–4 days	67–84	35–53
1 mo	73–94	36–56
3 mo	78–103	44–65
6 mo	82–105	46–68
1 yr	67–104	20–60
2 yr	70–106	25–65
7 yr	79–115	38–78
15 yr	93–131	45–85

* Females have slightly lower systolic blood pressures and slightly higher diastolic blood pressures when compared with males of the same age.
[1] From Ralston M, Hazinski M, Zaritsky A, et al. Pediatric assessment. *Pediatric Advanced Life Support, Provider Manual.* American Heart Association; 2006:1–32.

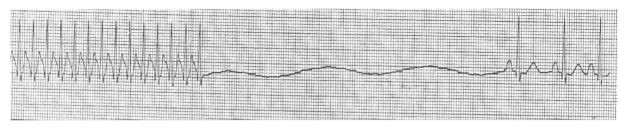

Figure 5.2. Asystole. This patient presented with supraventricular tachycardia and was administered adenosine. Adenosine administration resulted in a pharmacologically induced asystole followed by resumption of normal sinus rhythm. (Courtesy of CDR Jonathan T. Fleenor, MD, Naval Medical Center San Diego, San Diego, California.)

"LEAN": lidocaine, epinephrine, atropine, and Narcan (naloxone).[18]

Effective chest compressions are crucial to improve survival. Compressions provide blood flow to vital organs, such as the heart and brain, during resuscitation. The AHA now recommends "push hard and push fast." Interruptions in compressions should be limited to fewer than 10 seconds for interventions such as placing an advanced airway or defibrillation. Interruptions in compressions have shown to decrease the rate of return to spontaneous circulation. Rhythm checks should be performed every 2 minutes, or every 5 cycles of CPR. Once an advanced airway is in place, compressions and breaths should be performed continuously without interruption.

In those patients without a pulse or in newborns and children with a heart rate less than 60 beats per minute (BPM), compressions should be initiated (Figure 5.2). Bradycardia is often a terminal rhythm in children; therefore, it is not necessary to wait for pulseless arrest to initiate compressions. Compressions should be performed at a rate of 100 per minute for all ages, except newborns, in whom compressions should occur at a rate of 120 per minute. The compression to ventilation ratio is 30:2 for single rescuers, whereas the ratio is 15:2 for two-rescuer health provider resuscitations in children. These universal rates simplify guidelines for providers and are best for all victims of cardiac arrest, including hypoxic arrests. Furthermore, it allows for sufficient time for adequate chest recoil, in order to allow for adequate cardiac filling and venous return.[19]

In order to perform adequate compressions for children, the heel of one or two hands can be used to compress the lower half of the sternum to a depth of one half to one third of the chest diameter.[20] For infants, the AHA now recommends that two thumbs press on sternum, with the hands encircling the chest. In addition to compressing the sternum, the hands should squeeze the thorax. This improves coronary artery perfusion pressure, and may generate higher systolic and diastolic blood pressures.[21] When performing chest compressions, rescuers should be changed after 5 cycles of CPR or after 2 minutes, in order to decrease rescuer fatigue. This switch should be performed in less than 5 seconds in order to minimize interruptions in CPR.[22]

CIRCULATION: ADVANCED LIFE SUPPORT

The advanced cardiac evaluation and management includes the recognition of rhythm abnormalities and their targeted treatment, including defibrillation, and the pharmacologic treatment of rhythm disturbances.

The heart rhythm initially can be determined as being regular or irregular and too fast or too slow. In order to determine the specific rhythm, one must attach at least a 3-lead electrocardiogram (ECG). Various rhythm disturbances, or arrhythmias, can be recognized in order to initiate appropriate interventions. *Bradycardia* is defined as a heart rate slower than the lower limit of normal for the patient's age. Mechanisms of bradycardia include depression of the pacemaker in the sinus node and conduction system blocks. Complete heart block is a common cause of significant bradycardia in pediatric patients and may be acquired or congenital.

Evaluation: Bradycardia

Bradycardia in children may be attributable to vagal stimulation, hypoxemia, acidosis or an acute elevation of intracranial pressure. Other serious etiologies can include first-, second-, and third-degree heart block. Overall, the most common cause of bradycardia in the pediatric population is hypoxemia. It is important to correct hypoxemia prior to increasing the heart rate in children.

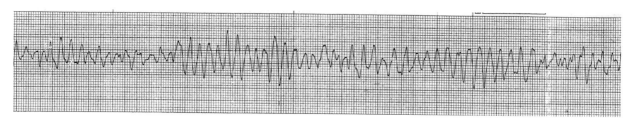

Figure 5.3. Rhythm strip of ventricular fibrillation (Torsades de pointes). This child had a history of dilated cardiomyopathy and returned to sinus rhythm after defibrillation. (Courtesy of CDR Jonathan T. Fleenor, MD, Naval Medical Center San Diego, San Diego, California.)

Management: Bradycardia

In patients presenting with a heart rate of fewer than 60 BPM, providers must support oxygenation and ventilation and perform CPR. Primary management is to search for and treat possible underlying causative abnormalities. Despite these measures, in those patients who have persistently poor perfusion, pharmacologic therapy should then be initiated. Initially, epinephrine (IV/IO, 0.01 mg/kg; ETT, 0.1 mg/kg) should be administered and can be repeated every 3 to 5 minutes. In situations of a primary atrioventricular block or increased vagal tone, atropine is recommended (initial dose, 0.02 mg/kg; minimum dose, 0.1 mg; max dose, 1 mg) and may be repeated.[23]

Evaluation: Pulseless Electrical Activity and Asystole

Pulseless Electrical Activity

Pulseless electrical activity (PEA) refers to a patient without a pulse that exhibits any organized electrical activity. This may be represented on ECG as normal or wide QRS complexes. However, PEA specifically does not include ventricular fibrillation, ventricular tachycardia or asystole.[23] It is important to expeditiously identify potential reversible underlying causes of PEA, and it may be remembered by the mnemonic "5 H's and 5 T's": 5 H's include hypovolemia, hypothermia, hypo/hyperkalemia, H⁺ (acidosis) and hypoxia; 5 T's include tamponade, tension pneumothorax, toxins and thromboembolism (pulmonary and cardiac).

Asystole

Asystole is defined as cardiac standstill with no visible electrical activity, which is otherwise known as a *flat line* (Figure 5.2). Causes of this terminal rhythm are submersion, hypothermia, sepsis and poisoning.[23] This diagnosis must be clinically correlated with the patient, as a loose ECG lead may cause the appearance of asystole.[1]

Management: Pulseless Electrical Activity and Asystole

In cases of asystole or PEA, one should initiate immediate CPR. This is followed by pharmacologic therapy of epinephrine (0.01 mg/kg IV/IO). Alternatively, atropine may be administered (1 mg IV/IO). For PEA in particular, it is important to identify and treat its underlying causes.

Evaluation: Tachycardias

Tachycardia is defined as a heart rate beyond the upper limit of normal for the patient's age. In adults, it is greater than 100 BPM. The vast majority of tachycardias are supraventricular in origin. Those that are ventricular in origin are typically associated with hemodynamic compromise. Upon recognition of a tachycardia, step-wise questioning can help evaluate the ECG tracing. Is it regular or irregular? Is the QRS narrow or wide? Does every P result in a single QRS? Once this is established, treatment options are considered, according to whether or not the patient has a pulse and the presenting rhythm on ECG. The important tachydysrhythmias to recognize are ventricular fibrillation, ventricular tachycardia, PEA, asystole and supraventricular tachycardia (SVT).

Ventricular Fibrillation

Ventricular fibrillation is an uncommon rhythm in the pediatric population, but it is certainly life threatening (Figure 5.3). Causes of ventricular fibrillation include postoperative complications from congenital heart disease

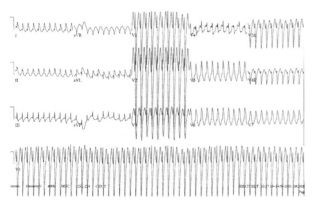

Figure 5.4. Ventricular tachycardia. This is an example of an extraordinarily fast ventricular tachycardia with a heart rate of almost 300 BPM. (Courtesy of CDR Jonathan T. Fleenor, MD, Naval Medical Center San Diego, San Diego, California.)

repair, severe hypoxemia, hyperkalemia, medications (digitalis, quinidine, catecholamines, and anesthesia), myocarditis and myocardial infarction.

The hallmark of ventricular fibrillation is chaotic irregular ventricular contractions without circulation to the body the rhythm. The ECG reveals a rapid rate; it has bizarre QRS complexes with varying sizes and configurations.

Ventricular Tachycardia

Ventricular tachycardia is an important rhythm to recognize and promptly treat (Figure 5.4). By definition, *ventricular tachycardia* is three or more consecutive premature ventricular contractions (PVCs), with heart rates ranging

from 120 to 200 BPM. The rate may be as rapid as 400 or 500 BPM.[24]

In those patients who are stable, pharmacologic intervention is appropriate. In the hemodynamically unstable patient, defibrillation must be initiated. There is great potential to decompensate into ventricular fibrillation, if left untreated.

Ventricular tachycardia may result from electrolyte disturbances (hyperkalemia, hypokalemia) and metabolic abnormalities, congenital heart disorders, myocarditis or drug toxicity. Other etiologies include cardiomyopathies, cardiac tumors, acquired heart disease, prolonged QT syndrome, and idiopathic causes.

On ECG, the QRS complexes have a wide configuration. The QRS duration is prolonged, ranging from 0.06 to 0.14 seconds. Complexes may appear monomorphic, with a uniform contour and absent or retrograde P waves. Alternatively, the QRS complexes may appear polymorphic or vary randomly as is seen in Torsades de pointes. ECG findings that further support the presence of ventricular tachycardia include the presence of atrioventricular dissociation with the ventricular rate exceeding the atrial rate.

Supraventricular Tachycardia

SVT is the most common type of tachyarrhythmia in childhood (Figure 5.5). Diagnosis often begins in triage, with the nurse reporting a heart rate that is "too fast to count." In newborns and infants with SVT, the heart rate is often

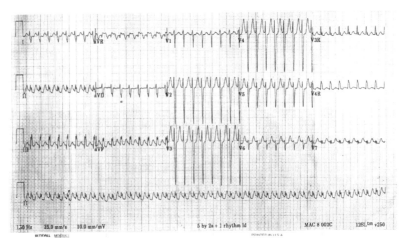

Figure 5.5. Supraventricular tachycardia with concomitant right ventricular hypertrophy. This 4-year-old boy was postoperative from repair of congenital heart disease (Fontan repair). He was eventually converted to normal sinus rhythm after multiple doses of adenosine.

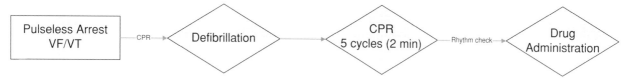

Figure 5.6. Sequence of resuscitation in pulseless arrest with ventricular fibrillation (VF) and ventricular tachycardia (VT).

between 220 and 280 BPM.[25] Typical ECG findings are a normal QRS interval with a heart rate that has little beat-to-beat variation. Most patients do not have an underlying cause to account for the tachycardia, such as fever, dehydration, fluid or blood loss, anxiety or pain. The most common type of SVT is the reentrant tachycardia, one cause of which is Wolff-Parkinson-White syndrome. In patients presenting with SVT, symptoms can vary from nonspecific, to florid heart failure. Upon presentation to the emergency department (ED), it is crucial to expeditiously distinguish the stable from unstable patients. The unstable patients require more aggressive, immediate intervention of cardioversion, whereas vagal maneuvers and adenosine are first-line treatments for the stable patients.

Management: Tachydysrhythmias, Defibrillation

In situations of sudden witnessed collapse, immediate defibrillation is warranted, followed by CPR, followed by drug administration (Figure 5.6). CPR provides some blood flow, delivering oxygen and substrate to the heart muscle, thereby making it more likely to abort ventricular fibrillation. A single shock should be administered at a dose of 2 J/kg, followed by immediate CPR. In at least 90% of cases, ventricular fibrillation is eliminated by the first shock.[26] In those cases in which the first shock does not terminate ventricular fibrillation, CPR is of greater value.

CPR is beneficial immediately post-defibrillation. This "primes" the heart for the next defibrillation attempt. In cases of prolonged ventricular fibrillation, it has been shown that giving CPR prior to defibrillation increased survival rates from 4% to 22%.[27] The dosages of defibrillation are now 2 J/kg followed by 4 J/kg for subsequent dosages, regardless of the type of defibrillator. It is important to note that stacked shocks are no longer recommended. A single shock is recommended followed by CPR largely due to the prolonged period of time to administer three shocks (see Figure 5.6). Do not interrupt CPR until 5 cycles or 2 minutes for a pulse/rhythm check.

More specifically, the treatment of each rhythm disturbance can be classified according to the tachycardia algorithm (Figure 5.7). The presence or absence of a pulse determines which arm of the algorithm to initiate. Of note, sinus tachycardia with adequate perfusion is no longer included in the algorithm. In addition, polymorphic ventricular tachycardia is now considered most likely to be an unstable rhythm. Therefore, it is recommended to use unsynchronized rather than synchronized shocks. In contrast to previous recommendations, low energy synchronized shocks have a high likelihood of provoking ventricular fibrillation.[6]

In the community, automated external defibrillators (AEDs) have been shown to increase survival rates. There has been sufficient evidence to show that AEDs can safely be used for those older than 1 year of age.[28] In a sudden witnessed collapse, the AED should be used as soon as it becomes available. If the collapse is unwitnessed, CPR should be performed for 5 cycles or 2 minutes prior to the use of the AED. Pediatric AED pads and energy levels should be used in those 1 to 8 years of age. If the pediatric dose is unavailable, the adult dose is a reasonable alternative.

Management: Tachydysrhythmias, Pharmacologic Therapy

For the most part, the algorithm drug dosages remain the same in the updated 2005 AHA Recommendations. Drug delivery should not interrupt CPR. The timing of drug delivery is less important than maximizing chest compressions. Amiodarone is the preferred drug for treatment for pulseless arrest because it is most effective. Lidocaine is recommended only when amiodarone is unavailable.[29] Additionally, lidocaine is no longer listed on the stable ventricular tachycardia algorithm (see Figure 5.7). Lidocaine has been replaced by amiodarone and procainamide.

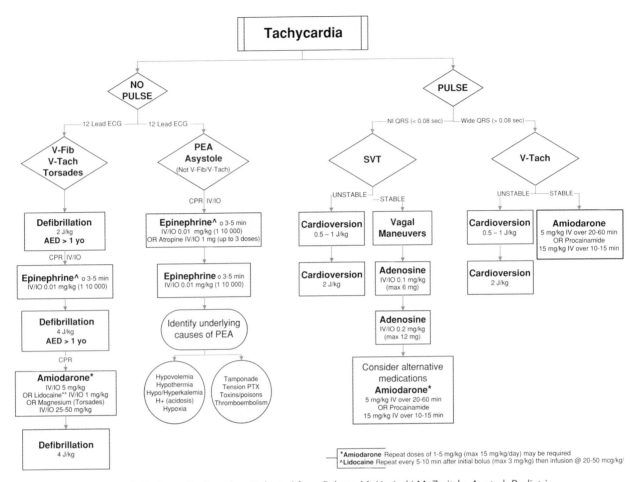

Figure 5.7. Tachycardia algorithm. (Adapted from Ralston M, Hazinski M, Zaritsky A, et al. Pediatric assessment. *Pediatric Advanced Life Support, Provider Manual.* American Heart Association; 2006:1–32.[1])

It is important to note that amiodarone and procainamide should not be administered together as they can lead to severe hypotension and prolongation of the QT interval.

High dose epinephrine (1:1000 concentration via IV) is not recommended in any age group and is actually associated with a worse outcome, especially in cases of asphyxia.[30] Therefore, the standard recommended dose is (0.01 mg/kg IV/IO) for all doses, which correlates to 0.1 cc/kg. Although the preferred routes of administration are IV and IO, it may be given via the ETT when such access is unable to be obtained (0.1 mg/kg ETT). In exceptional cases, such as β-blocker overdoses, high dose epinephrine may be considered.

CIRCULATION: NEONATES

Compressions and ventilations should be given in a 3:1 ratio of compressions to ventilations with 90 compressions and 30 breaths in 1 minute for a total of 120 events per minute. When compressions are given continuously, the rate should be 120 compressions per minute.

In newborn resuscitation, drug therapy is rarely indicated.[31] However, the 2005 AHA recommendations for drug therapy in the newborn focus on the indications for the use of epinephrine and naloxone. High-dose epinephrine is no longer recommended but rather epinephrine is recommended at a dose of 0.01 to 0.03 mg/kg/dose. The IV concentration is 1:10,000, and the IV route for epinephrine administration is preferred. Although the endotracheal route is unpredictable for drug delivery, it may be used when there is difficulty obtaining IV or IO access. The endotracheal concentration of epinephrine is 1:1000. Naloxone should not be given endotracheally due to the lack of clinical data in newborns. Further, naloxone is no longer recommended in primary resuscitative efforts. Heart rate and color must be restored through ventilatory support prior to naloxone administration.[5]

POST-RESUSCITATIVE CARE

In general, it is recommended to maintain a normal body temperature in post-resuscitative care of neonates and children. Recent evidence is insufficient to recommend the routine use of systemic or selective cerebral hypothermia after resuscitation. However, it is important to avoid hyperthermia, especially in very-low-birthweight infants and hypoxic-ischemic events. There are possible benefits of induced hypothermia (32°C–34°C) for 12 to 24 hours following successful resuscitation.[32]

In addition, new recommendations recognize the probable benefits of vasoactive medications, including inodilators (inamrinone, milrinone) to treat post-resuscitation myocardial depression. However, there may be adverse effects on cerebral circulation and hyperventilation Further studies are recommended prior to universal initiation of these agents.[33]

New evidence suggests that the length of resuscitation is not an adequate prognostic indicator of survival. Intact survival has been reported, even in those patients who have endured prolonged resuscitation and who have received 2 doses of epinephrine.[34]

Once the initial resuscitation has been performed or if a critically ill infant presents to the ED, the following mnemonic can be helpful in determining the etiology of the patient's condition. Each of these items will be discussed in detail in subsequent chapters.

THE MISFITS

T   Trauma, consider nonaccidental trauma

H   Heart, hypoxia, hematologic

E   Endocrine

M   Metabolic disturbances (congenital adrenal hyperplasia)

I   Inborn errors of metabolism

S   Sepsis

F   Formula dilution of overconcentration

I   Intestinal catastrophes

T   Toxins

S   Seizures

Neonates

Lastly, neonatal recommendations include guidelines regarding withholding and withdrawing resuscitative efforts. Such decisions are optimal when there are opportunities for parental agreement. It may be reasonable to withhold resuscitation in those conditions associated with an unacceptably high mortality. Such situations include extremely low birth weights (<400 g), young gestational age (<23 weeks) and certain congenital anomalies (anencephaly, trisomy 13).[5] Alternatively, resuscitation is indicated in those patients who have a high survival rate and an acceptable mortality. In other situations, the parental desires would dictate resuscitative efforts. This occurs in babies with an uncertain prognosis, borderline survival, a relatively high morbidity rate and a high anticipated burden to the child. Further, after 10 minutes of adequate continuous resuscitation, if there are still no signs of life (i.e., no heartbeat of respiratory effort), it is reasonable to discontinue resuscitation. This is due to evidence which shows that there is a high mortality rate and chance for severe neurodevelopmental disability.[35]

PITFALLS

- Failure to emphasize effective CPR while limiting interruptions "Push hard, push fast," at 100 compressions per minute
- Failure to reduce ventilation rate to 8 to 10 per minute once an advanced airway is in place
- Failure to recognize that the IV/IO route is preferable to ETT for drug administration
- Failure to know that stacked shocks are no longer recommended. Each defibrillation attempt should be followed by immediate resumption of CPR

REFERENCES

1. Ralston M, Hazinski M, Zaritsky A, et al. Pediatric assessment. *Pediatric Advanced Life Support, Provider Manual.* American Heart Association; 2006:1–32.
2. Ludwig S, Lavelle J. Resuscitation – pediatric basic and advanced life support. In: Fleisher G, Ludwig S, Henretig F, eds. *Textbook of Pediatric Emergency Medicine,* 5th ed. Philadelphia, PA: Lippincott Williams & Wilkins; 2006:3–33.
3. Donoghue A, Nadkarni V, Berg R, et al. Out-of-hospital pediatric cardiac arrest: an epidemiologic review and assessment of current knowledge. *Ann Emerg Med.* 2005;46(6):512–522.
4. Abella B, Alvarado J, Myklebust H, et al. Quality of cardiopulmonary resuscitation during in-hospital cardiac arrest. *JAMA.* 2005;293(3):363–365.
5. ECC Committee SaTFotAHA. 2005 American Heart Association Guidelines for Cardiopulmonary Resuscitation and Emergency Cardiovascular Care: Part 13: Neonatal Resuscitation Guidelines. *Circulation.* 2005;112:188–195.
6. ECC Committee SaTFotAHA. Highlights of the 2005 American Heart Association Guidelines for Cardiopulmonary

Resuscitation and Emergency Cardiovascular Care. *Currents*. Winter 2005–2006;15(4).

7. Newth C, Rachman B, Patel N, et al. The use of cuffed versus uncuffed endotracheal tubes in pediatric intensive care. *J Pediatr*. 2004;144(3):333–337.

8. Khine H, Corddry D, Kettrick R, et al. Comparison of cuffed and uncuffed endotracheal tubes in young children during general anesthesia. *Anesthesiology*. 1997;86:627–631.

9. Hoffman R, Parwani V, Hahn I. Experienced emergency medicine physicians cannot safely inflate or estimate endotracheal tube cuff pressure using standard techniques. *Am J Emerg Med*. 2006;24(2):139–143.

10. Park C, Bahk J, Ahn W, Do S, et al. The laryngeal mask airway in infants and children. *Can J Anaesth*. 2001;48(4):413–417.

11. Bhende M, Thompson A, Orr R. Utility of an end-tidal carbon dioxide detector during stabilization and transport of critically ill children. *Pediatrics*. 1992;89(6 Pt 1):1042–1044.

12. Sharieff G, Rodarte A, Wilton N, et al. The self-inflating bulb as an airway adjunct: is it reliable in children weighing less than 20 kilograms? *Acad Emerg Med*. 2003;41:623–629.

13. Aufderheide T, Lurie K. Death by hyperventilation: a common and life-threatening problem during cardiopulmonary resuscitation. *Crit Care Med*. 2004;32(9 Suppl):S345–351.

14. Allwood A, Madar R, Baumer J, et al. Changes in resuscitation practice at birth. *Arch Dis Child Fetal Neonatal Ed*. 2003;88:F375–F379.

15. Tan A, Schulze A, Davis P. Air versus oxygen for resuscitation of infants at birth. *Cochrane Database Syst Rev*. 2004;3:CD002273.

16. Vain N, Szyld E, Prudent L, et al. Oropharyngeal and nasopharyngeal suctioning of meconium-stained neonates before delivery of their shoulders: multicentre, randomised controlled trial. *Lancet*. 2004;364:597–602.

17. Efrati O, Ben-Abraham R, Barak A, et al. Endobronchial adrenaline: should it be reconsidered? Dose response and haemodynamic effect in dogs. *Resuscitation*. 2003;59(1):117–122.

18. Johnston C. Endotracheal drug delivery. *Pediatr Emerg Care*. 1992;8:94–97.

19. Aufderheide T, Pirrallo R, Yannopoulos D, et al. Incomplete chest wall decompression: a clinical evaluation of CPR performance by EMS personnel and assessment of alternative manual chest compression-decompression techniques. *Resuscitation*. 2005;64:355–362.

20. Stevenson A, McGowan J, Evans A, et al. CPR for children: one hand or two? *Resuscitation*. 2005;64:205–208.

21. Ishimine P, Menegazzi J, Weinstein D. Evaluation of two-thumb chest compression with thoracic squeeze in a swine model of infant cardiac arrest. *Acad Emerg Med*. 1998;5:397.

22. Ashton A, McCluskey A, Gwinnutt C, et al. Effect of rescuer fatigue on performance of continuous external chest compressions over 3 min. *Resuscitation*. 2002;55:151–155.

23. Ralston M, Hazinski M, Zaritsky A, et al. *PALS Provider Manual*. Dallas, TX: American Heart Association; 2006.

24. Garson A. Abnormalities of cardiac rate and rhythm. In: McMillan J, Deangelis C, Feigin R, et al, eds. *Oski's Pediatrics: Principles and Practice*. Philadelphia, PA: Lippincott Williams & Wilkins; 1999.

25. Perry J. Supraventricular tachycardia. In: Bricker J, Fisher D, Neish S, eds. *The Science and Practice of Pediatric Cardiology*, 2nd ed. Baltimore, MD: Williams & Wilkins; 1998.

26. Martens P, Russell J, Wolcke B, et al. Optimal response to cardiac arrest study: defibrillation waveform effects. *Resuscitation*. 2001;49:233–243.

27. Wik L, Kramer-Johansen J, Myklebust H, et al. Quality of cardiopulmonary resuscitation during out-of-hospital cardiac arrest. *JAMA*. 2005;293:299–304.

28. Atkinson E, Mikysa B, Conway J, et al. Specificity and sensitivity of automated external defibrillator rhythm analysis in infants and children. *Ann Emerg Med*. 2003;42:185–196.

29. Dorian P, Cass D, Schwartz B, et al. Amiodarone as compared with lidocaine for shock-resistant ventricular fibrillation. *N Engl J Med*. 2002;346:884–890.

30. Perondi M, Reis A, Paiva E, et al. A comparison of high-dose and standard-dose epinephrine in children with cardiac arrest. *N Engl J Med*. Apr 22 2004;350(17):1708–1709.

31. Perlman J, Risser R. Cardiopulmonary resuscitation in the delivery room. Associated clinical events. *Arch Pediatr Adolesc Med*. 1995;140:20–25.

32. Holzer M, Bernard S, Hachimi-Idrissi S, et al. Hypothermia for neuroprotection after cardiac arrest: systematic review and individual patient data meta-analysis. *Crit Care Med*. 2005;33(2):1449–1452.

33. Abdallah I, Shawky H. A randomised controlled trial comparing milrinone and epinephrine as inotropes in paediatric patients undergoing total correction of tetralogy of Fallot. *Egyptian H Anaesthesia*. 2003;19:323–329.

34. Lopez-Herce J, Garcia C, Dominguez P, et al. Characteristics and outcome of cardiorespiratory arrest in children. *Resuscitation*. 2004;63:311–320.

35. Haddad B, Mercer B, Livingston J, et al. Outcome after successful resuscitation of babies born with Apgar scores of 0 at both 1 and 5 minutes. *Am J Obstet Gynecol*. 2000;182:1210–1214.

6

Death of a Child in the Emergency Department

Phyllis L. Hendry

INTRODUCTION

Dealing with a child's death in the emergency setting is considered one of the most stressful situations encountered by physicians and other care providers. Advance preparation for death, and training programs, are important to have in place and must be based on current national epidemiology and local trends. Infant and neonatal deaths are particularly tragic and the cause of death often is not easily discernable in the emergency department (ED). This chapter focuses specifically on neonatal and infant death in the ED.

EPIDEMIOLOGY OF INFANT AND NEONATAL DEATH

The data found in annual U.S. vital statistic reports are based on death and birth statistics and adjusted for population growth. ICD-10 codes are used to report cause of death statistics, and periodically revisions are made to certificate of live birth or death forms. In recent years, some states began using a revised birth certificate during mid-year, which has led to difficulty in comparing national data. It is important for emergency physicians to use accurate terminology when completing death certificates, although sudden infant deaths are usually medical examiner's or coroner's cases.[1,2]

Historically, about half of the deaths in U.S. children happen in the first year of life with two thirds of those deaths occurring in the neonatal period. Not surprisingly, most infant deaths occur in the hospital or ED setting. The overall death rate in the United States continues to decrease annually; however, this decrease is not as significant in the infant and pediatric population.[1,2]

In 2004, the infant (0–12 months) mortality rate (IMR) was 6.79 infant deaths per 1000 live births (27,936 deaths).

In this same year, 25,325 children between the ages of 1 and 19 years died, with unintentional injuries and homicide as the two leading causes. There continues to be significant race differences in infant mortality, with non-Hispanic black infants more than twice as likely as white and Hispanic infants to die within 1 year of birth. The IMR had been declining steadily for 40 years until 2002 when the rate suddenly increased to 6.95.[1,2]

The *perinatal mortality rate* (PMR), which is defined as late fetal (>28 weeks of gestation) and early neonatal (<7 days) deaths per 1000 births plus fetal deaths, has continued to decline annually. Timely prenatal care has not shown recent improvement. The percentage of preterm births has risen 20% since 1990 and continues to rise, with a 2005 rate of 12.7%. This correlates with a continued rise of infants born with low birth weight (LBW) (<2500 g).[1,2]

More than half of all infant deaths in 2004 were attributable to five leading causes: congenital malformations (20%), disorders relating to short gestation and LBW not elsewhere classified (17%), sudden infant death syndrome (SIDS) (8%), maternal complications of pregnancy (6%) and unintentional injuries (4%).[1]

The position of the U.S. relative to other countries remains unfavorable for infant mortality. Possible reasons include the high percentage of LBW infants, heterogeneity of population and group health disparities.[1]

PRESENTATION

The ED physician must be alert for any clues that would explain the death, beginning at transfer of care from the parent or emergency medical services (EMS), going through resuscitation and continuing after declaration of death. Many larger communities have infant death scene investigation protocols or teams in place.

HISTORY

Details of the scene, if known, should be obtained in the history to include sleep position, bedding, clothing, type of ventilation or heating source, animals in the house, odors, chemicals, emesis, and so on. Details of the history are often obtained after the death is pronounced when caregivers are in a very distraught state. The ED team should make every effort to coordinate history taking with law enforcement and other agencies. The history should include details regarding recent illnesses or immunizations, medications, feeding history and other pertinent history. Family history of neonatal deaths, stillborns and sudden or unexplained child deaths should be explored.[3]

PHYSICAL EXAMINATION

In addition to a complete examination, particular attention should be given to body temperature, skin markings, pupil size and dysmorphic features. All clothing and body fluids should be saved and all equipment left in place until autopsy status determined.[3]

DIFFERENTIAL DIAGNOSIS

Clues to the most common differential diagnoses can be found by reviewing the epidemiology of neonatal and infant deaths in context with the individual history and exam. The following list shows differential diagnoses to consider[1]:

- Congenital malformations
- Disorders related to prematurity or complications of pregnancy and birth
- SIDS
- Unintentional injuries (motor vehicle accidents, falls, burns, drowning)
- Intentional injuries (abuse, suffocation, head trauma)
- Suffocation or asphyxia secondary to bedding items or cosleeping
- Inborn metabolic disorders
- Toxins or poisonings
- Sepsis, pneumonia or other infectious diseases

SIDS VERSUS CHILD ABUSE

Fatal child abuse has been mistaken for SIDS, prompting numerous scientific studies and consensus statements.[3–5]

The distinction between these two entities and the classification of unexpected infant deaths requires further discussion.

SIDS, also called *crib* or *cot death*, is the sudden death of an infant younger than 1 year of age that remains unexplained after thorough case investigation, including performance of a complete autopsy, examination of the death scene and a review of the clinical history. SIDS remains the third most common cause of death in infants despite educational sleep position campaigns. The incidence of SIDS peaks between 2 and 4 months of age. Despite extensive research, understanding of the etiology of SIDS remains incomplete.[3–5]

The rate of SIDS is two to three times higher in African American and some American Indian populations. SIDS has been associated with sleeping in a prone position, sleeping on a soft surface, maternal smoking during or after pregnancy, overheating, late or no prenatal care, young maternal age, prematurity, LBW and male gender.[3,5] Since 1992, national campaigns aimed at reducing prone sleeping during infancy have dramatically decreased the incidence of SIDS in the United States and in other countries. The overall post-neonatal mortality rate decreased by 27% and the SIDS rate by 55% between 1992 and 2001. However, from 1999 to 2001, there was no significant change in the overall postneonatal rate despite a SIDS rate decline by 17%. One proposed explanation is the increased tendency for infant deaths to be certified as undetermined, unspecified or suffocation.[2]

Recently, the benefits and harms of bed sharing with infants and the association with SIDS and undetermined infant death has been a topic of debate. A review of 40 observational studies concluded the following: there may be an association between bed sharing and SIDS among smokers, bed sharing may be more strongly associated with SIDS in younger infants (<12 weeks) and a positive association between bed sharing and breastfeeding was identified.[6] Although further study is needed, many countries and the American Academy of Pediatrics (AAP) stress the hazards of adults sleeping with infants in the same bed.[4]

The diagnosis of SIDS is one of exclusion and cannot be made until a comprehensive postmortem examination and death scene investigation are complete and autopsy findings are compatible with SIDS. The AAP recommends the following criteria be met before ruling an infant's death as "attributable to SIDS":

- There is no evidence of trauma or significant bone disease on skeletal radiological survey, in autopsy or in clinical history.
- Other causes of death are adequately excluded, including meningitis, sepsis, aspiration, pneumonia, myocarditis, trauma, dehydration, fluid and electrolyte imbalance, significant congenital lesions, inborn metabolic disorders, asphyxia, drowning or burns.
- There is no evidence of alcohol, drug or toxic exposure.
- A thorough death scene investigation and review of the clinical history are negative.[3]

Deaths without postmortem examination and death scene examination should not be attributed to SIDS. These deaths are often designated as "undetermined."

As the occurrence of cases of true SIDS has decreased, the proportion of unexplained infant deaths attributable to fatal child abuse may be increasing. It is very difficult to distinguish at autopsy between SIDS and accidental or deliberate asphyxiation with a soft object. The following findings indicate the possibility of intentional suffocation:

- Previous recurrent cyanosis, apnea or apparent life-threatening event (ALTE) while in the care of the same person
- Age at death older than 6 months
- Previous unexpected or unexplained deaths of one or more siblings
- Simultaneous or nearly simultaneous death of twins
- Previous death of infants under the care of the same unrelated person
- Discovery of blood on the infant's nose or mouth in association with ALTEs[3]

LABORATORY AND RADIOLOGY STUDIES

Laboratory and radiological studies are often key to determining the cause of unexplained infant and neonatal deaths. Communication among the ED, medical examiner's office, pathology and child protective services is important to ensure that appropriate testing is completed and documented without duplication.

Autopsy and perimortem sampling are important. Genetic disease is a major contributing factor in 15% to 25% of all infant deaths. More than 400 inborn errors of metabolism have been described in the pediatric literature, many with treatment. Unfortunately, many infants die before a diagnosis is made. Most inborn errors are

autosomal recessive, thus they indicate a 25% recurrence risk for future pregnancies. Postmortem examinations have been shown to alter recurrence risks for future pregnancies by 25%. This makes neonatal and infant autopsies of crucial importance. Fluid and tissue samples are often required to diagnose rare metabolic and genetic disorders. These studies are commonly performed at out of area specialty laboratories, and final results may take months.[7]

There is great variation among pathologists in the interpretation of infant postmortem exams. Inflammation of the respiratory tract is a common alternative diagnosis for SIDS or, in some cases, the SIDS label is applied too liberally, preventing investigation of another severe genetic or metabolic disorder.[3,5]

During resuscitation, every effort should be made to obtain electrolytes, blood cultures and other appropriate laboratory studies. All remaining laboratory specimens, body fluids and clothing should be saved and sent to the pathologist or medical examiner's office with the body.

Radiographic skeletal surveys are best performed before autopsy, particularly when intentional injury and abuse are suspected. Interpretation of radiographs in an unexpected neonatal or infant death is best performed by a pediatric radiologist.

MANAGEMENT

Management of neonatal and infant death in the ED is mainly focused on support of the family and the ED staff. Advance preparation, protocols and education are essential. Recently, there have been several practice guidelines, review articles and technical reports by national emergency-related organizations.[8–11]

Table 6.1 summarizes the organizational phases of dealing with death in the ED setting.[11] These phases were published after a panel of multidisciplinary experts in the field of emergency services was convened by the National Association of Social Workers to develop Bereavement Practice Guidelines. The phases are the basis of any ED death protocol and include the following:

1. Advance preparation of the ED to help the family of a child who dies
2. What to do when the family arrives in the ED
3. Issues to handle at the time of death
4. Follow-up after the death
5. Helping staff cope with ED child deaths

Table 6.1. Bereavement practice guidelines for health care professionals in the emergency department

Phase 1: Preparing the ED to Help the Family of a Critically Ill or Injured Child Who Dies

- Have protocols and procedures in place (media, police, medical examiner, family presence, death certificate, organ donation).
- Train all the ED staff (physicians, nurses, techs, students, clerks, security) about the needs of families, including expected reactions and cultural and religious differences.
- Designate a family room with a phone.
- Assign a trained family care provider (FCP), chaplain or other appropriate staff member to work with the family.

Phase 2: When the Critically Ill or Injured Child and the Family Arrive in the ED
- FCP prepares for the arrival of the family, if time permits.
- FCP greets the family upon arrival to the ED.
- FCP guides family to a private room.
- FCP acts as the liaison between family and staff and remains with family for the duration of their stay.

Phase 3: When a Child Dies in the ED
- Help the family with grief expressions: anger, sadness, fainting, violence, guilt.
- Review all procedures and "what was done" to help their child.
- Praise family and allay guilt.
- Explain role of medical examiner, autopsy, organ or tissue donation, law enforcement, child abuse and other agencies.
- Contact family religious or spiritual leader.
- Give the family the option of spending time with their deceased child if allowed by law enforcement or medical examiner.
- If appropriate, offer funeral resources.
- Offer informational and resource brochures to take home.

Phase 4: Follow-up After the Death of a Child in the ED
- Have a follow-up plan ready.
- Send a letter of condolence.
- Physician meeting with family to review autopsy or medical examiner results.
- Provide the family with time for questions.
- Provide a list of bereavement support groups.
- Direct the family toward programs and support networks offered by most hospice programs and children's hospitals.

Phase 5: Helping Staff Cope With Childhood Deaths
- Provide proper education and supervision.
- Hold debriefing sessions in some cases.
- Recognize outstanding work.

Adapted from Lipton H, Coleman M. Bereavement practice guidelines for health care professionals in the emergency department. *Int J Emerg Ment Health.* 2000;2(1):1–13.

Although there are many national resources and protocols for pediatric ED deaths, each case must be individualized, and local or state statutes must be followed. All families are unique and have different values, cultures and spiritual beliefs. Table 6.2 reviews cultural and religious aspects of death.[10] There remain wide variations in all cultures and religions. Most hospitals offer nondenominational chaplain services or a list of on-call counselors by type of religion and baptism or last rite procedures. It is important for the provider to be familiar with the practices of different cultures (Table 6.3).

Most families want the opportunity to hold their infant after death has been pronounced and treasure mementos such as foot or handprints, hair locks, clothing and so on.[12] Unfortunately, a large proportion of infant deaths are unexpected or unexplained and thus involve medical examiners and law enforcement. The ED must be aware of local protocols and statutes concerning family presence and contact after death pronouncement. Most cases involving law enforcement investigation do not allow ink on the body for prints or removal of hair, or clothing, for example. The ED may serve as a liaison for the family with law enforcement. One suggestion is to have an observer or staff member remain with the family and the body at all times in case questions regarding postmortem artifacts arise.

Special attention should be paid to siblings of the dead child. The ED protocol must address notification of the family pediatrician or primary care physician, subspecialists, home health or other services. The family pediatrician can monitor the bereavement response of the family and address needs of the siblings.[13] Table 6.4 lists bereavement

Table 6.2. Cultural concepts of grieving

Culture	Predominant religion	Grief expressions	Death rituals	Autopsy	Tissue/organ donation
Black	Protestants, Baptists, Methodists	No prohibitions	Big funerals strong family support	Acceptable	Acceptable
Black Muslim	Muslim	No prohibitions	Specific rituals: washing & shrouding the dead, specific funeral rites	Acceptable	Acceptable
American Indian	Various Native American sects	Stoic to dramatic, touching family members may be viewed as inappropriate	Some bury ≤24hr, some will not leave dead alone until the burial, Navajo do not touch the deceased or their belongings	High value on integrity of body, don't believe autopsy is helpful	Wide variation, decision individually broached
Chinese American	Buddhism, Taoism, Shamanism, Confucianism	No prohibitions	Strict rules regarding death announcement, preparing body, arranging funeral & burial	Acceptable	Acceptable
Latin American	Most Catholic	Possible emotional gathering	Many rites to assist dead with passage into the afterlife	Acceptable	Acceptable but usually a family decision
Japanese American	Majority Buddhists	No prohibitions	Death viewed as a passage, body must be prepared, cremation is common	Acceptable	Individual decision

Knazik SR, Gausche-Hill M, Dietrich AM, et al. *Ann Emerg Med.* 2003;42(4):519–529.

Table 6.3. Death practices by religion

Religion	Death practices
Buddhism	Body is left as found at death, gently covered with a sheet.
Catholicism	Before or after time of death, a priest should administer the sacrament of anointing the sick
Hinduism	Death should be peaceful, and the body must be attended until cremation
Islam	After death, eyes are closed, mouth is closed with a bandage, and arms/legs straightened
Judaism	Burial arranged ≤24hr. Body must be attended until burial. Cremation is not acceptable

resources that the family may wish to use. Most children's hospitals and hospice agencies provide bereavement programs and resources.

Table 6.4. Resource and Support Organizations

The Compassionate Friends, Inc.
PO Box 3696
Oak Brook, IL 60522-3696
630-990-0010; 877-969-0010
www.compassionatefriends.org
Offers support for bereaved parents, siblings and grandparents; chapters in all states.

American SIDS Institute
2480 Windy Hill Road, Suite 380
Marietta, GA 30067
770-612-1030; 800-232-SIDS
www.sids.org
Provides crises phone counseling, grief literature and referrals.

SIDS Alliance
1314 Bedford Avenue, Suite 210
Baltimore, MD 21208
410-653-8226; 800-221-SIDS
www.sidsalliance.org
Provides support to those affected by an infant death.

Pregnancy and Infant Loss Center
1421 East Wayzata Boulevard, Suite 30
Wayzata, MN 55391
612-473-9372
www.bloomington.in.us/socserv/mit/PREGNANCY_AND_INFANT_LOSS_CENTER.html
Offers support, resources and education on miscarriage, stillbirth and newborn death. Literature, keepsake items and sympathy cards available.

Partnership for Parents
www.partnershipforparents.org
Is a support network for parents of children with serious illnesses.

End-of-Life Care of Children
www.childendoflifecare.org
Website provides overviews of essential components for providing quality care, support and comfort at the end of a child's life.

Table 6.5. GRIEV_ING Mnemonic

G	Gather the family; ensure that all members are present.
R	Resources; call for support resources available to assist the family with their grief, i.e., chaplain services, ministers, family, and friends.
I	Identify; identify yourself, identify the deceased or injured patient by name, and identify the state of knowledge of the family relative to the events of the day.
E	Educate; briefly educate the family as to the events that have occurred in the ED, educate them about the current state of their loved one.
V	Verify; verify that their family member has died. Be clear! Use the words dead or died.
_	Space; give the family personal space and time for an emotional moment; allow the family time to absorb the information.
I	Inquire; ask if there are any questions and answer them all.
N	Nuts and bolts; inquire about organ donation, funeral services, and personal belongings. Offer the family the opportunity to view the body.
G	Give; give them your card and access information. Offer to answer any questions that may arise later. Always return their calls.

From Hobgood C, Harward D, Newton K, et al. The educational intervention "GRIEV_ING" improves the death notification skills of residents. *Acad Emerg Med.* 2005;12(4):296–301.

EDUCATIONAL PROGRAMS

Residency training programs in pediatrics and emergency medicine are beginning to address the educational needs in acute death and end-of-life training by offering role-playing scenarios, simulation cases, and other discussion-based training courses.[14] The Pediatric Advanced Life Support (PALS) course contains teaching modules and a video about coping with death.[15]

The GRIEV_ING mnemonic has been shown to improve ED physician competence and confidence in death notification skills (Table 6.5) and is a useful teaching tool for all ED staff.[16]

The education of all ED staff and communication skills is of utmost importance. Family members will never forget the words that were used and how they were treated when their child died.[12] Unlike illnesses in which there may be a second encounter to make a different diagnosis, with death notification there is no second chance to "get it right."

PITFALLS

- Failure to have an ED protocol for handling infant and neonatal deaths that includes a task checklist for issues such as medical examiner or law enforcement notification,

autopsy, organ donation, family bereavement resources and others
- Failure to give parents and family an adequate place or adequate time to say goodbye to their infant
- Failure to recognize signs of physician and staff grief after the death
- Failure to complete a detailed physical examination after death is pronounced to look for signs of abuse, congenital or genetic disorders
- Failure to understand that SIDS is a diagnosis of exclusion and must be distinguished from child abuse or suffocation

REFERENCES

1. Hamilton BE, Minino AM, Martin JA, et al. Annual summary of vital statistics: 2005. *Pediatrics.* 2007;119(2):345–360.
2. Malloy MH, MacDorman M. Changes in the classification of sudden unexpected infant deaths: United States, 1992–2001. *Pediatrics.* 2005;115:1247–1253.
3. American Academy of Pediatrics, Committee on Child Abuse and Neglect. Distinguishing sudden infant death syndrome from child abuse fatalities. *Pediatrics.* 2001;107(2):437–441.
4. American Academy of Pediatrics Task Force on Sudden Infant Death Syndrome. The changing concept of sudden infant death syndrome: diagnostic coding shifts, controversies regarding the sleeping environment, and new variables to consider in reducing risk. *Pediatrics.* 2005;116:1245–1255.
5. Beckwith JB. Defining the sudden infant death syndrome. *Arch Pediatr Adolesc Med.* 2003;157:286–294.
6. Horsley T, Clifford T, Barrowman N, et al. Benefits and harms associated with the practice of bed sharing. *Arch Pediatr Adolesc Med.* 2007;161:237–245.
7. Tifft CJ, Ramasethu J. Perimortem sampling. In: MacDonald MG, Ramasethu J, eds. *Atlas of Procedures in Neonatology*, 4th ed. Philadelphia, PA: Lippincott Williams & Wilkins; 2007:133–137.
8. Dobson JV, Smith MJ. Coping with unexpected pediatric death in the emergency department. *Pediatric Emergency Reports.* 2001;6:89–99.
9. Knapp J, Mulligan-Smith D, and the Committee on Pediatric Emergency Medicine. Death of a child in the emergency department. *Pediatrics.* 2005;115:1432–1437.
10. Knazik SR, Gausche-Hill M, Dietrich AM, et al. The death of a child in the emergency department. *Ann Emerg Med.* 2003;42(4):519–529.
11. Lipton H, Coleman M. Bereavement practice guidelines for health care professionals in the emergency department. *Int J Emerg Ment Health.* 2000;2(1):1–13.
12. Ahrens W, Hart R, Maruyama N. Pediatric death: managing the aftermath in the emergency department. *J Emerg Med.* 1997;15(5):601–603.
13. American Academy of Pediatrics. The pediatrician and childhood bereavement. Committee on Psychosocial Aspects of Child and Family Health. *Pediatrics.* 2000;105:445–446.
14. Bagatell R, Meyer R, Herron S, et al. When children die: a seminar for pediatric residents. *Pediatrics.* 2002;110:348–353.
15. American Heart Association. Textbook of Pediatric Advanced Life Support. Dallas, TX: American Heart Association. 2006.
16. Hobgood C, Harward D, Newton K, et al. The educational intervention "GRIEV_ING" improves the death notification skills of residents. *Acad Emerg Med.* 2005; 12(4):296–301.

PART II

CHIEF COMPLAINTS

7

Apparent Life-Threatening Events

Tonia J. Brousseau

INTRODUCTION

The term *apparent life-threatening event* (ALTE) was first described in 1986 by the National Institutes of Health Consensus Development Conference on Infantile Apnea and Home Monitoring. ALTE was defined by the consensus in the following manner:

> An episode that is frightening to the observer and is characterized by some combination of apnea (central or occasionally obstructive), color change (usually cyanotic or pallid, but occasionally erythematous or plethoric), marked change in tone (usually marked limpness), choking, or gagging. In some cases the observer fears that the infant has died.[1]

Before 1986, ALTEs were referred to as *near-miss SIDS* or *aborted crib deaths*. These terms were determined to be misleading because they implied there was a direct association between sudden infant death syndrome (SIDS) and ALTE. *SIDS* is defined as the sudden death of an infant younger than 1 year of age that remains unexplained after a thorough case investigation including a complete autopsy, examination of the death scene and review of the clinical history.[2]

Although it was once thought that infants with ALTE episodes were more likely to die of SIDS, less than 7% of patients who died of SIDS were described as having had a prior ALTE.[1] Several important differences in epidemiology of SIDS and ALTE include the following[3]:

- The greater than 40% decrease in SIDS deaths with the "back-to-sleep" campaign was not also accompanied by a decrease in the rate of ALTE episodes.
- SIDS deaths predominantly occur between midnight and 6:00 AM, whereas ALTEs usually occur during waking hours (8:00 AM–8:00 PM).

- When the risk factors for SIDS were evaluated, the only overlapping risk profile between ALTE and SIDS was smoking in pregnancy.

The true incidence of ALTEs is difficult to estimate not only because an ALTE may be the initial presentation of many different illnesses but also because an ALTE is often difficult to track because it is not included as the discharge diagnosis unless the ALTE was determined to have no other cause. Table 7.1 outlines the American Academy of Pediatrics (AAP) guidelines for SIDS prevention. An ALTE is estimated to occur in 0.5% to 6% of all infants, with 82% of these events occurring during the daytime hours.[4] ALTE is not a diagnosis but a term used to describe a clinical presentation of a very broad differential diagnosis.

Apnea is defined as the cessation of breathing for 20 seconds or for any length of time when also accompanied by a change in color, muscle tone or heart rate. Apnea may be the result of local airway abnormalities causing obstruction or central nervous system (CNS) influences on the respiratory drive.

Table 7.1. American academy of pediatrics recommendations on SIDS prevention

Do's	Don'ts
Back to sleep	Prone/side sleeping position
Pacifier use	Soft pillows or bedding
Sleeping in room in close proximity	Bed sharing/ co-sleeping
Immunizations	Overbundling/Overheating
Breastfeeding	Overfeeding
Tummy time when awake and observation to avoid plagiocephaly	Home monitoring as a strategy to reduce SIDS risk

SIDS, sudden infant death syndrome.

Table 7.2. Patient history to consider when diagnosing an apparent life-threatening event

Chief complaint	• Condition of child: Awake or asleep, body position, location of event, type of bedding used
	• Activity at time of event: Feeding, coughing, gagging, choking, vomiting
	• Length of time: Time to when infant regained normal respiratory effort
History of present illness HPI	• Recent illness or exposure, rash, fever
	• Weight loss, poor feeding, spitting up, wet burps
	• Irritability, lethargy
Interventions	• None
	• Gentle stimulation
	• Blowing air in face
	• Vigorous stimulation
	• Mouth-to-mouth breathing
	• Cardiopulmonary resuscitation by medically trained person
Past medical history	• Prior episodes
	• Home monitor: Heart rate or breathing alarms, frequency of alarms, lead placement, reason for monitor
	• Gastroesophageal reflux
	• Birth history
	• Prenatal history
	• Accidents
	• Previous hospitalizations/surgeries
Family history	• SIDS or other unexplained childhood deaths
	• Cardiac arrhythmias
	• Congenital diseases
Social history	• Smoking in the home
	• Caretakers
	• Medications in the home
Medication	• Prescriptions
	• Over-the-counter medications
	• Herbs, herbal teas or supplements

SIDS, sudden infant death syndrome.

PRESENTATION

Determining whether a true ALTE occurred is almost always based on the history obtained in the emergency setting. It may be difficult to obtain accurate historical data because of parental or caregiver anxiety. Although some patients may present in mild to severe distress requiring immediate interventions, most infants are well appearing and have no physical signs of illness. One study found that 83% of patients in the prehospital setting with a history consistent with an ALTE had no abnormalities on physical examination and therefore had no clinically reliable indicators to determine the severity of the event.[5]

Because the description of an ALTE is entirely based on the caregiver and his or her ability to recall details of the stressful event, it becomes the physician's responsibility to ascertain the necessary information about the severity of the event. The historical data need to include very specific details about the infant and event. One survey found that 10 of 76 infants who required mouth-to-mouth

resuscitation subsequently died.[6] In addition, the maternal history, prior pregnancy history and family history are important and also warrant close attention. The complete list of important historical information is listed in Table 7.2.

DIFFERENTIAL DIAGNOSIS

Although the differential diagnosis for ALTE is large and heterogeneous, the evaluation of these infants will yield a diagnosis only 50% of the time.[7] Lists of the causes of ALTE are available in Tables 7.3, 7.4 and 7.5.

GASTROINTESTINAL

Although gastroesophageal reflux disease (GERD) is the diagnosis given to the majority of ALTE events, other catastrophic events should be mentioned: volvulus, intussusception, rotavirus, esophageal atresia, and strangulated hernia.[8] *GERD* is a term used to describe reflux that is

Table 7.3. Differential diagnosis of obstructive apnea

Neonate/infant	Both	Toddler/young child
Stridor		
Vascular ring	Vocal cord paralysis	
	Foreign body	
	Croup/epiglottitis	
	Prematurity	
	Positional	Laryngeal web
	Laryngomalacia	Tracheostomy plug
	Tracheomalacia	Subglottic stenosis
	Bronchopulmonary dysplasia	
Abnormal Airway		
Choanal atresia/stenosis	Craniofacial abnormalities	Large tonsils/adenoids
Tracheoesophageal fistula		
Other		
	Gastroesophageal reflux	
	Hemangioma/lymphangioma	
	Pharyngeal/retropharyngeal mass	

potentially pathologic. GERD is thought to be the diagnosis of ALTE in 18% to 66% of cases.[9,10] This large range may reflect the controversy of GERD as a true cause of ALTE. A study of 25 infants with 527 total apneic events revealed no evidence of association between either acid or nonacid reflux and apnea.[11]

The gold standard for diagnosis of reflux, the 24-hour esophageal pH probe, typically is not useful in the diagnosis of uncomplicated reflux and does not record nonacid reflux, which may account for 50% of reflux.[12] The use of the pH probe together with the multi-channel intraluminal impedance (pH-MII) helps record both acid and nonacid reflux. In infants with apneic episodes, the pH probe is useful only when there is a temporal relationship established between reflux and documented apnea or bradycardia.[13]

One study suggested that gastroesophageal reflux (GER) is frequent in ALTE and that apnea preceded the GER in 90% of patient episodes.[14] Furthermore, ALTEs

may be related to reflux in situations in which gross emesis or oral regurgitation occurs at the time of the ALTE, the infant is awake and supine and the ALTE is characterized by obstructive apnea.[11]

The mechanism for apnea as a result of reflux includes both obstructive and central etiologies. The obstructive mechanism may be vagally induced, but it has been suggested that the stimulation of chemoreceptors around the larynx, which respond to gastric acid and water, may result in central apnea, bradycardia and hypertension.[15]

NEUROLOGIC

Seizures

Seizure activity has a high association with sudden death and ALTE. A history consistent with seizure activity often is not obvious; therefore, the clinician requires a high level of suspicion. The history of recurrent ALTE episodes

Table 7.4. Differential diagnosis of central apnea

Neonate/infant	Both	Toddler/young child
Central Nervous System		
Central nervous system immaturity	Seizures	Apneustic breathing (achondroplasia)
Aberrant thermoregulation	Brainstem tumor	
	Chiari type 1 malformation	
	Increased intracranial pressure	
	Vascular malformation/hemorrhage	
	Congenital central hypoventilation syndrome	

Table 7.5. Other causes of apnea

Neonate/infant	Neonate/infant and Toddler/young child
Cardiovascular	
	Shock
	Dysrhythmias
	Congenital heart disease
	Prolonged QT syndrome
Infectious Diseases	
Infant botulism	Sepsis
Respiratory syncytial	Pertussis
Virus	Meningitis
	Encephalitis
	Pneumonia
Miscellaneous	
	Anemia
	Trauma
	Poisoning
	Neuromuscular disorders
	Munchausen syndrome by proxy
	Metabolic disorders

has been associated with a higher incidence of seizures and likelihood of sudden death. Typically, seizure activity is accompanied by tachycardia rather than bradycardia; therefore, witnessed episodes of apnea with tachycardia should increase the suspicion of seizures. Diagnosis is typically made using an electroencephalogram (EEG), but a normal EEG recording does not exclude seizure activity because the patient may have a normal EEG between events.

Breath Holding Spells

Breath holding spells (BHSs) occur in up to 3% of children, and 25% of the time, the initial presentation occurs in infants younger than 6 months of age.[16,17] These episodes usually are preceded by a painful or undesirable event, resulting in an expiratory apnea. The infant may become rapidly cyanotic, have a change in overall tone and lose consciousness, typically for fewer than 30 seconds after onset of symptoms and, occasionally, followed by a generalized seizure.[18] If the infant becomes pale prior to the episode, this is actually vaso-vagal syncope rather than a BHS.

A history and clinical presentation that are consistent with a classic BHS may not require an extensive evaluation. Because an association between iron deficiency anemia and BHSs has been demonstrated, an evaluation of the patient's hemoglobin (Hb) and mean corpuscular volume (MCV) may be included in the workup of a BHS.[19]

Increased Intracranial Pressure

An elevation of intracranial pressure as a result of hydrocephalus or intracranial hemorrhage or mass may present as an ALTE. The physical examination may reveal a large head circumference; a full, bulging fontanelle; bradycardia; hypertension and even "sundown eyes."

ABUSE

Nonaccidental trauma should be considered in all infants with an ALTE. There must be a high index of suspicion because the abused infant may appear well and have no physical signs of injury.[20] Pitetti et al. found an incidence rate of 2.3% of physical abuse in patients with an ALTE.[21] Abuse is often not diagnosed on the initial physician visit and is associated with a high morbidity if it is not discovered. A fundoscopic examination may reveal occult head injury and should be included in the assessment of all patients with an ALTE who do not have a readily apparent diagnosis.[21]

Munchausen by proxy was first described in 1977 and is defined by DSM-IV in the following way:

> [I]ntentional production or feigning of physical or psychological signs or symptoms in another person who is under the individual's care, and the motivation of the perpetrator's behavior is to assume the sick role by proxy, external incentives for the behavior, such as economic gain, avoiding legal responsibility, or improving physical well-being are absent. A history that includes recurrent apneic or cyanotic episodes may be the result of intentional suffocation.[22]

Apnea is the presenting sign in Munchausen by proxy 19% of the time. One review found that the mean time to diagnosis of abuse was 14.9 months.[23] A missed diagnosis may be life-threatening because Munchausen by proxy is associated with a 10% morbidity rate.[24]

INFECTION

Respiratory Syncytial Virus

Respiratory syncytial virus (RSV) is the most common cause of brochiolitis and has been described to cause apnea in 20% of hospitalized patients with RSV.[25] There are several risk factors for apnea in RSV infections: full-term infants younger than 1 month of age, premature infants fewer than 48 weeks post-conception and infants in whom there have been witnessed apneic episodes prior to presentation.[26] Yet low-risk infants may have less than a 1% incidence of apnea.[26]

It is important to recognize that in RSV infections, apnea may be the only initial presenting symptom and may precede the development of other more classic respiratory symptoms.[27,28] The pathophysiology of apnea caused by RSV remains unclear. In animal studies, Lingren et al. demonstrated that RSV may alter the sensitivity of the laryngeal chemoreceptors, leading to laryngeal chemoreflux and central apnea.[29] Another study that used polysomnographies (PSGs) to evaluate apnea caused by RSV found all events to be central, resulting in oxygen desaturation and bradycardia.[30]

Bordetella Pertussis

Pertussis remains a threat to nonimmunized infants.[31] It has been suggested that pertussis is underdiagnosed because infants often have an atypical presentation.[32] There may be no history of the classic "whooping cough," and the initial presentation may be an ALTE.[32]

In addition, unless a polymerase chain reaction (PCR) test is used instead of a culture to identify pertussis as the pathogen, there may be only a 20% to 40% sensitivity of cultures.[33,34] In one study, an RSV and pertussis co-infection was found in 11 of 33 infants.[32]

Other Infections

Bacterial meningitis, sepsis, rotavirus, encephalitis and other respiratory infections also may present as an ALTE.[35] More recently, urinary tract infections (UTIs) were recognized as a cause of ALTE. A series of three case reports described the initial presenting symptom of UTIs as an ALTE.[36]

HEMATOLOGIC

Iron deficiency anemia has been hypothesized to cause apnea by a decreased oxygen-carrying capacity to the CNS or from a resulting decrease in blood volume and CNS perfusion pressure.[37] Pitetti compared Hb and MCV in ALTE patients with a control group and found that although patients with a single ALTE episode did not significantly vary from the patients in the control group, patients with recurrent ALTE events were 21.9% more likely to have an iron deficiency anemia than the controls.[19]

METABOLIC

Inborn errors of metabolism (IEMs) result from a deficiency or absence of an enzyme or co-factor leading to the accumulation of a toxic metabolite. An ALTE may be the initial presentation after acute metabolic decompensation. Fatty acid oxidation defects (medium chain acyl CoA dehydrogenase deficiency [MCAD]), disorders of amino acid metabolism and urea cycle and organic acidemias are the IEMs most likely to present as an ALTE.[38] A family history of SIDS, recurrent or severe ALTE, consanguinity or seizures should increase the suspicion of an IEM.[39] In addition, laboratory evidence of hypoglycemia, hyperammonemia, metabolic acidosis, elevated liver enzymes or abnormal hemostasis or a patient history of failure to thrive (FTT), developmental delay or seizures should prompt a full evaluation for an IEM.

CARDIAC

Although structural cardiac defects may play a role in ALTE, more data are available on the association of ALTE and cardiac arrhythmias. Prolongation of the QT is known to be associated with SIDS and has been suggested to play a role in ALTE. Goldhammer et al. evaluated 89 infants with ALTE and found the QTc to be significantly greater in the ALTE group.[40]

In another study, 62% of ALTE patients had cardiac arrhythmias and 30% of the 62% had QT intervals greater that 2 SD above the mean.[41] The QTc is calculated from measured intervals on the electrocardiogram (ECG) by the Bazett formula (QTc = QT/$\sqrt{\text{R-R}}$), with a normal value of fewer than 0.42 to 0.43 seconds.

A lack of heart rate variability (HRV) or autonomic dysfunction in response to stress also may be a cause of ALTE. In two studies, Edner et al. measured HRV. Each study found less HRV and more incidences of bradycardia in infants with ALTE, and the second study had more such instances in the male subjects.[42,43]

MECHANICAL/ANATOMICAL AIRWAY OBSTRUCTION

Mechanical airway obstruction has several different etiologies. Included in the causes are small mandibular size, facial dysmorphia, small airway patency, increased inspiratory effort and obstructive sleep apnea.[44–49] Determining obstructive apnea versus central apnea is only accurate using PSG, which evaluates nasal and oral air flow during apnea.

TOXINS

Toxins may cause apnea and be a result of accidental or intentional poisoning. In general, cough and cold preparations, especially those containing codeine, should be avoided in infants and neonates. ALTE as a result of respiratory depression in repetitive dosage of codeine has been reported.[50] A thorough medication history including a breastfeeding mother's prescription and nonprescription medications, including any homeopathic remedies, should be included in the historical data.

APNEA OF IMMATURITY

Apnea of immaturity is a respiratory pause lasting 20 seconds or more, or pauses lasting fewer than 20 seconds that are accompanied by pallor, cyanosis, bradycardia or hypotonia in a term infant. This phrase is reserved for infants with an ALTE who have had a thorough evaluation and in whom no other etiology is identified.

LABORATORY AND RADIOLOGY EVALUATION

Emergency department (ED) evaluation and interventions are usually directed by 1) the clinical appearance of the infant or neonate (<1 month of age) with an ALTE, and 2) historical data obtained from the caregiver. All patients should have their airway, breathing and circulation (ABCs) evaluated and immediately addressed if abnormalities are present. In addition, the physician should complete a rapid bedside blood glucose test and give careful attention to the infant's temperature control. Unless the history reveals a specific etiology, the initial ED evaluation should include a complete blood cell count; electrolytes including serum sodium, potassium, calcium and magnesium; renal and liver function tests; blood cultures; nasopharyngeal aspirates for RSV and pertussis PCR; an ECG and a chest radiograph. Cerebrospinal fluid also should be obtained in the hemodynamically stable patient if the infant is younger than 1 month of age or appears ill.

Additionally, if an IEM is suspected, then adjunctive studies should include an arterial blood gas; serum ammonia (obtained without a tourniquet and immediately placed on ice); prothrombin time (PT) and urine evaluation for color, odor and ketones.

One study that tried to determine the yield of different diagnostic tests in ALTE found that most tests in the ED had a low positive yield. The study did find a subset of tests that were helpful in the identification of occult causes of ALTE. These tests include the following[51]:

1. Screening for GER
2. Urinalysis and culture
3. Brain imaging
4. Pneumogram
5. White blood cell count

Nonaccidental trauma should be considered in all patients with an ALTE. Current recommendations for the evaluation of these patients should include a dilated fundoscopic examination for retinal hemorrhages. This examination also may increase the yield of occult causes of ALTE.[21,52]

MANAGEMENT

After initial ED evaluation and stabilization, the decision needs to be made whether to discharge the patient home or admit the patient to the hospital for further evaluation and monitored observation. One study looked at 59 patients and found that those infants who were younger than 1 month of age or who had multiple episodes of apnea were considered high risk and yielded a negative predictive value of 100% to identifying the need for hospital admission.[53] A second study by Piero evaluated 122 patients to determine the yield of positive ED diagnostic tests in infants after an ALTE. This study found the overall yield to be low and recommend that the majority of patients can be managed with a less extensive ED evaluation. Piero recommended that all patients be admitted after an ALTE because of the significant number of patients who required an intervention after admission.[54]

Although these studies suggest that low-risk infants may be discharged home, further investigation with larger numbers of patients is needed before this can be the standard of care. Infants who are febrile, ill-appearing or younger than 30 days of age should receive broad-spectrum antibiotics after cultures are drawn. Any electrolyte abnormalities should be corrected. A patient who has a recurrence of ALTE episodes requiring intervention or a patient who is hemodynamically unstable should be admitted to the pediatric intensive care unit. If there is a suspicion of Munchausen by proxy, then the patient should be admitted to an institution where covert video surveillance is available. In instances of suspected nonaccidental trauma, the proper child protection services should be notified. All infants with an ALTE who are admitted for observation and further testing should be admitted to a hospital bed with central monitoring.

HOME MONITORING

Home apnea monitors with memory are widely used to record respirations, heart rate and, occasionally, oxygen saturation. Despite 25 years of data about home apnea monitor use, there has been no evidence that they decrease SIDS deaths. A review of the literature suggests that apnea monitors may be warranted if they are used to document apnea, bradycardia or hypoxia in the high-risk preterm infant, infants with documented ALTEs and infants who are technologically dependent.[55]

PITFALLS

- Failure to obtain a complete, detailed, thorough history from the caregiver
- Failure to recognize that recurrent ALTE episodes are more common in undiagnosed epileptic seizures and intentional suffocation
- Failure to complete a fundoscopic examination
- Failure to not consider admission in all episodes of ALTE
- Failure to know the new AAP SIDS prevention guidelines (Table 7.1)

REFERENCES

1. National Institutes of Health Consensus Development Conference in Infantile Apnea and Home Monitoring, Sept 29 to Oct 1,1986: Consensus Statement. *Pediatrics.* 1987;79:292–299.
2. Willinger M, James LS, Catz C. Defining the sudden infant death syndrome (SIDS): deliberation of an expert panel convened by the National Institute of Child Health and Human Development. *Pediatr Pathol.* 1991;11:677–684.
3. Kiechl-Kohlendorfer U, Hof D, Pupp Peglow U, et al. Epidemiology of apparent life threatening events. *Arch Dis Child.* 2005;90:297–300.
4. Kahn A, Rebuffat E, Franco P, et al. Apparent life-threatening events and apnea of infancy. In: Beckerman RC, Brouillette RT, Hunt CE, eds. *Respiratory Control Disorders in Infants and Children.* New York, NY: Williams & Wilkins; 1992:178–189.
5. Stratton ST, Taves A, Lewis RJ, et al. Apparent life-threatening events in infants: high risk in the out-of-hospital environment. *Ann Emerg Med.* 2004;43:711–717.
6. Oren J, Kelly D, Shannon DC. Identification of a high risk group for sudden infant death among infants who were resuscitated for sleep apnea. *Pediatrics.* 1986;77:495–499.
7. Brooks JG. Apparent life-threatening events and apnea of infancy. *Clin Perinatol.* 1992;4:809–838.
8. Cozzi DA, Zani A, Conforti A, et al. Pathogenesis of apparent life-threatening events in infants with esophageal atresia. *Pediatric Pulmon.* 2006;41:488–493.
9. Davies F, Gupta R. Apparent life-threatening events in infants presenting to an emergency department. *Emerg Med J.* 2002;19(1):11–16.
10. Gray C, Davies F, Molyneux E. Apparent life-threatening events presenting to an emergency department. *Pediatr Emerg Care.* 1999:15(3):195–199.
11. Mousa H, Woodley FW, Metheney M, et al. Testing the association between gastroesophageal reflux and apnea in infants. *J Pediatr Gastroenterol Nutr.* 2005;41:169–177.
12. Candino AA, Sondheimer J, Pan Z, et al. Evaluation of gastroesophageal reflux in pediatric patients with asthma using impedance-pH monitoring. *J Pediatr.* 2006;149(2):216–219.
13. Colletti RB, Christie DL, Orenstein SR. Statement of the North American Society of Pediatric Gastroenterology and Nutrition (NASPGN). Indications for pediatric esophageal pH monitoring. *J Pediatr Gastroenterol Nutr.* 1995;21:253.
14. Arad-Cohen N, Cohen A, Tirosh E. The relationship between gastroesophageal reflux and apnea in infants. *J Pediatr.* 2000;137:321–326.
15. Johnson P, Salisbury DM, Storey AT. Apnoea induced by stimulation of sensory receptors in the larynx. In: Bosma JF, Showacre J, eds. Development of Upper Respiratory Anatomy and Function. Washington DC: US Department of Health, Education, and Welfare; 1975:160–178.
16. DiMario FJ Jr. Prospective study of children with cyanotic and pallid breath-holding spells. *Pediatrics.* 2001;107(2):265–269.
17. Weese-Mayer DE, Marazita ML, Berry-Kravis ME. Congenital hypoventilation syndrome. *Gene Review.* February 23, 2007 (Accessed March 1, 2007).
18. Steinschneider A, Richmond C, Ramaswamy V, et al. Clinical characteristics of an apparent life-threatening event (ALTE) and the subsequent occurrence of prolonged apnea or prolonged bradycardia. *Clin Pediatr.* 1998;37:223–230.
19. Pitetti RD, Lovallo A, Hickey R. Prevalence of anemia in children presenting with apparent life-threatening events. *Acad Emerg Med.* 2005;12:926–931.
20. Morris MW, Smith S, Cressman J, Ancheta J. Evaluation of infants with subdural hematoma who lack external evidence of abuse. *Pediatrics.* 2000;105:549–553.
21. Pitetti RD, Maffei F, Chang K, et al. Prevalence of retinal hemorrhages and child abuse in children who present with an apparent life-threatening event. *Pediatrics.* 2002;110(3):557–562.
22. Sheridan MS. Munchausen syndrome by proxy and apnea. *Neonatal Intensive Care.* 2003;16:25.
23. Brooks JG. Sudden infant death syndrome and apparent life-threatening events. In: Levin DL, Morris FL, eds. *Essentials*

of Pediatric Intensive Care. New York, NY: Churchill Livingstone; 1997:111–115.

24. Kato I, Groswasser J, Franco P, et al. Developmental characteristics of apnea in infants who succumb to sudden infant death syndrome. Am J Respir Crit Care Med. 2001;164:1464–1469.

25. Bruhn FW, Mokrohisky ST, McIntosh K. Apnea associated with respiratory syncytial virus infection in young infants. J Pediatr. 1977;90(3):382–386.

26. Willwerth BM, Harper MB, Greenes DS. Identifying hospitalized infants who have bronchiolitis and are at high risk for apnea. Ann Emerg Med. 2006;48(4):441–447.

27. Bruhn FW, Mokrohisky ST, McIntosh K. Apnea associated with respiratory syncytial virus infection in young infants. J Pediatr. 1977;90:382–386.

28. Kneyber MC, Brandenburg AH, de Groot R, et al. Risk factors for respiratory syncytial virus associated apnea. Eur J Pediatr. 1998;157:331–335.

29. Lingren C, Lin J, Graham BS, et al. Respiratory syncytial virus infection enhances the response to laryngeal chemostimulation and inhibits arousal from sleep in young lambs. Acta Pediatr. 1996;85:789–797.

30. Rayyan M, Naulaers G, Daniels H, et al. Characteristics of respiratory syncytial virus-related apnoea in three infants. Acta Pediatr. 2004;93:847–849.

31. Crowcraft NS, Andrews N, Rooney C, et al. Deaths from pertussis are underestimated in England. Arch Dis Child. 2002;86:336–338.

32. Crowcraft NS, Booy R, Harrison T, et al. Severe and unrecognized: pertussis in UK infants. Arch Child Dis. 2007;88:802–806.

33. Heininger U. Pertussis: an old disease that is still with us. Curr Opin Infect Dis. 2001;14:329–335.

34. Crowcraft NS, Britto J. Whooping cough-a continuing problem. BMJ. 2002;324:1537–1538.

35. Panitch HB, Callahan CW, Schidlow D. Bronchiolitis in children. Clin Chest Med. 1993;14:715–731.

36. Edwards KS, Gardner T, Altman RL. Urinary tract infection presenting as an ALTE: report of three cases. Clin Pediatr. 2004;43:375–377.

37. Kattwinkel J. Neonatal apnea: pathogenesis and therapy. J Pediatr. 1977;90:342–347.

38. Howat AJ, Bennett MJ, Variend S, et al. Deficiency of medium chain fatty acylcoenzyme A dehydrogenase presenting as the sudden infant death syndrome. Br Med J (Clin Res Ed) 1984;288:976.

39. Perkin RM. Apparent life-threatening events. Pediatr Emerg Med Rep. 2005;10(2).

40. Goldhammer EI, Zaid G, Tal V, et al. QT dispersion in infants with apparent life-threatening events syndrome. Pediatr Cardiol. 2002;23(6):605–607.

41. Woolf PK, Gewitz MH, Preminger T, et al. Infants with apparent life threatening events. Cardiac rhythm and conduction. Clin Pediatr (Phila). 1989;28(11):517–520.

42. Edner A, Katz-Salamon M, Lagercrantz M, et al. Heart rate variability in infants with apparent life-threatening events. Acta Pediatr. 2000;89:1326–1329.

43. Edner A, Ericson M, Milerad J, et al. Abnormal heart rate response to hypercapnia in boys with an apparent life-threatening event. Acta Pediatr. 2002;91:1318–1323.

44. Horn MH, Kinnamon DD, Ferraro N, et al. Smaller mandibular size in infants with a history of an apparent life-threatening event. J Pediatr. 2006;149:499–504.

45. McNamara F, Sullivan CD. Obstructive sleep apnea in infants: relation to family history of sudden infant death syndrome, apparent life-threatening events, and obstructive sleep apnea. J Pediatr. 2000;136:318–323.

46. McNamara F, Sulllivan CD. Obstructive sleep apnea in infants and its management with nasal continuous positive airway pressure. Chest. 1999;116:10–16.

47. Guilleminault C, Pelayo R, Leger D, et al. Apparent life-threatening events, facial dysmorphia and sleep-disordered breathing. Eur J Pediatr. 2000;159:444–449.

48. Hartman H, Seidenberg J, Noyes JP, et al. Small airway patency in infants with apparent life-threatening events. Eur J Pediatr. 1998;157:71–74.

49. Horemuzova E, Katz-Salamon M, Milerad J. Increased inspiratory effort in infants with a history of apparent life-threatening event. Acta Pediatr. 2002;91:280–286.

50. Tong TF, Ng KK. Codeine ingestion and apparent life-threatening event in a neonate. Pediatr Int. 2001;43:517–518.

51. Brand DA, Altman RL, Purtill K, et al. Yield of diagnostic testing in infants who have had an apparent life-threatening event. Pediatrics. 2005;115:885–893.

52. Altman RL, Brand DA, Forman S, et al. Abusive head injury as a cause of apparent life-threatening events in infancy. Arch Pediatr Adolesc Med. 2003;157(10):1011–1015.

53. Claudius I, Keens T. Do all infants with apparent iife-threatening events need to be admitted? Pediatrics. 2007;119:679–683.

54. Piero AD, Teach SJ, Chamberlain JM. ED evaluation of infants after an apparent life-threatening event. Am J Emerg Med. 2004;22:83–86.

55. Farrell PA, Weiner GM, Lemons JA. SIDS, ALTE, apnea, and the use of home monitors. Pediatr Rev. 2002;23(1):3–9.

8 The Crying Infant

Martin I. Herman and Audrey Le

[H]is face flushes, his brow furrows, and then he draws his legs up, clenches his fists and emits piercing, high-pitched screams, which do not stop when he is picked up, continuing unabated in his mother's arms. – Illingsworth[1]

INTRODUCTION

Crying is certainly a part of normal infant behavior. Intuitively, most providers know that babies cry for various reasons, including the desire for attention, hunger, discomfort and pain. It is only when their reasons for crying appear indiscernible or when the amount of crying is considered to be excessive that guardians become concerned and seek assistance. Excessive crying is one of the most frequent problems reported by mothers during the first 4 months of a child's life, and is a common reason families bring babies to medical attention.[2]

EPIDEMIOLOGY

The prevalence of excessive crying in the infant population has been estimated to be between 1.5% and 40%.[3–5] In England, caring for infants who are crying and have difficulty sleeping is estimated to cost $108 million annually.[6] Families with infants who are perceived to be crying excessively are subject to a considerable amount of stress. The entire family dynamic, including the interactions between infant and mother, between infant and father and between the two parents can be negatively affected.[7,8] Excessive infant crying has been found to be associated with maternal anxiety and depression.[9–11] It has served as a factor in the discontinuation of breastfeeding, and in the most extreme and tragic cases, it has been cited as a contributing factor to physical violence and infant homicide.[12–14]

Trying to determine whether or not the crying is normal versus excessive can be challenging to the most experienced clinicians. Further delineating whether excessive crying is physiologic and somewhat self-limiting, as in colic, or a manifestation of some organic pathological process can and will test the skills of every provider. Indeed, because of the seeming ordinariness of the complaint, clinicians may be inclined to trivialize it and dismiss the guardians as overanxious or excessively vigilant.

PATHOPHYSIOLOGY

To begin, one needs to understand the difference between normal, expected amounts of crying and excessive or abnormal crying. It was Brazelton who first codified normal infant crying in his work published in 1962.[15] He reported that infants in their second week of life cried and fussed for a median of $1^3/_4$ hours. The crying gradually increased to a peak median of $2^3/_4$ hours at 6 weeks of age, after which it decreased. Babies 3 weeks of age cried most often between 6:00 and 11:00 PM, with smaller groups crying between 4:00 and 7:00 AM and 9:00 and 11:00 AM. By $1^1/_2$ months, the babies were crying more between 3:00 PM and 12:00 AM. A month later, the study infants were crying to a lesser extent and that was mostly after waking in the early mornings or later in the afternoon and evenings. Thanks to the work of Brazelton and others, we now understand that normal or typical infant crying is characterized by a peak at 2 months of age and a decline thereafter until about 4 months, when it plateaus.[16,17] There even appears to be a circadian pattern, with crying occurring most in the late afternoon and evenings. Of course, considerable variability may exist within and between infants when it comes to their crying.[16,18] If the crying exceeds the norm, it is deemed excessive.

COLIC/EXCESSIVE CRYING

The terms *paroxysmal fussing, persistent crying,* and *infantile colic* have been used interchangeably to describe infants with nonorganic etiologies for excessive crying. A mid-20th century report by Illingsworth describing infants in the first 3 months of life with "rhythmic attacks of screaming" and no evident inciting cause was one of the first to address the topic of excessive crying.[1] In that landmark report, the episodes reportedly lasted 5 or more minutes and occurred predominately in the evenings. Because they lessened significantly by the time the infants reached the 3-month age mark, Illingsworth coined the phrase "3 months' colic" to describe the phenomenon.

During that same period, another group described a similar phenomenon and, in what has come to be known as the *rule of 3's,* defined infants as fussy when they cried or fussed for more than 3 hours in a day with episodes occurring on more than 3 days a week.[19] Even though this definition of excessive crying or colic has become the most commonly accepted, variations of it in the literature have led to studies comprised of such disparate groups that it is difficult to determine the true prevalence, find possible causes or assess any remedies for excessive crying.[4]

Several theories have been presented over the years to explain the colic syndrome. Early investigators postulated that some type of gastrointestinal (GI) dysfunction had to be playing a role. Cow's milk protein allergy, malabsorption and GI dysmotility have all been offered as explanations. Some investigators have blamed substances found in breast milk for the violent peristalsis in the GI tracts of colicky infants.[20] Others have suggested that a mother's milk made while she was consuming a diet rich in cow's milk somehow affected the infant. However, studies altering the breastfeeding mother's diet by eliminating cow's milk have yielded equivocal results.[21–23] Still other investigations have found that when cow's milk protein was eliminated from the diets of colicky formula-fed infants, the crying decreased.[24–26]

Excess colonic gas with its attendant abdominal cramping and discomfort from malabsorption has also been implicated as a cause of colic. There is some evidence to support this theory. When breath hydrogen was measured in 122 healthy infants after feedings containing lactose, colicky infants had more positive breath tests compared to noncolicky infants, and failure to produce hydrogen

gas throughout the breath test was more frequent in the latter group.[27] Yet another study of infants with colic found that the stool pH and reducing substances were normal, which indicates that intestinal absorption was normal.[28] These and other studies have led researchers to conclude that malabsorption may account only for a small subset of infants with colic.

During the past few decades, gastroesophageal reflux disease (GERD) has become a common diagnosis assigned to infants who cry excessively. It is so commonly invoked as a diagnosis that when infants are admitted with crying or irritability, a past history of GERD is elicited more than any other diagnosis.[29] That GERD may actually be a significant cause of infant crying was confirmed by esophageal pH determinations in 16 of 26 (61.5%) infants with colic referred to a pediatric gastroenterology clinic.[30] Of note, all of those infants experienced a reduction in crying 2 weeks after institution of treatment. Ironically, a resolution of the crying also occurred in the remaining infants without GERD, leading to speculation that the patients who received treatment might have improved even without intervention. More importantly, because the median age of the infants in the group was 4.8 months, which is outside the typical age range for infantile colic, it is likely that those investigators were not really dealing with prototypical colicky infants. Although GI disturbances cannot fully account for the colicky behavior in many infants, they might explain crying and irritability in at least a subgroup of patients. Obviously, feeding difficulties, excessive emesis, diarrhea, constipation or the passage of bloody stools does help support a GI etiology.[26,30,31]

No discussion of infantile colic would be complete without at least mentioning that infant temperament and the parental–infant unit also has been implicated as a cause of excessive crying. Sadly, colic was once thought to represent the pleas of an infant for the attention of an aloof or indifferent mother. Fortunately for today's mothers, that theory was tested and debunked. When caretaking styles of mothers of persistent criers at 6 weeks of age who cried 3 or more hours a day were compared with those of mothers of moderate criers and those of evening criers who cried fewer than 3 hours a day in total, there was no significant difference in maternal sensitivity or affection between the groups.[32] Health care providers should discard this premise as it can only serve to further damage the maternal–infant bond and does not help the infant. Whatever the cause of colic, our mission should be to alleviate the distress and soothe frazzled nerves of the baby's caretakers.

PRESENTATION

Illingsworth's eloquent description cited at the opening of this chapter represents the typical presentation of the colicky infant. More importantly, it may also represent the presentation of infants with any of the organic etiologies for crying. These patients and their distraught families typically present in the late evening or early morning hours. Unfortunately, those are the hours the babies are most likely to be crying. They are also the hours the parents are most likely to be exhausted. Hence the following conundrum emerges for practitioners, "Is it normal or excessive?" Furthermore, if the crying is excessive, how much of an investigation is warranted?

DIFFERENTIAL DIAGNOSIS

Normal Versus Excessive

The most basic challenge lies in distinguishing the many potentially serious causes of crying from the benign causes. In making that distinction, a provider has to balance the tendency to trivialize and dismiss the complaint against a desire to investigate causes that may lead to unnecessary and invasive testing. Even though organic disease accounts for less than 5% of infants whose guardians seek medical care for their excessive crying,[33] there remains the task of distinguishing organic disease from the more common and benign etiologies.

The traditional Socratic approach of taking a thorough history and performing a thorough physical examination will yield a diagnosis in a majority of the cases. This was borne out in a prospective emergency department study of 56 infants presenting with crying, in which it was determined that, based on the history alone, a diagnosis could be deduced in 20% of the infants.[34] Another 41% of the time, the physical examination provided the diagnoses and in 13% more, the clues to the diagnosis. Twenty-four percent of infants with conditions that were considered serious had unrevealing histories and physical examinations; however, all of them continued to cry excessively after the time of the initial assessment. For the harried practitioner, a thorough history and physical examination supplemented by an appropriate period of observation will go a long way in discerning the possible explanations for crying.

Differential Diagnosis of Pathological Crying

Once crying has been determined to be excessive either in quality or quantity, the etiology remains to be elucidated. The differential diagnosis for pathological causes of infant crying is considerable and can be overwhelming. The workup should be guided by the history and clinical presentation. This includes not only the history of present illness and physical examination but also a thorough review of systems, birth history, developmental history, past medical history, recent and current medications and immunizations. A complete head to toe physical examination should be performed with the child fully disrobed. Maintaining a broad differential that includes such problems as colic, trauma, abuse, starvation, respiratory system disease, cardiac pathologies, surgical disease and many other etiologies is essential to being thorough.

Although the differential is extensive (Table 8.1), using a mnemonic such as IT CRIES MA (Table 8.2) to help recall some of the more common and potentially serious sources for excessive crying might help the provider organize his or her thoughts and formulate a plan to arrive at a logical and accurate diagnosis.[35] Once normal crying or colic has been addressed and there is need to look for other explanations, a working knowledge of those possibilities is essential. To help readers organize their thoughts, we have enumerated many of the organic sources of crying by following the just mentioned mnemonic.

INFECTION

The immature immune systems of young infants render them more susceptible to communicable diseases. A history of fever, hypothermia, rash, concurrent illnesses such as an upper respiratory infection, and any contact with sick persons should be solicited from the guardians. In some cases, the examination will reveal the cause for irritability. A complete examination of the skin can reveal infectious lesions including cellulitis, abscesses and common dermatitides with or without bacterial superinfection (Figure 8.1). Otoscopy should be performed on every infant who presents with crying. Among the infants in Poole's study with unexplained excessive crying, otitis media was the most common diagnosis.[34] Using a tongue blade to

Table 8.1. Differential diagnosis for excessive crying in infants

Corneal abrasion	Urinary retention
Ocular/nasal/ear foreign body	Urinary tract infection
Glaucoma	Hair/synthetic fiber tourniquet
Otitis media	Fracture
Oral thrush/stomatitis/pharyngitis	Osteomyelitis
Palatal burns	Arthritis
Panniculitis	Rickets
Congestive heart failure	Vasoocclusive crisis (sickle-cell anemia)
Supraventricular tachycardia	Dactylitis
Endocarditis/myocarditis	Neonatal drug withdrawal
Myocardial infarction	Increased intracranial pressure
Upper respiratory infection	Hydrocephalus
Foreign body aspiration	Mass
Pneumothorax	Intracranial hemorrhage
Pneumonia	Cerebral edema
Constipation	Meningitis/encephalitis
Anal fissure	Burns
Hemorrhoids	Cellulitis
Bowel obstruction	Insect bites/urticaria
Intussusception	Atopic dermatitis
Malrotation/midgut volvulus	Mastocytosis
Hirschsprung's disease	Inborn errors of metabolism
Milk protein allergy	Hypoglycemia
Gastroesophageal reflux disease/esophagitis	Electrolyte abnormalities
Celiac disease	Hyperthyroidism
Appendicitis	Pheochromocytoma
Peritonitis	Carbon monoxide poisoning
Testicular torsion	Hunger
Incarcerated inguinal hernia	Infantile colic
Genital tourniquets	Immunizations
Balanitis/posthitis/balanoposthitis	Abuse
Hydrocele	

Herman MI, Le A. The crying infant. *Emerg Med Clin North Am.* 2007 Nov;25(4):1137–59, vii.

examine the oropharynx may reveal thrush, pharyngitis or vesicular lesions indicative of stomatitis. Palpate the neck for masses or tenderness that may indicate lymphadenitis or abscess. Auscultation of the lungs yielding abnormal sounds could suggest pneumonia and should prompt a chest radiograph. Early signs of inadequate oxygenation or ventilation from pneumonia or other pulmonary disease processes such as pneumothorax or indwelling foreign bodies resulting in air hunger include nonspecific symptoms such as irritability.

All bones and joints should be examined for warmth, swelling, tenderness or irritability that may be indicative of osteomyelitis or arthritis. These can present early in infants and especially neonates with nonspecific signs and symptoms such as irritability, decreased use of the affected limb, including pseudoparalysis, and fever. Children with septic arthritis may, in addition, maintain the affected

Table 8.2. IT CRIES MA mnemonic for infant crying

I	Infections (herpes stomatitis, urinary tract infection, meningitis, osteomyelitis, etc)
T	Trauma (accidental and nonaccidental), Toxins
C	Colic, Cardiac (congestive heart failure, supraventricular tachycardia, myocardial infarction)
R	Reflux, Reactions to medications, Reactions to formulas
I	Immunizations, Insect bites
E	Eye (corneal abrasions, ocular foreign bodies, glaucoma)
S	Surgical (volvulus, intussusception, inguinal hernia, testicular torsion)
(S)	Strangulation (hair/ fiber tourniquet)
M	Metabolic
A	Abuse

Modified from Herman MI, Nelson RA. Crying infants: what to do when babies wail. *Critical Decisions in Emergency Medicine.* 2006;20(5):2–10.

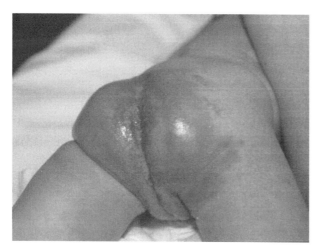

Figure 8.1. Diaper dermatitis.

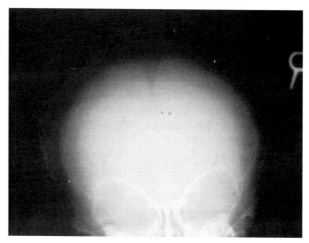

Figure 8.2. Skull fracture.

joint in the position that best maximizes intracapsular volume and comfort. Affected hips may be held naturally flexed, abducted and externally rotated, and affected knees may be moderately flexed.[36] In infants with sickle cell disease, dactylitis resulting from microinfarcts in the phalanges and metatarsal bones must be differentiated from osteomyelitis.

Although the physical examination may point at a number of etiologies for crying as noted previously, some may be more occult. A screening urinalysis for urinary tract infection in infants with a normal examination and continued unexplained crying can be helpful in some cases. Other life-threatening infections, including meningitis and encephalitis, are always considerations in the irritable infant. Young infants are known to present during the early course of systemic infections with nonspecific signs such as crying, irritability or fussiness without fever. This is not to say that all infants who present with unexplained excessive crying should undergo a spinal tap but rather that they should undergo an appropriate period of observation with prudent ancillary testing as becomes necessary. The infants in Poole's study were extremely unlikely to have a serious illness given a normal physical examination and a cessation of crying beyond the initial assessment.

TRAUMA/TOXINS

A history of trauma may direct the workup. However, even when the history does exist, it is often lacking in infants who are ambulatory, who interact with other young children, and who are under the care of multiple caretakers, some of whom may not be present at the time of

evaluation. Therefore, the index of suspicion should be high. Again, a head to toe examination is highly important.

When the head and scalp are palpated carefully, any existing soft tissue swelling, tenderness or skull depression can be discovered. Radiological testing should strongly be considered in this case, especially when there is lack of history or when it is inconsistent (Figure 8.2). Radiological testing is doubly important when a bulging fontanelle is found because this can signify increased intracranial pressure secondary to lesions such as hemorrhage and space-occupying masses, in addition to intracranial infections. Focal findings on the neurological examination may also suggest increased intracranial pressure.

Many times, unfortunately, the presentation is not so apparent. Infants with acute intracranial pathology can initially present with fussiness, irritability, decreased activity or feeding or lethargy. Those with chronic subdural hematomas, hydrocephalus, intracranial mass or Chiari malformation type I can, in addition, present with poor weight gain, failure to thrive or developmental delay.[37]

The skin should be examined thoroughly for abrasions and bruises. Palpate the abdomen and flank for tenderness. In addition, the chest, spine, all bony prominences and extremities should be examined for swelling and palpated for tenderness. Any abnormalities uncovered can direct the workup.

Toxic environmental exposures and ingestions are always a consideration, the latter particularly true in ambulatory infants. Carbon monoxide poisoning is the most frequent cause of asphyxiant poisoning in the United

States and should be considered especially in the winter months in households with indoor heaters or gas stoves. Although adults and older children in the acute stages complain of headache, dizziness, blurred vision, confusion, nausea/vomiting, chest pain, weakness, tachycardia and/or dyspnea, young infants can present merely with irritability or lethargy and vomiting.[38] More severe poisonings can cause apnea, seizures, cardiac dysrhythmias or even cardiopulmonary arrest. Although cherry-red lips, cyanosis and retinal hemorrhages are classic findings and helpful when present, they are, in actuality, seen only rarely. Also, pulse oximetry readings are often falsely elevated. In the end, the measurement of carboxyhemoglobin in the blood is required for diagnosis. The mainstay of treatment is supplemental oxygen along with supportive care.[39]

It is important to keep in mind that maternal medications can be significant in breastfeeding infants who may be exposed to medications that are excreted in the breast milk. Maternal medication information usually is not volunteered and must be specifically elicited. Similarly important for the very young infant, birth history should include a history of any maternal drug use. Neonates with in utero exposure may be in drug withdrawal and are often irritable, jittery and difficult to console.

CARDIAC/COLIC

Any infant with a history of preexisting congenital heart disease deserves increased consideration. Many of these infants are at increased risk for infective endocarditis in which case they can present with nonspecific symptoms such as fever, malaise, crying and irritability. Examination may reveal a new or changing murmur, splenomegaly or petechiae. Congestive heart failure can present at any time, both in infants with diagnosed and those with undiagnosed heart disease. Although cyanosis and/or shock are classic and do occur in more severe cases, many will have less obvious complaints and signs including fussiness, agitation and feeding difficulty. Myocardiac infarctions are extremely rare in the pediatric population, but they can occur in those with an anomalous left coronary artery. Supraventricular tachycardias should be considered in infants with persistently high heart rates, particularly if unvarying and incompatible with activity and state of hydration.[40]

Colic is added here just to remind the provider that it is a common cause of crying, especially if the crying has stopped or had been going on for 3 or more hours a day for 3 or more days for 3 or more weeks.

REFLUX, REACTION TO MEDICATION, AND REACTION TO FORMULA

It is important to obtain a detailed history of feeding, including type of feeding, changes in feeding, vomiting and stooling patterns and history of growth. Although controversial, gastroesophageal reflux and formula intolerance have been linked to excessive crying in at least a subgroup of infants. A history or physical examination consistent with these diagnoses includes feeding difficulties, excessive emesis, diarrhea, constipation or mucousy or bloody stools. In addition, the index of suspicion is increased when excessive crying occurs beyond 3 months of age or when there is worsening of crying at this point, although it must be noted that in some cases excessive crying has been shown to persist into the fifth month of life in otherwise healthy infants.[41]

The clinician will also want to enquire about current and recent medications. Reactions to medications can present with a variety of possible signs and symptoms. One may need to specify that this includes both prescribed as well as over-the-counter medications. Because over-the-counter medications often are viewed as irrelevant to the presentation, the infants' caretakers may not volunteer the information without prompting.

IMMUNIZATIONS AND INSECT BITES

A history of immunizations should be included when any infant presents with crying. This is important not only in determining the child's susceptibility to certain diseases but also in ascertaining possible reactions to recent immunizations. Symptoms of immunization reactions can range from major anaphylactic reactions to milder systemic symptoms including low grade fever or irritability and local irritation at the site of injection. Persistent crying associated with painful local reactions has been reported following administration of the diphtheria-tetanus-pertussis vaccine.[42]

A skin examination is again vital to the assessment of the crying infant. Infectious lesions or rashes can be diagnosed easily when one is thorough. Particularly during

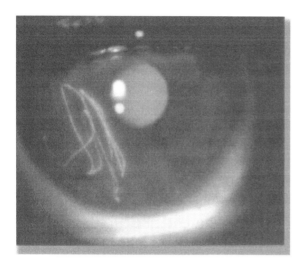
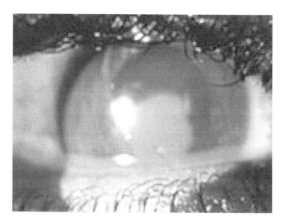

Figure 8.3. Corneal abrasions seen with fluorescein stain. (Courtesy of Edward Chaum, MD, PhD, Plough Foundation Professor of Ophthalmology, University of Tennessee, Hamilton Eye Institute, Memphis, TN.)

the warmer months with more outdoor activities, the skin examination may reveal papular urticaria from insect bites or spider bites. When lesions are present in the interdigital web spaces, infestation with *Sarcoptes scabiei*, or scabies, is a real possibility.

EYES

Examination of the eyes can provide a wealth of information. Retraction and or eversion of the lids can reveal foreign bodies. The presence of discharge or tearing could be a sign of lacrimal duct obstruction, infection, allergy or glaucoma.[43] Any suspicion for the latter should prompt urgent referral to a pediatric ophthalmologist. In the earlier stages, it characteristically presents with the triad of epiphora, blepharospasm and photophobia. Although corneal enlargement is the hallmark of pediatric glaucoma, any edema present may be subtle especially when both eyes are involved. The diagnosis is supported when there is an intraocular pressure greater than 20 mm Hg in a comfortably resting infant or an asymmetry of more than 5 mm Hg between eyes.[44]

Direct ophthalmoscopy can be performed to examine the red reflex, which should be symmetrical and bright reddish-yellow or light gray in brown-eyed individuals. A blunted or asymmetric reflex raises concerns about possible intraocular tumors, vitreous opacities, or retinal detachment.[43] Fluorescein stain of the cornea performed in an infant with unexplained crying may demonstrate corneal abrasions even in the absence of trauma history

and corneal redness or edema[34] (Figure 8.3). Retinal hemorrhages also may be seen (Figure 8.4).

SURGICAL

A number of potentially serious surgical problems can have occult presentations. Infants with GI pathology such as intussusception, midgut volvulus and Hirschsprung disease causing bowel obstruction often present early on with vague symptoms such as crying, irritability or vomiting. When the vomiting is bilious, it could indicate an obstructive process distal to the ampulla of vater, whereas nonbilious vomiting conversely suggests that there is a problem proximal to the ampulla. The incidence of

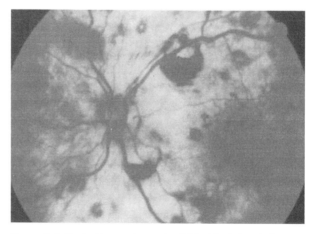

Figure 8.4. Retinal hemorrhages in child with shaken baby syndrome. (Courtesy of Edward Chaum, MD, PhD, Plough Foundation Professor of Ophthalmology, University of Tennessee, Hamilton Eye Institute, Memphis, TN.)

intussusception peaks between 3 and 9 months of age and appears to be concentrated during the warmer months. It may occur in conjunction with common childhood viral illnesses.[45] One retrospective chart review of 90 patients diagnosed with intussusception found that vomiting alone or in combination with other signs or symptoms was the most common clinical manifestation, and screaming attacks ranked a close second. The triad of vomiting, screaming attacks and lethargy was found in 38% of patients later diagnosed with intussusception. Only 30% of patients had bloody stools.[46]

Infants with intestinal malrotation during fetal development are at risk of developing midgut volvulus. Although they can present at any point in their lifetimes, most become symptomatic during the first year of life, particularly during the first month. A high index of suspicion is required for early diagnosis and management. Early signs can range from acute onset of abdominal pain and fussiness to bilious emesis. Later signs can include abdominal distension and tenderness, hematemesis and passage of blood from the rectum. Those with chronic intermittent midgut volvulus can have recurrent bouts of abdominal pain and malabsorption, constipation alternating with diarrhea, and intolerance to solid food. When suspicion is high in the stable patient, an upper GI series is required for diagnosis.[45]

Hirschsprung's disease is most commonly diagnosed in the newborn period. Classically, an afflicted infant does not pass any stool during the first 24 hours of life. When presenting at a later age, children can have a history of severe chronic constipation and irritability. The abdominal examination may illicit some degree of discomfort and reveal hard palpable stool. In addition, an empty rectal vault may be found on examination.[45]

Testicular torsion and incarcerated inguinal hernias are surgical emergencies that highlight the importance of a complete physical examination with the child uncovered. Testicular torsion occurs most commonly during the perinatal and peripubertal periods. In addition to acute scrotal pain, tenderness and swelling, patients can experience nausea and vomiting. Because there are a number of potential causes for scrotal swelling including trauma, orchitis, epididymitis and hydroceles, a Doppler ultrasound is required to differentiate testicular torsion from these causes. An incarcerated inguinal hernia presents as scrotal swelling that can extend to the inguinal area and is not invariably tender.[47]

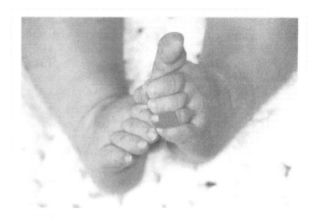

Figure 8.5. Digital hair tourniquet.

STRANGULATION

Small tourniquets may occur in young infants leading to strangulation injury if not relieved in a timely manner. All digits in the irritable crying infant should be examined closely for swelling. If swelling is present, digital tourniquets, which are not always readily apparent, should be carefully sought (Figure 8.5). Similarly, genital tourniquets can lead to ischemic injury to the organ if not promptly relieved.

METABOLIC

Metabolic disorders can be challenging to diagnose. Infants may often present with irritability or lethargy and vomiting and, in the more advanced stages, with a sepsis-like picture. The child with an inborn error of metabolism can come to medical attention either during the newborn period or later in life. Older infants and toddlers typically present during periods of stress such as when they have common viral illnesses. They may have histories of poor weight gain, developmental delay, or recurrent severe illnesses. Many of these metabolic disorders have common enzymatic or protein defects, which allow accumulation of toxic intermediates resulting in neurological dysfunction. These toxic intermediates are often acids, thus patients can have metabolic acidosis and tachypnea.[48]

Hypoglycemia is one of the more common metabolic abnormalities that is particularly relevant in the neonatal period. It can present in infants with any combination of symptoms including jitteriness, irritability, abnormal cry, poor feeding, respiratory distress, apnea, cyanosis, temperature instability, myoclonic jerks and seizures. Premature or small-for-gestational-age infants, because of poor glucose and fat stores as well as immature glucoregulatory mechanisms, are more prone to developing hypoglycemia than term or larger infants. This is usually a transient process that resolves over a matter of days. Transient hyperinsulinemia causing hypoglycemia can occur in infants born to diabetic mothers. This also resolves over a period of 3 to 5 days in most cases.[49]

Although hypoglycemia in infants can be simply the result of inadequate nutritional intake, other etiologies should be considered, especially with a history inconsistent with that process. When it occurs beyond the newborn period, hypoglycemia could be indicative of pituitary or adrenal dysfunction; inborn errors of glucose synthesis, storage or breakdown; errors in fatty acid oxidation or congenital hyperinsulinemia.[48] It can also be one of the many manifestations of serious systemic illness including infection when metabolic demand is increased.[50]

ABUSE

This subject of abuse deserves special consideration. It is perhaps during the period of infancy that children are most vulnerable as they have neither the benefit of language to communicate nor the motor skills to attempt escape. The average person may find it difficult to comprehend such occurrences, which could put it out of mind. However, those who care for children should always be alert to the risk. Although one should rely upon common sense and personal judgment, as a child advocate, it is important not to dismiss the possibility of abuse even in those who appear to originate from the best of families.

When infants present with the sole complaint of excessive crying, occult injury must be contemplated. It is essential to obtain a clear and detailed history of trauma that includes the time of injury occurrence as well as the mechanism of injury. Consider the developmental capabilities of the infant when determining the plausibility of the mechanism. The suspicion of abuse should be heightened with any injury that does not appear to fit with the stated mechanism.

Any child with bruises on the body should be evaluated thoroughly for occult injuries and for the possibility of abuse. Bruises are extremely rare occurrences in preambulatory infants younger than 6 months of age and are

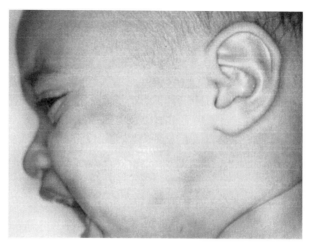

Figure 8.6. Facial and ear bruises.

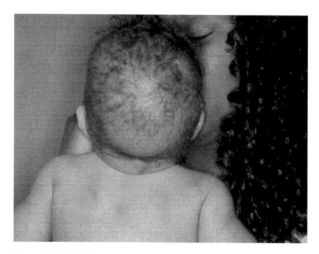

Figure 8.7. Back bruises.

still uncommon in those younger than 9 months of age. The distribution of bruises can alert the clinician to at-risk infants.

Accidental bruises characteristically occur over bony prominences at the front of the body in a newly ambulatory infant, whereas those that occur over the ears, on the face, genitourinary area, soft tissue of the upper back and buttocks regions are rarely the results of accidental injury, especially if the baby has not acquired the skills to pull to a stand or cruise around while holding onto the furniture[51] (Figures 8.6 and 8.7). Inflicted bruises can reflect the shape of the object used to inflict injury such as the linear marks left when the child has been struck with a belt or an open hand or the elliptical pattern of bite marks. Burn injuries can be approached in a likewise manner. When present over the bilateral lower extremities, buttocks, or perineal regions, the chances are much higher that they were purposefully inflicted. Similarly, when a pattern can be delineated such as that from hot objects like a cigarette or hand iron or immersion of a body area into hot liquid, the burns should be considered highly suspicious for abuse.[52]

The head and scalp should be examined carefully for swelling and tenderness as previously stated. Direct ophthalmoscopy may be performed to look for retinal hemorrhages, which can be seen with shaken baby syndrome (Figure 8.4). However, a complete external examination, although important, is not conclusive. Indeed, infants with inflicted traumatic brain injuries commonly present without any external signs of trauma and a wide spectrum of signs and symptoms. The neurological examination is often normal. Rubin et al. found that 19 of 51 (37%) of children under the age of 2 years with one or more criteria considered high risk (rib fractures, multiple fractures, facial fractures, age younger than 6 months) had occult head injuries diagnosed on computed tomography, although they had normal scalp and neurological examinations.[53]

Fractures are second only to bruises as the most common presentation of abuse, and in some series, up to 80% of fractures in infants younger than 1 year of age have been attributed to abuse. Classic metaphyseal lesions, posterior rib fractures, scapula fractures, spinous process fractures, and sternal fractures have high specificities for abuse.[54] The presenting complaint is often vague in such cases and may include fussiness, irritability, an acutely swollen extremity of unknown origin, or sudden refusal to move or use a limb. In children younger than 3 years of age, the likelihood of abuse is increased if a history of trauma is lacking, if the extent of injury is greater than expected with the given mechanism, if there is an extremity fracture (in an infant <1 year of age) or if there is fracture at the midshaft or metaphyseal humerus.[55]

LABORATORY AND RADIOLOGY EXAMINATIONS

When pursuing an etiology for crying, it is useful to obtain a urinalysis. In Poole's study, of all ancillary testing the urinalysis had one of the highest yields.[34] Other useful adjuncts include plain radiographs of long bones, skull, ribs and abdomen as dictated by the history, examination or index of suspicion. Computed tomographs of various body areas might also be helpful, if indicated. Sometimes a pulse oximetry reading or rhythm strip may be

illustrative. Complete blood cell counts may reveal undiagnosed sickle cell anemia, infections or even myelosuppresive processes. In some infants, the cause of the crying will not be determined until a needle is placed in the subarachnoid space of the back. Obviously, one should pursue the differential starting with the least risky and least expensive testing. However, no reasonable test should be avoided if the baby's condition warrants a comprehensive evaluation.

MANAGEMENT

Colic Treatments

Various pharmacologic remedies have been examined with respect to their efficacy in reducing crying in colic. Defoaming agents like simethicone have been used in the treatment of infantile colic for years, although their effectiveness has not been fully validated. In theory, simethicone prevents the formation and accumulation of gas bubbles, thereby accelerating the passage of gas from the GI tract. When empirically examined, the actual efficacy has been variable. Results have ranged from no benefit over placebo to possible improvement.[56,57] Effective or not, simethicone is so safe that the common practice of prescribing this agent to ameliorate the symptoms of colic is free of adverse effects.[58]

Anticholinergic medications such as dicyclomine and dicycloverine can relieve crying in colic by inhibiting GI smooth muscle spasm. Effectiveness has been reported by several investigators in randomized controlled trials.[59] Unfortunately adverse effects including drowsiness, constipation, diarrhea, shortness of breath, apnea, syncope, seizures, hypotonia and coma, which occurred in infants younger than 7 weeks of age, preclude their use in infants younger than 6 months of age.[60] Sucrose, which may be given via a pacifier dipped in concentrated sugar water (sucrose 12%–48%), has been studied in the treatment of infantile colic. In a double-blind double-crossover study, 12% sucrose given to 19 infants resulted in a positive response in 12 patients, although this effect only lasted 30 minutes to 1 hour.[61] In an even less compelling randomized controlled trial, 48% sucrose resulted in a brief (<3 minute) improvement.[62]

Several research efforts have tried modifying the type of formula by introducing lactase into the milk of infants with colic, substituting soy for cow's milk protein, or using a protein hydrolysate. A review that included four randomized controlled trials determined that the evidence for the use of lactase was such that one cannot draw firm conclusions.[58]

The efficacy of using soy-based as opposed to cow's milk–based formulas is also suspect. Even though there are studies that demonstrate some efficacy, most, unfortunately, have methodologic flaws such that one cannot find substantive evidence for the use of soy products to ameliorate colic.[57–59] Hypoallergenic formulas including casein hydrolysate and whey hydrolysate formulas are potentially promising treatments for colic.[57–59] In a comparison of casein hydrolysate formula to cow's milk formula, the infants randomized to the former group did significantly better in terms of reduction of distress. However, there were only 38 bottle-fed infants in the study, and the results were pooled with those of breastfed infants.[63] Forsythe et al. evaluated the effects of alternating casein hydrolysate and cow's milk formula on colic symptoms in a double-blind crossover randomized study with 17 infants.[64] Symptoms were significantly reduced when the infants were on the casein hydrolysate formula, but the beneficial effects diminished over time and half of the infants dropped out before completing the study. When a whey hydrolysate formula is compared with a cow's milk formula, infants cry an average of 63 minutes less compared with those receiving cow's milk formula.[65] Although the results were promising, this study has been criticized as the blinding may have been inadequate.

Other remedies for colic have included the recommendation that mothers who are breastfeeding alter their diets. The efficacy of using a low allergen diet in mothers of breastfeeding infants to reduce symptoms of colic has been evaluated and the findings were once again a disappointment. In a study of 77 breastfed and 38 bottle-fed infants, mothers of the breastfed infants were randomized to either a low allergen diet free of milk, egg, wheat and nut, or to a control diet free of artificial color, preservatives and additives.[63] Bottle-fed infants received either a hypoallergenic casein hydrolysate formula or a control cow's milk formula. Sixty-one percent of infants randomized to the low allergen or hypoallergenic feeds experienced a significant reduction in distress versus 43% of those on the control diets. However, the differences between the bottle-fed and breastfed groups were not significant. That altering the mother's diet may help if she has a history of atopy was demonstrated in small cross-over trial with 20 exclusively breastfed infants.[22] A maternal diet free of dairy products, soy, wheat, eggs, peanuts, tree nuts and fish did help 47 out of 90 colicky infants as opposed to the remaining 43 babies whose mothers were randomized to the control diet.[66] Overall, although there is some conflicting evidence, the studies suggest that some therapeutic benefit may be derived in colicky breastfed infants when their mothers maintain a low allergen diet.

Alternative and complementary medicine techniques also have been used in the treatment of colic. Chamomile tea, vervain, licorice, fennel and balm-milk were compared to placebo, and after 7 days of treatment, 57% of "treated" infants were crying fewer than 3 hours/day, fewer than 3 days a week. Only 27% of the placebo group had extinguished their crying.[67] As a word of caution, the long-term effects were not studied, and there is the potential for caloric or nutrient deficits if the herbal products displace the amount of milk consumed. No adverse effects were reported in that study, but not all herbal remedies may be considered safe. Star anise, a spice used among the Caribbean and Latino populations to make tea for the treatment of colic, and Chinese star anise may cause neurological symptoms if taken in large enough quantities. Japanese star anise has been reported to cause vomiting, jitteriness, myoclonus or clonus, nystagmus and seizures.[68,69]

Behavioral interventions such as increased infant carrying, car rides, decreasing stimulation, and infant swaddling for colicky infants are occasionally advised. Two systematic reviews found that increased infant carrying did not reduce the symptoms.[57,59] When it comes to the use of a car ride simulator, it was no better than counseling and reassurance in easing infant crying or maternal anxiety.[70] Reducing the amount of stimulation the baby is subjected to was assessed in at least one randomized controlled trial, which did find support for this advice.[71] Adding swaddling does not provide any additional benefit except to those infants younger than 8 weeks of age but even that effect is modest with a crying time reduction of 12 minutes per 24 hours.[72]

SUMMARY

Distinguishing normal crying from crying that is a symptom of colic or organic causes is a challenge. Fortunately, the majority of babies will not have serious problems. However, even those families seeking help with a baby whose crying does not stem from a serious problem present an opportunity for providers to play an important role in their well being. Taking a thorough history, doing a careful examination, and spending the time with a distraught parent may be the very thing that saves the infant's life. It certainly can impact how the mother–child unit develops. Teaching caregivers about normal infant crying or colic can empower them and give them the confidence to soothe the baby who is crying.

When the crying is due to a pathologic process, the provider again can be a life-saver. Put aside the obvious danger of neglecting to suspect child abuse and consider the potential for harm if a gut volvulus is mistaken for colic. Even a simple problem like a corneal abrasion can lead to permanent vision problems if missed. All one need do is maintain a healthy amount of intellectual curiosity regarding the possible cause of the crying. In addition, one will do well to understand that the baby is in distress and that the mother or other caregiver may be reaching the end of the ability to cope.

PITFALLS

- Failure to perform a thorough examination and assuming that every crying infant has colic
- Failure to look for causes of crying, such as corneal abrasions, ear infections, scalp hematomas, bruises, tourniquets, rectal fissures and hemorrhoids. The mnemonic IT CRIES MA can help with the differential diagnoses.
- Failure to fluorescein stain the cornea or look for an ocular foreign body under the lid.
- Failure to take a social history. Remember to survey for drug and alcohol use among the caregivers.
- Failure to assess the child's social situation and provide support for the caregiver. Blaming the crying on the parenting skills of the caregivers can further damage the bonds between the baby and its caregivers.
- Failure to fully document patient history and examination.

REFERENCES

1. Illingworth RS. Three months' colic. *Arch Dis Child.* 1984;29(145):165–174.
2. St. James-Roberts I, Conroy S, Wilsher K. Bases for maternal perceptions of infant crying and colic behavior. *Arch Dis Child.* 1996;75(5):375–384.
3. Wake M, Morton-Allen E, Poulakis Z, et al. Prevalence, stability, and outcomes of cry-fuss and sleep problems in the first 2 years of life: prospective community-based study. *Pediatrics.* 2006;117(3):836–842.
4. Reijneveld SA, Brugman E, Hirasing RA. Excessive infant crying: the impact of varying definitions. *Pediatrics.* 2001;108(4):893–897.
5. Van Der Wal MF, van den Boom DC, Pauw-Plomp H, et al. Mothers' report of infant crying and soothing in a multicultural population. *Arch Dis Child.* 1998;79(4):312–317.
6. Morris S, St. James-Roberts I, Sleep J, et al. Economic strategies for managing crying and sleeping problems. *Arch Dis Child.* 2001;84(1):15–19.
7. Raiha H, Lehtenon L, Huhtala V, et al. Excessively crying infant in the family: mother–infant, father–infant, and mother–father interaction. *Child Care Health Dev.* 2002;28(5):419–429.
8. Papousek M, von Hofacker N. Persistent crying in early infancy: a non-trivial condition of risk for the developing mother–infant relationship. *Child Care Health Dev.* 1998;24(5):395–424.
9. Akman I, Kuscu K, Ozdemir N, et al. Mother's post-partum psychological adjustment and infantile colic. *Arch Dis Child.* 2006;91(5):417–419.
10. Miller AR, Barr RG, Eaton WO. Crying and motor behavior of six-week-old infants and post-partum maternal mood. *Pediatrics.* 1993;92(4):551–558.
11. Beebe SA, Casey R, Pinto-Martin J. Association of reported infant crying and maternal parenting stress. *Clin Pediatr.* 1993;32(1):15–19.
12. Forsyth BW, McCarthy PL, Leventhal JM. Problems of early infancy, formula changes, and mother's beliefs about their infants. *J Pediatr.* 1985;106(6):1012–1017.
13. Levitzky S, Cooper R. Infant colic syndrome – maternal fantasies of aggression and infanticide. *Clin Pediatr.* 2000;39(7):395–400.
14. Reijneveld SA, van der Wal MF, Brugman E, et al. Infant crying and abuse. *Lancet.* 2004;364(9442):1340–1342.
15. Brazelton TB. Crying in infancy. *Pediatrics.* 1962;29:579–588.
16. Barr RG. The normal crying curve: what do we really know? *Dev Med Child Neurol.* 1990;32(4):356–362.
17. St. James-Roberts I. Persistent infant crying. *Arch Dis Child,* 1991;66(5):653–655.
18. St. James-Roberts I, Plewis I. Individual differences, daily fluctuations, and developmental changes in amounts of infant waking, fussing, crying, feeding, and sleeping. *Child Dev.* 1996;67(5):2527–2540.
19. Wessel MA, Cobb JC, Jackson EB, et al. Paroxysmal fussing in infancy, sometimes called "colic." *Pediatrics.* 1954;14(5):421–434.
20. Zahorsky J. Mixed feeding of infants. *Pediatrics.* 1901;11:208–215.
21. Jakobsson D, Lindberg T. Cow's milk as a cause of infantile colic in breast-fed infants. *Lancet.* 1978;2(8087):437–439.
22. Evans RW, Fergusson DM, Allardyce RA, et al. Maternal diet and infantile colic in breast-fed infants. *Lancet.* 1981;1(8234):1340–1342.
23. Jakobsson I, Lindberg T. Cow's milk proteins cause infantile colic in breast-fed infants: a double-blind crossover study. *Pediatrics.* 1983;71(2):268–271.
24. Lothe L, Lindberg T. Cow's milk whey protein elicits symptoms of infantile colic in colicky formula-fed infants: a

double-blind crossover study. *Pediatrics*. 1989;83(2):262–266.

25. Iacono G, Carrocio A, Montalto G, et al. Severe infantile colie and food intolerance: a long-term prospective study. *J Ped Gas Nutr*. 1991;12(3):332–335.

26. Lothe L, Lindberg T, Jakobsson I. Cow's milk formula as a cause of infantile colic: a double blind study. *Pediatrics*. 1982;70(1):7–10.

27. Moore DJ, Robb TA, Davidson GP. Breath hydrogen response to milk containing lactose in colicky and noncolicky infants. *J Pediatr*. 1988;113(6): 979–984.

28. Liebman WM. Infantile colic: association with lactose and milk intolerance. *JAMA*. 1981;245(7):732–733.

29. Armstrong KL, Previtera N, McCallum RN. Medicalizing normality? Management of irritability in babies. *J Paediatr Child Health* 2000;36(4):301–305.

30. Sutphen J. Is it colic or is it gastroesophageal reflux? *J Pediatr Gastroenterol Nutr*. 2001;33(2):110–111.

31. Treen WR. Infant colic: a pediatric gastroenterologist's perspective. *Pediatr Clin North Am*. 1994;41(5):1121–1138.

32. St. James-Roberts I, Conroy S, Wilsher K. Links between maternal care and persistent infant crying in the early months. *Child Care Health Dev*. 1998;24(5):353–376.

33. Gormally SM, Barr RG. Of clinical pies and clinical clues: proposal for a clinical approach to complaints of early crying and colic. *Ambulatory Child Health*. 1997;3:137–153.

34. Poole SR. The infant with acute, unexplained, excessive crying. *Pediatrics*. 1991;88(3):450–455.

35. Herman MI, Nelson RA. Crying infants: what to do when babies wail. *Critical Decisions in Emergency Medicine*. 2006;20(5):2–10.

36. Frank G, Mahoney HM, Eppes SC. Musculoskeletal infections in children. *Pediatr Clin North Am*. 2005;52(4):1083–1106.

37. Piatt JH. Recognizing neurosurgical conditions in the pediatrician's office. *Pediatr Clin North Am*. 2004;51(2):237–270.

38. Ernst A, Zibrak JD. Carbon monoxide poisoning. *N Engl J Med*. 1998;339(22):1603–1608.

39. Kao LW, Nañagas KA. Toxicity associated with carbon monoxide. *Clin Lab Med*. 2006;26(1):99–125.

40. Woods WA, McCulloch MA. Cardiovascular emergencies in the pediatric patient. *Emerg Med Clin North Am*. 2005;23(4):1233–1249.

41. Treen WR. Infant colic: a pediatric gastroenterologist's perspective. *Pediatr Clin North Am*. 1994;41(5):1121–1138.

42. Blumberg DA, Lewis K, Mink CA. Severe reactions associated with diphtheria-tetanus-pertussis vaccine: detailed study of children with seizures, hypotonic-hyporesponsive episodes, high fevers, and persistent crying. *Pediatrics*. 1993;91(6):1158–1165.

43. Swanson J, Yasuda K, France L, et al. Committee on Practice and Ambulatory Medicine, Section on Ophthalmology. Eye examination in infants, children, and young adults by pediatricians. *Pediatrics*. 2003;111(4 Pt 1):902–907.

44. Brandt JD. Congenital glaucoma. In: Yanoff M, Duker JS, Augsburger JJ, eds. *Ophthalmology*, 2nd ed. St. Louis, MO: Mosby; 2004:1475–1480.

45. Halter JM, Baesl T, Nicolette L, et al. Common gastrointestinal problems and emergencies in children. *Clinics in Family Practice*. 2004;6(3):731–754.

46. Eshel G, Barr J, Heyman E, et al. Intussusception: a nine-year survey (1986–1995). *J Pediatr Gastroenterol Nutr*. 1997;24(3):253–256.

47. Haynes JH. Inguinal and scrotal disorders. *Surg Clin North Am*. 2006;86(2):371–381.

48. Claudius I, Fluharty C, Boles R. The emergency department approach to newborn and childhood metabolic crisis. *Emerg Med Clin North Am*. 2005;23(3):843–883.

49. Sperling MA, Menon RK. Differential diagnosis and management of neonatal hypoglycemia. *Pediatr Clin North Am*. 2004;51(3):703–723.

50. Losek JD. Hypoglycemia and the ABC's (sugar) of pediatric resuscitation. *Ann Emerg Med*. 2000;35(1):43–46.

51. Sugar NF, Taylor JA, Feldman KW. Bruises in infants and toddlers: those that cruise rarely bruise. *Arch Pediatr Adolesc Med*. 1999;153(4):399–403.

52. Daria S, Sugar NF, Feldman KF, et al. Into hot water head first: distribution of intentional and unintentional immersion burns. *Pediatr Emerg Care*. 2004;20(5):302–310.

53. Rubin D, Christian CW, Bilaniuk LT, et al. Occult head injury in high-risk abused children. *Pediatrics*. 2003;111(6 Pt 1):1382–1386.

54. Pierce MH, Bertocci G. Fractures resulting from inflicted trauma: assessing injury and history compatibility. *Clin Pediatr Emerg Med*. 2006;7:143–148.

55. Leventhal JM, Thomas SA, Rosenfield NS, et al. Fractures in young children. Distinguishing child abuse from unintentional injuries. *Am J Dis Child*. 1993;147(1):87–92.

56. Metcalf TJ, Irons TG, Sher LD, et al. Simethicone in the treatment of infant colic: a randomized, placebo-controlled, multicenter trial. *Pediatrics*. 1994;94(1):29–34.

57. Garrison MM, Christakis DA. A systemic review of treatments for infant colic. *Pediatrics*. 2000;106(1):184–190.

58. Wade S. Infantile colic. *Clin Evid*. 2006;15:439–447.

59. Lucassen PL, Assendelft WJ, Gubbels JW, et al. Effectiveness of treatments for infantile colic: systemic review. *BMJ*. 1998;316(7144):1563–1569.

60. Williams J, Watkins-Jones R. Dicyclomine: worrying symptoms associated with its use in some small babies. *BMJ*. 1984;288(6421):901.

61. Markestad T. Use of sucrose as treatment for infant colic. *Arch Dis Child*. 1997;76(4):356–358.

62. Barr RG, Young SN, Wright JH, et al. Differential calming responses to sucrose taste in crying infants with and without colic. *Pediatrics*. 1999;103(5):e68.

63. Hill DJ, Hudson IL, Sheffield LJ, et al. A low allergen diet is a significant intervention in infantile colic: results of a community-based study. *J Allergy Clin Immunol*. 1995;96(6):886–892.

64. Forsyth BW. Colic and the effect of changing formulas: a double-blind, multiple-crossover study. *J Pediatr*. 1989;115(4):521–526.

65. Lucassen PL, Assendelft WJ, Gubbels JW, et al. Infantile colic: crying time reduction with a whey hydrolysate: a double-blind, randomized, placebo-controlled trial. *Pediatrics*. 2000;106(6):1349–1354.

66. Hill DJ, Roy N, Heine RG, Hosking CS, et al. Effect of a low-allergen diet on colic among breastfed infants: a randomized, controlled trial. *Pediatrics.* 2005;116(5):700–715.

67. Weizman Z, Alkrinawi S, Goldfarb D, et al. Efficacy of herbal tea preparation in infantile colic. *J Pediatr.* 1993;122(4):650–652.

68. Ize-Ludlow D, Ragone S, Bruck IS, et al. Neurotoxicities in infants seen with the consumption star anise tea. *Pediatrics.* 2004;114(5):e653–656.

69. Ize-Ludlow D, Ragone S, Bruck IS, et al. Chemical composition of Chinese star anise (*Illicium verum*) and neurotoxicities in infants. *JAMA.* 2004;291(5):562–563.

70. Parkin PC, Schwartz CJ, Manuel BA. Randomized controlled trial of three interventions in the management of persistent crying of infancy. *Pediatrics.* 1993;92(2):197–201.

71. Mckenzie S. Troublesome crying in infants: effect of advice to reduce stimulation. *Arch Dis Child.* 1991;66(12):1416–1420.

72. Van Sleuwen BE, L'Hoir MP, Engelberts AC, et al. Comparison of behavior modification with and without swaddling as interventions for excessive crying. *J Pediatr.* 2006;149(4):512–517.

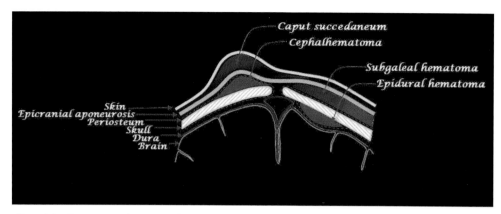

Plate 1.1. Caput succedaneum is the most common scalp injury due to birth trauma. Created by AMH Sheikh, Jan. 25, 2006. Used with permission.

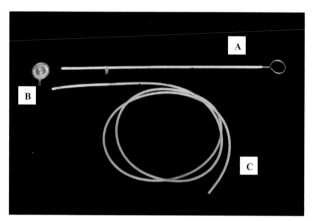

Plate 2.1. Components of a CSF shunt system. A, Ventricular catheter with stylet, B, Reservoir (palpable externally), C, Peritoneal catheter.

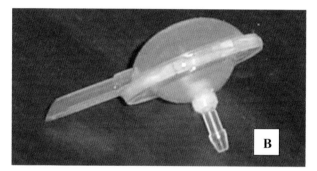

Plate 2.2. Close-up of reservoir.

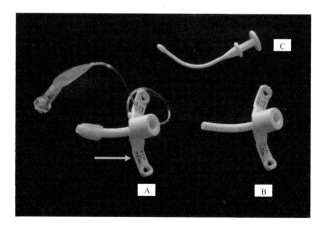

Plate 2.6. Tracheostomy tubes: cuffed (A), uncuffed (B) and obturator (C). *Arrow* indicates where the size is marked.

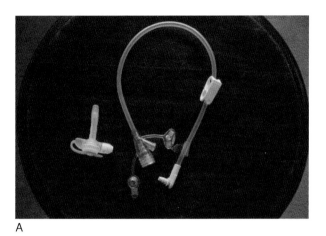
A

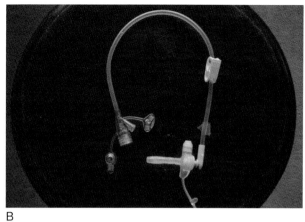
B

Plate 2.7. Mic-Key gastrostomy tube with attachment shown separately (A) and jointly (B).

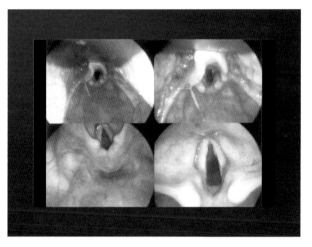

Plate 4.2. The progression of the pediatric airway: *top left*, infant; *top right*, toddler; *bottom left*, 8 year old; *bottom right*, teenager. (Courtesy of John Kanegaye, MD, Rady Children's Hospital, Emergency Care Center. San Diego, California.)

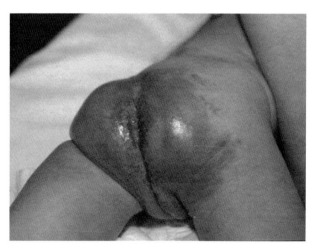

Plate 8.1. Diaper dermatitis.

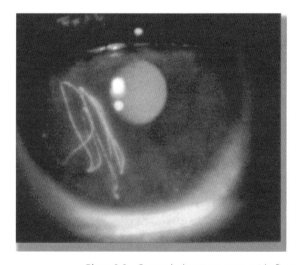

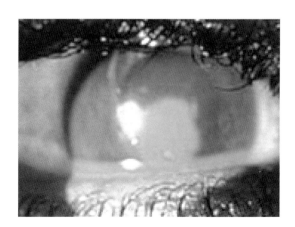

Plate 8.3. Corneal abrasions seen with fluorescein stain. (Courtesy of Edward Chaum, MD, PhD, Plough Foundation Professor of Ophthalmology, University of Tennessee, Hamilton Eye Institute, Memphis, TN.)

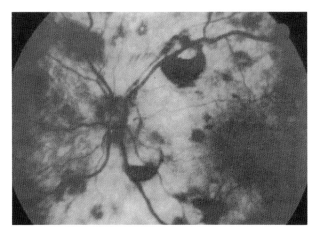

Plate 8.4. Retinal hemorrhages in child with shaken baby syndrome. (Courtesy of Edward Chaum, MD, PhD, Plough Foundation Professor of Ophthalmology, University of Tennessee, Hamilton Eye Institute, Memphis, TN.)

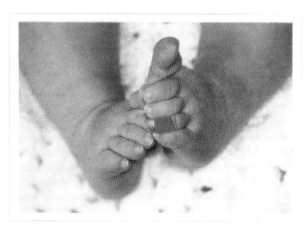

Plate 8.5. Digital hair tourniquet.

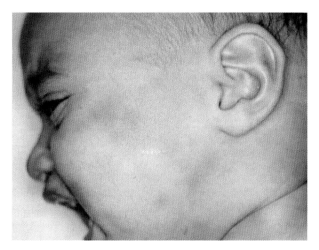

Plate 8.6. Facial and ear bruises.

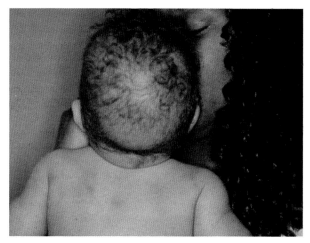

Plate 8.7. Back bruises.

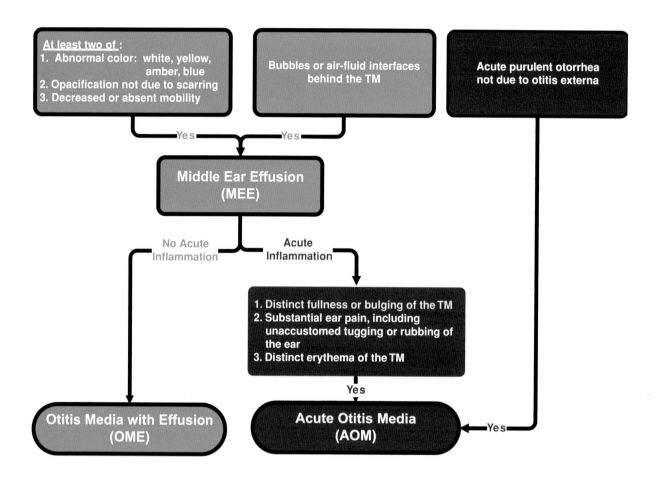

Plate 9.1. Approach to distinguishing between acute otitis media and otitis media with effusion. (Adapted from Hoberman A, Marchant CD, Kaplan SL, et al. Treatment of acute otitis media consensus recommendations. *Clin Pediatr.* 2002;41:373–390,[10] with permission.)

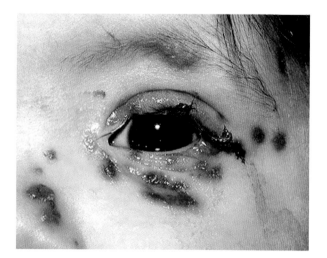

Plate 16.1. Herpes with corneal involvement requires consultation with an ophthalmologist.

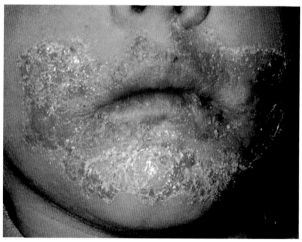

Plate 16.2. Example of the honey-colored crusty exudates of the bacterial infection Impetigo contagiosa.

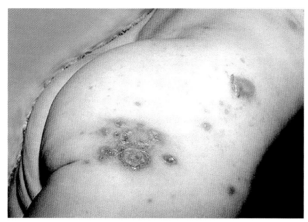

Plate 16.3. Bullous impetigo caused by certain strains of staph present as thin-walled pustules and bullae.

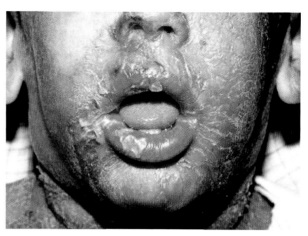

Plate 16.4. Staphylococcal scalded skin syndrome presents with a generalized painful red skin rash, fever and irritability.

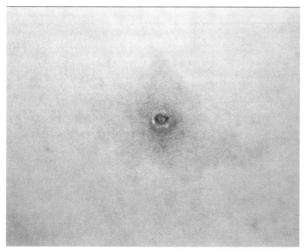

Plate 16.5. Classic lesion of Varicella. This image was published in Color Textbook of Pediatric Dermatology (4th ed.), Weston et al., 2007, copyright Elsevier.

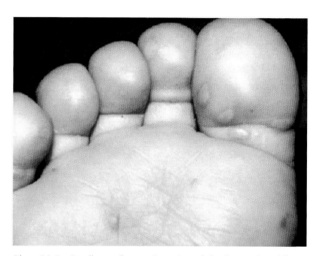

Plate 16.6. Small papules on the soles of the feet in hand-foot-mouth disease.

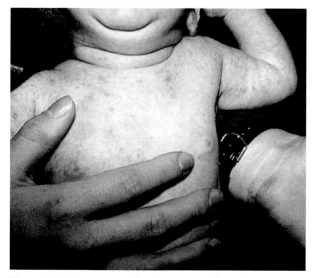

Plate 16.7. Presentation of scabies in an infant shows pustule-like lesions located on the trunk.

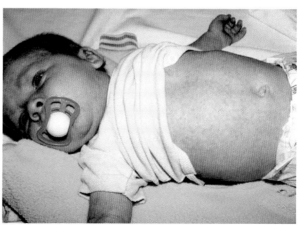

Plate 16.8. A rose-pink maculopapular exanthem appears in Roseola after 3 to 5 days of fever.

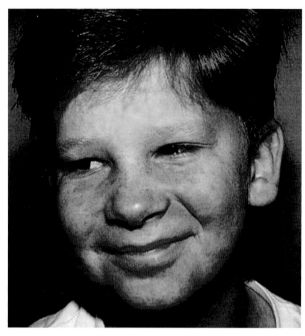

Plate 16.9. The blotchy erythematous rash, that is characteristic of measles.

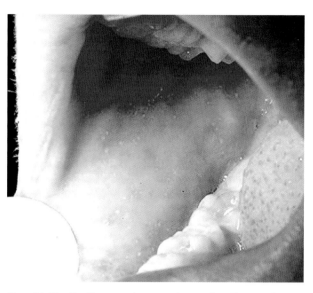

Plate 16.10. Koplik spots also occur in measles. The papules are evident in the mucous membranes of the mouth.

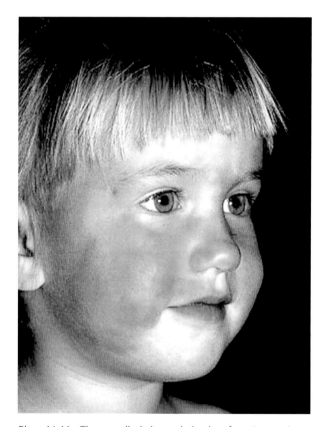

Plate 16.11. The so-called slapped cheeks of *Erythema infectiosum*, or *Fifth's disease.*

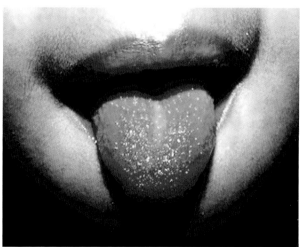

Plate 16.12. The strawberry tongue presentation of Kawasaki disease.

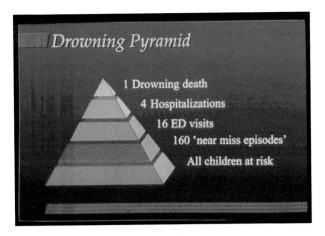

Plate 17.I.1. The Drowning Pyramid.

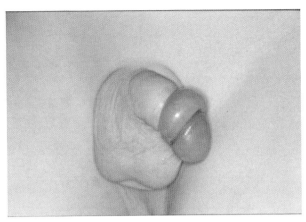

Plate 19.1. Paraphimosis with entrapment of the foreskin proximal to the glans.

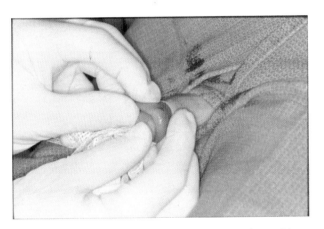

Plate 19.2. Reduction of a paraphimosis using index and long fingers to exert traction on the foreskin while the thumbs maneuver the glans under the constricting ring.

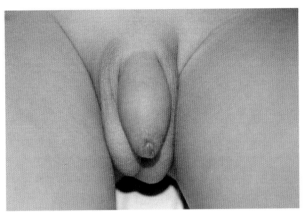

Plate 19.3. Balanoposthitis with erythema, edema and discharge.

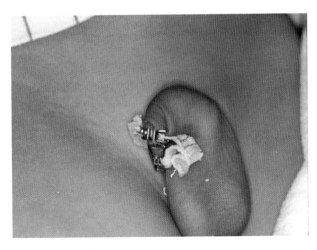

Plate 19.4. Penile zipper entrapment.

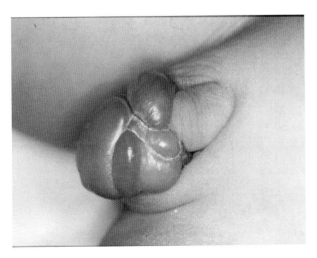

Plate 19.5. Extensive penile hair tourniquet.

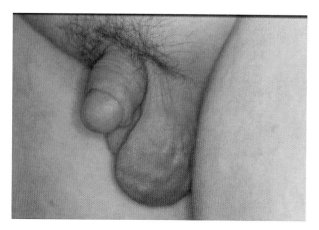

Plate 19.6. Varicocele.

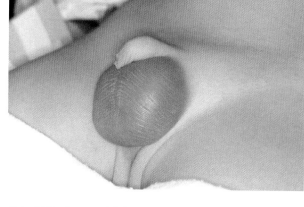

Plate 19.7. Acute painful scrotum.

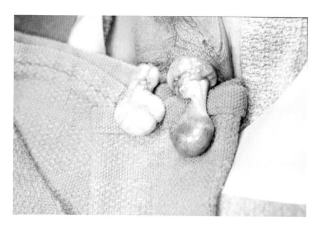

Plate 19.8. Scrotal exploration revealing ischemic left testis shortly following detorsion and normal right testis.

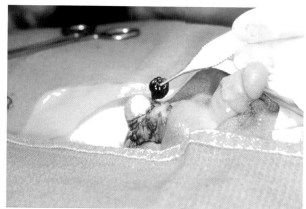

Plate 19.9. Scrotal exploration revealing torsion of testicular appendage.

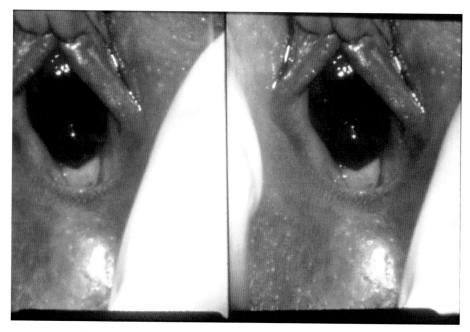

Plate 19.11. Urethral prolapse. (Courtesy of Marilyn Kaufhold, MD.)

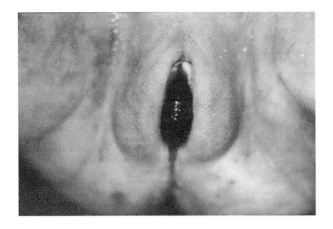

Plate 19.12. Interlabial mass, prolapsed ectopic ureterocele.

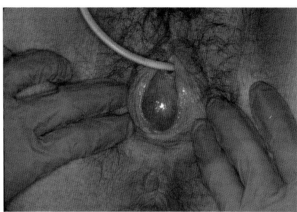

Plate 19.13. Preoperative view of bulging imperforate hymen.

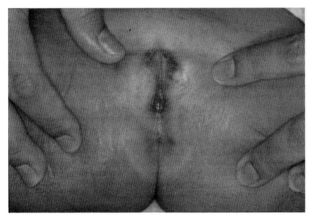

Plate 19.14. Lichen sclerosus with typical figure-eight configuration surrounding vulva and anus with hemorrhagic changes.

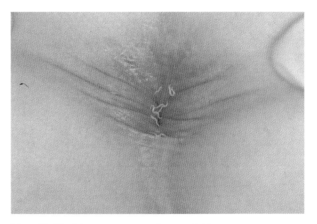

Plate 19.15. Pinworms exposed on anal skin.

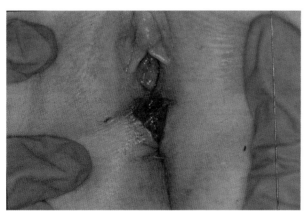

Plate 19.16. Extensive accidental straddle injury requiring repair of posterior fourchette and perineal body.

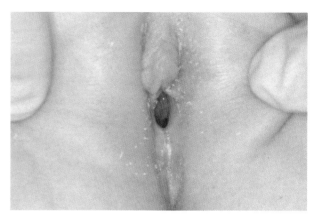

Plate 19.17. Partial labial adhesion (posterior) resulting in false-positive voided urine cultures.

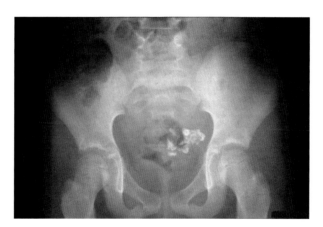

Plate 19.18. Calcified abdominal mass in a young girl presenting with lower abdominal pain. Ultimately, the mass was pathologically demonstrated to be a teratoma.

Acute Ear Pain

Melissa A. Vitale and Noel S. Zuckerbraun

ACUTE OTITIS MEDIA

INTRODUCTION

Ear infections are a leading reason for antibiotic prescriptions and acute care visits by infants and children. Acute otitis media (AOM) is most commonly diagnosed in children younger than 2 years of age, especially in those who attend daycare and experience frequent upper respiratory infections (URIs).[1] AOM is rare in the newborn period, but it should still be considered in the newborn presenting with fever or other AOM symptoms. Additional risk factors for AOM include smoke exposure, lack of breastfeeding in the first 6 months of life, pacifier use beyond the first 6 months of age and craniofacial anomalies (e.g., Down syndrome, cleft palate). Young children are prone to develop AOM secondary to their eustachian tube (ET) anatomy (short, narrow, horizontal and floppy), and their frequent acquisition of URIs cause ET dysfunction via inflammation/edema and decreased ciliary activity. This prevents physiologic drainage of middle ear secretions into the nasopharynx and creates a negative pressure that draws bacteria from the nasopharynx into the middle ear.

The most common pathogens are *Streptococcus pneumoniae* and nontypeable *Haemophilus influenzae* followed by *Moraxella catarrhalis*. Since the introduction of the heptavalent pneumococcal conjugate vaccine (PCV-7), the microbiology of AOM has shifted toward a predominance of *H. influenzae*, especially in patients with persistent AOM and those with treatment failure.[2] Although the proportion of penicillin-resistant *S. pneumoniae* has remained fairly consistent, ranging between 30% and 88% of isolates, there has also been a notable increase in β-lactamase–positive *H. influenzae* (50% of isolates).[3,4]

Nearly 100% of *M. cattarrhalis* are also β-lactamase positive.

Viruses also cause AOM and may be clinically indistinguishable from bacterial AOM; common viral etiologies include picornovirus, respiratory syncytial virus and enterovirus. Infants younger than 12 weeks of age with AOM most often have the typical pathogens, but they can also have Group B streptococcus and gram-negative bacilli.[5] Common pathogens such as *H. influenzae* and *S. pneumoniae* show antibiotic resistance patterns similar to those in older children. In children with tympanostomy tubes, *Staphylococcus aureus* and *Pseudomonas aeruginosa* are also common, with methicillin-resistant *S. aureus* becoming more prevalent.[6]

PRESENTATION

The symptoms of AOM have an acute onset, usually within 48 hours of clinical presentation, and include otalgia, fever, excessive crying or fussiness, restless sleep and decreased appetite. A small percentage of infants also may present with cough and signs of conjunctivitis.[5,7] Otalgia has the highest likelihood ratio in predicting the presence of AOM[8] but may not be apparent in young infants. Nonverbal infants may demonstrate ear discomfort by ear-pulling. The absence of fever does not rule out AOM. Studies including children of all ages have demonstrated that fever is present in less than half of all cases of AOM,[9] and in studies of children younger than 3 months of age, fever was present in only two thirds of those diagnosed with AOM.[5,7]

In an attempt to increase the diagnostic accuracy of AOM as well as decrease the unnecessary use of antibiotics, guidelines were published by the Subcommittee on Management of Acute Otitis Media (SMAOM) in 2004.[4]

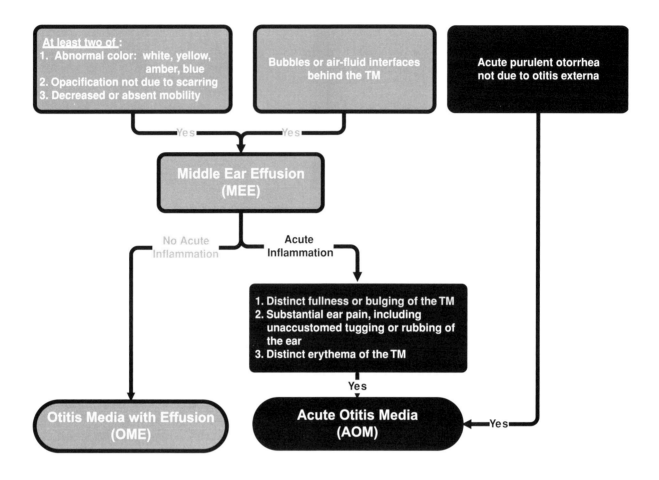

Figure 9.1. Approach to distinguishing between acute otitis media and otitis media with effusion. (Adapted from Hoberman A, Marchant CD, Kaplan SL, et al. Treatment of acute otitis media consensus recommendations. *Clin Pediatr.* 2002;41:373–390,[10] with permission.)

According to these guidelines, three key components are necessary for the diagnosis of AOM:

1. History of acute onset of symptoms
2. Signs of middle ear effusion (MEE)
3. Signs and symptoms of middle-ear inflammation

Examination of the tympanic membrane (TM) is facilitated by using the largest speculum that fits comfortably in the canal to allow proper visualization. Unfortunately, due to the small diameter of the external ear canal in young infants, viewing the TM can be technically challenging. Pneumatic otoscopy involves assessing TM mobility by insufflating air into the external ear canal. This technique can aid in confirming the presence of an MEE, in which case the TM is not mobile; however, this it is not successful unless the TM is adequately visualized and the speculum forms a tight seal on the ear canal. If the tympanic

membrane cannot be visualized because of cerumen, the cerumen can be removed with a curette or by gentle irrigation with warm water. Ceruminolytics can be instilled before irrigation.

A normal TM is intact, neutrally positioned (not retracted or bulging), pearly grey and translucent, and it moves easily with gentle positive and negative insufflating pressure. MEE is suggested by a bulging or retracted TM with limited-to-no mobility, visualization of an air-fluid level in the middle ear or frank otorrhea, indicative of a perforated TM. MEE can signify either AOM or otitis media with effusion (OME); it is the presence of inflammatory changes that distinguishes AOM from OME (Figure 9.1). It is important to note that although redness of the TM can represent inflammation, it can also be secondary to vascular engorgement caused by fever or crying. Relying on TM redness alone will result in the

Table 9.1. Evaluation and management of young infants with acute otitis media based on age and appearance

Age	Evaluation	Disposition and management
≤28 days with AOM *and* fever	Full sepsis workup*	Admit to hospital on parenteral antibiotics
29–60 days with AOM *and* fever	Full sepsis workup*	Observe at home on oral antibiotics if fulfills low-risk criteria[†]
		Admit to hospital on parenteral antibiotics if does not fulfill low-risk criteria[†]
61–90 days with AOM *and* fever; well-appearing	Blood and urine cultures	Observe at home on oral antibiotics if fulfills low risk criteria[†]
≤90 days with AOM and *no* fever; well-appearing	No further workup	Observe at home on oral antibiotics
Any age, toxic appearing	Full sepsis workup*	Admit to hospital on parenteral antibiotics

* Full sepsis workup includes blood, urine and cerebrospinal fluid cultures.

[†] Low risk criteria include the following: previously healthy; no additional focal bacterial infection on examination except acute otitis media; negative laboratory screen including white blood cell count (WBC) 5000–15,000; bands <1500/mm³; normal urinalysis and Gram stain; stool with <5 WBC/hpf; cerebrospinal fluid with <5 WBC/hpf.

over-diagnosis of AOM. This finding, combined with the acute onset of symptoms and evidence of MEE on examination, is more specific for AOM.

Complications of AOM *within the middle ear* include *cholesteatoma* (a white cystic mass behind or involving the TM) and peripheral facial nerve palsy. Nerve palsy is secondary to inflammation of the facial nerve as it traverses the inner and middle ear; it is treated by emergent myringotomy and tube placement. Case reports of facial nerve palsy associated with AOM have been documented in infants as young as 2 weeks of age.[11] AOM can extend *laterally* out of the middle ear space causing TM perforation and otorrhea. *Posterior* spread causes acute mastoiditis, which can be complicated by subperiosteal abscess. *Medial* spread can cause labyrinthitis. Rare, but potentially life-threatening, *superior* spread can cause intracranial complications that include sphenoid sinus thrombosis, intracranial or epidural abscess and meningitis.[12,13]

DIFFERENTIAL DIAGNOSIS

The differential diagnosis of AOM is broad among young infants in whom AOM is suspected because the presentation is often nonspecific and AOM can occur concomitantly with other infections. The spectrum ranges from viral URI, bronchiolitis and pneumonia, to urinary tract infection, bacteremia and meningitis. In older children in whom otalgia is clearly present but AOM is not, the most likely cause is referred pain from infection or trauma in regions with shared innervation, namely the pharynx, nares and teeth. Eustachian tube dysfunction causing negative pressure can also cause otalgia.

LABORATORY TESTS AND RADIOLOGY STUDIES

There are no specific laboratory tests or radiological studies that aid in the diagnosis of AOM. Diagnosis is based primarily on history and physical examination. *Tympanocentesis*, needle aspiration of MEE, is a useful method to establish a bacterial diagnosis. It should be considered in neonates and patients with immunosuppression, persistent treatment failure and/or suppurative complications.[4] Although routine culture of otorrhea is unnecessary, careful culturing with appropriately sized swabs after cleaning the ear canal can be helpful in those with persistent otorrhea.

MANAGEMENT

The primary goals of treatment are to relieve symptoms and to prevent complications. AOM should not be considered an isolated bacterial infection in children 0 to 90 days of age with fever; thus, the evaluation and management of fever in this age group should proceed as indicated by the patient's age and clinical appearance irrespective of the presence of AOM. This subject is covered in detail in Chapter 11. Additional factors that should be considered in management decisions include allergies, recent antibiotic exposure and the severity of the infection (Table 9.1, Figure 9.2).

Infants ages 28 days and younger who present with fever and AOM must undergo a full sepsis evaluation, including blood, urine and cerebrospinal fluid cultures, as they are still at significant risk for serious bacterial infection.[14–16]

Infants between 29 and 60 days of age who present with fever and AOM also warrant a full sepsis evaluation;

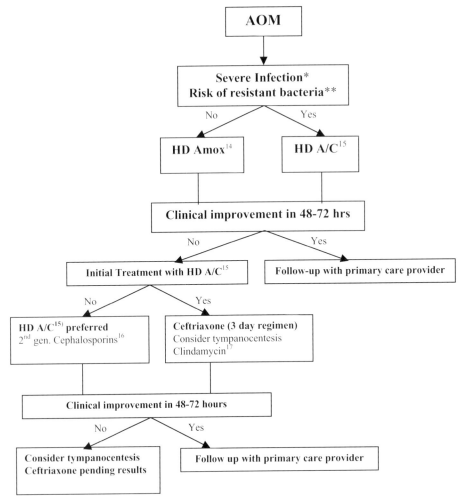

Figure 9.2. Algorithm for antibiotic choice in children with acute otitis media.[4] *Severe infection refers to patients with moderate to severe otalgia or fever >39° C (see text).**Risk of resistant bacteria refers to those with risk of β-lactamase positive M. catarrhalis, H. influenzae (e.g., recent antibiotic use, otitis-conjunctivitis).[14] HD Amox, high dose amoxicillin (see text)[15]; HD A/C, high dose amoxicillin-clavulanate (see text).[16] Selected second generation cephalosporins include cefuroxime, cefpodoxime and cefdinir.[17] Clindamycin should only be used if S. pneumoniae is highly suspected or confirmed by tympanocentesis.

however, infants in this age group may fulfill low risk criteria for observation at home on oral antibiotics if all laboratory and diagnostic studies are negative.[18]

Infants between 61 and 90 days of age with fever and AOM who are well-appearing may undergo a modified sepsis evaluation, which includes blood and urine cultures. If low-risk criteria are met, these infants also may be observed at home on oral antibiotics.

Infants 90 days and younger diagnosed with AOM *without* fever and well-appearing may be treated at home with oral antibiotics. As it is uncommon for infants in this age group to have AOM *without* fever or ill-appearance, the diagnosis should be certain and close follow-up should be ensured.

Certainly, an infant or child of any age who is diagnosed with AOM and who appears ill or toxic requires further workup and hospital admission for evaluation and treatment of sepsis and/or meningitis. Parenteral antibiotics, when indicated, should cover both *S. pneumoniae* and *H. influenzae*, as these are the most common pathogens causing AOM in children of all ages, including those fewer than 3 months of age.[5,7] However, parenteral antibiotic coverage also should take into account the most common pathogens causing serious bacterial infections in the patient's age group as well (see Chapter 11).

High-dose amoxicillin is the first-line agent in treating AOM (Table 9.2); 80% of children with AOM will respond to this therapy.[4] Risk factors identified for the

Table 9.2. Oral antibiotic treatment options for acute otitis media

Antibiotic	Dosage*
High-dose amoxicillin	90 mg/kg/day divided BID
High-dose amoxicillin/ clavulanate	90 mg/kg/day divided BID based on amoxicillin component, using ES preparation, see text
Cefuroxime	30 mg/kg/day divided BID
Cefpodoxime	10 mg/kg/day divided QD or BID
Cefdinir	14 mg/kg/day divided QD or BID
Azithromycin	10 mg/kg loading dose, then 5 mg/kg QD
Clarithromycin	15 mg/kg/day divided BID

* Standard duration of therapy is 10 days for all except azithromycin which is 5 days.

BID, twice daily; ES, extra strength; QD, once daily.

Table 9.3. Observation option for children with acute otitis media

Age	Certain diagnosis	Uncertain diagnosis
<6 months	Antibiotic therapy	Antibiotic therapy
6 months– 2 years	Antibiotic therapy	Severe illness: Antibiotic therapy Nonsevere illness*: Observation option

Adapted from Subcommittee on Management of Acute Otitis Media (SMAOM). (2004). Diagnosis and management of acute otitis media. *Pediatrics.* 113:1451–1465.[4]

* *Nonsevere illness* is defined as rectal temperature <39°C, absence of moderate or severe otalgia and signs of toxicity.

presence of bacterial species likely to be resistant to amoxicillin include attendance at child care, recent receipt of antibiotics (<30 days) and age younger than 2 years. Higher doses of amoxicillin are necessary to overcome the mechanism of *S. pneumoniae* penicillin resistance (mutations of the penicillin-binding protein resulting in less efficient binding kinetics). The SMAOM recommends a strategy of treatment based on the age of the patient, the severity of the AOM and the likely pathogens. For children with nonsevere AOM (mild otalgia or fever <39°C), high-dose amoxicillin is the recommended initial agent. For children with severe AOM (moderate to severe otalgia or fever >39°C) and in those for whom additional coverage for β-lactamase positive *M. catarrhalis and H. influenzae* is desired, high-dose amoxicillin-clavulanate is the recommended initial agent.[4] High-dose amoxicillin-clavulanate is an extra strength preparation, which allows high-dose amoxicillin dosing (90 mg/kg/day based on the amoxicillin component, divided BID) while keeping the clavulanate portion in a range less likely to cause diarrhea and other side effects. High-dose amoxicillin-clavulanate is also preferred for patients with concomitant conjunctivitis because of the association of nontypeable *H. influenzae* with conjunctivitis-otitis.[1]

A management strategy of "watchful waiting" with the avoidance of antibiotics has gained support in the United States but is only appropriate in certain patient populations.[19,20] When compared to those who successfully avoided antibiotics with watchful waiting, patients treated with antibiotics had higher rates of multidrug-resistant pathogens.[20] In addition to decreasing bacterial resistance, proponents also cite the high rate of spontaneous resolution of bacterial AOM. The SMAOM guidelines include an "observation option" for selected children (Table 9.3).[4] Observation is only an option for those older than 6 months of age with nonsevere illness and when the diagnosis of AOM is "uncertain." Exceptions in which antibiotics should be strongly considered are patients with bilateral AOM and patients with both AOM and otorrhea.[21] For all patients being observed, follow-up must be assured and antibiotics must be able to be initiated if symptoms worsen or fail to improve within 48 to 72 hours. In the emergency department setting, this may be facilitated by giving the parents a prescription to hold for 2 to 3 days; this prescription can then be filled if symptoms do not improve over this period.

If signs and symptoms fail to improve after 48 to 72 hours of outpatient therapy, or if the patient was treated with an antibiotic in the preceding month, second-line therapy should be started.[4] Second-line therapy should take into consideration the spectrum of the "failed" antibiotic, in order to provide coverage against the most likely organism(s) untreated by this regimen. Treatment failure with high-dose amoxicillin suggests β-lactamase–producing organisms; thus, options include high-dose amoxicillin-clavulanate, selected second-generation cephalosporins (cefdinir, cefuroxime or cefpodoxime) and ceftriaxone (Table 9.2, Figure 9.2).[22] Of these oral agents, high-dose amoxicillin-clavulanate is preferred because it is more biologically potent than the second-generation cephalosporins and proven highly effective against both β-lactamase–producing pathogens as well as penicillin-nonsusceptible *S. pneumoniae.*[23] Although a single injection of ceftriaxone (50 mg/kg intramuscularly) can be used for first-line therapy in patients that are vomiting or who cannot take oral antibiotics, a three-dose (3 day) regimen is recommended if the AOM was unresponsive to initial antibiotic therapy.[4] In cases that have failed high-dose amoxicillin-clavulanate as first-line therapy, the 3-day regimen of ceftriaxone is recommended; if high-dose amoxicillin-clavulanate was the second line of treatment, tympanocentesis should be considered for treatment failure.[4]

Most maculopapular rashes, often mislabeled *penicillin allergy*, are not mediated by immunoglobulin E (IgE). Patients with reactions that are not mediated by IgE can be safely given penicillin-containing (β-lactam) drugs and should be considered for standard first-line AOM therapy.[24] Alternatives to amoxicillin include cephalosporins. Patients with a true IgE-mediated penicillin allergy (anaphylaxis, urticaria) should not be given penicillin-containing drugs or cephalosporins (due to their potential cross-reactivity with β-lactams). Cephalosporins with a side chain similar to benzylpenicillin, such as cephalexin or cefazolin, are more likely to cross-react with penicillin. True penicillin allergies are only present in about 10% of the population.[24] For these patients, options include clarithromycin and azithromycin, and if *S. pneumoniae* is strongly suspected or can be confirmed, clindamycin.[4] It should be noted, however, that amoxicillin-clavulanate is superior to azithromycin in both pathogen eradication and time to clinical cure; therefore, azithromycin should not be used in cases in which penicillin allergy is not present.[25]

Children with AOM and otorrhea secondary to acute TM perforation are managed similarly to patients without a perforation; however, some clinicians advocate the concomitant use of ototopical agents to hasten the resolution of AOM and prevent the development of otitis externa (OE).[12] Because the perforation may seal before sterilization of the middle ear, topical agents cannot be used as monotherapy.

There is no standard therapy for children with tympanostomy tubes and otorrhea from AOM. Systemic antimicrobials are effective in reducing the duration of otorrhea and bacterial growth. However, monotherapy with topical agents, specifically ciprofloxacin-dexamethasone, is just as effective for the typical pathogens and is also effective for *P. aeruginosa*, a common pathogen in this setting for which no oral systemic antibiotic is approved for children.[26] Studies have shown that topical ciprofloxacin-dexamethasone compared with oral antibiotics results in more rapid resolution of symptoms.[26] Moreover, topical agents do not lead to bacterial resistance, have fewer side effects and are more convenient for the patient compared with systemic therapy. Ciprofloxacin-dexamethasone dosing for AOM with tympanostomy tubes is 4 drops twice daily for 7 days; this differs from ofloxacin dosing for AOM with tympanostomy tubes, which is 5 drops twice daily for 10 days. Pumping the tragus after the installation of ear drops can improve delivery through the tube. Concomitant treatment with systemic antibiotics is advocated by some clinicians for those children with systemic signs and symptoms or with copious exudate that may interfere with the administration of topical agents. In these cases, use of an agent with additional staphylococcal coverage, such as high-dose amoxicillin-clavulanate, is useful as *S. aureus* is common in those with chronic drainage.

An essential component of AOM therapy is pain management, which is most often adequately achieved with either acetaminophen or ibuprofen. In rare cases, opioids may be needed. There is not sufficient evidence to support the routine use of topical analgesics.[27] If needed, they should only be used in the presence of an intact TM. Other adjunctive medications, namely decongestants, antihistamines and systemic steroids, are not beneficial and are associated with increased side effects.

DISPOSITION

Children older than 28 days of age without evidence of serious systemic infection may be managed as outpatients. A follow-up appointment with the primary care physician should occur within 24 hours for infants younger than 3 months of age and in 2 to 3 weeks for older infants and children to monitor recovery of the MEE. Instruction should be given to parents for them to seek care for their child sooner if symptoms, including fever, do not resolve in 48 to 72 hours or signs of worsening infection develop. Children younger than 28 days of age and those with signs of toxicity, other serious systemic infections, intracranial complications or clinically significant immunodeficiencies should be hospitalized and placed on parenteral antibiotics.

MASTOIDITIS

Mastoiditis is a suppurative complication of AOM that most commonly affects children younger than 2 years of age.[28,29] The overall incidence of mastoiditis has decreased since the introduction of antibiotics for the treatment of AOM.[28] Mastoiditis is a spectrum of disease ranging from infectious inflammation of mastoid air cells to abscess development and subsequent spread to contiguous areas. Acute mastoiditis without periosteitis or osteitis is the initial subclinical stage involving inflammation of the lining of the mastoid air cells. Acute mastoiditis with periosteitis occurs when the infection spreads into the periosteum. Acute mastoiditis with osteitis occurs when the infection results in erosion of the bony septae that separate the mastoid air cells, resulting in an empyema.

Patients with clinically significant acute mastoiditis present with postauricular edema, erythema and tenderness. The postauricular crease may be absent. The auricle may be displaced downward and outward. Fever, ear pain and irritability are common, especially in younger children. Up to half of children presenting with mastoiditis may not have had AOM diagnosed within the preceding weeks; in addition, up to half of children with acute mastoiditis may have received treatment with antibiotics for AOM prior to presentation.[29,30] If symptoms and signs of mastoiditis are present, a computed tomography scan of the temporal bones and intracranial cavity should be performed to evaluate for a subperiosteal abscess or osteitis of the mastoid bone.[13]

The most common bacterial pathogens are *S. pneumoniae* and *S. pyogenes*, followed by *S. aureus*, *P. aeruginosa*, and nontypeable *H. influenzae*.[28] It is recommended that all patients with mastoiditis, especially those younger than 12 months, be admitted for parenteral antibiotics and otolaryngology consultation.[13] Fluoroquinolones are relatively contraindicated in young children because of theoretic, but unproven, concerns about cartilage toxicity. Ampicillin-sulbactam or second- and third-generation cephalosporins are acceptable for initial intravenous antibiotic therapy. Vancomycin may be added if there is a suspicion of penicillin-resistant *S. pneumoniae*. If *P. aeruginosa* is suspected, initial, empiric antipseudomonal coverage with ceftazidime or piperacillin-tazobactam can be used. When *Pseudomonas* is suspected, tympanocentesis can be helpful in directing therapy. Traditionally, treatment involved intravenous antibiotics and mastoidectomy with the removal of necrotic bone; however, more recently the use of myringotomy with or without the placement of tympanostomy tubes has allowed for the avoidance of mastoidectomy in many cases.

Table 9.4. Ototopical antibiotics for treatment of otitis externa

Antibiotic	Dose	Duration
Polymyxin B/neomycin	3 gtts TID-QID	10 days
Ofloxacin	1–12 years: 5 gtts QD	7 days
	>12 years: 10 gtt QD	7 days
Ciprofloxacin and dexamethasone	4 gtts BID	7 days

BID, twice daily; QD, once daily; QID, four times daily.

OTITIS EXTERNA

Otitis externa is a diffuse inflammation or infection of the external ear canal, which is most often acute in nature. It is commonly caused by recurrent exposure of the external ear canal to water while swimming (swimmer's ear) and thus is extremely uncommon in children younger than 2 years of age.[17] Although swimming is the most common precipitant, a break in the epithelial lining from any cause (e.g., trauma, foreign body and eczematous skin disorder) can result in otitis externa. The most common bacterial pathogen is *Pseudomonas aeruginosa* followed by *Staphylococcus aureus*.[31] The diagnosis of otitis externa in young children may be challenging.

Key examination findings are tenderness elicited by manipulation of the tragus or pinna and diffuse ear canal edema or erythema.[32] Isolated otitis externa can often be distinguished clinically from AOM by the presence of pain with manipulation of the outer ear. However, AOM with a perforated tympanic membrane should be considered in the differential diagnosis of otitis externa, especially in this age group, as purulent drainage from the middle ear also can cause a secondary otitis externa.

Topical antibiotics are recommended as first-line treatment for uncomplicated otitis externa (Table 9.4).[32] Polymyxin B-neomycin-hydrocortisone agents have been used extensively for years with good results. However, topical fluoroquinolones (ofloxacin and ciprofloxacin) are now used more frequently because they are proven to be as effective as the traditional agents and have decreased risk of ototoxicity and hypersensitivity.[33,34] Most children with otitis externa may be managed at home. The patient should be re-evaluated if symptoms do not improve in 48 to 72 hours. In young infants presenting with otitis externa, additional contributing factors should be investigated such as the presence of immunodeficiency.

PITFALLS

- Failure to consider other more serious co-existing diagnosis in toxic-appearing infants and children and infants younger than 90 days old
- Over-diagnosis of AOM secondary to failure to remove cerumen from ear canal
- Diagnosis based solely upon redness of the TM
- Failure to distinguish OME from AOM
- Failure to know that infants younger than 28 days of age who present with a fever should undergo a complete sepsis evaluation and hospital admission, regardless of the diagnosis of acute otitis media; infants between 28 and 90 days of age who present with fever and acute otitis media should also undergo evaluation for serious bacterial infections but may fulfill criteria for outpatient management
- Failure to use high-dose amoxicillin as the mainstay of first-line therapy for outpatient treatment of acute otitis media
- Failure to admit young patients with mastoiditis for parenteral antibiotics

REFERENCES

1. Corbeel L. What is new in otitis media? *Eur J Pediatr.* 2007;166:511–519.
2. Casey JR, Pichichero ME. Changes in frequency and pathogens causing acute otitis media in 1995–2003. *Pediatr Infect Dis J.* 2004;23:824–828.
3. McEllistrem MC, Adams JM, Patel K, et al. Acute otitis media due to penicillin-nonsusceptible *Streptococcus pneumoniae* before and after the introduction of the pneumococcal conjugate vaccine. *Clin Infect Dis.* 2005;40:1738–1744.
4. Subcommittee on Management of Acute Otitis Media (SMAOM). Diagnosis and management of acute otitis media. *Pediatrics.* 2004;113:1451–1465.
5. Turner D, Leibovitz E, Aran A, et al. Acute otitis media in infants younger than two months of age: microbiology, clinical presentation and therapeutic approach. *Pediatr Infect Dis J.* 2002;21:669–674.
6. Coticchia JM, Dohar JE. Methicillin-resistant *Staphylococcus aureus* otorrhea after tympanostomy tube placement. *Arch Otolaryngol Head Neck Surg.* 2005;131:868–873.
7. Sakran W, Makary H, Colodner R, et al. Acute otitis media in infants less than three months of age: clinical presentation, etiology and concomitant diseases. *Int J Otorhinolaryngol.* 2006;70:613–617.
8. Powers JH. Diagnosis and treatment of acute otitis media: evaluating the evidence. *Infect Dis Clin North Am.* 2007;21:409–426.
9. Pelton SI. Otitis media: re-evaluation of diagnosis and treatment in the era of antimicrobial resistance, pneumococcal conjugate vaccine, and evolving morbidity. *Pediatr Clin North Am.* 2005;52:711–728.
10. Hoberman A, Marchant CD, Kaplan SL, et al. Treatment of acute otitis media consensus recommendations. *Clin Pediatr.* 2002;41:373–390.
11. Rizk EB, El-Bitar MA, Matae GM, et al. Facial nerve palsy with acute otitis media during the first two weeks of life. *J Child Neurol.* 2005;20:452–454.
12. Bluestone CD, Klein JO. *Otitis Media in Infants and Children.* Philadelphia, PA: WB Saunders; 2001.
13. Smith JA, Danner CJ. Complications of chronic otitis media and cholesteatoma. *Otolaryngol Clin North Am.* 2006;39:1237–1255.
14. American College of Emergency Physicians Clinical Practices Committee and the Clinical Policies Subcommittee on Pediatric Fever (ACEP & CPSPF). Clinical policy for children younger than three years presenting to the emergency department with fever. *Ann Emerg Med.* 2003;42:530–545.
15. Baraff LJ. Management of fever without source in infants and children. *Ann Emerg Med.* 2000;36:602–614.
16. Baraff LJ, Bass JW, Fleisher GR, et al. Practice guideline for the management of infants and children 0-36 months of age with fever without a source. *Pediatrics.* 1993;92:1–12.
17. Beers SL, Abramo T. Otitis externa review. *Pediatr Emerg Care.* 2004;20:250–256.
18. King C. Evaluation and management of febrile infants in the emergency department. *Emerg Med Clin North Am.* 2003;21:89–99.
19. Marchetti R, Ronfani L, Nibali SC, et al. Delayed prescription may reduce the use of antibiotics for acute otitis media. *Arch Pediatr Adolesc Med.* 2005;159:679–684.
20. McCormick DP, Chonmaitree T, Pittman C, et al. Nonsevere acute otitis media: a clinical trial comparing outcomes of watchful waiting versus immediate antibiotic treatment. *Pediatrics.* 2005;115:1455–1465.
21. Rovers M, Glasziou P, Appelman CL, et al. Antibiotics for acute otitis media: a meta-analysis with individual patient data. *Lancet.* 2006;368:142–143.
22. Pichichero ME. Pathogen shifts and changing cure rates for otitis media and tonsillopharyngitis. *Clin Pediatr.* 2006;45:493–502.
23. Dagan R, Hoberman A, Johnson C, et al. Bacteriologic and clinical efficacy of high dose amoxicillin/clavulanate in children with acute otitis media. *Pediatr Infect Dis J.* 2001;20:829–837.
24. Pichichero ME. A review of evidence supporting the American Academy of Pediatrics recommendation for prescribing cephalosporin antibiotics for penicillin-allergic patients. *Pediatrics.* 2005;115:1048–1057.
25. Hoberman A, Dagan R, Liebovitz E, et al. Large dosage amoxicillin/clavulanate, compared with azithromycin, for the treatment of bacterial acute otitis media in children. *Pediatr Infect Dis J.* 2005;24:525–532.
26. Dohar J, Giles W, Roland P, et al. Topical ciprofloxacin/dexamethasone superior to oral amoxicillin/clavulanic acid in acute otitis media with otorrhea through tympanostomy tubes. *Pediatrics.* 2006;118:e561–e569.
27. Foxlee R, Johansson A, Wejfalk J, et al. Topical analgesia for acute otitis media. *Cochrane Database Syst Rev.* 2006;3:1–19.
28. Katz A, Leibovitz E, Greenberg D, et al. Acute mastoiditis in Southern Israel: a twelve year retrospective study (1990 through 2001). *Pediatr Infect Dis J.* 2003;22:878–882.

29. Spratley J, Silveira H, Alvarez I, et al. Acute mastoiditis in children: review of the current status. *Int J Pediatr Otorhinolaryngol.* 2000;56:33–40.

30. Butbul-Aviel Y, Miron D, Halevy R, et al. Acute mastoiditis in children: *Pseudomonas aeruginosa* as a leading pathogen. *Int J Pediatr Otorhinolaryngol.* 2003;67:277–281.

31. Roland PS, Stroman D. Microbiology of acute otitis externa. *Laryngoscope.* 2002;112:1166–1177.

32. Rosenfeld RM, Brown L, Cannon CR, et al. Clinical practice guideline: acute otitis externa. *Otolaryngol Head Neck Surg.* 2006;134:S4–S23.

33. Roland PS, Pien FD, Schultz CC, et al. Efficacy and safety of topical ciprofloxacin/dexamethasone versus neomycin/ polymyxin B/hydrocortisone for otitis externa. *Curr Med Res Opin.* 2004;20:1175–1183.

34. Schwartz RH. Once-daily ofloxacin otic solution versus neomycin sulfate/polymyxin B sulfate/hydrocortisone otic suspension four times a day: a multicenter, randomized, evaluator-blinded trial to compare the efficacy, safety, and pain relief in pediatric patients with otitis externa. *Curr Med Res Opin.* 2006;22:1725–1736.

10 Failure to Thrive

Robert Sapien

INTRODUCTION

Infants who are diagnosed with growth failure in the emergency department (ED) are greatly outnumbered by infants with growth failure cared for by primary and specialty care providers. There are many infants with failure to thrive (FTT) in other clinical settings whose situations may be subtle and more chronic. This chapter discusses several cases that illustrate some of the many faces of FTT in the ED. These cases are fairly severe in presentation and represent a subgroup of the larger FTT group.

PRESENTATION

Case 1

An 8-week-old male infant presents to the ED with a history of vomiting since birth that has worsened over the past 2 weeks; now, the baby vomits the entire feed. The baby is bottle-fed with cow's milk–based formula. He is described as having a vigorous suck and he "always seems hungry." He has not had a fever or diarrhea, but he has had a decrease in urine output for 24 hours. On physical examination, the baby is small, has sunken eyes and anterior fontanel with a wasted appearance. He is sluggish to respond and has tenting of the skin over his abdomen. Bowel activity is visible with peristaltic waves.

Diagnosis: FTT with superimposed dehydration secondary to pyloric stenosis

Case 2

An 8-month-old female infant with seizure activity is brought to the ED by emergency medical service (EMS) workers. Generalized seizure activity began 5 minutes before the mother called 911. En route to the ED, the baby was administered oxygen by nonrebreather mask and rectal diazepam per EMS protocol. EMS, however, had difficulty estimating the baby's weight because she looked very small for her age. Mom says the baby is not growing and weighs only 13 lb.

Upon arrival, the baby is having intermittent clonic jerks (about 4/minute) of all extremities. The baby's airway is positioned and cleared with suction, and oxygen is continued. Venous access is obtained, laboratory tests are run and lorazepam is administered. Normal saline is running through the venous catheter. The lorazepam dose is repeated 8 minutes later due to persistent clonic jerks. The bedside glucose is 107. The baby ultimately receives a 20 cc/kg bolus of normal saline.

The myoclonic jerks cease and the laboratory calls with a critical sodium value of 118. The mother is at the bedside during the stabilization efforts and overhears the sodium results. She says, "Again! She had seizures 2 months ago and had low sodium then also. No one was able to figure out why."

Diagnosis: Hyponatremic seizures and FTT due to water intoxication from Munchausen syndrome by proxy.

Case 3

A 6-month-old female infant is brought into the ED for increasing fussiness and possible fever over the past 24 hours. She is the product of a spontaneous vaginal delivery at home attended by a lay midwife. Although the parents do not know the baby's birth weight, they described her as a large baby who was difficult to deliver. The baby is breastfed and has received no vaccinations. This is the first visit to the health care system. The mother says that this baby feeds more slowly than her others and that it has been a challenge to get the baby to latch on. On physical examination, the baby is afebrile and alert with good perfusion, but she is floppy. The baby's tone is decreased throughout, and she does not grasp with her hands. On further questioning, you determine that the baby does not roll over yet.

Diagnosis: FTT secondary to poor feeding from developmental delay, perhaps due to birth trauma.

Case 4

An 8-month-old male infant is brought to the ED because he is pulling his right ear and the mother is concerned about a possible ear infection. On physical examination, the ED physician notes that the baby is thin and long. On questioning about feeding history and social history, the mother begins to sob. She tells the physician that the baby has always been a slow eater. She adds that she and the baby have been living with the grandfather because the baby's father is in the military and was recently deployed to Iraq. The grandfather convinced the mother that the baby may like diluted condensed milk more than formula and, besides, it is less expensive. The baby's birth weight was nearly 8 lb (3600 g). The baby's weight today is only 5000 g.

Diagnosis: FTT secondary to undernourishment and multifactorial developmental and social issues, including poor child response to food and possible maternal depression.

FTT is one of many symptoms that has become a diagnosis, at least for hospital admission records in emergency medicine. There is even an International Classification of Diseases (ICD-9) code for FTT: 783.41. FTT may be the symptom that enables the child to be admitted to the hospital, but the ultimate diagnosis is actually the processes that result in or lead to the growth failure. Infants with FTT do not commonly present to the ED with a chief complaint of poor weight gain; instead, they present with other complaints such as fever, congestion, fussiness or cough. An astute ED physician will note that the infant appears smaller than expected, thin and long or "just not right." It is at this point that further investigation begins. This investigation should include a careful measurement of growth parameters and a detailed dietary history (what

food is offered, when it is offered and what the baby does take) as well as evaluation of developmental milestones.

PATHOPHYSIOLOGY

FTT not only comes to the attention of the ED provider through many presentations and levels of acuity but also is known by many names such as growth failure, growth retardation, pediatric undernutrition and child malnourishment. Incidence and prevalence in the emergency setting are not well established.

Although any chronic disease can lead to growth failure, FTT is a symptom or sign indicating that the infant's growth has been affected. FTT may be an isolated disease process, but more likely its causes are multifactorial. There may be a chronic disease as the root, but there are social, developmental and environmental aspects that contribute to the FTT. Conversely, the social, developmental and environmental aspects may be the primary causes, independent of any chronic disease processes. One can see that FTT is a compilation of factors leading to inadequate infant growth, some medical, some physiological and others social and environmental.

To better evaluate abnormal growth, normal growth must be understood. Infants normally lose 1% to 8% of their birth weight in the first few days of life. This weight is regained within the first 7 to 14 days of life. Formula-fed babies gain more weight, more quickly.

General parameters for breastfed baby weight gain is 2 lb/month for 3 months, 1 lb/month for the next 3 months, then $\frac{1}{2}$ lb/month for the remainder of the first year.[1] Other sources report normal weight gain to be at least $\frac{1}{2}$ oz (15 g)/day or 1 lb (454 g)/month for the first 4 months[2] or 4 to 7 oz/week for 1 month and 0.5 to 1 kg/month for the first 6 months.[3] Normal growth is reported to be 1 inch/month in length for first 6 months and $\frac{1}{2}$ inch/month for months 6 through 12.[3] Basically, a baby's age roughly matches his or her weight in kilograms by 9 months (i.e., 50th percentile for a 9 month old is 9 kg).

The baby's weight, length, weight-for-length and head circumference should be graphed on the growth charts of the Centers for Disease Control and Prevention (CDC) National Center for Health Statistics (NCHS). These charts are percentile-based and gender specific, and they indicate growth trends, including ranges from the 3rd to the 97th percentile (Figures 10.1 through 10.4). The charts combine data for both breastfed and formula-fed babies.[4]

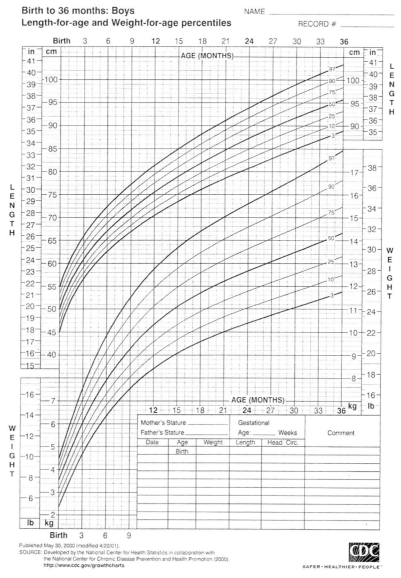

Figure 10.1. CDC-NCHS growth chart for infant males, length for age and weight for age.

The isobars indicate growth trends with the hope that an infant will grow along an isobar. For example, a baby boy may be born at 3.5 kg, which is the 30th percentile. Normally, a baby will continue to grow along the same isobar; hence, this same baby should weigh 5.8 kg at 3 months of age, 9.2 kg at 9 months and so on to remain at the 30th percentile. Head circumference and length growth trends are similar to the weight-gain pattern.

Babies who start life small may not be diagnosed with FTT if they continue to grow along their chosen isobars. For example, the baby in Figure 10.5 is below the 3rd percentile, the first of the criteria to consider in FTT, but the baby demonstrates a normal growth trend along that isobar. Second, this baby's length growth also follows a reasonable growth trend. Third, the baby's head circumference is growing at a reasonable rate (Figure 10.6). Most importantly, when the baby's weight is graphed according to length, the baby, although small, is growing normally (see Figure 10.6).

This is in contrast to the child whose growth is illustrated in Figure 10.7. Her length continues to gain along a determined isobar, but she begins to not gain sufficient weight to remain on the isobar from 2 to 3 months, and ultimately she falls two isobars (from 2-4 months). This is an obvious pattern of FTT. Although not graphed, her weight for length percentile would be abnormal.

It is when these growth patterns are disrupted that FTT becomes of concern. Definitions and criteria to secure the

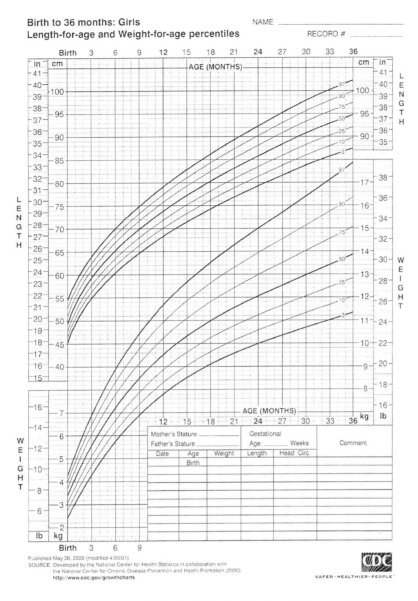

Figure 10.2. CDC-NCHS growth chart for infant females, length for age and weight for age.

condition of growth failure vary, but generally they are stated as a decrease in growth leading to a fall by two isobars (two major percentile lines) for weight or a weight that is less than the 3rd percentile on the NCHS growth charts.

There are other anthropometric measurements that can be performed, such as skinfold thickness, middle upper arm circumference[5] and body mass index, none of which are very practical in an emergency setting. Unfortunately, there is no one measurement that will confirm growth failure[6]; however, in the ED, weight, length and head circumference measurements are the most practical. Trends from prior measurements in the child's medical record or history help confirm the condition.

DIFFERENTIAL DIAGNOSIS

Determining the causes of the growth failure can be challenging in the primary care setting and even more so in the emergency setting. The basic premise in growth failure is that the caloric intake does not meet the metabolic demands of the child. This can happen through a variety of mechanisms: inadequate intake, intake of insufficient calories or increased usage. Inadequate intake can be caused by caregiver factors, infant factors or environmental factors. Increased usage usually is from physiological factors. It is important to remember that the condition of FTT usually results from a constellation of factors in the medical, physiological, social and

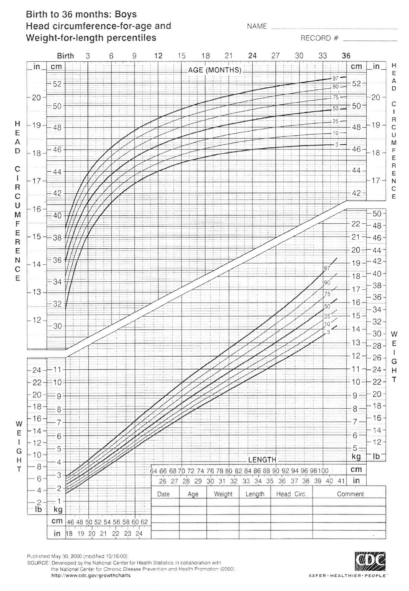

Figure 10.3. CDC-NCHS growth chart for infant males, head circumference and weight for length.

environmental realms. Prior nomenclature differentiated FTT as originating from organic (medical or physiological) compared with nonorganic (social or environmental) causes. The more the constellation of factors and their interaction in the child's condition are considered, however, the more archaic this nomenclature becomes. A standard definition of FTT is still controversial.[7]

Although any chronic disease can affect growth, chronic diseases that may lead to FTT (specifically poor weight gain) include cardiac diseases (congenital and acquired heart disease or failure), glycogen storage diseases, renal tubular acidosis, cystic fibrosis, thyroid disease, tuberculosis, human immunodeficiency virus, hepatitis, diencephalic syndrome, cerebral palsy, developmental delay, milk allergies and gastroesophageal reflux.[8–17]

Combine these chronic diseases with the social and environmental impact they have on families such as feelings of stress, guilt, depression and inadequacy; economic hardship; medical expenses; and lack of familial and community support, and one can begin to appreciate the complexity of FTT as a symptom.

Specific social and environmental conditions that may result in FTT include those stemming from the infant and those originating with the caregivers. Examples of infant-based factors include quality of the infant–parent interaction and bond, fussy disposition, poor or inadequate sucking mechanisms, poorly coordinated chewing and swallowing mechanisms, food aversion and pickiness. Examples of caregiver factors include maternal depression, mental illness, Munchausen syndrome by

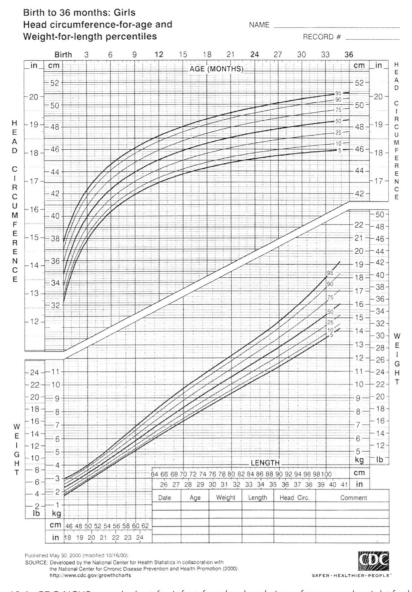

Figure 10.4. CDC-NCHS growth chart for infant females, head circumference and weight for length.

proxy, neglect, abuse, interpersonal violence in the home, parental impression of infant feeding, parental feelings of inadequacy, parent–infant interaction and bond.[18–25] There are conflicting reports as to the impact of maternal depression on infant growth failure,[26–30] but again, understanding that FTT is multifactorial in origin does not support the attempt to assign to it a single social or environmental etiology.[31]

LABORATORY AND RADIOLOGY

Even though there are many potential differential diagnoses, casting a wide net and ordering exhaustive laboratory tests is not warranted. After a careful history and physical, specific tests may be helpful in determining biochemical stability of the infant, leaving the more esoteric laboratory tests to be ordered by the infant's primary or specialty physician. Consequently, specific laboratory workup of the infant usually proceeds in a stepwise fashion by the primary or specialty provider. Although there are rare occasions, as shown in Cases 1 and 2, in which laboratory values may help make the diagnosis, they usually do not add much to the emergency management of children with FTT nor do they add to the likelihood of determining a single cause for the undernutrition.

General, routine screening tests do help assure the provider of the infant's biochemical stability, general

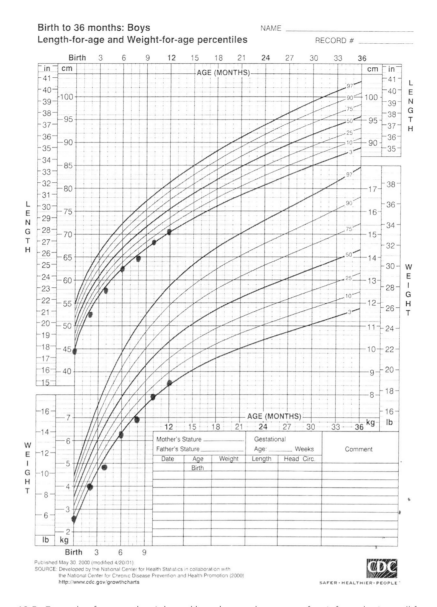

Figure 10.5. Example of a normal weight and length growth pattern of an infant who is small for age. The pattern of growth is not consistent with FTT.

nutrition and hydration status. These routine screening laboratory tests include the following[9]:

1. A complete blood cell count to assess for cytopenia and anemia
2. Electrolytes to partly assess hydration status (although this is better determined with the physical examination) and acid-base status
3. Albumin and total protein, which may be determiners of advanced nutritional compromise
4. Urinalysis with culture and sensitivity
5. Calcium and phosphorous

It has been reported, however, that especially as the workup pertains to renal tubular acidosis as an etiology for FTT, venous blood gas is a more accurate determiner of acid-base status than routine chemistry tests.[32] Normal values in these tests are reassuring, especially in determining disposition of the infant. Social factors aside, is the child stable to be discharged with close follow-up? If the child is to be admitted to the hospital, is the child stable enough for a general hospital ward or does he or she need close monitoring?

Radiological studies have limited value in the care of these children; however, there are specific indications for radiological applications. For example, if it has been determined that the child is the victim of specific abuse or has been in a potentially abusive social environment, then obtaining a skeletal or long bone series of x-rays may

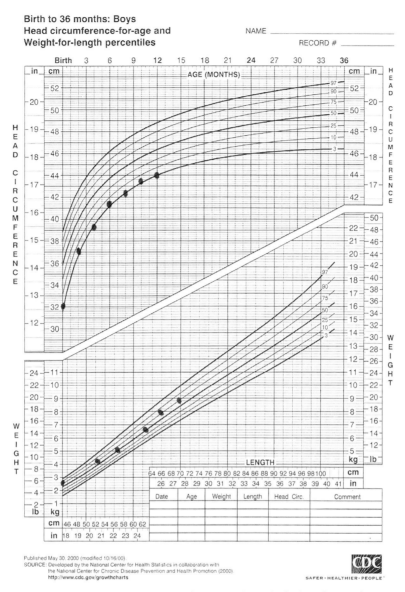

Figure 10.6. Example of a normal head circumference and weight for length growth pattern of the infant in Figure 10.5. The pattern is not consistent with FTT.

be warranted. This series will help determine if there are new, old or healing fractures, adding to the evidence that abuse has occurred. Chest x-rays of an infant suspected of growth failure due to cystic fibrosis or chronic pneumonia also may be helpful, but these x-rays are not routine tests for all infants with FTT. Bone age can be assessed with radiographs, and this helps the provider determine the impact a chronic disease may have on the child's growth.[9] These radiographs are not a routine part of the ED workup, however. Also, as in Case 1, with this history and physical examination, if pyloric stenosis is considered, then an abdominal ultrasound is a logical approach. However, if there is a palpable "olive," then many surgeons do not require any further confirmatory studies. As with laboratory tests, radiological studies should not be routinely ordered in the workup of an infant with FTT. They should be directed at specific disease processes, determined by history and physical evaluation.

MANAGEMENT

The approach to medically managing the infant with FTT is much like the approach to most children in the ED. First, assess for medical stability (Figure 10.8). In severe cases, in which hydration and acid-base status are affected, even airway and breathing problems may present as the child

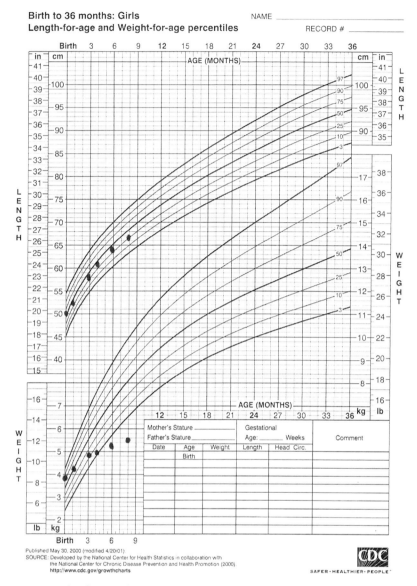

Figure 10.7. Example of a growth pattern indicating FTT by two parameters in an infant (e.g., fall in weight growth pattern of at least two isobars and to a weight of ≤3rd percentile).

deteriorates acutely. Although these severe presentations are rare, supplemental oxygen and respiratory management (respiratory support with bag valve mask or even endotracheal intubation) may be necessary. Once medical stability has been addressed, depending on the baby's hydration and acid-base balance, the baby's circulation may need to be supported. Obtaining intravenous access and administering isotonic fluid boluses in 20 mL/kg aliquots is the usual approach. Active and diligent reassessment of the child's airway, breathing and circulation (ABCs) to determine response to the interventions or deterioration is prudent.

Children with FTT more commonly present to the ED in stable condition, sometimes with chief complaints directly linked to the growth failure (e.g., poor feeding [in the neonate] or vomiting) but sometimes not directly linked to the growth failure (e.g., fussiness, suspected infection, etc.). Growth failure is almost an incidental finding in the baby's assessment. Once the ED physician becomes aware that growth failure may exist, there are components in the history and physical examination that help direct management and, ultimately, disposition.

In most EDs, infants are weighed and vital signs are taken early in the course of treatment. The remaining

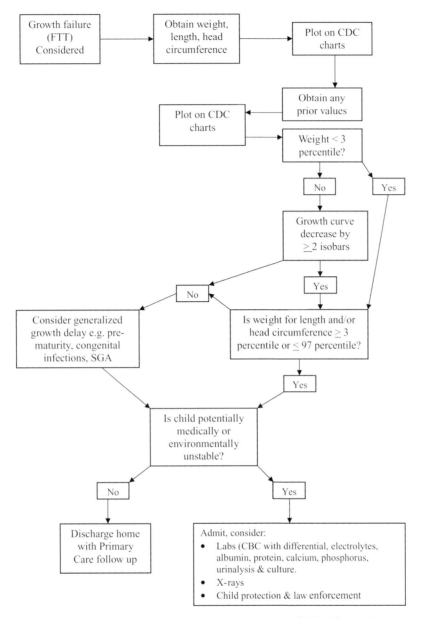

Figure 10.8. Algorithm for the ED evaluation and management of FTT (after addressing airway, breathing and circulation stabilization).

growth parameters also must be determined, including the baby's length and head circumference. The weight, length and head circumference should be graphed on standardized growth charts shown in Figures 10.1 and 10.2, which are downloadable from the CDC and NCHS website (http://www.cdc.gov/growthcharts/).[33] Because the ED measurements are single point-in-time measurements and FTT is verified by growth trends, reviewing the medical record for previous growth values is helpful. At a minimum, the parents may be able to provide the baby's birth weight, which will enable two values to be charted

on the weight graph. It is important to remember that the weights probably have been obtained on different scales, which introduces error in measurement and may affect comparability of the values.

Once it is determined that the infant does indeed have growth failure, a careful history is paramount, starting from the prenatal period through social and environmental history. For the prenatal history, the provider would ask about prenatal care and issues (e.g., maternal weight gain), gravidity and parity, gestational age, prior miscarriages, substance use (medications, alcohol, tobacco, illicit drugs), planned pregnancy, maternal medical problems, as well as genetic and infection screenings. Labor and delivery history should include length of labor, maternal and infant fever, prolonged labor or delivery, birth anoxia, Apgar scores, feeding difficulties including latching on and strength of suck, feeding instruction or education received, bonding at birth, prematurity, birth weight and length of hospitalization. The baby's medical history should include primary and medical home, developmental milestones, immunizations and feeding behavior (what the baby is fed, how it is prepared and how often and how much the baby eats). Breastfeeding patterns should also be assessed, including maternal diet, maternal breast discomfort, milk production and understanding of the process.[8] A review of the baby's symptoms, including mental status, difficulty taking food (fluids or solids), stool pattern, vomiting, fevers and appetite is also helpful. These children also may have a history of recurrent infections, indicating a relative immune deficiency.[8] The social history helps assess the baby's risk for neglect or abuse as well as maternal and other caregiver depression or mental illness. This includes life stresses, age and occupation of parents and socioeconomic support structure (friends, community, religious, governmental support programs).[34]

Specific physical examination abnormalities may be clues of specific etiologies of growth failure. For example, abnormal vital signs such as hypotension or hypertension could indicate adrenal, thyroid or renal disease. Head, eyes, ears, neck and throat examinations might reveal thyroid enlargement, cataracts (from congenital infections or galactosemia) or bottle caries of the teeth, indicating neglect.

Abnormal chest examination findings, which may require further workup, include cardiac murmurs and wheezing. Abnormal bowel sounds or abdominal distention may hint at malabsorption syndromes, and hepatosplenomegaly may indicate liver disease or glycogen storage diseases. Genitourinary findings, such as structural abnormalities, may indicate renal disease or endocrine diseases. Significant and uncared for diaper rashes or poor hygiene in this area could be a result of neglect. Extremities may be edematous in patients with hypoalbuminemic conditions, and obvious deformity or tenderness may indicate a fracture, either acute or healing, indicating abuse or pathological fracture from significant malnutrition.

Neurological examination should include deep tendon reflexes, infant reflexes and especially muscle tone. Abnormalities in any of these may indicate cerebral palsy or other neurological condition leading to the growth failure. Examination of the skin may reveal signs of neglect and abuse (bruising, poor hygiene, scarring), allergies (eczema), or anemia (pallor). Finally, examination by and evaluation of the feeding activities and interactions on the part of the mother and infant can provide much insight into the growth difficulties. This can be done by the physicians or nurses in the ED.

Historically, infants with FTT have been admitted to the hospital. Deciding on the ultimate disposition, however, as with any ED patient, depends on determining medical, social and environmental stability. No recent studies have looked at the efficacy of hospitalization in these children, but older studies report two findings:

1. Only 31% of these children who were hospitalized were found to have a clear medical diagnosis; 33% had no diagnosis and 32% were of a social or environmental etiology[35]
2. Growth of the admitted child who has social or environmental challenges was improved as an inpatient with only modest impact on the psychosocial aspects of the child's life.[10,36]

Of course, these studies took place during an era when children with FTT were predominantly admitted to the hospital. It is important to keep in mind that children whose FTT is predominately of a medical etiology will gain weight in the hospital as will children whose weight gain challenge is social or environmental in nature.[11] In other words, hospitalization does not differentiate between medical or social or environmental etiologies.

Medically unstable or potentially unstable infants obviously must be admitted to the hospital. Questions of social and environmental instability should prompt early involvement of hospital social services and new mother support services (lactation, occupational therapy and nutritional support).[37] In those patients with social instability for whom there is concern regarding possible child abuse or neglect, child protective services and local law enforcement agencies must be notified. If the child ultimately is discharged, ensuring medical home, primary and specialty care follow-up is essential. A mechanism for the ED to confirm that the family actually kept their appointments is also helpful. Home visits by nurses have also been shown to be effective in improving outcomes in these infants.[38]

- Failure to recognize the unit of measure for the reported weight (e.g., pounds versus kilograms)
- Failing to recognize that the infant is small for age, that is, failing to recognize that there is growth failure
- Failure to consider child abuse risks based on the child's presentation or environmental assessment
- Failure to review the infant's previous weight
- Failure to secure an adequate follow-up plan for the infant, should he or she be discharged

REFERENCES

1. Lawrence RA. Infant nutrition. *Pediatr Rev.* 1983;5(5):133–140.
2. www.healthsystem.virginia.edu/uvahealth/peds-newborn/diffslow.cfm. Accessed August 12, 2007.
3. www.AskDrSears.com/html/2/T023600.asp. Accessed August 12, 2007.
4. Radcliffe B, Payne JE, Porteous H, et al. "Failure to thrive" or failure to use the right growth chart? *Med J Aust.* 2007;186(12):560–561.
5. Shah MD. Failure to thrive in children. *J Clin Gastroenterol.* 2002;35(5):371–374.
6. Olsen EM, Petersen J, Skovgaard AM, et al. Failure to thrive: the prevalence and concurrence of anthropometric criteria in a general infant population. *Arch Dis Child.* 2007;92:109–114.
7. Olsen EM. Failure to thrive: still a problem of definition. *Clin Pediatr (Phila).* 2006;45:1–6.
8. Schwartz ID. Failure to thrive: an old nemesis in the new millennium. *Pediatr Rev.* 2000;21:257–264.
9. Zenel JA. Failure to thrive: a general pediatrician's perspective. *Pediatr Rev.* 1997;18:371.
10. Gahagan S. Failure to thrive: a consequence of undernutrition. *Pediatr Rev.* 2006;27:e1–e11.
11. Adam HM. Weight loss/failure to thrive. *Pediatr Rev.* 2000;21(7):238–239.
12. Ozen H. Glycogen storage diseases: new perspectives. *World J Gastroenterol.* 2007;13(18):2541–2553.
13. Moissidis I, Chaidaroon D, Vichyanond P, et al. Milk-induced pulmonary disease in infants. *Pediatr Allergy Immunol.* 2005;16(6):545–552.
14. Ozbek OY, Canan O, Ozcay F, et al. Cow's milk protein enteropathy and granulomatous duodenitis in a newborn. *J Pediatr Child Health.* 2007;43:494–496.
15. Maloney J, Nowak-Wegrzyn A. Educational clinical case series for pediatric allergy and immunology: allergic proctocolitis, food protein-induced enterocolitis syndrome and allergic eosinophilic gastroenteritis with protein-losing gastroenteropathy as manifestations of non-IgE-mediated cow's milk allergy. *Pediatr Allergy Immunol.* 2007;18:360–367.
16. Logan LK, Zheng XT, Disikes GS, et al. Failure to thrive in Chicago. *Lancet.* 2007;369:2132.
17. Huber J, Sovinz P, Lackner H, et al. Diencephalic syndrome: a frequently delayed diagnosis in failure to thrive. *Klin Pediatr.* 2007;219(2):91–94.
18. Chatoor I, Surles J, Ganiban J, et al. Failure to thrive and cognitive development in toddlers with infantile anorexia. *Pediatrics.* 2004;113:e440–e447.
19. Moldavsky M, Stein D. Munchausen syndrome by proxy: two case reports and an update of the literature. *Int J Psychiatry Med.* 2003;33:411–423.
20. Stirling J Jr. Beyond Munchausen syndrome by proxy: identification and treatment of child abuse in a medical setting. *Pediatrics.* 2007;119:1026–1030.
21. Bair-Merritt MH, Blackstone M, Feudner C. Physical health outcomes of childhood exposure to intimate partner violence: a systematic review. *Pediatrics.* 2006;117:e278–e290.
22. Block RW, Krebs NF. Failure to thrive as a manifestation of child neglect. *Pediatrics.* 2005;116:1234–1237.
23. Wright CM, Weaver LT. Image or reality: why do infant size and growth matter to parents? *Arch Dis Child.* 2007;92:98–100.
24. Wright CM, Parkinson KN, Drewett RF. How does maternal and child feeding behavior relate to weight gain and failure to thrive: data from a prospective birth cohort. *Pediatrics.* 2006;117:1262–1269.
25. Am Drewett EA, Blair P, et al. Weak infant sucking in the first 8 weeks, reliance on breastfeeding for ≥9 months, small feeds, and difficulties in weaning were associated with failure to thrive. *Arch Dis Child.* 2007;92:115–119.
26. Ramsay M, Gisel EG, McCusker J, et al. Infant sucking ability, non-organic failure to thrive, maternal characteristics, and feeding practices: a prospective cohort study. *Develop Med Child Neurol.* 2002;44:405–414.
27. Wright CM, Parkinson KN, Drewett RF. The influence of maternal socioeconomic and emotional factors on infant weight gain and weight faltering (failure to thrive): data for a prospective birth cohort. *Arch Dis Child.* 2006;91:312–317.
28. Drewett R, Blair P, Emmett P, et al. Failure to thrive in the term and preterm infants of mothers depressed in the postnatal period: a population-based birth cohort study. *J Child Psychol Psychiatry.* 2004;45:359–366.
29. O'Brien LM, Heycock EG, Hanna M, et al. Postnatal depression and faltering growth: a community study. *Pediatrics.* 2004;113:1241–1247.
30. Stewart RC. Maternal depression and infant growth – a review of recent evidence. *Maternal Child Nutrition.* 2007;3:94–107.
31. Black MM, Dubowitz H, Krishnakumar A, et al. Early intervention and recovery among children with failure to thrive: follow-up at age 8. *Pediatrics.* 2007;120:59–69.
32. Adeoyin O, Gottlieb B, Frank R, Vento S, et al. Evaluation of failure to thrive diagnostic yield of testing for renal tubular acidosis. *Pediatrics.* 2003;112:e463–e466.
33. National Center for Health Statistics. www.cdc.gov. Accessed August 12, 2007.
34. Kleinman RE, ed. *Pediatric Nutrition Handbook,* 5th ed. Elk Grove Village, IL: The American Academy of Pediatrics; 2004:443–457.

35. Berwick DM, Levy JC, Kleinerman R. Failure to thrive: diagnostic yield of hospitalization. *Arch Dis Child.* 1982;57:347–351.

36. Fryer GE Jr. The efficacy of hospitalization of nonorganic failure-to-thrive children: a meta-analysis. *Child Abuse Negl.* 1988;12:375–381.

37. Stewart KB, Meyer L. Parent-child interactions and everyday routines in young children with failure to thrive. *Am J Occup Ther.* 2004;58(3):342–346.

38. Black MM, Dubowitz H, Casey PH, et al. Failure to thrive as distinct from child neglect. *Pediatrics.* 2006;117:1456–1458.

11   Approach to the Infant with Fever

Paul Ishimine

INTRODUCTION

Febrile young children frequently present to the emergency department (ED) for evaluation. As emergency physicians, we have been taught to be concerned about young children who have higher fevers but no clear source for that fever as this puts them at higher risk for occult infections such as bacteremia or urinary tract infections (UTIs). In 2005, fever of unclear source was the second most common ED discharge diagnosis in children younger than 1 year of age, representing nearly 10% of all ED visits by children in this age range.[1] Despite the frequency of this complaint, however, the approach to fever in the child younger than 1 year of age remains controversial, and evaluation and treatment of these patients varies considerably.[2–4]

This variability in the approach to the febrile young child arises in part because of the broad differential diagnosis of fever without obvious source (FWS). Younger children, especially infants, present a particularly vexing group when compared with older children; young children are unable to verbalize their symptoms, the physical examination may be unrevealing and they are more likely to develop serious bacterial infections (SBIs) than older children (Figure 11.1).

Attempts have been made to standardize the approach to the young febrile child.[5–7] Although the majority of febrile young children have self-limited viral infections, the ED approach to the young child who has FWS has traditionally emphasized detection of SBIs such as meningitis, pneumonia, UTI, bacterial gastroenteritis osteomyelitis and bacteremia. This emphasis on detecting SBIs is not unfounded as children with SBIs are more likely to develop serious sequelae if these infections are untreated.

HISTORY AND PHYSICAL EXAMINATION

The history and physical examination is invaluable in the assessment of the febrile child. A *fever* is defined as temperature of 38.0°C (100.4°F). Rectal thermometry is considered the gold standard for noninvasive temperature measurement, as this route is thought to most closely represent the core temperature.[8–12] Bundling a young child may increase the skin temperature but probably does not increase the core temperature.[13] The subjective determination of fever by parents at home is moderately accurate[14–16] but may be the only indicator of a potential SBI in a child who is afebrile in the ED.[17] A patient with a fever measured rectally at home should undergo the same evaluation as a child who has a fever in the ED.

Certain characteristics of the fever should be noted. There is an increase in the rate of pneumococcal bacteremia with an increase in temperature, and this is more pronounced in young children.[18] Some studies suggest that the incidence of SBIs in young children is higher in patients with hyperpyrexia.[19,20] The duration of the fever itself at the time of ED presentation does not predict whether a child has occult bacteremia.[21] The use of antipyretics should be noted; however, a response (or lack thereof) to antipyretic medications does not predict whether the underlying cause is bacterial or viral.[22–26] Additional important data include associated signs and symptoms, underlying medical conditions, and exposure to ill contacts. Inquiring about a patient's immunization status is important; however, parental recall of a child's immunization history is frequently inaccurate.[27]

An assessment of the child's overall appearance is critical. Although there is an imperfect correlation between physical examination findings and SBIs, ill-appearing children are more likely than well-appearing children to

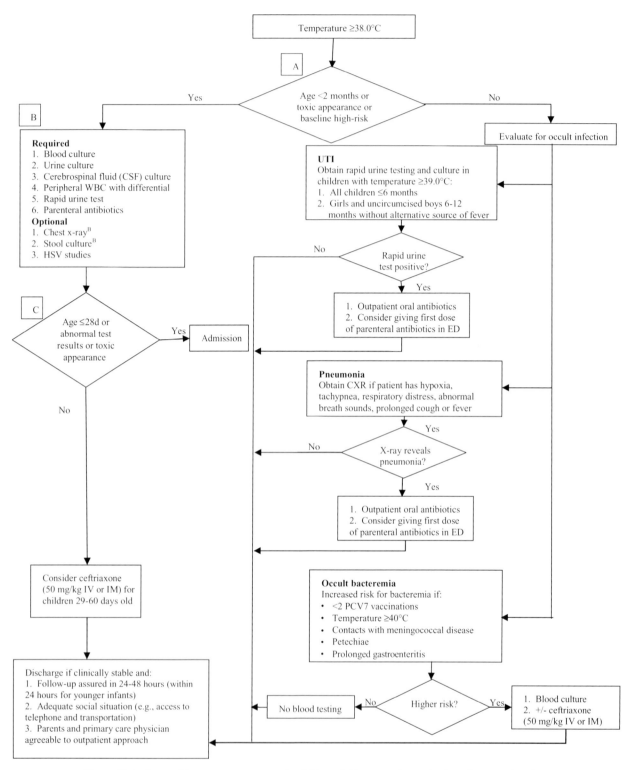

Figure 11.1. Fever without apparent source in children A, Young patients who have increased under-lying risk include children who were born prematurely, had prolonged hospital stays after birth, have underlying medical conditions, have indwelling medical devices, have fever lasting more than 5 days, or are already on antibiotics.

B, Urine testing can be accomplished by microscopy, Gram stain or urine dipstick. Chest x-rays (CXRs) are indicated in patients with hypoxia, tachypnea, abnormal lung sounds or respiratory distress. Stool studies are indicated in patients with diarrhea. Herpes simplex virus (HSV) testing should be con-sidered in the presence of risk factors (see text for details). HSV testing is best accomplished by polymerase chain reaction or viral culture. Neonates should receive both ampicillin (50 mg/kg IV; 100 mg/kg IV if concern for meningitis) and cefotaxime (50 mg/kg; 100 mg/kg IV if concern for have SBIs, and most well-appearing children do not have SBIs.[28–31] If a child has a toxic appearance, this mandates an aggressive workup, antibiotic treatment and hospitalization, regardless of age or risk factors.

The physical examination may often reveal obvious sources of infection, and the identification of a focal infection may decrease the need for additional testing. For example, febrile patients with clinically recognizable viral conditions (e.g., croup, chicken pox and stomatitis) have lower rates of bacteremia than patients with no obvious sources of infection.[32]

With the exception of neonates and very young infants, if a child has a nontoxic appearance, a more selective approach can be undertaken. When a child who has a febrile illness has an obviously identifiable cause, the treatment and disposition should generally be tailored to this specific infection. The approach to all febrile children younger than 2 months of age and the approach to older infants and children without an identifiable source for the fever are discussed.

APPROACH TO FEBRILE CHILDREN YOUNGER THAN 2 MONTHS OF AGE

Overview

Neonates, defined as children younger than 1 month old, are at particularly high risk for SBIs. Approximately 12% to 28% of all febrile neonates presenting to a pediatric ED have serious bacterial illness.[33–35] Neonates are infected typically by more virulent bacteria such as group B Streptococcus, *Escherichia coli* and *Listeria monocytogenes.* Group B streptococcus, a common bacteria pathogen in this age group, is associated with high rates of meningitis, nonmeningeal foci of infection and sepsis.[36] The most common sources for bacterial infections in this

group are UTIs and occult bacteremia[33,35]; neonates are more likely to develop serious sequelae from viral infections (e.g., herpes simplex virus [HSV] meningitis).

Children between 1 and 2 months of age are also at significant risk for SBIs but at lower rates than infants younger than 1 month old. As with neonates, the information obtained from the physical examination is still limited.[37] In the past, young infants with fever routinely underwent sepsis evaluations (blood, urine and cerebrospinal fluid [CSF] testing), received antibiotics and were admitted to the hospital.[38]

In the late 1980s and early 1990s, several decision rules were created for use in evaluation of the febrile young infant. The first of these were the "Rochester criteria," which stratified children younger than 60 days old into high- and low-risk groups. The children who met the low-risk criteria appeared well, had been previously healthy and had no evidence of skin, soft tissue, bone, joint or ear infection. Additionally, these children had normal peripheral white blood cell (WBC) counts (5000–15,000/mm^3), normal absolute band counts ($\leq$1500/mm^3), less than or equal to 10 WBC/high-power field (hpf) of centrifuged urine sediment and, for those patients with diarrhea, less than or equal to 5 WBC/hpf on stool smear.[39,40] The low-risk group identified children who were unlikely to have SBIs, with a negative predictive value of 98.9%.[41]

The "Boston criteria" was derived for febrile children between 1 and 3 months of age who presented to the ED with temperatures $\geq$38.0°C. Infants were discharged after an intramuscular (IM) injection of ceftriaxone, 50 mg/kg, if they generally appeared to be well (not strictly defined) and had no ear, soft tissue, joint or bone infections on physical examination. Furthermore, these patients had to have CSF with less than or equal to 10 WBC/hpf, microscopic urinalysis (UA) with less than or equal to 10 WBC/hpf or urine dipstick negative for leukocyte

---

Figure 11.1. (*continued*)
meningitis) or gentamicin (2.5 mg/kg IV). Older children should receive ceftriaxone (50 mg/kg IV; 100 mg/kg IV if concern for meningitis). Patients who may have HSV infection should receive 20 mg/kg of IV acyclovir.
C, Abnormal laboratory studies:
Peripheral white blood cell (WBC) count: <5000/mm^3 or >15,000/mm^3 or band-to-neutrophil ratio >0.2
Urine testing: $\geq$5 WBC/hpf, bacteria on Gram stain, or positive leukocyte esterase or nitrite
Cerebrospinal fluid: $\geq$8 WBC/mm^3 or bacteria on Gram stain
Stool specimen: $\geq$5 WBC/hpf
Chest x-ray: infiltrate on chest x-ray
CSF, cerebrospinal fluid; ED, emergency department; hpf, high-power field; PCV7, 7-valent pneumococcal conjugate vaccine; WBC, white blood cell.

esterase, a peripheral WBC count of less than or equal to 20,000/mm^3 and normal findings in patients in whom a chest radiograph was obtained (all tests except the chest radiograph were performed on all patients). Twenty-seven of 503 children (5.4%) were later found to have SBI (bacterial gastroenteritis, UTI and occult bacteremia).[42]

The "Philadelphia criteria" similarly sought to identify low-risk patients between 29 and 56 days old with temperatures of greater than or equal to 38.2°C. Patients who appeared to be *well* (as defined by an Infant Observation Score of ≤10) had a peripheral WBC count of less than or equal to 15,000/mm^3, a band-to-neutrophil ratio of less than or equal to 0.2, a UA with fewer than 10 WBC/hpf, few or no bacteria on a centrifuged urine specimen, CSF with fewer than 8 WBC/mm^3, a gram-negative stain, negative results on chest radiographs (obtained on all patients) and stool negative for blood and few or no WBCs on microscopy (ordered on those patients with watery diarrhea) were considered to have a negative screen and were not treated with antibiotics. Of the 747 consecutively enrolled patients, 65 (8.7%) had SBIs. All 65 patients who had SBIs were identified using these screening criteria. In a follow-up study of 422 consecutively enrolled febrile young infants (in which *fever* was defined as ≥38.0°C rectally), 43 (10%) had SBIs, and all 101 patients who were identified as low risk had no SBIs. All 43 patients who had SBIs were identified prospectively as high risk using the Philadelphia criteria.[43]

Evaluation

Neonates are difficult to assess clinically. In addition to fever, other findings seen with neonatal infections are frequently nonspecific and include increased sleepiness, increased crying and poor feeding. Physical examination findings may be similarly nonspecific and may include lethargy, irritability or poor tone. (Hypothermia can also be seen in neonates with bacterial infection.)

Because of the inability of the history and physical examination to accurately predict serious infections in neonates, ancillary testing is warranted. These patients need blood cultures, rapid urine testing (e.g., urine dipstick, standard UA or enhanced UA), urine cultures and CSF studies. A peripheral WBC count is often ordered in the evaluation of febrile neonates, but the discriminatory value of the WBC count is insufficient to differentiate between patients with SBIs and patients with nonbacterial infection.[44,45] Because of the inability of the WBC count

to predict bacteremia, blood cultures should be ordered on all patients.

Although various options for rapid testing for UTI exist (e.g., urine dipstick, standard UA and enhanced UA), no test detects all cases of UTI; therefore, urine cultures must be ordered in all of these patients.[46,47] Urine should be collected by bladder catheterization or suprapubic aspiration because bag urine specimens are associated with unacceptably high rates of contamination.[48–51] Because the peripheral WBC count is a poor screening test for meningitis,[52] a lumbar puncture (LP) should be performed in all febrile neonates, and the CSF should be sent for analysis and bacterial culture. CSF should also be sent for HSV testing if initial CSF studies are abnormal or if there is a concern for HSV infection. Chest radiographs are indicated only in the presence of respiratory symptoms, and stool analyses are indicated only in the presence of diarrhea. In neonates, the presence of signs suggestive of viral illness does not negate the need for a full diagnostic evaluation. Unlike older children, in whom documented respiratory syncytial virus (RSV) infections decrease the likelihood of SBI, RSV-infected neonates have the same rate of SBI compared with RSV-negative neonates.[53]

In children 1 to 2 months of age, relying solely on the clinical examination still results in a substantial number of missed SBIs; therefore, laboratory testing is also required in this age group. A catheterized urine specimen and blood and urine cultures should be obtained in all patients. Although an abnormally high or low WBC count increases the concern for bacteremia or meningitis, the WBC count is an imperfect screening tool and the decision to obtain blood cultures and spinal fluid should not depend on the results of the WBC.[44,45,52] Stool studies for WBC counts and stool cultures should be ordered in patients with diarrhea. Chest radiographs should be obtained only in young febrile infants with signs of pulmonary disease (tachypnea ≥50 breaths/minute, rales, rhonchi, retractions, wheezing, coryza, grunting, nasal flaring, cough or low pulse oximetry reading).[54,55]

The results of these tests help to risk-stratify these children 1 to 2 months of age. Using evidence from the Rochester, Boston and Philadelphia criteria, the WBC count is considered abnormal if the count is higher than 15,000/mm^3 or lower than 5000/mm^3 or if the band-to-neutrophil ratio is greater than 0.2. There should be fewer than 8 WBC/mm^3 and no organisms on Gram stain of the CSF. The urine is considered abnormal if the urine dipstick is positive for nitrite or leukocyte esterase, if there are greater than or equal to 5 WBC/hpf on microscopy or if organisms are seen on a Gram-stained sample of uncentrifuged urine. If obtained, there should be fewer than 5 WBC/hpf on the stool specimen and no evidence of pneumonia on chest x-ray.[5]

The need for LP is controversial in this age group. Although the Boston and Philadelphia criteria require CSF analysis, the Rochester criteria does not mandate LP. The rarity of bacterial meningitis contributes to the controversy surrounding the utility of the LP. However, the prevalence of bacterial meningitis in febrile infants younger than 3 months old is 4.1 per 1000 patients, and neither the clinical examination nor the peripheral WBC count is reliable in diagnosing meningitis in this age group.[44,52] Therefore, an LP should be strongly considered in febrile children between 1 and 2 months of age.

The presence of a documented viral infection lowers but does not eliminate the likelihood of SBIs in this age group. Young infants classified as high-risk patients using the Rochester criteria who had test-proven viral infection (enterovirus, respiratory virus, rotavirus and HSV) were at lower risk for SBI compared with patients who did not have an identified source (4.2% versus 12.3%).[56] A subgroup analysis of 187 febrile infants 28 to 60 days old from the largest prospective multicenter study of RSV infection in young infants showed a significantly lower rate of SBI in RSV-positive patients compared with RSV-negative patients (5.5% versus 11.7%),[53] confirming the results of similar studies in young infants who had bronchiolitis. Most of these bacterial infections were UTIs.[57,58] These studies were underpowered to detect differences in rates of bacteremia and meningitis between RSV-positive and RSV-negative patients, that is, based on available data, it remains unclear if the clinician can forgo blood and spinal fluid testing in RSV-positive infants. Patients younger than 90 days old who have enteroviral infections have a similar rate of concurrent SBIs (mostly UTIs) of 7%.[59]

Treatment and Disposition

Even with the help of laboratory testing, it is difficult to accurately predict which neonates have SBIs. Clinical prediction rules that are very accurate when applied to older infants miss a significant portion of neonates with SBIs, even when they meet "low risk" criteria.[35,60] Therefore, all febrile neonates should receive antibiotics and be admitted to the hospital. Typically, these patients are treated with a third-generation cephalosporin or

gentamicin. Ceftriaxone is not recommended for neonates who are jaundiced because of the concern of inducing unconjugated hyperbilirubinemia.[61,62] Other third-generation cephalosporins, such as cefotaxime, 50 mg/kg intravenously (IV) (100 mg/kg if there is a concern for meningitis based on CSF results), or gentamicin, 2.5 mg/kg IV, are used in this age group. Additionally, although the incidence of L. monocytogenes is quite low,[63] ampicillin, 50 mg/kg IV (100 mg/kg IV if there is a concern for meningitis) is still recommended in the empiric treatment of these patients[64]; ampicillin treats enterococcal infections as well. Acyclovir is not recommended routinely for empiric treatment in addition to standard antibiotics in febrile neonates[65] but should be considered in neonates with risk factors for neonatal HSV.

Screening laboratory tests sent from the ED do not detect all culture-proven infections, and neonates with bacterial infections are at high risk for serious complications. Therefore, hospitalization is mandatory for all febrile neonates, regardless of test results.

Most infants aged 1 to 2 months with FWS who are otherwise healthy and born at full-term and who are well appearing and have normal laboratory values can be managed on an outpatient basis. If the patient undergoes a reliable follow-up within 24 hours, the parents have a way of immediately accessing health care if there is a change in the patient's condition, and the parents and the primary care physician understand and agree with this plan of care, then the patient may be discharged home. Controversy surrounds the need for antibiotics in patients who are identified as low risk. Patients identified as low risk by the Philadelphia criteria were not given antibiotics, whereas patients enrolled in the Boston studies were given IM ceftriaxone, 50 mg/kg IV. Published recommendations state that parenteral antibiotics should be considered if an LP is performed.[5] Parenteral antibiotics should not be given if blood, urine and CSF cultures are not obtained. Patients who did not undergo LP in the ED should not receive antibiotics because this will confound the evaluation for meningitis if the patient is still febrile on follow-up examination. There is no role for presumptive treatment with oral antibiotics in the absence of a documented infection.

Infants between 1 and 2 months of age who have abnormal test results or who appear ill need antibiotics and should be hospitalized. Ceftriaxone, 50 mg/kg IM or IV (100 mg/kg if meningitis is suspected) is commonly used for these patients. Additional antibiotics should be considered in select circumstances (e.g., ampicillin or vancomycin for suspected infection by *Listeria*, gram-positive cocci or *Enterococcus*). Some studies suggest that patients in this age group who have UTIs may be treated on an outpatient basis[66,67]; however, there are no large prospective studies that provide evidence as to safety of outpatient management in this age range. Young infants who are RSV-positive are at higher risk of serious complications, such as apnea.[68] The clinician must evaluate this concern, in addition to the risks of SBI, and consider them when making a disposition decision.

APPROACH TO FEBRILE CHILDREN 2 MONTHS TO 1 YEAR OF AGE

Overview

A temperature of 38.0°C defines a *fever* and is the usual threshold at which diagnostic testing is initiated in the neonate and young infant. However, in febrile children 2 months of age and older, a temperature of 39.0°C is commonly used as the temperature for initiating further evaluation. This higher temperature cutoff is used because of the increasing risk of occult bacterial infections with increasing temperatures[18] and because large studies of occult bacteremia, widely referenced in the medical literature, use this temperature as the study entry criteria.[69–71]

Evaluation

Patient history is often helpful in this age group. Patients are more likely to have specific symptoms, and the physical examination is more informative. Clinical assessment as to whether a child appears to be well, ill or toxic is important and helps guide the assessment and treatment of these patients.[72] As stated earlier, a source for the fever, such as croup or stomatitis, often can be identified by history and physical examination alone. If no identifiable source for the fever can be found, then possible occult infections, such as bacteremia, UTIs and possibly pneumonia, should be considered. Selective diagnostic testing should be performed to identify these occult bacterial infections.

MOST COMMON INFECTIONS IN YOUNG CHILDREN

Occult Bacteremia

In the era before 7-valent pneumococcal conjugate vaccine (PCV7), the children at greatest risk for occult bacteremia

were 6 to 24 months old, and the most common pathogen was *Streptococcus pneumoniae*.[69,71] However, in the era of universal PCV7 vaccination, the overall incidence of pneumococcal bacteremia (and, accordingly, the total overall incidence of bacteremia) has dropped substantially. Maximum individual protection against the seven serotypes covered by this vaccine occurs after completion of the four-dose immunization regimen (the standard immunization regimen entails doses at age 2 months, 4 months, 6 months and 12–15 months).[73] However, declines in the rate of invasive disease occur even when the four-dose regimen is incomplete, and even one dose of PCV7 offers some protection.[74] Although similarly high rates of vaccine efficacy in protecting against serotype disease also were noted in two- and three-dose immunization regimens, one immunization with PCV7 in younger children provides only limited protection.[74,75] Among the seven serotypes, the amount of disease reduction is variable.[76–78] Furthermore, although the overall rate of invasive pneumococcal disease is declining, the rates of invasive disease caused by nonvaccine serotypes appear to be stable but may be increasing.[79–82]

The shifting epidemiology of bacteremia has prompted cost-effectiveness analyses of various testing strategies. This changing epidemiology has added to the confusion regarding the utility of blood testing in the identification of occult bacteremia. Although there is an increased risk of pneumococcal bacteremia with an increasing WBC count, the sensitivity and specificity of a WBC count greater than or equal to 15,000/mm³ is only 74% to 86% and 55% to 77%, respectively.[71,83–85] Similarly, patients with *E. coli* bacteremia were more likely to have elevated WBC counts when compared with control subjects without bacteremia. However, the WBC counts in patients with *Salmonella*,[85] *Staphylococcus aureus*[85] and *Neisseria meningitidis*[86] bacteremia do not differ from control patients without bacteremia. Using an elevated WBC count as a surrogate marker for occult bacteremia means that many patients will unnecessarily receive antibiotics, and a substantial number of patients with bacteremia will go untreated. Using pre-PCV7 data, Lee et al. analyzed five strategies for the 3- to 36-month-old febrile child who did not have an identifiable source of infection. In their sensitivity analysis, the authors found that when the prevalence rate of pneumococcal bacteremia dropped to 0.5% (essentially the current rate of pneumococcal bacteremia in EDs),[85,87–89] clinical judgment (e.g. patients who were deemed to be at low risk clinically for occult pneumococcal bacteremia received no testing or antibiotics) was the most cost-effective testing strategy.[90]

In addition to pneumococcus, another common cause of bacteremia is *E. coli*. *E. coli* bacteremia is more common in children younger than 12 months and is most common in children 3 to 6 months of age. *E. coli* bacteremia is commonly associated with a concomitant UTI,[91] and in one recent study, all 27 patients identified with *E. coli* bacteremia had UTIs.[85] *Salmonella* causes 4% to 8% of occult bacteremia, occurring in 0.1% of all children 3 to 36 months old who have temperatures higher than or equal to 39.0°C.[69–71,85] Although the majority of patients with *Salmonella* bacteremia have gastroenteritis, 5% will have primary bacteremia.[92] One large retrospective study of children with non–Typhi *Salmonella* bacteremia showed that 54% of bacteremic children had temperatures lower than 39.0°C (29% of patients were afebrile) and a median WBC count of 10,000/mm^3. These children had a 41% rate of persistent bacteremia on follow-up cultures, and the rates of persistent bacteremia were the same in patients who were treated with antibiotics at the initial visit and those who were not. Among immunocompetent patients, 2.5% of patients with *Salmonella* bacteremia had focal infections, and no differences in rates of focal infection were noted between children younger than 3 months of age and older children.[93]

Meningococcal infections are infrequent causes of bacteremia but are associated with high rates of morbidity and mortality.[94] *Neisseria meningitidis* is a leading cause of bacterial meningitis.[95] Combining the data from two large occult bacteremia studies, 0.02% of children who appeared to be nontoxic and had temperatures higher than or equal to 39.0°C had meningococcal disease.[69,71] Usually, these patients are overtly sick; however, 12% to 16% of patients with meningococcal disease have unsuspected bacteremia.[86,96] Although there is an association between younger age and elevated band count with meningococcal disease, routine screening for all young febrile children with CBCs for meningococcal bacteremia is not useful given the low prevalence of disease.[86] Patients who had unsuspected meningococcal disease who were treated empirically with antibiotics had fewer complications than patients who were untreated, but there were no differences in rates of permanent sequelae or death.[97] However, testing and empiric treatment may be warranted for children at higher risk for meningococcal disease. Risk factors for meningococcal bacteremia include

contact with patients with meningococcal disease, periods of meningococcal disease outbreaks and presence of fever and petechiae (although the majority of children with fever and petechiae do not have invasive bacterial disease).[98–100] A tetravalent meningococcal conjugate vaccine was licensed for use in the United States in 2005. Although clinical trials in infants and young children are in progress, this vaccine has been licensed and recommended for routine administration only in children 11 years old and older.[101]

The role of antibiotics in children believed to be at high risk for bacteremia is controversial as well. There is conflicting evidence demonstrating that the use of either oral or parenteral antibiotics prevents significant, adverse infectious sequelae in febrile children.[102,103] A meta-analysis has shown that although ceftriaxone prevents SBIs in patients with proven occult bacteremia, 284 patients at risk for bacteremia would need to be treated with antibiotics to prevent one case of meningitis.[104] Complicating this analysis is the fact that in a majority of patients with pneumococcal bacteremia, the bacteremia will resolve spontaneously,[69] and a minority of patients with bacteremia develop focal bacterial infections.[104,105] These analyses were conducted on data obtained in the pre-PCV7 era, and similar risk-benefit analyses have not been conducted after the introduction of PCV7. Nonetheless, it is clear that with the significant decrease in invasive pneumococcal disease,[82,106,107] many more children will be treated unnecessarily with antibiotics in order to prevent a single serious outcome. Furthermore, contaminated blood cultures are common, and in younger children, the rate of contaminated cultures frequently exceeds the rate of true positive cultures.[69,71,85,88,89,108]

Given the observed decline in invasive pneumococcal disease, the inconsistent relationship between height of fever and rates of bacteremia, the strong association between *E. coli* UTIs and *E. coli* bacteremia, the relative infrequency of meningococcemia and *Salmonella* bacteremia and the limited value of the WBC count in predicting the latter two diseases, the need for routine complete blood cell counts, blood cultures and empiric antibiotics has been called into question in fully immunized children.[85,89,109,110] If the clinician decides to obtain blood testing, the most important test is the blood culture, as this is the gold standard test for bacteremia. At best, the WBC is a limited screening tool and a relatively poor surrogate marker for bacteremia. It is reasonable to address parental preferences when devising an approach to these children because parental perceptions and preferences regarding risk may differ from those of the treating clinician.[111–113]

Children who have positive blood cultures need to be reexamined. A child with a positive blood culture with any pathogen who appears ill needs a repeat blood culture, LP, IV antibiotics and hospital admission. Because the rates of spontaneous clearance of pneumococcal bacteremia are high, patients with pneumococcal bacteremia who are afebrile on repeat evaluation can be followed on an outpatient basis[114] after repeat blood cultures are obtained and these patients are given antibiotics. Children who have pneumococcal bacteremia and who are persistently febrile need repeat blood cultures and generally should undergo LP and require hospital admission. The treatment and disposition for well-appearing children with *Salmonella* bacteremia are less clear, but patients with meningococcal bacteremia should be hospitalized for parenteral antibiotics.[84] A patient with an *E. coli* UTI who later grows *E. coli* in a blood culture needs a repeat assessment and blood culture, and strong consideration should be given to LP and admission.

Occult Urinary Tract Infection

UTIs are common sources of fever in young children, and children are at risk for permanent renal damage from UTIs. In older children, historical and examination features such as dysuria, urinary frequency, and abdominal and flank pain may suggest UTI. However, in young children, symptoms are usually nonspecific. Although the overall prevalence in children is 2% to 5%,[115–117] certain subgroups of children are at higher risk for UTIs. White race, female sex, uncircumcised boys, children with no alternative source of fever, and temperatures of 39.0°C or higher were associated with a higher risk of UTI; 16% of white girls younger than 2 years with temperatures 39.0°C or higher and FWS had UTIs.[116,117] UTIs were found in 2.7% to 3.5% of febrile children, even when there were other potential sources of fever (e.g., gastroenteritis, otitis media, upper respiratory tract infection and nonspecific rash).[116,117]

Gorelick et al. derived a clinical decision rule that has been subsequently validated for febrile girls with temperatures 38.3°C or higher who are younger than 24 months of age. Urine testing is indicated in girls who meet these criteria if two or more of the following risk factors are present[118]:

- Age less than 12 months
- Fever for 2 or more days
- Temperature 39.0°C or higher
- White race
- No alternative source of fever

This rule has a sensitivity of 95% to 99% and a false-positive rate of 69% to 90% in detecting UTIs in girls.[118,119] No similar clinical decision rules exist for boys, but because the prevalence in boys younger than 6 months old is 2.7%,[117] urine should be collected in all boys in this age group. The prevalence of UTIs in uncircumcised boys is eight to nine times higher than circumcised boys, so uncircumcised boys younger than 12 months old should also undergo urine testing.[117,120,121]

Several rapid urine tests have very good sensitivity for detecting UTIs. Enhanced UA ($\geq$10 WBC/hpf or bacteria on Gram stained, uncentrifuged urine)[46,122] or a combination of greater than or equal to 10 WBC/hpf and bacteriuria (on either centrifuged or uncentrifuged urine)[123] are both excellent screening tests. The more readily available urine dipstick (positive for either leukocyte esterase or nitrites) has a sensitivity of 88%.[46] Importantly, however, because no rapid screening test detects all UTIs, urine cultures should be ordered on all of these patients.[49] Any positive test results from a rapid test should lead to a presumptive diagnosis of a UTI, and antibiotic treatment should be initiated. Most patients with UTIs who appear well can be treated on an outpatient basis. Empiric antibiotic therapy should be tailored to local bacterial epidemiology, but reasonable outpatient medications include cefixime (8 mg/kg twice on the first day of treatment, then 8 mg/kg/day, starting on the second day) or cephalexin (25–100 mg/kg/day, divided into four doses). The duration of therapy should be from 7 to 14 days.

Occult Pneumonia

Young children commonly develop pneumonia, and the most common pathogens are viruses and (based on pre-PCV7 data) *S. pneumoniae*.[124] The diagnosis of pneumonia based on clinical examination can be difficult.[125] Multiple attempts have been made at deriving clinical decision rules for the accurate diagnosis of pneumonia, but none has been successfully validated.[126–128] The presence of any pulmonary findings on examination (e.g., tachypnea, crackles, respiratory distress or decreased breath sounds) increases the likelihood of pneumonia, and, conversely, the absence of these findings decreases the likelihood of pneumonia.[129–131] The role of pulse oximetry in detecting pneumonia is unclear,[132,133] and although the chest radiograph is often believed to be the gold standard, there is variability in the interpretation of radiographs even by pediatric radiologists.[134] Furthermore, radiographic findings cannot be used to distinguish reliably between bacterial and nonbacterial causes,[135,136] and there is some question as to whether chest x-rays affect the outcomes in children with symptoms of lower respiratory tract infections.[137]

Some cases of pneumonia are likely to be clinically occult. In the pre-PCV7 era, Bachur et al. found that 19% to 26% of children younger than 5 years old who had a temperature of 39.0°C or higher, a WBC count 20,000/mm^3 or higher, and no other source or only a "minor" bacterial source on examination had a pneumonia infection as seen on a chest radiograph.[138] However, a retrospective study at the same institution after universal PCV7 vaccination showed a 5% *occult* (i.e., no respiratory distress, no tachypnea or hypoxia and no lower respiratory tract abnormalities on examination) pneumonia rate in patients selected to receive chest radiographs.[139] A clinical policy by the American College of Emergency Physicians states that there is insufficient evidence to determine when a chest x-ray is required, but the clinician is advised to consider a chest x-ray in children older than 3 months who have a temperature 39°C or higher and a WBC count greater than or equal to 20,000/mm^3 and that a chest radiograph is usually not indicated in febrile children older than 3 months who have a temperature lower than 39°C without clinical evidence of acute pulmonary disease.[54] These recommendations may change based on the decline of the prevalence of pneumococcal pneumonia.[140] A chest x-ray should be obtained in all febrile children regardless of height of fever if there are physical examination findings suggestive of pneumonia such as tachypnea, increased work of breathing, asymmetric or abnormal breath sounds or hypoxia.

No decision rules exist that help with disposition decisions in children who have pneumonia, but the majority of patients are treated on an outpatient basis. Many different antibiotic regimens are acceptable.[141,142] Both amoxicillin (80 mg/kg/day divided three times daily) and macrolide antibiotics (e.g., azithromycin 10 mg/kg by mouth on the first day, then 5 mg/kg/day for 4 more days) are acceptable. Treatment duration is usually from 7 to 10 days (with the exception of azithromycin), but no definitive evidence supports a specific duration of therapy.[143]

OTHER SELECTED INFECTIONS IN YOUNG CHILDREN

Meningitis

Meningitis is the inflammation of the meninges covering the brain and spinal cord and is commonly caused by bacteria and viruses and, less frequently, fungi and parasites. Young children in particular are at higher risk for bacterial meningitis. Causes of meningitis vary by age. Neonates are most commonly infected with group B streptococcus, *E. coli* and *L. monocytogenes*. Neonates are also at risk for central nervous system infection with HSV. Children older than 2 months develop meningitis caused by *S. pneumoniae* and *Neisseria meningitidis*, and young infants between 1 and 2 months of age are commonly infected with both neonatal pathogens, and *S. pneumoniae* and *N. meningitidis*. Viral meningitis is most frequently caused by enteroviruses. Other causes of meningitis include tuberculosis and Lyme disease.

The diagnosis of meningitis can be difficult because the clinical findings in meningitis are frequently nonspecific. Caregivers may note that patients are irritable, lethargic, feeding poorly and vomiting. Children are frequently febrile and may paradoxically become more irritable when they are picked up. The fontanels may be bulging. Young children with meningitis usually do not have neck stiffness, Kernig or Brudzinski signs.

Blood testing is of some value in patients with suspected meningitis. Blood cultures should be obtained because the bacteria causing meningitis may be isolated. An abnormal peripheral WBC count is a poor screening test for meningitis and should not be used to decide whether an LP is indicated.[52] Meningitis may lead to a coagulopathic state, leading to abnormalities of platelets and elevated prothrombin or partial thromboplastin times. Meningitis can lead to the syndrome of inappropriate antidiuretic hormone secretion, so serum sodium levels should be measured.

A computed tomography (CT) scan of the head should be obtained only if the patient has signs of increased intracranial pressure, such as bulging fontanelle, cranial nerve palsy, abnormal pupils, papilledema, focal neurologic signs, obtundation or decorticate or decerebrate posturing.

The definitive study for detection of meningitis is the LP with CSF analysis. An elevated opening pressure (>20 cm H_2O) may be seen with meningitis but is difficult to accurately measure in young children. Glucose levels in the CSF should be one half to two thirds of the serum glucose, and a low CSF glucose level can be seen in meningitis. The CSF protein in children should be less than 40 mg/dL (neonates can have higher protein levels, up to 170 mg/dL).[144] Red blood cells should not be seen in normal CSF and suggest a traumatic LP or intracranial hemorrhage; an exception is hemorrhagic CSF seen with herpes infection. Some WBC counts may be seen in normal CSF, and the upper limit of normal depends on the infant's age. Neonates can have fewer than 22 WBC/mm^3 CSF, and older children can have fewer than 7 WBC/mm^3 CSF.[144] Rarely, in neonates and young infants, patients may have meningitis despite having a normal number of WBCs in the CSF.[145,146] CSF should be sent for Gram stain and culture. Additional testing should be considered as well. This includes polymerase chain reaction testing for HSV and enteroviruses, cryptococcal antigen and India ink staining for suspected cryptococcal meningitis and serology for Lyme disease or syphilis.

Patients with suspected meningitis need antibiotic therapy. Because the causative agent in patients with meningitis is frequently unknown until an organism is identified on CSF culture, broad-spectrum antibiotic therapy should be initiated until these results are known. Neonates should receive ampicillin (100 mg/kg IV) and cefotaxime (100 mg/kg IV) or gentamicin (2.5 mg/kg IV). Older children should receive ceftriaxone (100 mg/kg); vancomycin (15 mg/kg) should be considered as well when there is a concern for resistant strains of *S. pneumoniae*. When there is a significant delay in obtaining CSF (e.g., the patient needs to have a CT performed), blood cultures should be obtained and antibiotics should be given as soon as possible[147] with the understanding that administration of parenteral antibiotic therapy can rapidly sterilize the CSF, which can complicate making the diagnosis of bacterial meningitis.[148]

Dexamethasone (0.15 mg/kg IV every 6 hours for 2 days) may decrease the neurological sequelae, especially hearing loss, in children with *Haemophilus influenza*

type B meningitis if given immediately prior to, or simultaneously with, antibiotic therapy.[149] Dexamethasone may have some benefit in patients with pneumococcal meningitis as well.[150] The use of dexamethasone (0.15 mg/kg IV) in children with suspected pneumococcal meningitis can be considered.[151] If dexamethasone is given to a child with suspected pneumococcal meningitis, it should given immediately before or simultaneously with antibiotic therapy.[147] There are insufficient data to recommend the use of steroids in neonates with meningitis.

Children with CSF abnormalities have traditionally been admitted to the hospital awaiting CSF culture results, but some studies suggest that there are subsets of children with abnormal CSF who are at very low risk for bacterial infection who can be identified at the time of the ED visit.[95,152]

Herpes Simplex Virus Meningoencephalitis

Neonates with central nervous system HSV infection usually present during the second and third weeks of life. The most common risk factor for neonatal HSV infection is birth to an HSV-infected mother. This risk is highest with vaginal delivery in mothers with primary genital infection (women may not have the typical genital herpes lesions during periods of active infection, thus a maternal history of HSV infection may be absent). Other risk factors include prolonged rupture of membranes at delivery; the use of fetal scalp electrodes; skin, eye or mouth lesions; seizures (especially focal seizures); and CSF pleocytosis.[153–155] Neonates with HSV infection can present with temperature instability, changes in behavior and focal neurologic findings. Only a minority of infected children have fever,[65] and cutaneous manifestations are frequently absent. CSF results commonly reveal a pleocytosis, and red blood cells are often seen in the CSF as well. The diagnostic study of choice is HSV viral culture, although HSV PCR is an acceptable alternative. Treatment with acyclovir (20 mg/kg IV) should be started, and all patients with suspected HSV infection should be admitted to the hospital.

Bone and Joint Infections

Bone and joint infections in neonates and young children usually result from hematogenous seeding in patients with bacteremia, leading to osteomyelitis and septic arthritis. Bones and joints are at particular risk for infection in the setting of bacteremia because of the rich blood supply to these areas. Less commonly, these infections can also arise from direct inoculation of bone and joint spaces from trauma or surgery or from a contiguous infection. In patients with osteomyelitis, the pathogen bacterial typically travels into the metaphyseal capillaries, leading to localized inflammation. The rapidly growing ends of the femur and the tibia are the most commonly affected areas in osteomyelitis.[156] Septic arthritis typically starts with hematogenous infection of the vascular synovium, leading to an inflammatory response and rapid destruction of the articular cartilage. The hips and the knees are the most commonly affected septic joints.

Most bone and joint infections are caused by *S. aureus*.[157,158] Methicillin-resistant *S. aureus* (MRSA) is a more common pathogen than methicillin-sensitive *S. aureus* in some centers.[159,160] Group B streptococcus and gram-negative enteric bacteria also cause infection in neonates. Group A streptococcus[161] and *S. pneumoniae* are rarer causes of bone and joint infections.[162] *Salmonella* species are the most common pathogens causing infections in patients with sickle cell disease,[163] and *Pseudomonas aeruginosa* is the most frequent cause of osteomyelitis in patients hospitalized for puncture wounds of the foot.[164] Other pathogens include *Kingella kingae*[165] and *Borrelia burgdorferi*.[166] In many children with bone infections, a pathogen cannot be isolated on culture.[167]

Fever is commonly (but not uniformly) seen. Patients will often refuse to move the affected area, resulting in pseudoparalysis; children who are normally ambulatory may not want to walk because of pain. Patients with infected joints tend to keep these joints in positions that maximize the joint space (e.g., patients with septic hips tend to have their hips flexed, abducted and externally rotated). Swelling or redness may be seen overlying the affected bone or joint.

The WBC can be elevated with bone and joint infections but is frequently normal. The erythrocyte sedimentation rate and the C-reactive protein are more consistently elevated in bone and joint infections.[168,169] Blood cultures should be sent in children with suspected bone and joint infections.

Plain radiographs may be normal early in the course of osteomyelitis. Soft tissue changes may be seen in early osteomyelitis, but bony changes, such as elevation of the periosteum or lytic changes in the bone, may not be seen until 10 to 14 days into the course of the illness.[170] Nuclear bone scans are more sensitive in detecting osteomyelitis, but the best modality is magnetic resonance imaging. A bone biopsy may be needed for definitive diagnosis.

Patients with septic arthritis will develop joint effusions that may be seen on x-rays. Ultrasonography is useful in confirming the presence of a joint effusion but cannot be used to determine if the effusion is from a septic joint or from transient synovitis. The definitive diagnosis of septic arthritis is made by analysis of joint fluid, and joint aspiration can be both diagnostic and therapeutic.

Patients with suspected septic arthritis require rapid drainage, given the risks of complications with delayed diagnosis and treatment. Successful treatment of joint infection depends on timely joint decompression, and orthopedic consultation should occur early in the evaluation of these children.

Patients with bone and joint infections need IV antibiotic therapy. All children with suspected bone and joint infections need antibiotics to cover *S. aureus*. Because of the increasing prevalence of MRSA, empiric antibiotic therapy should include medicines directed at MRSA, such as clindamycin, vancomycin or trimethoprim-sulfamethoxazole. Furthermore, young infants (<2 months of age) need antibiotics to cover group B streptococci and *E. coli* (e.g. cefotaxime). Patients with osteomyelitis and septic arthritis should be admitted to the hospital.

FUTURE DIRECTIONS AND QUESTIONS

The pneumococcal vaccine has already had a significant impact on the epidemiology of bacterial infection in young children, and this vaccine already seems to have had some impact on physician practice patterns.[85,171] However, although the decline in invasive pneumococcal disease has been dramatic, the rise in nonvaccine serotype pneumococcal disease raises concerns.[79,172] Likewise, there is an increase in antibiotic resistance in nonvaccine serotype pneumococci.[81,173,174] Newer pneumococcal conjugate vaccines with increased serotype coverage are in development.[175]

Despite the use of the PCV7 vaccine, patients will still develop bacteremia, thus there is still a need for better tests to diagnose invasive bacterial disease. Several additional tests are being studied as potential surrogate markers for bacterial disease in young children: procalcitonin, C-reactive protein and interleukin-6.[176–184]

The role of rapid viral testing will likely continue to evolve as well. Rapid influenza testing may result in a decreased need for additional diagnostic testing[185]; febrile children between 3 and 36 months who are influenza A–positive are less likely to have SBIs than those children who are influenza A–negative.[186]

KEY POINTS

- Febrile neonates (rectal temperature ≥38.0°C) are at high risk for SBI and therefore need blood, urine, and CSF testing. These patients should receive empiric antibiotic therapy and be admitted to the hospital.
- Young infants (1–2 months) with fever also need blood, urine and CSF testing but may be discharged home if these tests are normal.
- A febrile child between 2 and 12 months of age may undergo more selective testing but may have infections that are not evident clinically, such as bacteremia, UTI or pneumonia.

REFERENCES

1. Nawar EW, Niska RW, Xu J. National Hospital Ambulatory Medical Care Survey: 2005 emergency department summary. *Adv Data.* 2007;(386):1–32.
2. Belfer RA, Gittelman MA, Muniz AE. Management of febrile infants and children by pediatric emergency medicine and emergency medicine: comparison with practice guidelines. *Pediatr Emerg Care.* 2001;17(2):83–87.
3. Isaacman DJ, Kaminer K, Veligeti H, et al. Comparative practice patterns of emergency medicine physicians and pediatric emergency medicine physicians managing fever in young children. *Pediatrics.* 2001;108(2):354–358.
4. Wittler RR, Cain KK, Bass JW. A survey about management of febrile children without source by primary care physicians. *Pediatr Infect Dis J.* 1998;17(4):271–277; discussion 7–9.
5. Baraff L. Management of fever without source in infants and children. *Ann Emerg Med.* 2000;36(6):602–614.
6. Steere M, Sharieff GQ, Stenklyft PH. Fever in children less than 36 months of age–questions and strategies for management in the emergency department. *J Emerg Med.* 2003;25(2):149–157.
7. Ishimine P. Fever without source in children 0 to 36 months of age. *Pediatr Clin N Am.* 2006;53:167–194.
8. Craig JV, Lancaster GA, Taylor S, Williamson PR, Smyth RL. Infrared ear thermometry compared with rectal thermometry in children: a systematic review. *Lancet.* 2002;360(9333):603–609.
9. Craig JV, Lancaster GA, Williamson PR, et al. Temperature measured at the axilla compared with rectum in children and young people: systematic review. *BMJ.* 2000;320(7243):1174–1178.
10. Greenes DS, Fleisher GR. When body temperature changes, does rectal temperature lag? *J Pediatr.* 2004;144(6):824.

11. Greenes DS, Fleisher GR. Accuracy of a noninvasive temporal artery thermometer for use in infants. *Arch Pediatr Adolesc Med.* 2001;155(3):376–381.
12. Jean-Mary MB, Dicanzio J, Shaw J, et al. Limited accuracy and reliability of infrared axillary and aural thermometers in a pediatric outpatient population. *J Pediatr.* 2002;141(5):671–676.
13. Grover G, Berkowitz CD, Thompson M, et al. The effects of bundling on infant temperature. *Pediatrics.* 1994;94(5):669–673.
14. Banco L, Veltri D. Ability of mothers to subjectively assess the presence of fever in their children. *Am J Dis Child.* 1984;138(10):976–978.
15. Graneto JW, Soglin DF. Maternal screening of childhood fever by palpation. *Pediatr Emerg Care.* 1996;12(3):183–184.
16. Hooker EA, Smith SW, Miles T, et al. Subjective assessment of fever by parents: comparison with measurement by noncontact tympanic thermometer and calibrated rectal glass mercury thermometer. *Ann Emerg Med.* 1996;28(3):313–317.
17. Pantell RH, Newman TB, Bernzweig J, et al. Management and outcomes of care of fever in early infancy. *JAMA.* 2004;291(10):1203–1212.
18. Kuppermann N, Fleisher G, Jaffe D. Predictors of occult pneumococcal bacteremia in young febrile children. *Ann Emerg Med.* 1998;31(6):679–687.
19. Stanley R, Pagon Z, Bachur R. Hyperpyrexia among infants younger than 3 months. *Pediatr Emerg Care.* 2005;21(5):291–294.
20. Trautner BW, Caviness AC, Gerlacher GR, et al. Prospective evaluation of the risk of serious bacterial infection in children who present to the emergency department with hyperpyrexia (temperature of 106°F or higher). *Pediatrics.* 2006;118(1):34–40.
21. Teach SJ, Fleisher GR. Duration of fever and its relationship to bacteremia in febrile outpatients three to 36 months old. The Occult Bacteremia Study Group. *Pediatr Emerg Care.* 1997;13(5):317–319.
22. Baker MD, Fosarelli PD, Carpenter RO. Childhood fever: correlation of diagnosis with temperature response to acetaminophen. *Pediatrics.* 1987;80(3):315–318.
23. Baker RC, Tiller T, Bausher JC, et al. Severity of disease correlated with fever reduction in febrile infants. *Pediatrics.* 1989;83(6):1016–1019.
24. Huang SY, Greenes DS. Effect of recent antipyretic use on measured fever in the pediatric emergency department. *Arch Pediatr Adolesc Med.* 2004;158(10):972–976.
25. Torrey SB, Henretig F, Fleisher G, et al. Temperature response to antipyretic therapy in children: relationship to occult bacteremia. *Am J Emerg Med.* 1985;3(3):190–192.
26. Yamamoto LT, Wigder HN, Fligner DJ, et al. Relationship of bacteremia to antipyretic therapy in febrile children. *Pediatr Emerg Care.* 1987;3(4):223–227.
27. Williams ER, Meza YE, Salazar S, et al. Immunization histories given by adult caregivers accompanying children 3–36 months to the emergency department: are their histories valid for the *Haemophilus influenzae B* and pneumococcal vaccines? *Pediatr Emerg Care.* 2007;23(5):285–288.

28. Bonadio WA. The history and physical assessments of the febrile infant. *Pediatr Clin North Am.* 1998;45(1):65–77.

29. Bonadio WA, Hennes H, Smith D, et al. Reliability of observation variables in distinguishing infectious outcome of febrile young infants. *Pediatr Infect Dis J.* 1993;12(2):111–114.

30. McCarthy PL, Lembo RM, Fink HD, et al. Observation, history, and physical examination in diagnosis of serious illnesses in febrile children less than or equal to 24 months. *J Pediatr.* 1987;110(1):26–30.

31. McCarthy PL, Lembo RM, Baron MA, et al. Predictive value of abnormal physical examination findings in ill-appearing and well-appearing febrile children. *Pediatrics.* 1985;76(2):167–171.

32. Greenes DS, Harper MB. Low risk of bacteremia in febrile children with recognizable viral syndromes. *Pediatr Infect Dis J.* 1999;18(3):258–261.

33. Baker MD, Bell LM. Unpredictability of serious bacterial illness in febrile infants from birth to 1 month of age. *Arch Pediatr Adolesc Med.* 1999;153(5):508–511.

34. Chiu CH, Lin TY, Bullard MJ. Identification of febrile neonates unlikely to have bacterial infections. *Pediatr Infect Dis J.* 1997;16(1):59–63.

35. Kadish HA, Loveridge B, Tobey J, et al. Applying outpatient protocols in febrile infants 1–28 days of age: can the threshold be lowered? *Clin Pediatr (Phila).* 2000;39(2):81–88.

36. Pena BM, Harper MB, Fleisher GR. Occult bacteremia with group B streptococci in an outpatient setting. *Pediatrics.* 1998;102(1 Pt 1):67–72.

37. Baker MD, Avner JR, Bell LM. Failure of infant observation scales in detecting serious illness in febrile, 4- to 8-week-old infants. *Pediatrics.* 1990;85(6):1040–1043.

38. DeAngelis C, Joffe A, Willis E, et al. Hospitalization v outpatient treatment of young, febrile infants. *Am J Dis Child.* 1983;137(12):1150–1152.

39. Dagan R, Powell KR, Hall CB, et al. Identification of infants unlikely to have serious bacterial infection although hospitalized for suspected sepsis. *J Pediatr.* 1985;107(6):855–860.

40. Dagan R, Sofer S, Phillip M, et al. Ambulatory care of febrile infants younger than 2 months of age classified as being at low risk for having serious bacterial infections. *J Pediatr.* 1988;112(3):355–360.

41. Jaskiewicz JA, McCarthy CA, Richardson AC, et al. Febrile infants at low risk for serious bacterial infection – an appraisal of the Rochester criteria and implications for management. *Pediatrics.* 1994;94(3):390–396.

42. Baskin MN, O'Rourke EJ, Fleisher GR. Outpatient treatment of febrile infants 28 to 89 days of age with intramuscular administration of ceftriaxone. *J Pediatr.* 1992;120(1):22–27.

43. Baker MD, Bell LM, Avner JR. The efficacy of routine outpatient management without antibiotics of fever in selected infants. *Pediatrics.* 1999;103(3):627–631.

44. Bonsu BK, Harper MB. A low peripheral blood white blood cell count in infants younger than 90 days increases the odds of acute bacterial meningitis relative to bacteremia. *Acad Emerg Med.* 2004;11(12):1297–1301.

45. Bonsu BK, Harper MB. Identifying febrile young infants with bacteremia: is the peripheral white blood cell count an accurate screen? *Ann Emerg Med.* 2003;42(2):216–225.

46. Gorelick MH, Shaw KN. Screening tests for urinary tract infection in children: a meta-analysis. *Pediatrics.* 1999;104(5):e54.

47. Shaw KN, McGowan KL, Gorelick MH, et al. Screening for urinary tract infection in infants in the emergency department: which test is best? *Pediatrics.* 1998;101(6):e1.

48. Al-Orifi F, McGillivray D, Tange S, et al. Urine culture from bag specimens in young children: are the risks too high? *J Pediatr.* 2000;137(2):221–226.

49. Committee on Quality Improvement, Subcommittee on Urinary Tract Infection. Practice parameter: the diagnosis, treatment, and evaluation of the initial urinary tract infection in febrile infants and young children. *Pediatrics.* 1999;103(4):843–852.

50. McGillivray D, Mok E, Mulrooney E, et al. A head-to-head comparison: "clean-void" bag versus catheter urinalysis in the diagnosis of urinary tract infection in young children. *J Pediatr.* 2005;147(4):451–456.

51. Schroeder AR, Newman TB, Wasserman RC, et al. Choice of urine collection methods for the diagnosis of urinary tract infection in young, febrile infants. *Arch Pediatr Adolesc Med.* 2005;159(10):915–922.

52. Bonsu BK, Harper MB. Utility of the peripheral blood white blood cell count for identifying sick young infants who need lumbar puncture. *Ann Emerg Med.* 2003;41(2):206–214.

53. Levine DA, Platt SL, Dayan PS, et al. Risk of serious bacterial infection in young febrile infants with respiratory syncytial virus infections. *Pediatrics.* 2004;113(6):1728–1734.

54. Clinical policy for children younger than three years presenting to the emergency department with fever. *Ann Emerg Med.* 2003;42(4):530–545.

55. Bramson RT, Meyer TL, Silbiger ML, et al. The futility of the chest radiograph in the febrile infant without respiratory symptoms. *Pediatrics.* 1993;92(4):524–526.

56. Byington CL, Enriquez FR, Hoff C, et al. Serious bacterial infections in febrile infants 1 to 90 days old with and without viral infections. *Pediatrics.* 2004;113(6):1662–1666.

57. Liebelt EL, Qi K, Harvey K. Diagnostic testing for serious bacterial infections in infants aged 90 days or younger with bronchiolitis. *Arch Pediatr Adolesc Med.* 1999;153(5):525–530.

58. Titus MO, Wright SW. Prevalence of serious bacterial infections in febrile infants with respiratory syncytial virus infection. *Pediatrics.* 2003;112(2):282–284.

59. Rittichier KR, Bryan PA, Bassett KE, et al. Diagnosis and outcomes of enterovirus infections in young infants. *Pediatr Infect Dis J.* 2005;24(6):546–550.

60. Ferrera PC, Bartfield JM, Snyder HS. Neonatal fever: utility of the Rochester criteria in determining low risk for serious bacterial infections. *Am J Emerg Med.* 1997;15(3):299–302.

61. Martin E, Fanconi S, Kalin P, et al. Ceftriaxone – bilirubin-albumin interactions in the neonate: an in vivo study. *Eur J Pediatr.* 1993;152(6):530–534.

62. Robertson A, Fink S, Karp W. Effect of cephalosporins on bilirubin-albumin binding. *J Pediatr.* 1988;112(2):291–294.

63. Sadow KB, Derr R, Teach SJ. Bacterial infections in infants 60 days and younger: epidemiology, resistance, and implications for treatment. *Arch Pediatr Adolesc Med.* 1999;153(6):611–614.

64. Brown JC, Burns JL, Cummings P. Ampicillin use in infant fever: a systematic review. *Arch Pediatr Adolesc Med.* 2002;156(1):27–32.

65. Kimberlin DW, Lin CY, Jacobs RF, et al. Natural history of neonatal herpes simplex virus infections in the acyclovir era. *Pediatrics.* 2001;108(2):223–229.

66. Dayan PS, Hanson E, Bennett JE, et al. Clinical course of urinary tract infections in infants younger than 60 days of age. *Pediatr Emerg Care.* 2004;20(2):85–88.

67. Hoberman A, Wald ER, Hickey RW, et al. Oral versus initial intravenous therapy for urinary tract infections in young febrile children. *Pediatrics.* 1999;104(1 Pt 1):79–86.

68. American Academy of Pediatrics Subcommittee on the Diagnosis and Management of Bronchiolitis. Diagnosis and management of bronchiolitis. *Pediatrics.* 2006;118(4):1774–1793.

69. Alpern ER, Alessandrini EA, Bell LM, et al. Occult bacteremia from a pediatric emergency department: current prevalence, time to detection, and outcome. *Pediatrics.* 2000;106(3):505–511.

70. Fleisher GR, Rosenberg N, Vinci R, et al. Intramuscular versus oral antibiotic therapy for the prevention of meningitis and other bacterial sequelae in young, febrile children at risk for occult bacteremia. *J Pediatr.* 1994;124(4):504–512.

71. Lee GM, Harper MB. Risk of bacteremia for febrile young children in the post-*Haemophilus influenzae* type b era. *Arch Pediatr Adolesc Med.* 1998;152(7):624–628.

72. Bergman DA, Mayer ML, Pantell RH, et al. Does clinical presentation explain practice variability in the treatment of febrile infants? *Pediatrics.* 2006;117(3):787–795.

73. CDC. Recommended immunization schedules for persons aged 0–18 years – United States, 2007. *MMWR.* 2006;55(51 & 52):Q1–Q4.

74. Whitney CG, Pilishvili T, Farley MM, et al. Effectiveness of seven-valent pneumococcal conjugate vaccine against invasive pneumococcal disease: a matched case-control study. *Lancet.* 2006;368(9546):1495–1502.

75. Mahon BE, Hsu K, Karumuri S, et al. Effectiveness of abbreviated and delayed 7-valent pneumococcal conjugate vaccine dosing regimens. *Vaccine.* 2006;24(14):2514–2520.

76. Hsu K, Pelton S, Karumuri S, et al. Population-based surveillance for childhood invasive pneumococcal disease in the era of conjugate vaccine. *Pediatr Infect Dis J.* 2005;24(1):17–23.

77. Kaplan SL, Mason EO Jr, Wald E, et al. Six year multicenter surveillance of invasive pneumococcal infections in children. *Pediatr Infect Dis J.* 2002;21(2):141–147.

78. Whitney CG, Farley MM, Hadler J, et al. Decline in invasive pneumococcal disease after the introduction of protein-polysaccharide conjugate vaccine. *N Engl J Med.* 2003;348(18):1737–1746.

79. Kyaw MH, Lynfield R, Schaffner W, et al. Effect of introduction of the pneumococcal conjugate vaccine on drug-resistant *Streptococcus pneumoniae. N Engl J Med.* 2006;354(14):1455–1463.

80. Singleton RJ, Hennessy TW, Bulkow LR, et al. Invasive pneumococcal disease caused by nonvaccine serotypes among Alaska native children with high levels of 7-valent pneumococcal conjugate vaccine coverage. *JAMA.* 2007;297(16):1784–1792.

81. Steenhoff AP, Shah SS, Ratner AJ, et al. Emergence of vaccine-related pneumococcal serotypes as a cause of bacteremia. *Clin Infect Dis.* 2006;42(7):907–914.

82. Poehling KA, Talbot TR, Griffin MR, et al. Invasive pneumococcal disease among infants before and after introduction of pneumococcal conjugate vaccine. *JAMA.* 2006;295(14):1668–1674.

83. Bass JW, Steele RW, Wittler RR, et al. Antimicrobial treatment of occult bacteremia: a multicenter cooperative study. *Pediatr Infect Dis J.* 1993;12(6):466–473.

84. Kuppermann N. Occult bacteremia in young febrile children. *Pediatr Clin North Am.* 1999;46(6):1073–1109.

85. Herz AM, Greenhow TL, Alcantara J, et al. Changing epidemiology of outpatient bacteremia in 3- to 36-month-old children after the introduction of the heptavalent-conjugated pneumococcal vaccine. *Pediatr Infect Dis J.* 2006;25(4):293–300.

86. Kuppermann N, Malley R, Inkelis SH, et al. Clinical and hematologic features do not reliably identify children with unsuspected meningococcal disease. *Pediatrics.* 1999;103(2):E20.

87. Carstairs KL, Tanen DA, Johnson AS, et al. Pneumococcal bacteremia in febrile infants presenting to the emergency department before and after the introduction of the heptavalent pneumococcal vaccine. *Ann Emerg Med.* 2007.

88. Sard B, Bailey MC, Vinci R. An analysis of pediatric blood cultures in the postpneumococcal conjugate vaccine era in a community hospital emergency department. *Pediatr Emerg Care.* 2006;22(5):295–300.

89. Stoll ML, Rubin LG. Incidence of occult bacteremia among highly febrile young children in the era of the pneumococcal conjugate vaccine: a study from a children's hospital emergency department and urgent care center. *Arch Pediatr Adolesc Med.* 2004;158(7):671–675.

90. Lee GM, Fleisher GR, Harper MB. Management of febrile children in the age of the conjugate pneumococcal vaccine: a cost-effectiveness analysis. *Pediatrics.* 2001;108(4):835–844.

91. Bonadio WA, Smith DS, Madagame E, et al. *Escherichia coli* bacteremia in children. A review of 91 cases in 10 years. *Am J Dis Child.* 1991;145(6):671–674.

92. Yang YJ, Huang MC, Wang SM, et al. Analysis of risk factors for bacteremia in children with nontyphoidal *Salmonella* gastroenteritis. *Eur J Clin Microbiol Infect Dis.* 2002;21(4):290–293.

93. Zaidi E, Bachur R, Harper M. Non–typhi *Salmonella bacteremia* in children. *Pediatr Infect Dis J.* 1999;18(12):1073–1077.

94. Kaplan SL, Schutze GE, Leake JA, et al. Multicenter surveillance of invasive meningococcal infections in children. *Pediatrics.* 2006;118(4):e979–984.

95. Nigrovic LE, Kuppermann N, Macias CG, et al. Clinical prediction rule for identifying children with cerebrospinal

fluid pleocytosis at very low risk of bacterial meningitis. *JAMA.* 2007;297(1):52–60.

96. Wang VJ, Kuppermann N, Malley R, et al. Meningococcal disease among children who live in a large metropolitan area, 1981–1996. *Clin Infect Dis.* 2001;32(7):1004–1009.

97. Wang VJ, Malley R, Fleisher GR, et al. Antibiotic treatment of children with unsuspected meningococcal disease. *Arch Pediatr Adolesc Med.* 2000;154(6):556–560.

98. Mandl K, Stack A, Fleisher G. Incidence of bacteremia in infants and children with fever and petechiae. *J Pediatr.* 1997;131(3):398.

99. Nelson DG, Leake J, Bradley J, Kuppermann N. Evaluation of febrile children with petechial rashes: is there consensus among pediatricians? *Pediatr Infect Dis J.* 1998;17(12):1135–1140.

100. Wells LC, Smith JC, Weston VC, et al. The child with a non-blanching rash: how likely is meningococcal disease? *Arch Dis Child.* 2001;85(3):218–222.

101. Committee on Infectious D. Prevention and control of meningococcal disease: recommendations for use of meningococcal vaccines in pediatric patients. *Pediatrics.* 2005;116(2):496–505.

102. Jaffe DM, Tanz RR, Davis AT, et al. Antibiotic administration to treat possible occult bacteremia in febrile children. *N Engl J Med.* 1987;317(19):1175–1180.

103. Harper MB, Bachur R, Fleisher GR. Effect of antibiotic therapy on the outcome of outpatients with unsuspected bacteremia. *Pediatr Infect Dis J.* 1995;14(9):760–767.

104. Bulloch B, Craig WR, Klassen TP. The use of antibiotics to prevent serious sequelae in children at risk for occult bacteremia: a meta-analysis. *Acad Emerg Med.* 1997;4(7):679–683.

105. Baraff LJ, Oslund S, Prather M. Effect of antibiotic therapy and etiologic microorganism on the risk of bacterial meningitis in children with occult bacteremia. *Pediatrics.* 1993;92(1):140–143.

106. Haddy RI, Perry K, Chacko CE, et al. Comparison of incidence of invasive *Streptococcus pneumoniae* disease among children before and after introduction of conjugated pneumococcal vaccine. *Pediatr Infect Dis J.* 2005;24(4):320–323.

107. Black S, Shinefield H, Baxter R, et al. Postlicensure surveillance for pneumococcal invasive disease after use of heptavalent pneumococcal conjugate vaccine in Northern California Kaiser Permanente. *Pediatr Infect Dis J.* 2004;23(6):485–489.

108. Bandyopadhyay S, Bergholte J, Blackwell CD, et al. Risk of serious bacterial infection in children with fever without a source in the post-*Haemophilus influenzae* era when antibiotics are reserved for culture-proven bacteremia. *Arch Pediatr Adolesc Med.* 2002;156(5):512–517.

109. Baraff LJ. Clinical policy for children younger than three years presenting to the emergency department with fever [editorial]. *Ann Emerg Med.* 2003;42(4):546–549.

110. Kuppermann N. The evaluation of young febrile children for occult bacteremia: time to reevaluate our approach? *Arch Pediatr Adolesc Med.* 2002;156(9):855–857.

111. Madsen KA, Bennett JE, Downs SM. The role of parental preferences in the management of fever without source among 3- to 36-month-old children: a decision analysis. *Pediatrics.* 2006;117(4):1067–1076.

112. Bennett JE, Sumner IW, Downs SM, et al. Parents' utilities for outcomes of occult bacteremia. *Arch Pediatr Adolesc Med.* 2000;154(1):43–48.

113. Oppenheim PI, Sotiropoulos G, Baraff LJ. Incorporating patient preferences into practice guidelines: management of children with fever without source. *Ann Emerg Med.* 1994;24(5):836–841.

114. Bachur R, Harper MB. Reevaluation of outpatients with *Streptococcus pneumoniae* bacteremia. *Pediatrics.* 2000;105(3 Pt 1):502–509.

115. Bachur R, Harper MB. Reliability of the urinalysis for predicting urinary tract infections in young febrile children. *Arch Pediatr Adolesc Med.* 2001;155(1):60–65.

116. Hoberman A, Chao HP, Keller DM, et al. Prevalence of urinary tract infection in febrile infants. *J Pediatr.* 1993;123(1):17–23.

117. Shaw KN, Gorelick M, McGowan KL, et al. Prevalence of urinary tract infection in febrile young children in the emergency department. *Pediatrics.* 1998;102(2):e16.

118. Gorelick MH, Shaw KN. Clinical decision rule to identify febrile young girls at risk for urinary tract infection. *Arch Pediatr Adolesc Med.* 2000;154(4):386–390.

119. Gorelick MH, Hoberman A, Kearney D, et al. Validation of a decision rule identifying febrile young girls at high risk for urinary tract infection. *Pediatr Emerg Care.* 2003;19(3):162–164.

120. Schoen EJ, Colby CJ, Ray GT. Newborn circumcision decreases incidence and costs of urinary tract infections during the first year of life. *Pediatrics.* 2000;105(4 Pt 1):789–793.

121. Task Force on C. *Circumcision Policy Statement. Pediatrics.* 1999;103(3):686–693.

122. Zorc JJ, Kiddoo DA, Shaw KN. Diagnosis and management of pediatric urinary tract infections. *Clin Microbiol Rev.* 2005;18(2):417–422.

123. Huicho L, Campos-Sanchez M, Alamo C. Metaanalysis of urine screening tests for determining the risk of urinary tract infection in children. *Pediatr Infect Dis J.* 2002;21(1):1–11, 88.

124. Wubbel L, Muniz L, Ahmed A, et al. Etiology and treatment of community-acquired pneumonia in ambulatory children. *Pediatr Infect Dis J.* 1999;18(2):98–104.

125. Margolis P, Gadomski A. Does this infant have pneumonia? *JAMA.* 1998;279(4):308–313.

126. Jadavji T, Law B, Lebel MH, et al. A practical guide for the diagnosis and treatment of pediatric pneumonia. *CMAJ.* 1997;156(5):S703–711.

127. Lynch T, Platt R, Gouin S, et al. Can we predict which children with clinically suspected pneumonia will have the presence of focal infiltrates on chest radiographs? *Pediatrics,* 2004;113(3 Pt 1):e186–189.

128. Rothrock SG, Green SM, Fanelli JM, et al. Do published guidelines predict pneumonia in children presenting to an urban ED? *Pediatr Emerg Care.* 2001;17(4):240–243.

129. Leventhal JM. Clinical predictors of pneumonia as a guide to ordering chest roentgenograms. *Clin Pediatr (Phila).* 1982;21(12):730–734.

130. Taylor JA, Del Beccaro M, Done S, et al. Establishing clinically relevant standards for tachypnea in febrile children younger than 2 years. *Arch Pediatr Adolesc Med.* 1995;149(3):283–287.

131. Zukin DD, Hoffman JR, Cleveland RH, et al. Correlation of pulmonary signs and symptoms with chest radiographs in the pediatric age group. *Ann Emerg Med.* 1986;15(7):792–796.

132. Mower WR, Sachs C, Nicklin EL, et al. Pulse oximetry as a fifth pediatric vital sign. *Pediatrics.* 1997;99(5):681–686.

133. Tanen DA, Trocinski DR. The use of pulse oximetry to exclude pneumonia in children. *Am J Emerg Med.* 2002;20(6):521–523.

134. Davies HD, Wang EE, Manson D, et al. Reliability of the chest radiograph in the diagnosis of lower respiratory infections in young children. *Pediatr Infect Dis J.* 1996;15(7):600–604.

135. Courtoy I, Lande AE, Turner RB. Accuracy of radiographic differentiation of bacterial from nonbacterial pneumonia. *Clin Pediatr (Phila).* 1989;28(6):261–264.

136. McCarthy PL, Spiesel SZ, Stashwick CA, et al. Radiographic findings and etiologic diagnosis in ambulatory childhood pneumonias. *Clin Pediatr (Phila).* 1981;20(11):686–691.

137. Swingler GH, Zwarenstein M. Chest radiograph in acute respiratory infections in children. *Cochrane Database Syst Rev.* 2005;(3):CD001268.

138. Bachur R, Perry H, Harper MB. Occult pneumonias: empiric chest radiographs in febrile children with leukocytosis. *Ann Emerg Med.* 1999;33(2):166–173.

139. Murphy CG, van de Pol AC, Harper MB, et al. Clinical predictors of occult pneumonia in the febrile child. *Acad Emerg Med.* 2007;14(3):243–249.

140. Black SB, Shinefield HR, Ling S, et al. Effectiveness of heptavalent pneumococcal conjugate vaccine in children younger than five years of age for prevention of pneumonia. *Pediatr Infect Dis J.* 2002;21(9):810–815.

141. Kabra SK, Lodha R, Pandey RM. Antibiotics for community acquired pneumonia in children. *Cochrane Database Syst Rev.* 2006;3:CD004874.

142. Rojas MX, Granados C. Oral antibiotics versus parenteral antibiotics for severe pneumonia in children. *Cochrane Database Syst Rev.* 2006;(2):CD004979.

143. British Thoracic Society of Standards of Care C. BTS guidelines for the management of community acquired pneumonia in childhood. *Thorax.* 2002;57(90001):1i-24.

144. Robertson J. Body chemistries and body fluids. In: Robertson JSN, ed. The *Harriet Lane Handbook: A Manual for Pediatric House Officers.* Philadelphia, PA: Elsevier; 2005.

145. Bonsu BK, Harper MB. Accuracy and test characteristics of ancillary tests of cerebrospinal fluid for predicting acute bacterial meningitis in children with low white blood cell counts in cerebrospinal fluid. *Acad Emerg Med.* 2005;12(4):303–309.

146. Garges HP, Moody MA, Cotten CM, et al. Neonatal meningitis: what is the correlation among cerebrospinal fluid cultures, blood cultures, and cerebrospinal fluid parameters? *Pediatrics.* 2006;117(4):1094–1100.

147. Tunkel AR, Hartman BJ, Kaplan SL, et al. Practice guidelines for the management of bacterial meningitis. *Clin Infect Dis.* 2004;39(9):1267–1284.

148. Kanegaye JT, Soliemanzadeh P, Bradley JS. Lumbar puncture in pediatric bacterial meningitis: defining the time interval for recovery of cerebrospinal fluid pathogens after parenteral antibiotic pretreatment. *Pediatrics.* 2001;108(5):1169–1174.

149. McIntyre PB, Berkey CS, King SM, et al. Dexamethasone as adjunctive therapy in bacterial meningitis. A meta-analysis of randomized clinical trials since 1988. *JAMA.* 1997;278(11):925–931.

150. van de Beek D, de Gans J, McIntyre P, et al. Corticosteroids for acute bacterial meningitis. *Cochrane Database Syst Rev.* 2007;(1):CD004405.

151. American Academy of Pediatrics. Pneumococcal infections. In: *Red Book: 2006 Report of the Committee on Infectious Diseases,* 27 ed. Elk Grove Village, IL: American Academy of Pediatrics; 2006:525–537.

152. Bonsu BK, Harper MB. Differentiating acute bacterial meningitis from acute viral meningitis among children with cerebrospinal fluid pleocytosis: a multivariable regression model. *Pediatr Infect Dis J.* 2004;23(6):511–517.

153. Brown ZA, Wald A, Morrow RA, et al. Effect of serologic status and cesarean delivery on transmission rates of herpes simplex virus from mother to infant. *JAMA.* 2003;289(2):203–209.

154. Kimberlin D. Herpes simplex virus, meningitis and encephalitis in neonates. *Herpes.* 2004;11(Suppl 2):65A–76A.

155. Kimberlin DW. Neonatal herpes simplex infection. *Clin Microbiol Rev.* 2004;17(1):1–13.

156. Caksen H, Ozturk MK, Uzum K, et al. Septic arthritis in childhood. *Pediatr Int.* 2000;42(5):534–540.

157. Wang CL, Wang SM, Yang YJ, et al. Septic arthritis in children: relationship of causative pathogens, complications, and outcome. *J Microbiol Immunol Infect.* 2003;36(1):41–46.

158. Yuan HC, Wu KG, Chen CJ, et al. Characteristics and outcome of septic arthritis in children. *J Microbiol Immunol Infect.* 2006;39(4):342–347.

159. Martinez-Aguilar G, Avalos-Mishaan A, Hulten K, et al. Community-acquired, methicillin-resistant and methicillin-susceptible *Staphylococcus aureus* musculoskeletal infections in children. *Pediatr Infect Dis J.* 2004;23(8):701–706.

160. Arnold SR, Elias D, Buckingham SC, et al. Changing patterns of acute hematogenous osteomyelitis and septic arthritis: emergence of community-associated methicillin-resistant *Staphylococcus aureus. J Pediatr Orthop.* 2006;26(6):703–708.

161. Ibia EO, Imoisili M, Pikis A. Group A beta-hemolytic streptococcal osteomyelitis in children. *Pediatrics.* 2003;112(1 Pt 1):e22–26.

162. Bradley JS, Kaplan SL, Tan TQ, et al. Pediatric pneumococcal bone and joint infections. *Pediatrics.* 1998;102(6):1376–1382.

163. Burnett MW, Bass JW, Cook BA. Etiology of osteomyelitis complicating sickle cell disease. *Pediatrics.* 1998;101(2):296–297.

164. Laughlin TJ, Armstrong DG, Caporusso J, et al. Soft tissue and bone infections from puncture wounds in children. *West J Med.* 1997;166(2):126–128.

165. Kiang KM, Ogunmodede F, Juni BA, et al. Outbreak of osteomyelitis/septic arthritis caused by *Kingella kingae* among child care center attendees. *Pediatrics.* 2005;116(2): e206–213.

166. Gerber MA, Zemel LS, Shapiro ED. Lyme arthritis in children: clinical epidemiology and long-term outcomes. *Pediatrics.* 1998;102(4):905–908.

167. Floyed RL, Steele RW. Culture-negative osteomyelitis. *Pediatr Infect Dis J.* 2003;22(8):731–736.

168. Unkila-Kallio L, Kallio MJT, Peltola H, et al. Serum C-reactive protein, erythrocyte sedimentation rate, and white blood cell count in acute hematogenous osteomyelitis of children. *Pediatrics.* 1994;93(1):59–62.

169. Khachatourians AG, Patzakis MJ, Roidis N, et al. Laboratory monitoring in pediatric acute osteomyelitis and septic arthritis. *Clin Orthop Relat Res.* 2003(409):186–194.

170. Blickman JG, van Die CE, de Rooy JW. Current imaging concepts in pediatric osteomyelitis. *Eur Radiol.* 2004;14(Suppl 4):L55–64.

171. Lee KC, Finkelstein JA, Miroshnik IL, et al. Pediatricians' self-reported clinical practices and adherence to national immunization guidelines after the introduction of pneumococcal conjugate vaccine. *Arch Pediatr Adolesc Med.* 2004;158(7):695–701.

172. Peters TR, Poehling KA. Invasive pneumococcal disease: the target is moving. *JAMA.* 2007;297(16):1825–1826.

173. Farrell DJ, Klugman KP, Pichichero M. Increased antimicrobial resistance among nonvaccine serotypes of *Streptococcus pneumoniae* in the pediatric population after the introduction of 7-valent pneumococcal vaccine in the United States. *Pediatr Infect Dis J.* 2007;26(2):123–128.

174. Kaplan SL, Mason EO Jr, Wald ER, et al. Decrease of invasive pneumococcal infections in children among 8 children's hospitals in the United States after the introduction of the 7-valent pneumococcal conjugate vaccine. *Pediatrics.* 2004;113(3):443–449.

175. Oosterhuis-Kafeja F, Beutels P, Van Damme P. Immunogenicity, efficacy, safety and effectiveness of pneumococcal conjugate vaccines (1998–2006). *Vaccine.* 2007;25(12): 2194–2212.

176. Carrol ED, Newland P, Riordan FA, et al. Procalcitonin as a diagnostic marker of meningococcal disease in children presenting with fever and a rash. *Arch Dis Child.* 2002;86(4):282–285.

177. Fernandez Lopez A, Luaces Cubells C, Garcia Garcia JJ, et al. Procalcitonin in pediatric emergency departments for the early diagnosis of invasive bacterial infections in febrile infants: results of a multicenter study and utility of a rapid qualitative test for this marker. *Pediatr Infect Dis J.* 2003;22(10):895–903.

178. Galetto-Lacour A, Zamora SA, Gervaix A. Bedside procalcitonin and C-reactive protein tests in children with fever without localizing signs of infection seen in a referral center. *Pediatrics.* 2003;112(5):1054–1060.

179. Gendrel D, Raymond J, Coste J, et al. Comparison of procalcitonin with C-reactive protein, interleukin 6 and interferon-alpha for differentiation of bacterial vs. viral infections. *Pediatr Infect Dis J.* 1999;18(10):875–881.

180. Hsiao AL, Baker MD. Fever in the new millennium: a review of recent studies of markers of serious bacterial infection in febrile children. *Curr Opin Pediatr.* 2005;17(1):56–61.

181. Isaacman DJ, Burke BL. Utility of the serum C-reactive protein for detection of occult bacterial infection in children. *Arch Pediatr Adolesc Med.* 2002;156(9):905–909.

182. Pulliam PN, Attia MW, Cronan KM. C-reactive protein in febrile children 1 to 36 months of age with clinically undetectable serious bacterial infection. *Pediatrics.* 2001;108(6):1275–1279.

183. van Rossum AM, Wulkan RW, Oudesluys-Murphy AM. Procalcitonin as an early marker of infection in neonates and children. *Lancet Infect Dis.* 2004;4(10):620–630.

184. Hsiao AL, Chen L, Baker MD. Incidence and predictors of serious bacterial infections among 57- to 180-day-old infants. *Pediatrics.* 2006;117(5):1695–1701.

185. Abanses JC, Dowd MD, Simon SD, et al. Impact of rapid influenza testing at triage on management of febrile infants and young children. *Pediatr Emerg Care.* 2006;22(3):145–149.

186. Smitherman HF, Caviness AC, Macias CG. Retrospective review of serious bacterial infections in infants who are 0 to 36 months of age and have influenza A infection. *Pediatrics.* 2005;115(3):710–718.

Head and Neck Emergencies

Joyce C. Arpilleda

INTRODUCTION

Head and neck lesions are commonly encountered in children. A painless mass present at birth or shortly thereafter is consistent with a congenital lesion. Congenital lesions are common and include branchial cleft anomalies; cystic hygromas; hemangiomas; preauricular pits, sinuses, and cysts; and neonatal torticollis. Table 12.1 lists the common characteristics that are associated with congenital neck cysts. Unlike adults, most head and neck lesions in children are benign. History taking should include changes in the size of the mass over time with a child's growth. Most large neck masses grow laterally. However, emergencies can occur if neck masses compromise the airway or blood vessels.

The initial evaluation should rapidly assess airway, breathing or vascular compromise and level of consciousness. Drooling, hoarseness or stridor implies the presence of respiratory compromise. After assessing for emergent issues, the clinician should further examine the mass. Figure 12.1 shows areas where congenital neck masses can be found. It is important to palpate for other lesions, as 10% to 20% of branchial lesions are bilateral.[1] Ultrasononography might be useful in differentiating a cystic from a solid mass, detecting abscesses and guiding fine-needle aspiration (FNA). Computed tomography (CT) might detect involvement of surrounding structures. Congenital head and neck lesions usually require excision.

Neonatal torticollis may be caused by birth trauma and have bleeding into the sternomastoid muscle. These patients may present with a neck mass at several weeks of age.

At about 8 weeks of gestation, a diverticulum of dura extends through the fonticulus frontalis into the prenasal space.[2] An embryologic anomaly (e.g., dermoid, encephalocele or glioma) occurs if regression of this diverticulum is incomplete.

Inflammatory lesions are also common in pediatrics. Inflammatory lesions in the neck are usually of the lymph nodes.

Infection of a cystic lesion can present as a recurrent unilateral neck mass. Rarely, acute infection of a cyst can lead to mediastinitis or sepsis. FNA or intraoperative cultures and histopathology can identify pathogens and developmental anomalies. Oral antibiotics (e.g., amoxicillin-clavulanate, first-generation cephalosporins and clindamycin) may be used for mild cases. Parenteral antibiotics are used to treat more severe cases. Incision and drainage are indicated for abscesses or failed medical therapy. After resolution of an infection, surgical intervention is recommended to prevent recurrences.[3] This chapter discusses the common causes of neck masses in infants.

BRANCHIAL CLEFT ANOMALIES

Human embryos develop four pairs of branchial arches with intervening clefts during the fourth through eighth weeks of gestation that give rise to mature structures of the head and neck. Abnormal development of the first branchial arch results in cleft lip and palate, abnormal external ear and malformed internal ossicles. Abnormal development of the first branchial cleft is rare and results in microtia and aural atresia. Most branchial cleft anomalies are from the second branchial cleft. About 10% of these are bilateral.[4]

Branchial cleft sinuses and fistulae usually are identified in infancy; branchial cleft cysts more commonly present in childhood or early adulthood. An ostium of a second branchial cleft sinus tract or fistula is found along the

Table 12.1. Common congenital neck cysts in neonates and infants

Type	Location	Age	Signs
Branchial cleft	Anterior neck triangle, lateral	Childhood through adulthood	Associated with draining sinus
Cystic hygroma	Posterior neck triangle	Birth through infancy	Soft, enlarges in first few weeks of life
Dermoid	Midline	Birth through adulthood	Cyst may move with swallowing

anterior border of the middle to lower third of the sternocleidomastoid muscle. These have drainage and are painless. A blocked sinus can lead to an infected cyst.

Branchial cleft cysts present along the anterior border of the sternocleidomastoid muscle. Branchial cleft cysts are fluctuant, mobile and nontender. Ultrasonography may be useful in identifying these cysts. In addition, a contrast swallow study or endoscopy may be of use in confirming pyriform sinuses and cysts. Excision of the sinus tract and cyst soon after diagnosis is the treatment of choice. Recurrence in most series is less than 7%.[5] Infected cysts and sinus tracts should be treated with appropriate antibiotics and warm soaks before excision.

CERVICAL LYMPHADENITIS

Cervical lymphadenitis is an inflammation of the lymph nodes. *Staphylococcus aureus* and group A streptococcus are common bacterial pathogens. These pathogens initially colonize the nasopharynx or, less commonly, are introduced through the skin. The bacteria can spread to and proliferate in lymph nodes, leading to an inflammatory response if not contained by the immune system. Acute bilateral cervical lymphadenitis often has a viral cause but can also be caused by *Streptococcus pyogenes*. Viral infections typically resolve within 1 to 2 weeks without sequelae.

Bacterial infections are usually unilateral, whereas viral infections are typically bilateral. Fever can occur in children younger than 1 year old. The infected, tender lymph node might range from 2 cm up. Initially firm, fluctuance can later develop. There is overlying skin erythema and warmth and, at times, edema may be present. In patients with viral infections, the lymph nodes are generally rubbery, small, mildly erythematous and mildly warm to touch.

Lymphadenopathy is an enlargement of a lymph node as a reaction to a concurrent viral infection or as a reaction to bacterial disease in adjacent structures.

Unlike acute lymphangitis, tumors and congenital anomalies generally are present for weeks and are often midline.

The white blood cell (WBC) count may be elevated in patients who present acutely. Aspiration for Gram stain and aerobic and anaerobic cultures can help to identify the causative organism. Purified protein derivative (PPD) skin testing can reveal infection from *Mycobacterium tuberculosis*. Acid-fast stain and a mycobacterial culture also may be helpful. Ultrasonography or CT scan may be warranted to determine if there is abscess formation.

Antibiotic therapy against *S. aureus* and group A streptococcus is recommended (e.g., oral therapy with cephalexin, clindamycin or amoxicillin-clavulanic acid for 10–14 days[6]). Patients who are toxic, fail to improve after 36 to 48 hours, or have a positive PPD skin test require hospitalization for parenteral therapy with FNA or incision and drainage.

In neonates, acute unilateral cervical lymphadenitis is generally caused by *S. aureus*. Group B streptococci are

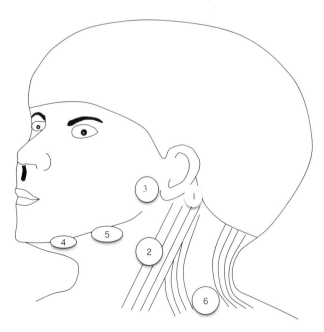

Figure 12.1. Congenital neck masses in neonates and infants by location. *Branchial cleft cyst:* 1, postauricular; 2, anterior sternocleidomastoid. *Cystic hygroma:* 3, parotid; 4, submental; 5, submandibular; 6, supraclavicular. *Hemangioma:* 3, parotid.

involved in the cellulitis-adenitis syndrome. Infant males are more affected than females. Patients present with facial or submandibular cellulitis, fever and ipsilateral otitis media. The organism can be isolated from blood and lymph node. A septic workup is recommended in this age group and the patient should be hospitalized for parenteral antibiotic therapy.

CYSTIC HYGROMAS

Cystic hygromas are benign lesions that are thought to come from the congenital failure of lymphatic primordial buds establishing drainage into the venous system.[4] They are lined by endothelial cells and produce lymph fluid. They are reported in 1 in 12,000 births.[7] About 50% to 60% of cystic hygromas are identified at birth; 80% to 90% are identified before 3 years of age.[8]

Cystic hygromas develop near large veins or the lymphatic system; 75% are found in the neck, particularly the posterior triangle of the neck.[9,10] The incidence of occurrence on the left side of the neck is 2:1.[4] Cystic hygromas are multiloculated lymphatic malformations that are discrete, mobile, nontender and soft, and they may transilluminate. Cystic hygromas usually grow in proportion to the infant, although they are characterized by gradual to rapid enlargement and vary in size from a few millimeters to several centimeters in diameter. Large lesions may compress the airway, for example, with extrinsic compression. Infection is less common.

An ultrasound study will detect whether the mass is truly cystic in nature. Cystic hygromas characteristically have linear septations. A CT scan with intravenous contrast will determine involvement of other structures. Cystic hygromas do not normally regress; therefore, complete excision is the treatment of choice.

DERMOID CYSTS

Dermoid cysts are congenital, subcutaneous nodules, arising from ectoderm. They are lined by epithelium and might contain bone, glands, hair, keratin, neural tissue, papillae, sebaceous glands and teeth. Malignant transformation is rare.

Dermoid cysts usually present as firm, noncompressible, nontender, round, smooth, solitary, subcutaneous nodules. They might feel doughy or rubbery with normal overlying skin. Dermoid cysts tend to be slow

growing and are commonly found on the lateral brow, nasal bridge, midline neck, scalp or anterior margin of the sternocleidomastoid. An external ostium may or may not be present.

Epidermoid cysts do not contain connective tissue, hair follicles, papillae and sebaceous glands. Dermoid cysts might be found in the midline of the neck and be confused with thyroglossal duct cysts. Compared to thyroglossal duct cysts, dermoid cysts are usually more superficial and contain sebaceous material and are not connected to the tongue. Midline dermoid cysts usually have deep attachments into the intracranium. All patients with midline lesions should undergo a magnetic resonance imaging (MRI)scan.[11] Complete surgical excision is the treatment of choice and is used to confirm the diagnosis.

ENCEPHALOCELES

Encephaloceles are made of neural tissue that herniates through a congenital defect in the midline of the calvarium. They always have an intracranial communication.

Encephaloceles are soft, sometimes pulsatile, and they enlarge with crying, straining or compression of the jugular veins (Furstenberg test). Nasal encephaloceles might present with a rounded mass at the nasal bridge and overt craniofacial deformities at birth. A nasopharyngeal encephalocele might be the only presentation, with signs of persistent nasal obstruction.

MRI is the study of choice in differentiating encephaloceles from other midline nasal masses and in studying size and extension. Nasopharyngoscopy might reveal a grape-like mass.

Neurosurgical evaluation and management are indicated. Ruling out significant intracranial involvement allows an endonasal approach versus craniotomy.[2]

GLIOMAS

Gliomas are derived from neuroectoderm and are benign lesions. They are composed of neural and fibrous tissue covered by nasal mucosa. Gliomas are usually firm, gray or red-gray nodules. They are 1 to 5 cm in diameter. About 60% of gliomas are found on the nasal bridge: 30% are intranasal and 10% are intranasal and extranasal.[1] It is important to note that gliomas do not have intracranial involvement. Gliomas can often be mistaken for hemangiomas. Surgical excision is the treatment of choice to prevent distortion of surrounding tissue.

HEMANGIOMAS

Hemangiomas are common head and neck tumors of infancy with an incidence of 10% to 20% in children younger than 1 year old and double this in preterm infants who weigh less than 1000 g.[12] Hemangiomas are vascular tumors that grow by proliferation of endothelial cells. At birth, they appear as small, erythematous or pale macules or patches, or telangiectasias. They are more common in females with a 4:1 ratio.[13] Most hemangiomas appear in the first 6 weeks of life. They can be seen in 4% to 10% of Caucasian newborns, with less frequency in non-Caucasian.[14,15] The head and neck are involved in 60% of cases.[13] Hemangiomas occur focally in 3:1 of cases.[16]

Hemangiomas typically enlarge in the first 18 months of life and involute over several years after this time. By 10 to 12 years of age, about half of the children with hemangiomas will have normal appearing skin.[13] Superficial lesions are characteristically red, raised and strawberry-like. Hemangiomas are soft, mobile, nontender and warm. During the proliferative phase, they may be pulsatile with an audible bruit. Deeper lesions in the dermis or subcutaneous tissue can be unnoticeable or have a bluish hue.

Hemangiomas can be differentiated from other vascular malformations by their rapid proliferation. Venous malformations are characterized by increase in size while crying. Sometimes it is difficult to differentiate hemangiomas from hypervascular soft-tissue tumors, which have less defined margins, irregular vessels with neovascularity and encasement.[13]

Thrombocytopenia is not associated with the common hemangioma of infancy. Common infantile hemangioma markers Glut1 and Lewis antigen Y are not present in Kasabach-Merritt phenomenon vascular tumors.[17] The Kasabach-Merritt phenomenon occurs with a more invasive infantile vascular tumor called *kaposiform hemangioendothelioma* or *tufted angioma*.[18-20]

Dermatologic conditions of early infancy can be confused with an infantile hemangioma. Nevus flammeius neonatorum – angel's kiss, stork bite or salmon patch – is a nonevolving macular stain that disappears by 1 year of age. Hemangiomas can look like port-wine stains or capillary malformations or silent arteriovenous malformations. Hemangiomas can be confused with the fruitlike pyogenic granuloma, which is a cutaneous vascular lesion. Nasal gliomas might look like hemangiomas.

Deeper hemangiomas might require ultrasound with Doppler imaging to differentiate them from soft-tissue malignancies and vascular malformations. The hallmark of hemangiomas on imaging is a homogeneous, solid, parenchymal mass with increased vascularity.[13] CT shows hemangiomas as similar or lower in density than muscle, with uniformly dense contrast enhancement and vessels around the lesion.[13] MRIs are helpful if deep, intracranial lesions are suspected. Magnetic resonance angiograms are not currently useful.

Preliminary data show that measuring the cellular marker basic fibroblast growth factor levels in the urine can aid in the diagnosis of proliferating hemangiomas.[21]

About 20% of hemangiomas are symptomatic and may require treatment.[22] Hypertrophy of the epidermis and subcutaneous tissue can result in ulceration in up to 5% of hemangiomas.[23] Infection or bleeding might occur. The psychologic impact of cosmetic impairment in the head and neck is something to consider. Earlier intervention by surgical excision, laser and embolization, in selected cases, is possible.[13,24] Potent topical steroids (e.g., clobetasol cream) have been used in the treatment of periorbital hemangiomas.[13] If a good early surgical excision is not possible, treatment is usually conservative management, as most hemangiomas involute.

Rare complications occur in about 1% of cases,[13] including airway obstruction, hemorrhage, infection, necrosis, disseminated intravascular coagulation and ulceration. Rapidly growing lesions can impair vision or hearing. Central nervous system involvement is rare.

NEONATAL TORTICOLLIS OR CONGENITAL MUSCULAR TORTICOLLIS

Neonatal torticollis is due to fibrosis and shortening of the sternocleidomastoid muscle. The etiology is unclear. It presents at birth or in the first 3 weeks of life.[25] Neonatal torticollis has an incidence of 0.4% to 1.3%.[26] The infant holds his or her chin away from the affected side. The mass is firm and feels attached to muscle. Neonatal torticollis might lead to plagiocephaly, or skull and facial asymmetry.[27]

Ultrasonography can differentiate postural torticollis from the sternomastoid mass of neonatal torticollis.[28-30] Physical therapy by passive and active stretching of the affected sternocleidomastoid muscle is the treatment of choice, resulting in complete resolution in most cases.[28,31,32] Prognosis is excellent if physical therapy is initiated before 6 weeks of age.[28] Surgery is rarely indicated.

If a neck mass persists after 6 weeks of age, patients need to be monitored for other deformities and persistent torticollis.

PREAURICULAR PITS, SINUSES, CYSTS AND TAGS

Preauricular pits, sinuses, cysts and tags are ectodermal inclusions lined by stratified squamous epithelium related to abnormal development of the auditory tubercles. They tend to be familial, are usually bilateral and present at birth or shortly thereafter. They are typically located anterior to the tragus. Preauricular cysts might contain hair. Occasionally, they may drain sebaceous material; these preauricular cysts are most likely to develop a secondary infection due to staphylococcus. Cutaneous tags, or accessory auricles, are pedunculated and skin-colored.

Excision is the treatment of choice. Infection should first be treated with appropriate antibiotics and warm soaks before excision. Needle aspiration or incision and drainage are performed as needed. Recurrence is uncommon.[4] Some preauricular tags with narrow bases may be tied off with sutures.

STURGE-WEBER SYNDROME

Sturge-Weber syndrome consists of a facial capillary malformation with ipsilateral ocular and leptomeningeal vascular abnormalities (e.g., capillary malformations, venous malformations or arteriovenous malformations). The capillary malformation can involve the ophthalmic, maxillary or mandibular regions.[33]

Small leptomeningeal involvement can be silent, but larger leptomeningeal vascular lesions can cause refractory seizures, contralateral hemiplegia and variable delayed development. Involvement of the ophthalmic region can lead to glaucoma, retinal detachment and blindness.

If the ophthalmic region is involved, periodic fundoscopic examination and tonometry are recommended every 6 months until 2 years of age and then yearly.[34]

Management of the capillary malformation is with cosmetics and laser photocoagulation. Occasionally, excision and grafting are performed. Significant lightening occurs in about 80% of patients, especially of the lateral face.[34]

PITFALLS

- Failure to recognize that congenital lesions may become secondarily infected
- Failure to recognize that neck masses may compromise the airway or blood vessels
- Failure to recognize that congenital nasal masses often present with airway obstruction in infants.

REFERENCES

1. Fleisher GR, Ludwig S, eds. *Textbook of Pediatric Emergency Medicine*. Philadelphia, PA: Lippincott Williams & Wilkins; 2000.
2. Manning SC, Blood DC, Perkins JA, et al. Diagnostic and surgical challenges in the pediatric skull base. *Otolaryngol Clin North Am*. 2005;38:773–794.
3. Brook I. Microbiology and management of infected neck cysts. *J Oral Maxillofac Surg*. 2005;63(3):392–395.
4. Brown RL, Azizkhan RG. Pediatric head and neck lesions. *Pediatr Clin North Am*. 1998;45(4):889–905.
5. Rowe MI. Neck lesion. In: O'Neill JA, Grasfeld JL, Fonkalsrud EW, et al, eds. *Essentials of Pediatric Surgery*. St. Louis, MO: Mosby-Year Book; 1995.
6. Al-Dajani N, Wootton SH. Cervical lymphadenitis, suppurative parotitis, thyroiditis, and infected cysts. *Infect Dis Clin North Am*. 2007;21:523–541.
7. Stringel G. Hemangiomas and lymphangiomas. In: Ashcraft KW, Holder TM, eds. *Pediatric Surgery*, 2nd ed. Philadelphia, PA: WB Saunders; 1993:802–822.
8. Bill AHJ, Sumner DS. A unified concept of lymphangioma and cystic hygroma. *Surg Gynecol Obstet*. 1965;120:79–86.
9. Kennedy TL. Cystic hygroma-lymphangioma: a rare and still unclear entity. *Laryngoscope*. 1989;99:1–10.
10. Stal S, Hamilton S, Spira M. Hemangiomas, lymphangiomas, and vascular malformations of the head and neck. *Otolaryngol Clin North Am*. 1986;19:769–797.
11. Davenport M. Lumps and swelllings of the head and neck. *BMJ*. 1996;312:368–371.
12. Amir J, Metzker A, Krikler R, et al. Strawberry hemangioma in preterm infants [abstract]. *Pediatr Dermatol*. 1986;3:331–332.
13. Song JK, Yasunari N, Berenstein A. Endovascular treatment of hemangiomas. *Neuroimaging Clin N Am*. 2007;17(2):165–173.
14. Jacobs AH, Walton RG. The incidence of birthmarks in the neonate [abstract]. *Pediatrics*. 1976;58:218–222.
15. Hidano A, Nakajima S. Earliest features of the strawberry mark in the newborn. *Br J Dermatol*. 1972;87:138–144.
16. Waner M, North PE, Scherer KA, et al. The nonrandom distribution of facial hemangiomas [abstract]. *Arch Dermatol*. 2003;139:869–875.

17. Lyons LL, North PE, Mac-Moune LF, et al. Kaposiform hemangioendothelioma: a study of 33 cases emphasizing its pathologic, immunophenotypic, and biologic uniqueness from juvenile hemangioma. *Am J Surg Pathol.* 2004;28(5):559–568.

18. Enjolras O, Wassef M, Mazoyer E, et al. Infants with Kasabach-Merritt syndrome do not have "true" hemangiomas. *J Pediatr.* 1997;130:631–640.

19. Sarkar M, Mulliken JB, Kozakewich HP, et al. Thrombocytopenia coagulopathy (Kasabach-Merritt phenomenon) is associated with kaposiform hemangioendothelioma and not with common infantile hemangioma. *Plast Reconstr Surg.* 1997;100:1377–1386.

20. Jones EW, Orkin M. Tufted angioma (angioblastoma): a benign progressive angioma, not to be confused with Kaposi's sarcoma or low grade angiosarcoma. *J Am Acad Dermatol.* 1989;20:214–225.

21. Takahashi K, Mulliken JB, Kozakewich HP, et al. Cellular markers that distinguish the phases of hemangioma during infancy and childhood. *J Clin Invest.* 1994;98(6):2357–2364.

22. Enjolras O, Riche MC, Merland JJ, et al. Management of alarming hemangiomas in infancy: a review of 25 cases [abstract]. *Pediatrics.* 1990;85(4):491–498.

23. Margileth AM, Museles M. Cutaneous hemangiomas in children: diagnosis and conservative management. *JAMA.* 1965;194:523.

24. Waner M, Suen JY. Treatment options for the management of hemangiomas. In: Waner M, Suen JY, ed. *Hemangiomas and Vascular Malformations of the Head and Neck.* New York, NY: Wiley-Liss; 1999:233–261.

25. Canale ST, Griffin DW, Hubbard CN. Congenital muscular torticollis. *J Bone Joint Surg.* 1982;64A:810–816.

26. Cheng JCY, Au AWY. Infantile torticollis: a review of 624 cases. *J Pediatr Orthop.* 1994;14:802–808.

27. Robin NH. Congenital muscular torticollis. *Pediatr Rev.* 1996;17:374–375.

28. Tatli B, Aydinli N, Caliskan M, et al. Congenital muscular torticollis: evaluation and classification. *Pediatr Neurol.* 2006;34:41–44.

29. Lin JN, Chou ML. Ultrasonographic study of the sternocleidomastoid muscle in the management of congenital muscular torticollis. *J Pediatr Surg.* 1997;32:1648–1651.

30. Dudkiewicz I. Congenital muscular torticollis in infants: ultrasound-assisted diagnosis and evaluation. *Pediatr Orthop.* 2005;25(6):812–814.

31. Cheng CY, Tang SP, Chen TMK, Wong MWN, Wong EMC. The clinical presentation and outcome of treatment of congenital muscular torticollis in infants: a study of 1086 cases. *J Pediatr Surg.* 2000;35:1091–1096.

32. Emery C. The determinants of treatment duration for congenital muscular torticollis. *Phys Ther.* 1994;74:921–929.

33. Enjolras O, Riche MC, Merland JJ. Facial port-wine stains and Sturge-Weber syndrome. *Pediatrics.* 1985;76:48–51.

34. Marler JJ, Mulliken JB. Current management of hemangiomas and vascular malformations. *Clin Plastic Surg.* 2005;32:99–116.

13 Hyperbilirubinemia in the Newborn

Dale P. Woolridge and James E. Colletti

INTRODUCTION

Hyperbilirubinemia, commonly referred to as *jaundice*, is a yellowish-greenish pigmentation of the sclera and skin caused by an increase in bilirubin production or a defect in bilirubin elimination. *Neonatal hyperbilirubinemia* (defined by a serum bilirubin concentration >5 mg/dL) is estimated to occur in the majority of term infants (60%) in the first week of life, and approximately 2% will reach total serum bilirubin (TSB) levels in excess of 20 mg/dL.[1–3] In the full-term infant, the TSB normally rises during the first 3 to 5 days of life and then begins to decline.[3] As such, it is important that bilirubin levels are interpreted based on the infant's age in hours.[4]

The feared complication of neonatal hyperbilirubinemia is bilirubin encephalopathy, the result of prolonged unconjugated hyperbilirubinemia. Acute bilirubin encephalopathy can eventually develop into chronic bilirubin encephalopathy (kernicterus). Kernicterus has been called the ultimate adverse manifestation of severe hyperbilirubinemia[5] and was rarely seen in the decades following the introduction of phototherapy and exchange transfusion. Unfortunately, recent reports suggest it is reemerging[3]; a worrisome number of cases have been reported in healthy term and near-term neonates.[6] Between 1990 and 1999, the Pilot Kernicterus Registry identified kernicterus in more than 120 near-term and term infants who had been discharged as healthy from the hospital.[7] This reemergence of kernicterus has been attributed partially to earlier hospital discharge (before the natural peak of bilirubin in the infant) as well as a result of relaxation of treatment criteria.[3,8]

Newborns are often discharged from the hospital within 48 hours of birth (before hyperbilirubinemia reaches its peak); as a result, hyperbilirubinemia is not as often detected before discharge as it had been previously. The practice of early newborn discharge has transformed neonatal hyperbilirubinemia from an inpatient issue to an outpatient one.[9] Currently, hyperbilirubinemia is one of the most common reasons for readmission of a newborn.[10,11] As such, emergency physicians should remain well educated in the diagnosis, evaluation and management of hyperbilirubinemia in the newborn.

EPIDEMIOLOGY

Hyperbilirubinemia is one of the most common presentations of neonates to the emergency department (ED) and one of the major causes for hospital readmission. Overall, hyperbilirubinemia is observed in the first week of life in 60% of term infants and 80% of preterm infants.[1] In a case control review, Maisels et al. concluded that hyperbilirubinemia is the major reason for hospital readmission in the first 2 weeks of life (incidence, 4.2 per 1000 discharges).[11] Although the percentage of infants with hyperbilirubinemia is higher among preterm infants, the majority of studies of assessment, evaluation and management of hyperbilirubinemia have been performed on term infants with birth weights of 2500 g or greater.

PATHOPHYSIOLOGY

Bilirubin is produced from the breakdown of hemoglobin. Hemoglobin is degraded by heme oxygenase, resulting in the release of iron and the formation of carbon monoxide and biliverdin. Biliverdin is then converted to bilirubin by biliverdin reductase.

Unconjugated bilirubin (also known as *indirect bilirubin*) is lipid soluble and is subsequently bound by albumin in the blood stream; therefore, any substance competing for binding sites, such as organic acids or drugs, can cause displacement and increase the levels of free bilirubin. In this lipophilic (unconjugated) state, bilirubin is difficult to excrete and can easily pass the blood–brain barrier, where it can precipitate and can produce kernicterus.

Unconjugated bilirubin is taken up by the liver hepatocytes where it is conjugated within the cell by the enzyme uridine diphosphate-glucuronosyltransferase (UDPGT) to its conjugated form. This conjugated form (referred to as *direct bilirubin*) is water soluble, nontoxic and unable to cross the blood–brain barrier. Conjugated bilirubin, as opposed to its unconjugated (indirect) counterpart, can be excreted into bile and transported through the biliary system into the intestinal tract. Once in the intestinal tract, it is either excreted in stool or deconjugated by bacteria, after which it may reenter the circulation (entero-hepatic circulation). Unconjugated bilirubin is poorly excreted in the urine and stool.

From a simple kinetic standpoint, there are three main causes of hyperbilirubinemia in the neonate:

1. Increase in hemolysis (increased production)
2. Delay in maturation or inhibition of conjugating mechanisms in the liver (decreased conjugation)
3. Impaired excretion

Neonates are particularly prone to the first two in the list. Major factors are a high red blood cell (RBC) volume at birth, shortened RBC survival (and therefore increased breakdown) and relative immaturity of the neonatal liver.

CLINICAL PRESENTATION

The emergency physician should be familiar with historical clues that put the neonate at increased risk for severe hyperbilirubinemia. Risk factors to consider are hyperbilirubinemia in the first 24 hours, visible hyperbilirubinemia before hospital discharge, fetal–maternal blood type incompatibility, prematurity (infants <35 weeks' gestational age), exclusive breastfeeding as well as significant weight loss associated with breastfeeding, maternal age greater than or equal to 25 years of age, male sex, delayed meconium passage and excessive birth trauma such as bruising or cephalohematomas.[5,12] The parents should be asked specifically about poor feeding, urine output (including dark urine), stooling (delayed passage of meconium, light-colored stool), vomiting or any changes in behavior (lethargy, changes in cry pattern, cries becoming more shrill, arching of the body).[13]

Family history is important as well. Pertinent family history includes ethnicity as well as siblings with hyperbilirubinemia, anemia, liver disease and splenectomy (implies a history of RBC abnormality). Ethnicity is a factor in determining likelihood of hyperbilirubinemia. Individuals of East Asian descent, people from certain tribes of Native Americans such as the Navajo, and Greeks have a higher incidence of hyperbilirubinemia.[14] Even though some inherent diseases cause an increase in bilirubin levels due to an increase in RBC breakdown such as glucose-6-phosphate dehydrogenase deficiency (G6PD) and spherocytosis, there is a 12.5 times greater risk for severe hyperbilirubinemia in infants who have had one or more siblings effected with hyperbilirubinemia when compared to individuals who do not have any sibling involvement.[15]

Physical assessment begins with the clinical appearance of the infant. Hyperbilirubinemia is assessed through blanching the skin with digital pressure, revealing the underlying color of the skin and subcutaneous tissue. The clinical assessment of hyperbilirubinemia is best undertaken in a well-lit room in order to maximize the ability to determine true skin color.[12] Hyperbilirubinemia in term and preterm infants typically follows a cephalo-caudal progression.[16] Visual estimation of the severity of hyperbilirubinemia can be unpredictable and imprecisely related to actual serum bilirubin levels. This is especially the case in infants with dark skin pigmentation and in those with hyperbilirubinemia that has extended to the lower legs and feet.[4,17,18] Moyer et al. evaluated 122 healthy infants who underwent examination by two observers followed by measurements of serum bilirubin. The authors determined that infants without hyperbilirubinemia below the nipple line had bilirubin levels lower than 12 mg/dL.[18] Otherwise, the investigation concluded that visual estimation of infantile hyperbilirubinemia is not reliable and prediction of serum bilirubin concentration by clinical examination is not accurate.

After assessing the skin, it is important to look for other signs indicative of pathologic hyperbilirubinemia such as pallor, petechiae, hydration, and weight status. Signs of blood loss or blood sequestration such as excessive bruising, hepatosplenomegaly or cephalhematoma should be sought out as well.[19]

A review of the birth history should be performed. First, it is important to establish if the child was large for gestational age (LGA), average for gestational age (AGA) or small for gestational age (SGA). Babies who are SGA have associated complications such as hypoglycemia, polycythemia and abnormal neurologic symptoms. Although hyperbilirubinemia is not a direct link to SGA infants, polycythemia can lead to an increased bilirubin level secondary to increased RBC destruction.[20,21]

Infants who were LGA have an increased incidence of birth trauma due to their size. Excessive bruising and cephalohematomas can be acquired from birth trauma and, because blood from hematomas and contusions is degraded to bilirubin, can be a source for hyperbilirubinemia.[22] One study determined over a 10-year period that 2.5% of all breech births had an associated cephalohematoma.[23] Forceps and vacuum extraction deliveries can also cause bruising and cephalohematomas.[21] Other injuries such as clavicle fractures and brachial plexus injury are also associated with hyperbilirubinemia. Clavicle fractures are most often due to shoulder dystocia in LGA babies.

As mentioned previously, certain medications taken by the mother before and during pregnancy can result in an increased incidence of hyperbilirubinemia. Turnball et al. found that mothers who received oxytocin had babies with higher bilirubin levels than babies born to mothers who did not receive oxytocin.[24] Therefore, a complete medication list should be sought from the mother when evaluating a newborn with elevated bilirubin levels.

The evaluating physician should be aware of other serious symptoms that can present as hyperbilirubinemia. Some of these are listed in Table 13.1. For example, if the patient has apnea or temperature instability, the clinician should entertain a diagnosis of sepsis. Similarly, galactosemia presents as feeding intolerance manifested by persistent vomiting, an enlarged liver, seizures and lethargy.[25]

DIFFERENTIAL DIAGNOSIS

Physiologic and Pathologic Hyperbilirubinemia

As mentioned previously, elevated bilirubin levels should be expected and is considered physiologic in normal newborns. This is owed to the high RBC turnover and relatively immature livers in these patients. The clinician therefore must understand the difference between physiologic and pathologic hyperbilirubinemia. *Physiologic hyperbilirubinemia* is the transient elevation of serum bilirubin during the first week of life. Hallmarks of *pathologic hyperbilirubinemia* are any of the following: occurs in

Table 13.1. Causes of conjugated and unconjugated hyperbilirubinemia

Unconjugated hyperbilirubinemia (elevated indirect bilirubin)	Conjugated hyperbilirubinemia (elevated direct bilirubin)
Physiologic hyperbilirubinemia	Sepsis
Rh or ABO incompatibility	TORCH infections
Polycythemia	Syphilis
Excessive bruising from birth trauma	Cystic fibrosis
G6PD	Meconium ileus
Breast milk hyperbilirubinemia	Biliary atresia
High intestinal obstruction	Hepatitis
Duodenal atresia	Inborn errors of metabolism
Congenital hypothyroidism	
Poor feeding	

G6PD, glucose-6-phosphate dehydrogenase deficiency; TORCH, toxoplasmosis, other infections, rubella, cytomegalovirus, herpes simplex virus.
Adapted from American Academy of Pediatrics Subcommittee on Hyperbilirubinemia. Management of hyperbilirubinemia in the newborn infant 35 or more weeks of gestation. *Pediatrics.* 2004;114:316–397.[12]

the first 24 hours of life, occurs in the presence of anemia or hepatosplenomegaly, has a rapidly rising serum bilirubin (>5 mg/dL/day) as well as prolonged hyperbilirubinemia (>7–10 days in a full-term infant) or has an elevated conjugated bilirubin concentration (>2 mg/dL or >20% of TSB). See Table 13.2 for more information.

It is important to rule out hemolytic disease as the cause of increased indirect bilirubin levels. Many conditions can cause hemolysis, and factors that will predict hemolysis and subsequent hyperbilirubinemia early need to be identified. The development of hyperbilirubinemia in the newborn before 24 hours of life is an indicator of possible hemolytic disease.[1] Another clue might be a positive family history relayed by the parents. In cases in which the history is not fully known, this may simply be reported as significant hemolytic disease in a family member or early and severe hyperbilirubinemia in a previous child. A poor response to therapy may also be indicative of ongoing hemolysis. For example, a child undergoing phototherapy whose bilirubin levels remain the same or continue to rise may have ongoing RBC breakdown.

Blood Group Incompatibility

Blood group incompatibility is the leading cause of increased bilirubin load and results from hemolysis. ABO

Table 13.2. High risk features in the newborn with hyperbilirubinemia

Findings suggestive of nonphysiologic causes of hyperbilirubinemia

Hyperbilirubinemia in first 24 hours of life
Total serum bilirubin rising >5 mg/dL/24 hr
Total serum bilirubin >15 mg/dL in full-term infant
Hyperbilirubinemia persisting after first week of life
Direct bilirubin >1 mg/dL or >20% of total at any time
Family history of hemolytic disease
Pallor, hepatomegaly, splenomegaly
Failure of phototherapy to lower bilirubin
Excessive weight loss
Risk Factors in Hyperbilirubinemia
Sibling with hyperbilirubinemia in newborn period
Prematurity, perinatal depression, decreased Apgar score at
    5 minutes
Inadequate or ineffective breastfeeding
Significant weight loss after birth
Maternal diabetes
Race (Asian, Native American)
Drug exposure – oxytocin, sulfonamides, aspirin
Altitude
Polycythemia
Blood group incompatibility, known hemolytic disease
    G6PD deficiency
Male gender
Bruising, cephalohematoma
Delayed stooling
Trisomy 21
Early discharge with inadequate follow up and poor feeding
Hyperbilirubinemia observed within first 24 hours of life

Data from American Academy of Pediatrics Subcommittee on Hyperbilirubinemia. Management of hyperbilirubinemia in the newborn infant 35 or more weeks of gestation. *Pediatrics.* 2004;114:316–397[12] and Porter LM, Dennis BL. Hyperbilirubinemia in the term newborn. *Am Fam Phys.* 2002;65(4):599–605.[19]

blood group incompatibility is the most common of these. This phenomenon occurs when a mother with blood type O carries a fetus with blood type A or B. This causes the mother's anti-A and anti-B antibodies to attack the blood within the fetus. The resultant reaction is an antibody-dependent cell mediated cytotoxicity. Approximately one third of these infants with ABO incompatibility will have a positive direct antiglobulin test (DAT or Coombs test), indicating that they have anti-A or anti-B antibodies attached to their RBCs.[26] Of this third, 20% will have a peak TSB of greater than 12.8 mg/dL.[26] Therefore, although ABO-incompatible, DAT-positive infants are more likely to develop moderate hyperbilirubinemia, severe hyperbilirubinemia is uncommon. Interestingly, 15% of all births are a set-up for ABO incompatibility,

but only 0.33% to 2.2% of all neonates have some manifestation of this disease.[27]

A mechanism similar to that of ABO incompatibility exists for Rh incompatibility. Rh incompatibility was at one time the most common cause of antigen-mediated hemolysis of the newborn. In Rh incompatibility, a mother does not have the Rh factor (Rh-negative) but the baby does (Rh-positive), thus allowing the mother's immunologic system the potential to develop antibodies against the baby's blood. Fortunately, mothers do not normally carry the Rh antibody and must be sensitized to develop them. Here, simple prevention of maternal sensitization has drastically reduced this disease. Similar manifestations are seen with many other minor blood group incompatibilities.

Enzyme Deficiencies

Enzyme deficiencies in the glycolysis pathway such as glucose-6-phosphate dehydrogenase deficiency (G6PD) and pyruvate kinase deficiency (PKD) also increase the indirect bilirubin load. G6PD mainly affects the RBCs and can cause acute hemolysis. G6PD affects somewhere between 200 and 400 million people worldwide and is a leading cause of hyperbilirubinemia in certain population subtypes such as African Americans, those of Mediterranean descent and some Far East populations.[28] Multiple studies have shown that infants with G6PD who are affected by hyperbilirubinemia have the same clinical course and clinical indicators as infants who do not have G6PD. For this reason it is prudent to have G6PD on the differential diagnosis if there is a family history of G6PD or if the patient fits into at risk demographic.[29]

PKD is the second leading cause of RBC enzyme deficiency in North America and an uncommon hemolytic cause of hyperbilirubinemia, but it is one cause that should still be on the differential diagnosis. In one study, of 217 infants with indirect hyperbilirubinemia, 3.21% were diagnosed with PKD.[30]

Red Blood Cell Membrane Abnormalities

Other diseases that can cause an increase in indirect bilirubin levels through hemolysis are abnormalities in the RBC membranes such as hereditary spherocytosis (HS) and elliptocytosis or ovalocytosis. In HS there is a defect in the RBC membrane, causing an increase in RBC breakdown and abnormal RBCs. Passi et al. reported that 50% of individuals with HS state they had significant hyperbilirubinemia as a newborn. The physical characteristics that this study found included early onset of hyperbilirubinemia or marked increase in bilirubin beyond what was expected with physiologic hyperbilirubinemia. If suspicious, a peripheral blood smear may show spherocytes, but this finding may not be present in neonates; therefore, the gold standard of an osmotic fragility test should be performed to confirm diagnosis.[31]

Elliptocytosis or ovalocytosis is an RBC membrane defect that makes RBCs have an oval appearance. Usually, this disease is asymptomatic in the newborn, but there have been case reports of this disease causing indirect hyperbilirubinemia. Inheritance is autosomal dominant; therefore, family history is key and certain ethnic groups (Southeast Asian and Mediterranean populations) are more commonly affected.[32]

Increased indirect bilirubin can also be caused by decreased bilirubin excretion. Newborns will clear much of their bilirubin via the stool, and bilirubin contributes to the dark color of meconium. Therefore, any condition that gives rise to decreased bowel motility will delay clearance and prolong hyperbilirubinemia. This causes an increased retention of bilirubin in the enterohepatic circulation and, in turn, leads to increased indirect bilirubin.[19,33] Examples of such conditions that cause decreased bilirubin excretion include sepsis, duodenal atresia, meconium ileus, dehydration, cystic fibrosis (CF) and poor feeding.

Crigler-Najjar Syndrome

One of the more life-threatening causes of hyperbilirubinemia by impaired bilirubin excretion is Crigler-Najjar syndrome, which is a defect in the enzyme that conjugates bilirubin: uridine diphosphate glucuronyl transferase (UDPGT).

There are two types of Crigler-Najjar syndrome. Type I is the more severe form in which there is no enzyme activity and which, without treatment, can lead to kernicterus and death by the age of 1 to 2 years. Type II has some enzyme activity (typically less than 10%) and for that reason is milder with severity based on the amount of enzyme present.

Without UDPGT, unconjugated bilirubin accumulates in the body and the threshold of albumin and other tissue phospholipids to bind is surpassed. Once this occurs,

unconjugated bilirubin begins to precipitate in the tissues. Precipitation in the brain results in kernicterus (discussed later). The disease is rare and inherited in an autosomal recessive fashion. The clinical presenting factor is high bilirubin levels; other possible symptoms include kernicterus, regardless of phototherapy.[34]

Congenital Hypothyroidism

Patients with congenital hypothyroidism can present with prolonged hyperbilirubinemia. Other clinical symptoms will also be present, such as lethargy, constipation, poor feeding, hypotonia and enlarged fontanelles. It is important to follow up with thyroid levels or the newborn genetic screen of individuals who have hyperbilirubinemia with other concerns of hypothyroidism.[35]

Increased indirect bilirubin levels can be the result of breastfeeding.

Breastfeeding-Associated Neonatal Hyperbilirubinemia

When compared with formula feeding, breastfeeding has been associated with neonatal hyperbilirubinemia that lasted longer and reached higher peaks.[36] This type of hyperbilirubinemia can present in two ways.

The first type, termed *human milk hyperbilirubinemia*, is a delayed course in which the bilirubin level rises on day 4 to 7 after physiologic hyperbilirubinemia is waning. A peak in the bilirubin level (15–25 mg/dL) occurs at about 2 weeks of life and may stay in this range for 2 weeks before a decrease is observed.[37]

The second type, termed *breastfeeding hyperbilirubinemia*, has also been described as an exaggerated physiologic hyperbilirubinemia. In this case, bilirubin levels are elevated above 10 mg/dL at day 3 or 4 of life.

The exact mechanism by which breastfeeding contributes to hyperbilirubinemia is not known. There is suggestive evidence that caloric deprivation results in hyperbilirubinemia. It may take anywhere from 2 to 5 days for breast milk to come in. As a result, a breastfed infant may experience a calorie deficiency. Furthermore, it has been shown that human breast milk contains a substance that inhibits hepatic UDPGT (the enzyme that conjugates bilirubin), which, in turn, leads to hyperbilirubinemia.[38] The American Academy of Pediatrics (AAP) stated that even when breastfeeding hyperbilirubinemia is suspected, it is still better to breastfeed then switch to a formula.[1]

Human milk hyperbilirubinemia syndrome or breastfeeding-associated hyperbilirubinemia should be distinguished from breastfeeding hyperbilirubinemia. Human milk hyperbilirubinemia appears later than breastfeeding hyperbilirubinemia, with an onset on day 4 to 7 of life, and is associated with a more prolonged course of hyperbilirubinemia than breastfeeding hyperbilirubinemia.[26] It is important to recognize the timeline within which the hyperbilirubinemia has occurred, as important clues to the etiology of hyperbilirubinemia include the time of onset and how long it lasts. When hyperbilirubinemia occurs in the first 24 hours of life, other causes such as those mentioned previously should be entertained. The first diagnoses that should come to mind are blood type incompatibilities such as ABO and Rh. Sepsis should be considered as well, as many investigations have described an association with proven bacterial infection and neonatal hyperbilirubinemia.[1] Studies have shown that a higher incidence of urinary tract infections (UTIs) occurred in infants who had hyperbilirubinemia.[1,39] Oftentimes, these infants had other symptoms as well to indicate a UTI.[39,40] A few studies have concluded that hyperbilirubinemia as the only symptom of sepsis is rare, especially in a well appearing infant.[1,39,40]

Duration of Hyperbilirubinemia

The duration of hyperbilirubinemia is a key feature to diagnosing the underlying cause. Hyperbilirubinemia appearing during day 2 to 3 of life is most likely physiologic and will dissipate by day 5 to 6 of life. If the child is breastfeeding, he or she may develop breastfeeding hyperbilirubinemia that can be present until the 14th day of life. The clinician needs to start thinking of pathologic reasons if the hyperbilirubinemia persists for longer than 14 days because it is at this time that direct hyperbilirubinemia is the major cause of hyperbilirubinemia. As mentioned earlier, direct hyperbilirubinemia should always be considered pathological. One prospective study showed that most newborns admitted for indirect hyperbilirubinemia are healthy, breastfed infants, but the newborns who had late onset hyperbilirubinemia, direct hyperbilirubinemia or a sepsis red flag in the history, physical or laboratory investigation needed a careful screening.[40]

Hyperbilirubinemia that persists for more than 14 days should stimulate the evaluating physician to entertain the idea of neonatal hepatitis syndrome (NHS) in the

Table 13.3. Suggested management of unconjugated hyperbilirubinemia in the full-term newborn

Age (days)	Consider photoTx	photoTx	X-Transfusion if photoTx fails	X-Transfusion and photoTx
1–2	>12	>15	>20	>25
2–3	>15	>18	>25	>30
>3	>17	>20	>25	>30

Photo Tx, phototherapy; X–Transfusion, exchange transfusion.
Adapted from American Academy of Pediatrics Subcommittee on Hyperbilirubinemia. Management of hyperbilirubinemia in the newborn infant 35 or more weeks of gestation. *Pediatrics.* 2004;114:316–397.[12]

differential diagnosis. *NHS* is a broad term that applies to a state in the newborn period in which there is accumulation of substances in the liver, blood, and extra-hepatic tissues that should be excreted in bile acid but are not secondary to decreased bile flow. This implies an increase in bile acids (i.e., direct bilirubin levels). The incidence of NHS can be anywhere from 1 in 2500 to 1 in 7000 births.[41] The various diseases that can cause NHS can be divided into multiple subgroups: infective, structural, metabolic, genetic, neoplastic, vascular, toxic, immune and idiopathic.

Conjugated Hyperbilirubinemia

Conjugated hyperbilirubinemia, although it lacks the toxicity of unconjugated hyperbilirubinemia, should always raise concern because it typically represents serious underlying disease. Etiologies of conjugated hyperbilirubinemia are summarized in Table 13.1. Associated findings of conjugated hyperbilirubinemia, although not always present in the newborn, are pale, acholic stools, dark urine or urine positive for bilirubin.[1] For a differential diagnosis of conjugated hyperbilirubinemia, see Table 13.1.

There are many infectious etiologies that can cause a patient to have a conjugated hyperbilirubinemia. The first and most important etiologies to rule out are the TORCH infections:

T Toxoplasmosis
O Other infections (e.g., syphilis, coxsackievirus, Epstein-Barr virus, varicella-zoster virus and parvovirus)
R Rubella
C Cytomegalovirus
H Herpes simplex virus

It is critical to diagnose these infections early due to their long-term sequelae if not treated. Typically, one sees enlargement of the liver and hyperbilirubinemia with each of these causative agents. Common findings in patients with toxoplasmosis include chorioretinitis, hydrocephaly or microcephaly and intracranial calcifications. Patients with rubella may present with intrauterine growth delay, anemia, thrombocytopenia, congenital heart defects, cataracts, salt and pepper chorioretinitis and sensorineural deafness. Patients with cytomegalovirus (CMV) clinically can present with a petechial rash, splenomegaly, microcephaly, intracranial calcifications, chorioretinitis and progressive sensorineural deafness. Clinically, patients with herpes simplex virus present with or without vesicular lesions, encephalitis, coagulopathy and an overall profound multisystem disorder. Syphilis can manifest as intrauterine growth delay, anemia, thrombocytopenia, nephrotic syndrome, periostitis, nasal discharge and skin rash.[42]

Biliary Atresia

The next subgroup that can cause NHS is structural in nature. Biliary atresia is the second most common diagnosis for children who present with liver disease (second to idiopathic neonatal hepatitis). The incidence of this disease ranges from 1 in 8000 to 1 in 21,000.[41,43] *Biliary atresia* is a progressive destruction of the extrahepatic bile ducts that causes scarring, obliteration and concomitant damage to the small- and medium-sized intrahepatic bile ducts.[42] This disease leads to liver failure by the age of 2 to 3 years. It is important to identify this disease so that intervention can be started early (within the first 60 days of life). Otherwise, long-term damage will ensue.[44] Other signs and symptoms to look for to identify biliary atresia are scleral icterus, significant hepatosplenomegaly and acholic stools.[44]

Choledochal Cysts

Choledochal cysts, a cystic dilation of the biliary tree, should be considered in children with increased direct hyperbilirubinemia. The incidence of choledochal cysts is lower than biliary atresia; this disease is present in 1 in 100,000 to 150,000 live births. Other than persistent hyperbilirubinemia, the clinical findings associated with this disease are a palpable abdominal mass and abdominal pain. It is important to identify this cause early by abdominal ultrasound so that spontaneous perforation, cholangitis and secondary biliary cirrhosis do not occur. This condition usually presents after the neonatal period but is still important to keep in the differential diagnosis.[45]

Alagille Syndrome

Alagille syndrome is a genetic syndrome that is transmitted in an autosomal dominant fashion. In this syndrome, a paucity of small bile ducts results in compromised biliary flow and hyperbilirubinemia. Many other clinical features present with this disease, such as broad forehead, mild hypertelorism, small pointed chin, posterior embryotoxon of the eye, peripheral pulmonary artery stenosis as well as other congenital heart defects, and vertebral anomalies.[46]

Several metabolic entities can cause NHS (alpha-1 antitrypsin deficiency, CF, and various inborn errors of metabolism). Alpha-1 antitrypsin disease is the most common inherited form of NHS. In this disease, there is a mutation in the alpha-1 antitrypsin gene that produces an enzyme that binds and inactivates leukocyte elastase. The incidence has been reported to be between 1 in 1600 to 1 in 2000 live births. These children present with prolonged hyperbilirubinemia and acholic stools, which indicates severe cholestasis. These patients may also have intrauterine growth retardation and vitamin K responsive coagulopathy. Diagnosis can only be confirmed by determining the alpha-1 antitrypsin level.[41]

Cystic Fibrosis

CF more commonly causes liver disease later in life but can sometimes cause NHS. Here, patients can present in a multitude of ways. Some may have a delayed passage of meconium, some may have hepatic steatosis without conjugated hyperbilirubinemia and some may present with NHS or neonatal cholestasis. Fortunately, the incidence is small.[42] One study showed that over a 35-year period at one hospital, 1474 children had neonatal cholestasis and only 9 of those children had CF.[47]

Other Inborn Errors of Metabolism

Other various inborn errors of metabolism (although more rare) that must be considered due to their short life expectancy are galactosemia (discussed earlier), tyrosinemia type I, fructosemia, Niemann-Pick disease and progressive familial intrahepatic cholestasis. A more thorough discussion of these diseases exceeds the scope of this chapter.

If a general workup has not determined the cause of hyperbilirubinemia, these specific enzyme deficiencies should be tested to rule out these rare causes of prolonged direct hyperbilirubinemia.

EMERGENCY DEPARTMENT EVALUATION

Evaluation should be guided by the clinical appearance of the infant and the timing of hyperbilirubinemia. A full-term, well-appearing, asymptomatic infant with no risk factors (see Table 13.2) who presents within a time frame that is consistent with physiologic hyperbilirubinemia is at low risk of complications. To aid in the assessment of the neonate with hyperbilirubinemia, serum bilirubin levels (including fractionation for direct and indirect bilirubin levels) and a hemoglobin measurement should be routinely ordered. With this, the evaluating physician can differentiate conjugated from unconjugated hyperbilirubinemia. Bilirubin measurements have a notoriously wide range, and these measurements are associated with a tremendous amount of inter-laboratory variability.[48] Nonetheless, inaccuracy between the physician's clinical estimation and actual serum bilirubin levels is well documented, as is poor inter-rater reliability, and physical examination alone should not be relied upon.

In a well-appearing, afebrile infant more than 3 days old with unconjugated hyperbilirubinemia lower than 15 mg/dL and normal hemoglobin, no further tests are needed. One should keep in mind that the threshold of concern is lower in younger infants (Table 13.3). Patients should be evaluated on the following day to reassess and determine if levels are continuing to rise.

Some practitioners would obtain a UA and urine culture.[2] Obtaining a UA may prove helpful in the infant with physiologic hyperbilirubinemia, as several investigations indicate this may be associated with asymptomatic UTIs and may be one of the earliest signs of an underlying UTI.[49] Furthermore, infants presenting with an onset of hyperbilirubinemia after 8 days of age and neonates with an elevated conjugated bilirubin fraction were more likely to have a UTI. One should therefore consider testing for a

UTI as part of the evaluation in the asymptomatic infant with hyperbilirubinemia who presents to the ED.[49]

In cases of significant hyperbilirubinemia (total bilirubin levels >15 mg/dL) or in patients in whom anemia is present, a complete blood count (CBC) with peripheral smear, DAT, reticulocyte count, and maternal and fetal blood types should be analyzed (ABO and Rh[D] typing).[2] DAT-positive infants are approximately twice as likely as their comparable peers to have a serum bilirubin of more than 12 mg/dL. In the presence of a positive DAT test, ABO or Rh incompatibility is the most likely cause of hyperbilirubinemia as the majority of other causes of hemolysis will be Coombs' negative.[2] Furthermore, a G6PD level has been recommended for any infant undergoing phototherapy with an appropriate genetic or geographic background, or for any infant who does not respond well to phototherapy.[2]

In patients with significant hyperbilirubinemia (serum bilirubin >15 mg/dL) or symptoms of underlying medical illness (fever, poor feeding, inconsolability, apnea, dehydration, etc.), the following should be obtained: direct and indirect bilirubin levels, CBC, peripheral blood smear, reticulocyte count, liver function tests, thyroid function tests and an evaluation for sepsis (cultures of blood, urine and cerebral spinous fluid). If an exchange transfusion is anticipated, a type- and cross-match must be obtained. Indirect hyperbilirubinemia, reticulocytosis and a smear consistent with RBC destruction is suggestive of hemolysis. Infants with hemolysis as cause of their hyperbilirubinemia are at a greater risk of kernicterus[50] and should be admitted.

For conjugated hyperbilirubinemia, evaluation efforts should be directed toward determining the underlying etiology.[2] Most commonly, conjugated hyperbilirubinemia is infectious in origin, and these cases should be treated accordingly with a sepsis workup and antibiotic therapy until the exact etiologic agent is identified. One should also consider other infectious causes, such as the TORCH infections, as being the causative agents. Testing includes a TORCH infection panel, hepatitis B serology and UA for CMV. Although less common, hyperbilirubinemia may be the presenting complaint in infants with inborn errors of metabolism, CF, alpha-1 antitrypsin deficiency and iron storage deficiencies. When any of these processes are suspected, investigative studies should be broad and include liver function tests, ammonia, albumin and total protein levels and a complete chemistry panel. Examining urine for reducing substances, testing sweat chloride and measuring RBC galactose-1 phosphate uridyltransferase activity (enzyme defect in galactosemia) may be required.

Obstructive causes may be more difficult to identify due to their insidious and often intermittent presentation. Abdominal ultrasound and hepatobiliary scintigraphy to assess for biliary atresia or choledochal cyst may provide a diagnosis that, when reached promptly, improves outcomes due to early surgical intervention.

KERNICTERUS

Kernicterus (bilirubin encephalopathy) is a rare but catastrophic bilirubin-induced brain injury and is one of the known causes of cerebral palsy. It is one of a few causes of brain damage occurring in the infant period that is preventable with current diagnostic and treatment regimens.[1] The link between hyperbilirubinemia and brain damage was first established in the early 1950s when Mollison and Hsia et al. demonstrated that the risk of kernicterus in infants with hemolytic disease of the newborn dramatically increased with bilirubin level and that exchange transfusion could dramatically decrease that risk.[51] Ultimately, the likelihood of kernicterus depends on the bilirubin level as well as the age of the child and the child's co-morbidities.

A schema for grading the severity of acute bilirubin encephalopathy has been described.[52] Earliest signs are often subtle and therefore may be missed but include early alterations in tone (hypotonia or hypertonia) of the extensor muscles with *retrocollis* (backward arching of the neck) and *opisthotonus* (backward arching of the trunk) as well as poor sucking.[53] The hypertonia and retrocollis often will increase in severity and may be accompanied by a shrill cry as well as unexplained irritability alternating with lethargy and fever.[53] Prompt and effective therapy during the early phase of bilirubin-induced neurologic dysfunction (BIND) can prevent chronic kernicteric sequelae.

Advanced signs of kernicterus are cessation of feeding, bicycling movements, irritability, seizures, fever and altered mental status. These late findings are predictors of severe kernicteric sequelae. The final stage is chronic irreversible bilirubin encephalopathy. The classic tetrad of this final stage is athetoid cerebral palsy, deafness or hearing loss, impairment of upward gaze and enamel dysplasia of the primary teeth.

Kernicterus was rarely seen in the decades following the introduction of phototherapy and exchange transfusion but recent reports suggest it is reemerging despite virtual elimination of Rh disease.[3] The majority of cases reported in the past decade have not occurred in infants with ABO, Rh or other hemolytic disease but in apparently healthy near-term and term infants with significantly elevated bilirubin levels (well above 30 mg/dL).[54]

Bhutani performed a review in which he defined steps to facilitate a safer experience with newborn hyperbilirubinemia and prevent the feared manifestation of severe hyperbilirubinemia and subsequent kernicterus.[5] A root cause analysis of cases of kernicterus was performed by the AAP subcommittee on neonatal hyperbilirubinemia, and they identified a series of recommendations to promote prevention.[53] These physician recommendations are listed[53]:

- Always have an increased level of concern.
- Assess for the presence or absence of hyperbilirubinemia through objective measures (rather than clinical estimation).
- Identify potential severe underlying disease.
- Pay close attention to parental concern regarding hyperbilirubinemia.
- Address poor feeding or lethargy.
- Intervene in a timely manner in infants with TSB greater than the 95th percentile.

EMERGENCY DEPARTMENT MANAGEMENT AND DISPOSITION

Management of hyperbilirubinemia in the term newborn is challenging as the clinician must balance the risks of aggressive versus conservative management. Careful consideration must be given to the risk-benefit ratio of each therapeutic intervention. Clinical decision-making is aided by weighing variables such as the infant's age, clinical appearance and bilirubin level and the etiology and timing of the hyperbilirubinemia.

The typical scenario an ED physician is confronted with is that of a child who is brought in by parents who noticed jaundice after the child was discharged from the nursery. Most often, these are infants who are already 3 to 4 days old. Less frequently, the ED physician evaluates younger children. Yet with the rise of home birth practices, situations may be encountered in which the ED physician will evaluate infants who have not received a nursery evaluation at all.

In the treatment of unconjugated hyperbilirubinemia, the ultimate goal is the prevention of kernicterus and its potentially devastating effects. The full-term, well-appearing and afebrile infant with no significant risk factors and a bilirubin less than 17 mg/dL may be observed only, monitoring closely for increasing hyperbilirubinemia. Dehydration should be corrected according to weight with normal saline boluses, and frequency of feeds may be increased to aid in the excretion of bilirubin. Frequent feeds and frequent stools aid in bilirubin excretion; therefore, frequent feeding should be encouraged.

The issue of continuing breastfeeding often arises. The AAP does not recommend the discontinuation of breastfeeding in healthy term newborns and encourages frequent breastfeeding, at least 8 to 10 times per 24-hour period.[1,2] The major risk of interrupting breastfeeding is that the interruption may result in a permanent discontinuation, thus the baby will lose the considerable benefits of breastfeeding. However, a temporary cessation (24–48 hours) may be considered to augment phototherapy. Upon cessation, a rapid drop in bilirubin levels will serve to confirm the diagnosis. Once breastfeeding is reinstated, serum levels will rise again but rarely to the extent prior to cessation. The adequacy of intake is then monitored to ensure proper hydration. For breastfed infants, supplemental feeds in the form of water or dextrose solution are not found to assist in lowering serum bilirubin levels, nor are they preventative against the development of hyperbilirubinemia.

Depending on the preference of the parents and the physician, several options for feeding exist (with or without phototherapy).[2] A candid conversation with the infant's parents will outline the risks and benefits of feeding options, each of which may be implemented with or without phototherapy:

1. Continuation of breastfeeding with close, objective monitoring
2. Supplementation of breastfeeding with formula
3. Brief substitution of breastfeeding with formula

Ultimately, feeding options for newborns with hyperbilirubinemia who are sufficiently healthy to be monitored on an outpatient basis depend upon both the parents' and physician's preferences.[2] In cases in which breast milk hyperbilirubinemia is most likely, one consideration is the temporary cessation of breastfeeding with reintroduction after the bilirubin has fallen to a safe level.

Phototherapy, one of the mainstays of therapy for the infant with hyperbilirubinemia, is a blue-green light that causes photoconversion of the bilirubin molecule in the skin to a water-soluble product that can be secreted into the bile or urine without the need for conjugation. The effect of phototherapy is therefore directly related to the amount of surface area exposed to the light. To optimize this, the treating physician may use an overhead light, photo blanket or both. The use of both devices (double phototherapy) ensures photo exposure to the child's back by lying on the photo blanket and to his or her front by using an overhead light. During the use of phototherapy, the infant should be naked and wear eye shields to avoid excessive exposure to the retina. In addition, the use of phototherapy may lead to greater insensible water loss; therefore, fluid intake must be increased by 20% and breastfeeding may be continued. Phototherapy should be avoided in the presence of a direct bilirubinemia due to the formation of a gray-brown discoloration of the skin (bronze baby syndrome). Other risks of phototherapy include dehydration, retinal damage, burns and loose stools. Appropriate phototherapy should decrease the TSB level by 1 to 2 mg/dL in 4 to 6 hours. In the absence of such a decline, consider ongoing hemolysis in the infant.

A general rule of thumb regarding when to initiate phototherapy for a full-term healthy infant is to begin phototherapy at a bilirubin of 17 mg/dL or higher and discontinue once bilirubin is lower than 12 mg/dL. It should be stressed that thresholds to initiate therapy will vary, based on the patient's age and the presence of associated risk factors. Table 13.3 demonstrates levels to initiate therapy in low risk infants. For example, phototherapy should be started at lower levels (15 mg/dL) for infants with a rapid rise in bilirubin levels (higher levels at younger ages), when ABO or Rh incompatibility exists, in the preterm infant and in the near-term infant.[1] *Near-term* is a phrase used to describe infants who do not meet the World Health Organization's definition of 38 to 42 weeks' gestation but weigh more than 2500 g at birth.[53,55]

A commentary by the AAP Subcommittee on Neonatal Hyperbilirubinemia concluded that infants who are near-term are at significant risk of severe hyperbilirubinemia.[53] A prospective investigation by Sarici et al. determined that infants of 35 to 42 weeks' gestation are 2.4 times more likely to develop significant hyperbilirubinemia.[55] The authors stated near-term infants should be considered in the high-risk group as one of four near-term infants require phototherapy for hyperbilirubinemia. For a full graphic layout of therapy guidelines by age and risk factor, refer to the recommendations outlined by the AAP Subcommittee on Neonatal Hyperbilirubinemia.[12]

Exchange transfusion should be initiated for emergent treatment of markedly elevated bilirubin (see Table 13.3). A body of literature exists that suggests that exchange transfusions to maintain a bilirubin level below 20 mg/dL prevent kernicterus in infants with severe hemolytic disease of the newborn.[51,52] An exchange transfusion is recommended for term infants with hemolysis if phototherapy is unable to maintain the total bilirubin level below 17.5 to 23.4 mg/dL or for any child showing signs of kernicterus.[1] Newman et al. similarly found that when high TSB levels were treated with phototherapy or exchange transfusion, there was not an association with adverse neurodevelopment.[56] An exchange transfusion will reduce the bilirubin concentration by approximately 50% and should be used with concurrent phototherapy.

Pharmacologic therapy also may be considered in conjunction with a neonatologist. Phenobarbital and ursodeoxycholic acid have been used to promote bilirubin conjugation, improve bile flow and lower bilirubin levels.[26] Tin mesoporphyrin decreases bilirubin production by inhibiting heme oxygenase and is awaiting Food and Drug Administration approval.[26]

Admission is indicated for all ill-appearing infants, those found to be anemic, those with bilirubin levels in the range of phototherapy or exchange requirements and those with pathologic or conjugated hyperbilirubinemia.[1] The latter always conceals serious underlying disease, and although conjugated bilirubin lacks the neurotoxicity of the unconjugated form, steps should be taken immediately to identify and treat the precipitating disorder. As outlined earlier, it is well documented that hyperbilirubinemia can be an early indicator of sepsis or UTI. If such an infectious etiology is suspected, antibiotics should be started immediately. The anatomic causes of biliary atresia or obstruction due to choledochal cyst must be identified early and surgical evaluation should be prompt.[2]

PROGNOSIS

For the majority of patients who are treated early and appropriately, the prognosis is good. This is evidenced by an investigation by Newman et al. that determined that when high TSB levels were treated with phototherapy or exchange transfusion, there was not an association with adverse neurodevelopment.[56]

CONCLUSION

Neonatal hyperbilirubinemia is estimated to occur in the majority of term infants in the first week of life and approximately 2% will reach a TSB greater than 20 mg/dL.[1–4] Secondary to early hospital discharge, neonatal hyperbilirubinemia has been transformed from an inpatient to an outpatient issue that is often dealt with by the ED physician. Consequently, the ED physician needs to be very comfortable with the presentation, evaluation and management of the newborn with hyperbilirubinemia. Kernicterus, a rare but catastrophic complication of neonatal hyperbilirubinemia, is preventable and, until recently, was thought to be extinct. The role of the ED physician is to balance the risks and benefits of diagnostic evaluation and management in the care of the neonate with hyperbilirubinemia.

PITFALLS

- Failure to recognize that hyperbilirubinemia may be an indication of sepsis. If risk factors exist, the patient should receive a full sepsis workup, and antibiotics should be started immediately. Assessing for hyperbilirubinemia in the newborn requires quantification of direct (conjugated) and indirect (unconjugated) bilirubin levels.
- Failure to recognize that direct hyperbilirubinemia should always be considered pathologic and that the infant should be admitted for further evaluation. *Hyperbilirubinemia* is defined by a serum bilirubin concentration greater than 5 mg/dL. *Direct hyperbilirubinemia* is defined as a direct bilirubin level greater than 2 mg/dL or a fraction greater than 20%. It should always be considered pathologic.

REFERENCES

1. American Academy of Pediatrics, Subcommittee on Neonatal Hyperbilirubinemia. Practice parameter: management of hyperbilirubinemia in the healthy term newborn. *Pediatrics.* 1994;94:55–565.
2. Claudius I, Fluharty C, Boles R. The emergency department approach to newborn and childhood metabolic crisis. *Emerg Med Clin N Am.* 2005;23:843–883.
3. Chou S-C, Palmer RH, Ezhuthachan S, et al. Management of hyperbilirubinemia in newborns: measuring performance by using a benchmarking model. *Pediatrics.* 2003;112(6):1264–1273.

4. Bhutani VK, Johnson L, Sivieri EM. Predictive ability of a predischarge hour-specific serum bilirubin for subsequent significant hyperbilirubinemia in healthy term and near-term newborns. *Pediatrics*. 1999;103:6–14.

5. Bhutani VK, Donn SM, Johnson LH. Risk management of severe neonatal hyperbilirubinemia to prevent kernicterus. *Clin Perinatol*. 2005;32(1):125–139.

6. Eggert LD, Wiedmeiser SE, Willson J, et al. The effect of instituting a prehospital–discharge newborn bilirubin screening program in an 18- hospital health system. *Pediatrics*. 2006;117:855–862.

7. Johnson L, Brown AK. A pilot registry for acute and chronic kernicterus in term and near-term infants. *Pediatrics*. 1999;104:736.

8. Tiker F, Gulcan H, Kilicdag H, et al. Extreme hyperbilirubinemia in newborn infants. *Clin Pediatr (Phila)*. 2006;45(3):257–261.

9. Newman TB, Xiong B, Gonzales VM, et al. Prediction and prevention of extreme hypobilirubinemia in a mature health maintenance organization. *Arch Pediatr Adolesc Med*. 2000;154:1140–1147.

10. Seidman DS, Stevenson DK, Ergaz Z, et al. Hospital readmission due to neonatal hyperbilirubinemia. *Pediatrics*. 1995;96:727–729.

11. Maisels MJ, Kring E. Length of stay, hyperbilirubinemia, and hospital readmission. *Pediatrics*. 1998;101:995–998.

12. American Academy of Pediatrics Subcommittee on Hyperbilirubinemia. Management of hyperbilirubinemia in the newborn infant 35 or more weeks of gestation. *Pediatrics*. 2004;114:316–397.

13. Bhutani VK, Johnson LH, Keren R. Diagnosis and management of hyperbilirubinemia in the term neonate: for a safer first week. *Pediatr Clin N Am*. 2004;51:843–861.

14. Kaplan M, Hammerman C. Understanding and preventing severe neonatal hyperbilirubinemia: is bilirubin neurotoxicity really a concern in the developed world? *Clin Perinatol*. 2004;31(3):555–575.

15. Khoury MJ, Calle EE, Joesoef RM. Recurrence risk of neonatal hyperbilirubinemia in siblings. *Am J Dis Child*. 1988;142(10):1065–1069.

16. Knudsen A, Ebbesen F. Cephalocaudal progression of hyperbilirubinemia in newborns admitted to neonatal intensive care units. *Biol Neonate*. 1997;71:357–361.

17. Bhutani VK, Gourley GR, Adler S, et al. Noninvasive measurement of total serum bilirubin in a multiracial predischarge newborn population to assess the risk of severe hyperbilirubinemia. *Pediatrics*. 2000;106(2):e17.

18. Moyer VA, Ahn C, Sneed S. Accuracy of clinical judgment in neonatal hyperbilirubinemia. *Arch Pediatr Adolesc Med*. 2000;154:391–394.

19. Porter LM, Dennis BL. Hyperbilirubinemia in the term newborn. *Am Fam Phys*. 2002;65(4): 599–605.

20. Tenovuo A. Neonatal complications in small-for-gestational age neonates. *J Perinat Med*. 1988;16:197–201.

21. Keren R, Bhutani VK, Luan X, et al. Identifying newborns at risk of significant hyperbilirubinemia: a comparison of two recommended approaches. *Arch Dis Child*. 2005;90:415–421.

22. Perlow JH, Wigton T, Hart J, Strassner HT, et al. Birth trauma: a five-year review of incidence and associated perinatal factors. *J Reprod Med*. 1996;41(10):754–760.

23. Thacker KE, Lim T, Drew JH. Cephalhaematoma: a 10-year review. *Aust N Z J Obstet Gynecol*. 1987;27(3):210–212.

24. Davies DP, Gomersall R, Robertson R, et al. Neonatal hyperbilirubinemia and maternal oxytocin infusion. *BMJ*. 1973;3:476–477.

25. Chung MA. Galactosemia in infancy: diagnosis, management, and prognosis. *Pediatr Nurs*. 1997;23(6):563–568.

26. Maisels M. Neonatal hyperbilirubinemia. *Pediatr Rev*. 2006;27(12):443–454.

27. Waldron P, de Alarcon P. ABO hemolytic disease of the newborn: a unique constellation of findings in siblings and review of protective mechanisms in the fetal–maternal system. *Am J Perinatol*. 1999;16(8):391–398.

28. Iranpour R, Akbar MR, Haghshenas I. Glucose-6-phosphate dehydrogenase deficiency in neonates. *Indian J Pediatr*. 2003;70(11):855–857.

29. Atay E, Bozaykut A, Ipek IO. Glucose-6-phosphate dehydrogenase deficiency in neonatal indirect hyperbilirubinemia. *J Trop Pediatr*. 2006;52(1):56–58.

30. Kedar PS, Warang P, Colah RB, et al. Red cell pyruvate kinase deficiency in neonatal hyperbilirubinemia cases in India. *Indian J Pediatr*. 2006;73(11):985–988.

31. Passi GR, Saran S. Neonatal hyperbilirubinemia due to hereditary spherocytosis. *Indian Pediatr*. 2004;41:199.

32. Laosombat V, Dissaneevate S, Peerapittayamongkol C, et al. Neonatal hyperbilirubinemia associated with southeast Asian ovalocytosis. *Am J Hematol*. 1999;60:136–139.

33. Gartner LM, Herschel M. Hyperbilirubinemia and breast-feeding. *Pediatr Clin North Am*. 2001;48(2):389–399.

34. Strauss KA, Robinson DL, Vreman HJ, et al. Management of hyperbilirubinemia and prevention of kernicterus in 20 patients with Crigler-Najjar disease. *Eur J Pediatr*. 2006;165(5):306–319.

35. LaFranchi SH, Murphey WH, Foley TP, et al. Neonatal hypothyroidism detected by the northwest regional screening program. *Pediatrics*. 1979;63(2):180–191.

36. Schneider AP. Breast milk hyperbilirubinemia in the newborn: a real entity. *JAMA*. 1986;255(23):3270–3274.

37. Brown LP, Arnold A, Allison D, et al. Incidence and pattern of hyperbilirubinemia in healthy breast-fed infants during the first month of life. *Nurs Res*. 1993;42(2):106–110.

38. Poland RL. Breast-milk hyperbilirubinemia. *J Pediatr*. 1981;99(1):86–88.

39. Chavalitdhamrong PO, Escobedo MB, Barton LL, et al. Hyperbilirubinemia and bacterial infection in the newborn. *Arch Dis Child*. 1975;50(8):652–654.

40. Maisels MJ, Kring E. Risk of sepsis in newborns with severe hyperbilirubinemia. *Pediatrics*. 1992;90(5):741–743.

41. McKiernan PJ. Neonatal cholestasis. *Semin Neonatol*. 2002;7:153–165.

42. Roberts EA. Neonatal hepatitis syndrome. *Semin Neonatol*. 2003;8:357–374.

43. Emerick KM, Whittington PF. Neonatal liver disease. *Pediatr Ann*. 2006;35(4):281–286.

44. Bates MD, Bucuvalas JC, Alonso MH, et al. Biliary atresia: pathogenesis and treatment. *Semin Liver Dis.* 1998;18(3):281–293.

45. Poddar U, Thapa BR, Chhabra M, et al. Choledochal cysts in infants and children. *Indian Pediatr.* 1998;35:613–618.

46. Emerick KM, Rand EB, Goldmuntz E, et al. Features of Alagille syndrome in 92 patients: frequency and relation to prognosis. *Hepatology.* 1999;29(3):822–829.

47. Lykavieris P, Bernard O, Hadchouel M. Neonatal cholestasis as the presenting feature in cystic fibrosis. *Arch Dis Child.* 1996;75:67–70.

48. Vreman HJ, Verter J, Oh W, et al. Interlaboratory variability of bilirubin measurements. *Clin Chem.* 1995;42:869–873.

49. Garcia FJ, Nager AL. Hyperbilirubinemia as an early sign of urinary tract infection in infancy. *Pediatrics.* 2002;109(5):846–851.

50. MacDonald MG. Hidden risks: early discharge and bilirubin toxicity due to glucose 6-phosphate dehydrogenase deficiency. *Pediatrics.* 1995;96(4): 734–738.

51. Mollison Pl, Cutbush M. Haemolytic disease of the newborn. *Recent Advances in Pediatrics.* 1954;110.

52. Volpe J. Bilirubin and brain injury. *Neurology of the Newborn*, 4th ed. Philadelphia, PA: WB Saunders; 2001:521–546.

53. American Academy of Pediatrics, Subcommittee on Neonatal Hyperbilirubinemia. Neonatal hyperbilirubinemia and kernicterus. *Pediatrics.* 2001;108:763–765.

54. Maisels MJ, Newman TB. Predicting hyperbilirubinemia in newborns: the importance of timing. *Pediatrics.* 1999;103:493–494.

55. Sarici SU, Serdar MA, Korkmaz A, et al. Incidence, course and prediction of hyperbilirubinemia in near-Term and term newborns. *Pediatrics.* 2004;113(4):775–780.

56. Newman TB, Liljestrand P, Jeremy RJ, et al; the Hyperbilirubinemia and Infant Feeding Study Team. Outcomes among newborns with total serum bilirubin levels of 25 mg per deciliter or more. *N Engl J Med.* 2006; 354(18):1889–1900.

14 Seizures

Michelle D. Blumstein and Marla J. Friedman

INTRODUCTION

A *seizure* is a paroxysmal electrical discharge of neurons in the brain resulting in an alteration of behavior or function. A seizure is not a diagnosis itself but rather a symptom of many different pathologic processes (Table 14.1). The clinical manifestations of a seizure are dependent on multiple factors, including the age of the child, the cortical location of neuronal discharge and the direction and speed of the electrical impulse. Most seizures are followed by a postictal period characterized by fatigue, confusion or irritability.[2] Some seizures are self-limited, whereas others require medical intervention. The annual incidence of first-time unprovoked seizures in children is 150,000, making seizures the most common neurologic disorder in children. Overall, 4% to 10% of children will experience a seizure before the age of 16 years.[3,4] The incidence is highest in children younger than 3 years and decreases with increasing age. Seizures account for 1% of all emergency department (ED) visits in children.[3,4]

Up to 30,000 children who experience a first-time unprovoked seizure will go on to receive a diagnosis of epilepsy.[3] *Epilepsy* is defined as the susceptibility to recurrent seizures. An *epileptic syndrome* is one in which a specific set of signs and symptoms are associated with characteristic neurologic and encephalographic (EEG) abnormalities. *Status epilepticus* refers to continuous seizure activity lasting longer than 30 minutes or failure to return to baseline level of consciousness between two or more consecutive seizures.

The body's metabolic demands increase during seizure activity. Cerebral oxygen and glucose consumption increase as does the production of lactate and carbon dioxide. Simultaneously, cerebral blood flow increases as a compensatory mechanism. Brief seizures rarely result in neurologic sequelae. If ventilation is inadequate or if the

Table 14.1. Etiology of seizures[1]

Infectious
Febrile seizure
Meningitis
Encephalitis
Brain abscess
Neurocysticercosis
Neurologic/Developmental
Birth injury
Hypoxic-ischemic encephalopathy
Neurocutaneous syndromes
Ventriculoperitoneal shunt malfunction
Congenital anomalies
Degenerative cerebral disease
Metabolic
Hypoglycemia
Hypoxia
Hypomagnesemia
Hypocalcemia
Hypercarbia
Inborn errors of metabolism
Pyridoxine deficiency
Traumatic/Vascular
Child abuse
Head trauma
Intracranial hemorrhage
Cerebral contusion
Cerebrovascular accident
Toxicologic
Alcohol, amphetamines, antihistamines, anticholinergics
Cocaine, carbon monoxide
Isoniazid
Lead, lithium, lindane
Oral hypoglycemics, organophosphates
Phencyclidine, phenothiazines
Salicylates, sympathomimetics
Tricyclic antidepressants, theophylline, topical anesthetics
Withdrawals (alcohol, anticonvulsants)
Idiopathic/Epilepsy
Obstetric (eclampsia)
Oncologic

From Friedman M, Sharieff G. Seizures in children. *Pediatr Clin North Am.* 2006;53:257;277.

Table 14.2. Seizure types

Generalized	Partial
Tonic	Simple
Clonic	Complex
Tonic-clonic (grand mal)	
Myoclonic	
Atonic (drop attacks)	
Absence (petit mal)	
• Simple (typical)	
• Complex (atypical)	

seizure is prolonged, this cerebral compensation fails and neurologic damage may result.

Tachycardia, hypertension and hyperglycemia may result from the increase in sympathetic discharge. Failure to maintain a patent airway can result from a decreased level of consciousness and may lead to hypoxia, hypercarbia and respiratory acidosis. The risks of lactic acidosis, hyperthermia, rhabdomyolysis, hyperkalemia and hypoglycemia increase with prolonged seizure activity.

SEIZURE TYPES

Classification of seizure type is an important step in seizure management (Table 14.2). When seizure activity involves both cerebral hemispheres, the seizure is referred to as *generalized*. These seizures may be either convulsive or nonconvulsive. Motor activity, when present, is bilateral. Types of generalized seizures include tonic-clonic (grand mal), tonic, clonic, myoclonic, atonic (drop attacks) and absence (petit mal).[2,5,6] The most common type of seizure in children is a generalized tonic-clonic seizure. The initial tonic phase lasts between 10 and 30 seconds and is marked by muscle contraction, pallor, eye deviation and mydriasis. Bowel or bladder incontinence may occur. A clonic phase follows, including jerking movements and flexor spasms. These seizures usually occur without warning, but an aura precedes the seizure in 20% to 30% of patients.[2,5] A postictal phase follows these seizures. A transient localized weakness or paralysis (Todd's paralysis) also may occur.[2] This finding requires only supportive treatment and resolves on its own. *Myoclonic seizures* are characterized by "jackknifing" (sudden arm flexion and head drop) and may occur hundreds of times daily. A sudden, abrupt loss of consciousness and muscle tone characterizes *atonic seizures* (drop attacks). *Absence* (petit mal) *seizures* are sudden, brief (5–30 seconds) lapses in

awareness. *Simple* (typical) *absence seizures* are not accompanied by a postictal phase or a loss in postural tone. Eye blinking is sometimes present. Increased myoclonic activity in the face or extremities, more gradual onset and resolution and prolonged seizure activity are associated with *complex* (atypical) *absence seizures.*[5]

In contrast to generalized seizures, *partial* (focal, local) *seizures* initially involve only one cerebral hemisphere. These seizures may have motor, sensory, autonomic and psychic components. Often, these seizures are preceded by an alteration in perception or hallucination known as an *aura.*[2] They are subclassified as simple or complex based on whether or not consciousness is impaired. A *complex partial seizure* is associated with an alteration in consciousness. Either simple or complex partial seizures may subsequently generalize; this occurs in approximately 30% of children.[5]

EPILEPSY SYNDROMES

Epilepsy syndromes can be classified by etiology in addition to clinical presentation. These syndromes are divided into symptomatic, cryptogenic and idiopathic epilepsy types. Symptomatic epilepsy accounts for approximately one quarter of epilepsy syndromes and refers to those syndromes with a preceding neurologic cause. In cryptogenic syndromes, an occult cause is suspected although one has not been identified. Idiopathic epilepsy or genetic syndromes refer to cases in which no cause has been determined, but multiple family members are affected.[7] Most epilepsy syndromes present during childhood and are diagnosed based on age at presentation, seizure type and EEG findings (Table 14.3).

Infantile spasms (West's syndrome) present between the ages of 4 and 18 months with jerking movements, which occur in clusters. These movements manifest as sudden contractions of the extremities, head, neck and trunk, which rarely occur during sleep. Twenty-five percent of patients with West's syndrome also have tuberous sclerosis and 95% have mental retardation. The syndrome is associated with a 20% mortality rate. The EEG characteristically demonstrates *hypsarrhythmia* (random, high-voltage, slow waves with multi-focal spikes).[5] Adrenocorticotropic hormone (ACTH) and prednisone are the most common treatments.[4,8,9] Some seizure control has been reported with valproic acid, lamotrigine, topiramate, vigabatrin and zonisamide.[8,10,11]

Table 14.3. Childhood epilepsy syndromes

Syndrome	Age	EEG findings	Presentation	Treatment
Infantile spasms (West's syndrome)	4–18 mo	Hypsarrhythmia (random high-voltage slow waves with multifocal spikes)	• Jerking of extremities, head, neck, trunk • Clusters • MR in 95%, TS in 25%, 20% mortality	ACTH, prednisone, valproate, lamotrigine, topiramate, vigabatrin, zonisamide
Lennox-Gastaut Syndrome	3–5 y	Irregular slow, high voltage spike pattern	• Intractable, mixed type seizures • MR, behavioral problems	Valproate, felbamate, topiramate, lamotrigine, zonisamide, ketogenic diet
Benign rolandic epilepsy	3–13 y	Perisylvian spiking	• Clonic activity of face • Wake child from sleep • Spontaneous resolution	• Usually not indicated • Carbamazepine, if severe
Juvenile myoclonic epilepsy of Janz	12–18 y	Fast spike and wave discharges	• Myoclonic jerks on awakening • Provoked by alcohol, stress, fatigue, hormones	Valproate, lamotrigine, topiramate, felbamate, zonisamide

ACTH, adrenocorticotropic hormone; MR, mental retardation; TS, Tuberous sclerosis.

Lennox-Gastaut syndrome presents with mixed seizure types (tonic, myoclonic, atonic and absence) between 3 and 5 years of age and is frequently accompanied by mental retardation. These seizures are quite difficult to control, although multiple medications have been used. Valproic acid is used most commonly; alternatives include zonisamide, lamotrigine, felbamate and topiramate.[8,10] This syndrome has also been treated successfully with the ketogenic diet.[12] The EEG shows an irregular, slow, high-voltage spike pattern.[5]

Nighttime seizures occur between the ages of 3 and 13 years in children with *benign rolandic epilepsy*. These seizures begin with facial grimacing and vocalizations that wake the child from sleep. The syndrome is inherited in an autosomal dominant fashion. EEG shows a pattern of perisylvian spiking. Treatment is usually unnecessary as the syndrome usually resolves on its own by early adulthood. Carbamazepine may be used if seizures are frequent.[3,5,8]

Juvenile myoclonic epilepsy of Janz is another syndrome that is inherited in an autosomal dominant fashion. Seizures begin in adolescence, between the ages of 12 and 18 years. Hormonal changes, alcohol, lack of sleep and stress can result in an increase in seizure activity. This syndrome presents with myoclonic jerks on awakening. Eighty percent of these patients have tonic-clonic seizures and 25% have absence seizures in addition to the myoclonic jerks. Characteristic fast, spike-and-wave discharges are seen on EEG. Valproic acid is the most commonly used antiepileptic, but zonisamide, topiramate, lamotrigine and felbamate are alternatives.[3,5,8]

SPECIAL CONSIDERATIONS

Febrile Seizures

A febrile seizure occurs in association with a febrile illness in children between the ages of 6 months and 5 years. The peak age of occurrence is 18 months. Febrile seizures occur in 25% of children, which makes these seizures the type most commonly found in young children.[3,13] Febrile seizures are classified as either simple or complex (Table 14.4). A simple febrile seizure is brief (<15 min), generalized and only occurs once during a febrile illness. If the convulsion lasts longer than 15 minutes, recurs during the same febrile illness or has focal features, it is classified

Table 14.4. Febrile seizures

Simple	Complex
Brief ($\leq$15 min)	Sustained (>15 min)
Single	Recurs during single febrile illness
Generalized	Focal

as complex. Simple febrile seizures account for 80% of all febrile seizures.

Although fever lowers the seizure threshold in some children, the exact pathophysiology of these seizures is unknown. A genetic predilection does exist, and 25% to 40% of children who experience a febrile seizure have a family history of febrile seizures. Approximately 33% of children who have a febrile seizure will experience a recurrence. Recurrences are most likely in children whose first seizure occurred prior to 1 year of age.[14] When they occur, recurrences tend to occur soon after the initial seizure, with 50% occurring within 6 months, 73% within the first year, and 90% within the first 2 years.[14] Less than 10% of these children will have three seizures in their lifetime.[15] It is unclear whether the rate of temperature rise or the absolute height of the temperature is more related to seizure activity.[13,15,16] Children who have their first febrile seizure at a higher temperature have fewer recurrences. There is no association between seizure type and recurrence.[3,17]

Most often, febrile seizures have no complications or long-term neurologic consequences.[13,15,16] The incidence of epilepsy in children who have experienced a febrile seizure is slightly higher (1%–2%) than the general population. In the general population, the incidence of epilepsy falls between 0.5% and 1%.[15] Patients with a family history of epilepsy, abnormal neurologic findings prior to the febrile seizure or a complex febrile seizure have a 10% to 13% chance of developing epilepsy.[14,15]

Frequently, children either are in the postictal period or have returned to baseline neurologic status by the time they present to the ED. In these situations, the evaluation should include a thorough history and physical exam as well as an age-appropriate search for the fever source.[13–17] The most common cause of fever in children with febrile seizures is a viral illness. Both influenza A and human herpes virus 6 (roseola infantum) have been associated with an increased incidence of febrile seizures.[18] The occurrence of a febrile seizure is not associated with a higher incidence of serious bacterial illness.[16,19] In children who have returned to baseline, have a normal physical exam and have no risk factors for epilepsy, routine examinations of electrolytes and glucose are unnecessary.[13,14]

The need for routine lumbar puncture (LP) in all children with a first-time febrile seizure is controversial. The American Academy of Pediatrics recommends the strong consideration of LP following a febrile seizure in children younger than 12 months of age and the consideration of LP in those younger than 18 months.[13] Some advocate basing the decision to perform an LP on clinical findings rather than age criteria alone, but the physical exam is often unreliable in young or postictal children.[16] Children younger than 18 months of age should have an LP if they have a history of irritability, lethargy or poor oral intake. Those with mental status changes, slow return from postictal period, bulging fontanelle or other meningeal signs should also have an LP. LP should be considered in children with complex febrile seizures or those who have been pretreated with antibiotics.[16]

The initial management of febrile seizures is the same as that of any other seizure type. Stabilization of the airway, breathing and circulation (ABCs) are initial priorities, followed by therapy to abort seizure activity. Benzodiazepines are the first-line therapy followed by fosphenytoin and phenobarbital. Antipyretics and cooling measures should be initiated as well.[16]

EEG is not necessary after a febrile seizure, but may be useful in patients with an underlying neurologic disorder.[14] Emergent neuroimaging is not necessary in a well appearing child following a first-time simple febrile seizure. Children with a complex febrile seizure may require emergent or nonemergent neuroimaging.[17]

Antiepileptic drug therapy is rarely indicated in children with febrile seizures. Exceptions include children with focal or prolonged seizures, neurologic deficits or a strong family history of epilepsy. Phenobarbital has been effective in the prevention of future febrile seizures. Phenobarbital cannot be administered at the onset of fever but must be taken continuously to be effective. Its use is limited by behavioral and cognitive side effects. Valproic acid is also effective, but its use is associated with pancreatitis and hepatotoxicity in young children. Neither carbamazepine nor phenytoin has shown any success in the prevention of febrile seizures. Diazepam (0.5 mg/kg/day) taken either rectally (PR) or orally (PO) divided into two daily doses from the onset of fever is effective in preventing febrile seizures, but its use is associated with lethargy, irritability and ataxia.[14] Although these medications decrease the recurrence of febrile seizures, none decrease the risk of future development of epilepsy. Early prophylactic use of antipyretics does not prevent future febrile seizures.

Patients with prolonged seizure activity, with complex febrile seizures or who required medications to stop the seizure activity should be admitted to the hospital for observation. Children with a normal physical exam following a spontaneously resolved simple febrile seizure can be safely discharged home with appropriate follow-up and parental reassurance.

Neonatal Seizures

Seizures are the most common manifestation of impaired brain function in neonates. From 2 to 3.5 of 1000 newborns will experience a seizure as the seizure threshold is lower in neonates than in older children. Neonatal seizures cause little direct brain injury; however, these children may be predisposed to learning difficulties and seizure activity later in life.[20] Poorer outcomes are seen in low birth weight infants, but it is unclear if this is due to seizure activity or to another initial cerebral insult.[20] The differential diagnosis of neonatal seizures is listed in Table 14.5. From 50% to 65% of neonatal seizures are the result of intrauterine or perinatal hypoxia. An additional 15% result from intracranial hemorrhages, whereas infections, metabolic abnormalities and toxins cause approximately 5% to 10% of neonatal seizures.[21] Neonatal seizures are frequently subtle and often difficult to discern from normal neonatal

Table 14.5. Causes of neonatal seizures

Perinatal or intrauterine hypoxia or anoxia
Intracranial hemorrhage
Intraventricular
Subdural
Subarachnoid

Infection
Group B Streptococcus
Escherichia coli
TORCH
● Toxoplasmosis
● Other (syphilis, hepatitis B, coxsackievirus, Ebstein-Barr virus, varicella zoster virus, human parvovirus)
● Rubella
● Cytomegalovirus
● Herpes simplex virus

Metabolic Abnormalities
Hypoglycemia
Hypocalcemia
Hypomagnesemia
Pyridoxine deficiency
Inborn errors of metabolism

Other
Toxins/drug withdrawal
Central nervous system abnormalities
Neurocutaneous diseases

movements because the immature brain is unable to sustain organized epileptiform activity. Lip smacking, apneic events, eye deviations or autonomic alterations may be the only manifestation of seizure activity. True seizure activity cannot be stopped with passive restraint and cannot be elicited by moving or startling the infant.[22]

When seizures are suspected in the neonate, EEG and cerebral imaging including head ultrasound, computed tomography (CT) or magnetic resonance imaging (MRI) may be indicated. Initial laboratory evaluation includes a complete blood cell count, blood culture, glucose, electrolytes including calcium and magnesium, urinalysis, urine culture and toxicology screens. Additionally, cerebrospinal fluid (CSF) cell counts, culture and herpes simplex virus polymerase chain reaction (HSV PCR) should be considered. If inborn errors of metabolism are suspected, urine organic acids, blood amino acids, lactate, pyruvate and ammonia also should be performed.

Two seizure syndromes unique to the neonatal period include benign familial neonatal convulsions (BFNCs) and benign idiopathic neonatal convulsions (BINCs). Both of these seizure types have an unknown etiology but carry a favorable prognosis. BINCs present on day of life 5 and are known as the *fifth day fits*. These resolve spontaneously by day of life 15.[23] BFNCs present within the first 3 days of life and resolve by 6 months. These patients usually have a family history of neonatal seizures.[23]

The initial treatment of neonatal seizures includes attention to the ABCs. The next therapeutic goal is cessation of seizure activity. Hypotension and respiratory depression may result from benzodiazepines, and these should be used with caution in this age group.[21,23,24] Phenobarbital and phenytoin are equally effective in neonatal seizure treatment; however, neither is particularly successful.[20] Phenytoin is variably metabolized by neonates and may cause myocardial depression. As a result, phenobarbital is most often used as the first-line agent.[21,23] Pyridoxine deficiency is an autosomal recessive disorder and a rare cause of neonatal seizures presenting in the first 1 to 2 days of life. A trial of pyridoxine is indicated in neonates who do not respond to conventional therapy.[23] Any electrolyte abnormalities should be corrected and infectious causes of seizures should be treated as soon as they are identified. Long-term antiepileptic therapy generally includes phenobarbital or fosphenytoin; however, topiramate and zonisamide have also been effective.[22]

Table 14.6. Differential diagnosis of seizures

Disorders with altered levels of consciousness
Breath-holding spells
Syncope
Cardiac dysrhythmias
Migraines
Apparent life-threatening event (ALTE)
Paroxysmal Movement Disorders
Tics
Shuddering attacks
Benign myoclonus
Pseudoseizures
Spasmus nutans
Acute dystonia
Paroxysmal choreoathetosis
Sleep Disorders
Night terrors
Sleepwalking
Narcolepsy
Nightmares
Sleep apnea or hypersomnia
Gastrointestinal Disorders
Sandifer's syndrome
Abdominal migraines
Cyclic vomiting
Psychiatric Disorders
Attention deficit hyperactivity disorder (ADHD)
Panic attacks
Hyperventilation
Hysteria
Daydreaming
Head Trauma

DIFFERENTIAL DIAGNOSIS

Many paroxysmal events in childhood mimic seizures. Disorders involving altered consciousness, abnormal movements, certain sleep disorders or psychiatric disorders may appear like seizure activity and must be differentiated from seizures (Table 14.6). Descriptions of the event as well as the time period preceding and following the event are invaluable when making these diagnoses. True seizure activity cannot be stopped with passive restraint, and most nonepileptic events are not followed by a postictal period.[22]

Approximately 5% of children between the ages of 6 months and 5 years experience breath-holding spells, either pallid or cyanotic. In *pallid breath-holding spells,* the child becomes pale and experiences a loss of consciousness and muscle tone. These episodes generally follow minor trauma. *Cyanotic breath-holding spells* occur after a short period of vigorous crying. The child becomes cyanotic and limp and loses consciousness. Shaking of the extremities may occur. Both types of breath-holding spells are brief, with a rapid return to normal activity. Neither is associated with a postictal period. These episodes resolve spontaneously with age and require no treatment.[5,25]

A *syncopal event* may result from a variety of causes that lead to a brief, sudden loss of muscle tone and consciousness. These events are more common in adolescents. The event is often preceded by a feeling of nausea, dizziness or lightheadedness. Mydriasis, pallor and diaphoresis may also occur.[5,25,26] *Tics* are brief, repetitive movements that may be induced by stress and are partially repressible. *Benign shuddering attacks* last a few seconds and are characterized by a rapid shaking of the head and arms before a return to baseline activity. The constellation of back arching, writhing and crying associated with vomiting is known as *Sandifer's syndrome.* It is a manifestation of gastroesophageal reflux disease that may mimic seizure activity. *Dystonic reactions* are most commonly a side effect of medication. They manifest with facial grimacing, sustained contractures of the trunk and neck muscles, and abnormal posturing and may be confused with a tonic seizure. These children experience no postictal period. *Spasmus nutans* presents between the ages of 4 and 12 months and is characterized by nystagmus, head tilting and nodding.[5,25]

Preschool aged children may experience *night terrors.* During these episodes, the child awakens suddenly – crying, confused and frightened. He or she has no recollection of the event, which lasts only a few minutes. *Somnambulism* (sleepwalking) is seen in school aged children who wake from sleep and walk around briefly before returning to bed. *Narcolepsy* is a rare disorder that presents in adolescence. Sudden, uncontrollable periods of sleep during waking hours are the hallmark of disease. It is associated with cataplexy, a sudden loss of muscle tone following an emotional outburst in 50% of patients. This event may be mistaken for an atonic type seizure.[5,25,27]

In patients with a personal or family history of seizure disorder, it is important to consider *pseudoseizures* in the differential diagnosis. Features that may suggest the diagnosis of pseudoseizures include moaning or talking during the seizure and suggestibility. These are often difficult to differentiate from true seizure activity, but EEG or video telemetry may be helpful.[5,25]

EVALUATION AND MANAGEMENT

History and Physical Exam

A thorough history and physical exam may provide significant insight into the type of seizure and the underlying cause of the seizure activity. It may also help differentiate between true seizure activity and other disorders that mimic seizures. The history should include questions regarding precipitating factors of seizure activity. It is helpful to know if the child has had fever, recent illness or trauma, or immunizations; taken medications; possibly ingested something; or has a history of neurologic disease or previous seizures. In children with a history of seizures, additional historic features should include the type of previous seizures, prior and current antiepileptic therapy, any recent medication changes, the child's baseline seizure frequency and how the current seizure compares to prior seizures. The history should also include questions regarding comorbid conditions such as autism, attention deficit hyperactivity disorder (ADHD), and mental retardation, which are associated with a higher incidence of seizure disorder.[28]

A detailed description of the event from a reliable witness is invaluable. History should include the length of the event, types of movements, eye involvement, level of consciousness and presence or absence of incontinence. The child's behavior or symptoms just prior to the event, including the presence or absence of an aura, should be reviewed. Additionally, symptoms following the event, including the presence and length of any postictal period, should be noted.[5]

A thorough physical exam should be performed in all patients with suspected seizure activity. A complete set of vital signs including temperature should be obtained immediately. Special attention should be paid to the neurologic exam looking for focal neurologic deficits, evidence of elevated intracranial pressure (vital sign changes, bulging fontanelle), head trauma (retinal hemorrhages, bruising), infection or meningeal irritation. Less obvious physical exam findings may also be present and represent diseases that are associated with seizures. Café au lait spots, ash leaf spots and port wine stains are associated with neurocutaneous diseases, whereas hepatosplenomegaly may be associated with glycogen storage diseases.[5]

Laboratory Testing

The history and physical exam findings should guide laboratory analysis and should aim to identify a treatable cause of seizure activity. A rapid glucose level should be performed in all patients following a seizure; however, a full electrolyte evaluation is not always necessary. Children younger than 1 month of age, those with hypothermia ($< 36.5°C$) and those who are actively seizing are more likely to have an electrolyte abnormality.[29] An electrolyte evaluation is also useful in patients with dehydration, excess free water intake, diabetes mellitus or other metabolic disorders, altered level of consciousness and prolonged seizure activity, and those who are younger than 6 months of age. If an infectious cause is suspected, measurement of the white blood cell (WBC) count may be useful. In certain clinical situations, urine amino acids, serum organic acids, ammonia levels and toxicology screens also may be useful.[26] In children with a known seizure disorder, serum anticonvulsant levels should be measured. Subtherapeutic anticonvulsant levels are a common cause of increased seizure activity in these children.[6]

An LP is not routinely necessary in evaluating seizure activity. Well appearing children who have made a complete return to baseline do not need an LP as part of their evaluation. CSF evaluation should be performed in any child with meningeal signs, altered mental status or a prolonged postictal period. LP should be considered in neonatal seizures as well.[26]

Neuroimaging

Emergent neuroimaging is not required in all patients following a first-time seizure. Patients with a history of trauma, a ventriculoperitoneal (VP) shunt, a hypercoagulable state (e.g., sickle cell disease), bleeding disorder, immunocompromise (e.g., human immunodeficiency virus, malignancy), neurocutaneous disorder or exposure to cysticercosis should have cranial imaging performed.[30] Patients with focal seizures, focal neurologic deficits, a prolonged postictal period or physical exam evidence of increased intracranial pressure should also be imaged.[30] CT scanning is often more readily available and is frequently performed in the emergency setting. MRI may be more sensitive for vascular malformations and certain tumors; however, it is not always available

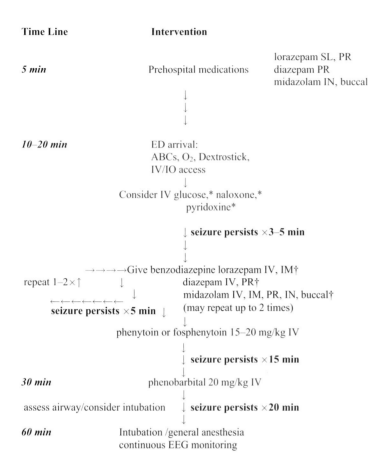

Figure 14.1. Status epilepticus management algorithm.
ABC, airway, breathing, circulation; EEG, electro-encephalogram; IM intramuscular; IN, intranasal; IO, intraosseous; IV, intravenous; PR, rectal; SL, sublingual.
∗Dextrose 2–4 mL/kg/dose D25W IV.
Naloxone 0.1 mg/kg/dose IV/IM/SC/ETT if <20 kg, 2 mg/dose if >20 kg.

emergently.[5,6] Well appearing children without any historical or physical exam risk factors can be safely discharged home without emergent neuroimaging.[26]

Electroencephalography

An emergent EEG is not necessary in well appearing children following a first-time afebrile seizure. These patients should, however, receive an outpatient EEG as part of their evaluation. An EEG during seizure activity is most useful but not often feasible. One performed in sleep states, in wake states and during stimulation yields significant information.[5,6] An emergent EEG is warranted in patients with refractory seizure activity or when non-convulsive status epilepticus is suspected. A negative EEG does not rule out a seizure disorder, but positive findings may help predict the risk of future seizures. Patients with an abnormal EEG have a 2-year seizure recurrence rate of 58%. The rate decreases to 28% in those with normal EEG findings.[31]

INITIAL MANAGEMENT

Because most seizures are brief and self-limited, the vast majority of patients present to the ED after a seizure has stopped. In patients who are actively seizing on presentation to the ED, the diagnosis of status epilepticus must be considered. After 10 minutes, seizure activity is unlikely to cease without medical intervention, and antiseizure medications become less effective with increasing length of seizure activity.[32]

Evaluation and stabilization of the ABCs are primary priorities when caring for a seizing patient (Figure 14.1). Airway positioning and, occasionally, a nasal or oral airway are frequently all that is needed to effectively control a patient's airway in these cases. Supplemental oxygen should be provided to all seizing patients. Intubation medications and equipment should be available at the patient's bedside. The need for intubation becomes more likely after the administration of certain antiseizure medications, and frequent re-evaluation of airway patency is necessary. Vascular access, either intravenous (IV) or intraosseous (IO), should be obtained as quickly as possible. The patient should also be protected from secondary injury.

Certain causes of seizure activity can be quickly and easily corrected, and these should be considered early in seizure management. A 25% dextrose bolus (2–4 mL/kg/dose D25W IV) should be administered to all patients with documented hypoglycemia. In cases in which rapid bedside glucose testing is unavailable, dextrose should be given prophylactically. It is important to note that if glucose is given to patients on the ketogenic diet, seizure activity may actually worsen secondary to the interruption of the ketogenic state. Naloxone (0.1 mg/kg/dose or 2 mg/dose if >20 kg IV/intramuscular [IM]/subcutaneous [SC]/via endotracheal tube [ETT]) should be administered to patients in whom opioid intoxication is suspected. Lastly, pyridoxine (50–100 mg/dose IV/IM) should be given to neonates and patients suspected of isoniazid toxicity.[32,33]

The next step in seizure management is the administration of benzodiazepines. These medications are frequently administered by family members or paramedics in the prehospital setting. Close attention to the airway is essential when benzodiazepines are administered as these medications may result in sedation, respiratory depression and occasionally hypotension. Administration of multiple doses increases the risk of these effects.

Lorazepam (Ativan) can be administered via an IV or IM route. A dose of 0.05 to 1 mg/kg/dose (maximum 4 mg/dose) may be administered every 5 to 15 minutes, as needed. Its effectiveness decreases, however, with repeated doses.[4,12] The rapid onset of action (2–5 min) and half-life of 12 to 24 hours make it the widely preferred agent.

Diazepam (Valium) has an onset of action similar to that of lorazepam but has a half-life of fewer than 30 minutes. It may be administered via IV, IO or PR at a dose of 0.2 to 0.4 mg/kg IV/IO (maximum 10 mg/dose) or 0.5 to 1 mg/kg PR.[12,14,15] A preformed gel suppository is available for PR administration, but the IV formulation may be instilled PR at the same dose if the gel formulation is unavailable.[34,35] PR-administered diazepam has a longer onset of action and is less effective than the IV form at controlling seizures.[36] Because of its short half-life, a longer acting antiseizure medication may be needed when diazepam is used. Midazolam (Versed) has multiple possible routes of administration including IV, IM, PR, intranasal (IN), PO, and buccal.[35,37,38] IN administration is as effective as IV midazolam and more effective than PR diazepam.[36] These alternate routes of administration are especially useful in the prehospital setting or when IV access cannot be readily obtained. Midazolam dosing varies depending on the route of administration (see Figure 14.1 for dosing information).

If benzodiazepines are ineffective, phenytoin or fosphenytoin should be administered. The loading dose of phenytoin is 10 to 20 mg/kg IV. Patients on chronic phenytoin therapy should receive 5 to 10 mg/kg. These patients require smaller loading doses in order to reach therapeutic serum drug levels. For each milligram per kilogram of drug administered, the serum drug level increases by approximately 1 mg/mL. Phenytoin must be administered slowly at a rate of less than 50 mg/minute. Administration may result in hypotension and cardiac dysrhythmias, and patients should have continuous cardiac monitoring. Local tissue damage can result if extravasation of the drug occurs. Additionally, when administered with a dextrose-containing solution, phenytoin will precipitate into the IV tubing. Fosphenytoin is a prodrug that is rapidly metabolized into phenytoin, yet it is not associated with the same side effects as phenytoin. The dose is calculated using phenytoin equivalents (10–20 PE/kg), and it can be given as fast as 150 mg/minute. It may also be given IM if needed. It does not precipitate if given in dextrose-containing solution and does not cause cardiac dysrhythmias or local tissue destruction. Neither drug results in sedation or respiratory depression.[6,32]

If seizure activity persists, phenobarbital should be added next. Its use may result in respiratory depression, sedation and hypotension, especially when used concurrently with benzodiazepines. Airway management, likely intubation, is essential at this stage. A loading dose of 20 mg/kg IV is given over 5 to 10 minutes. It may be administered via IM if necessary. It has an onset of action of 15 to 20 minutes and a duration of action lasting between 12 and 24 hours.[6,33]

In status epilepticus, valproic acid (25 mg/kg/dose) may be considered as an alternative to phenytoin or phenobarbital. This may be especially useful in patients on chronic valproate therapy. These patients require only 10 mg/kg/dose to raise their serum drug levels within the therapeutic range.[2]

IV levetiracetam has recently been approved by the Food and Drug Administration for use in nonconvulsive status epilepticus. Adult studies show that it is as effective and well tolerated as the orally administered form in patients with partial onset seizures.

If seizure activity persists for longer than 30 to 60 minutes despite these interventions, a continuous infusion of propofol, midazolam or pentobarbital may be required. Occasionally, neuromuscular blockade or general anesthesia may be required to prevent the development of rhabdomyolysis. Continuous EEG monitoring is required in these patients. Medications should be titrated to a goal of flat line or suppression pattern on EEG.[5,33] The decision to begin these therapies is most often made in conjunction with a neurologist.

LONG-TERM MANAGEMENT

Long-term antiepileptic medications are not indicated following a first-time afebrile seizure in well appearing children. They are not frequently prescribed in the ED. Long-term treatment goals in epileptic patients primarily focus on seizure control. Minimization of side effects and improvement in quality of life are additional factors that should not be overlooked.[28] The seizure type, risk of recurrence, the patient's age and co-morbid conditions should be considered when beginning antiepileptic therapy.[26,39] If the decision is made to begin antiepileptic drugs in the ED, it should be made in conjunction with the pediatrician or neurologist who will provide follow-up care.

There are many antiepileptic medications available for long-term seizure control (Table 14.7). If several drugs are appropriate for the patient's seizure type, the drug with the most favorable side effect profile should be the initial choice. Twenty-five percent of patients will not attain seizure control with a single medication.[27] Of those who do, dosage or medication changes may be necessary before seizure control occurs. Dosing should begin at the low end of the dosing range and be titrated up, if necessary. The dose should be increased until seizures are controlled or until side effects become intolerable. A second drug can be added if a single medication fails to control seizure activity.[5] Certain antiseizure medications may have either positive or negative effects on the patient's comorbid conditions, and these should be considered when choosing an antiepileptic drug.[28]

Carbamazepine (Tegretol)

Carbamazepine is useful in the treatment of generalized tonic-clonic seizures, both simple and complex partial seizures and benign rolandic epilepsy. Dosing begins at 10 mg/kg/day and is increased by 5 mg/kg/day to a maintenance dose of 10 to 40 mg/kg/day divided two to four times daily. Therapeutic serum drug levels range from 4 to 12 μg/mL. Multiple medications including diltiazem, verapamil, cimetidine, isoniazid and macrolide antibiotics may interfere with carbamazepine metabolism and result in toxic serum drug levels. Carbamazepine interferes with the efficacy of oral contraceptive medications.[39] Side effects include leukopenia, aplastic anemia, rash and hepatotoxicity. Drowsiness, lethargy and diplopia are dose related. Its use may have positive effects on mood stabilization.[40]

Phenytoin (Dilantin)

Phenytoin is effective therapy for generalized tonic-clonic and both simple and complex partial seizures. It is also useful in status epilepticus and may be used in neonatal seizures. Dosing ranges from 4 to 8 mg/kg/day divided one to three times daily. For most patients, the therapeutic range falls between 10 and 20 μg/mL, but some patients may require higher levels. Large fluctuations in serum drug levels may result from small changes in dosage or in form of the drug (between generic and trade). Serum drug levels of phenytoin may be increased with the concomitant use of chlorpromazine, chloramphenicol, isoniazid, anticoagulants and estrogens.

Phenytoin use affects the metabolism of other antiepileptic drugs, increasing phenobarbital levels and decreasing serum drug levels of carbamazepine, clonazepam and primidone. Side effects include gingival hyperplasia, acne, hirsutism, blood and liver toxicity and Stevens-Johnson syndrome. Nausea, vomiting, drowsiness, ataxia and nystagmus may occur at supratherapeutic levels.[7,39]

Phenobarbital (Luminal)

Phenobarbital can be used to treat both simple and complex partial seizures, generalized tonic-clonic seizures and status epilepticus. It is the treatment of choice in neonatal seizures. The dose ranges from 2 to 6 mg/kg/day divided

Table 14.7. Common anticonvulsant agents[1]

Drug	Indication	Side effects	Maintenance (mg/kg/day)	Miscellaneous
Carbamazepine (Tegretol)	Generalized tonic-clonic, partial, benign rolandic	Rash, hepatitis, diplopia, aplastic anemia, leukopenia	10–40	Mood stabilization, inexpensive, drug interactions
Clonazepam (Klonopin)	Myoclonic, akinetic, partial, absence, infantile spasms, Lennox-Gastaut	Fatigue, behavior problems, salivation, ataxia	0.05–0.3	
Ethosuximide (Zarontin)	Absence	N/V, weight gain, lethargy, SLE, rash	20–40	
Felbamate (Felbatol)	Refractory severe epilepsy	Aplastic anemia, hepatotoxicity	15–45	
Gabapentin (Neurontin)	Partial and secondarily generalized seizures	Fatigue, dizziness, diarrhea, ataxia, weight gain	20–70	
Lamotrigine (Lamictal)	Simple/complex partial, atonic, myoclonic, absence, tonic-clonic, Lennox-Gastaut, infantile spasms	Headache, nausea, rash, diplopia, Stevens-Johnson syndrome, GI upset	5–15	Mood stabilization
Levetiracetam (Keppra)	Adjunctive therapy for refractory partial seizures	Headache, anorexia, fatigue, infection, behavior problems	10–60	IV formulation available
Oxcarbazepine (Trileptal)	Adjunctive therapy for partial seizures	Fatigue, low Na, nausea, ataxia, rash	5–45	Mood stabilization, drug interactions
Phenobarbital (Luminal)	Generalized tonic-clonic, partial, myoclonic, neonatal	Sedation, behavior/sleep problems, rash, hypersensitivity	2–6	Inexpensive, readily available
Phenytoin (Dilantin)	Generalized tonic-clonic, partial, atonic, myoclonic, neonatal	Gum hyperplasia, hirsutism, acne, ataxia, Stevens-Johnson, lymphoma	4–8	Inexpensive, readily available, drug interactions
Primidone (Mysoline)	Generalized tonic-clonic, partial	Rash, ataxia, behavior problems, sedation, anemia	10–25	Metabolized to phenobarbital
Tiagabine (Gabitril)	Adjunctive therapy for refractory complex partial seizures	Fatigue, headache, tremor, dizziness, anorexia, loss of concentration	0.1–1 Average dose, 6 mg/day	
Topiramate (Topamax)	Refractory complex partial seizures, adjunctive therapy for temporal lobe epilepsy	Fatigue, headache, N/V, nephrolithiasis, acidosis, weight loss, tremor, behavior/sleep problems	1–9	Prevents migraines
Valproic acid (Depakote)	Generalized tonic-clonic, absence, myoclonic, partial, akinetic, infantile spasms	N/V, liver/pancreas problems, tremor, alopecia, sedation, weight gain, menstrual irregularities, thrombocytopenia	10–60	Inexpensive, readily available, mood stabilization, prevents migraines
Vigabatrin (Sabril)	Infantile spasms, adjunctive therapy for refractory partial seizures	Weight gain, behavior changes, visual field constriction	50–150	
Zonisamide (Zonegran)	Adjunctive therapy for partial seizures, atonic, infantile spasms	Fatigue, ataxia, anorexia, N/V, headache, rash, weight loss	2–8	

GI, gastrointestinal; Na, sodium; N/V, nausea and vomiting; SLE, systemic lupus erythematous.

once or twice daily, with a therapeutic range between 10 and 40 μg/mL. It is inexpensive, but up to 30% to 50% of children experience side effects, including hypersensitivity reactions, rash, hyperactivity, lethargy, sleep and behavioral disorders.[7,39]

Primidone (Mysoline)

Because this drug is metabolized into phenobarbital, the side effect profiles of the two drugs are similar. Primidone can be used to treat generalized tonic-clonic seizures and both simple and complex partial seizures. The maintenance dose is from 10 to 25 mg/kg/day divided between two and four times daily. Therapeutic drug levels range between 5 and 12 μg/mL and are followed using serum phenobarbital levels.[39]

Valproate (Depakote)

Valproate is effective treatment for generalized tonic-clonic and partial (simple and complex) seizures. It is primarily used in the treatment of myoclonic and absence seizures. It can also be used in Lennox-Gastaut syndrome, infantile spasms and juvenile myoclonic epilepsy of Janz.[10] Maintenance dosing ranges from 10 to 60 mg/kg/day divided into two to four doses per day. The initial dose is 10 mg/kg/day and is increased by 10 mg/kg weekly to obtain therapeutic serum levels between 50 and 100 μg/mL. Nausea, vomiting, alopecia, weight gain, menstrual irregularities and drowsiness can occur with valproate use. Children younger than 2 years of age are at risk of developing idiosyncratic pancreatitis or hepatic failure with valproate use. Dose-related side effects include tremors, thrombocytopenia and platelet dysfunction. It may aid in mood stabilization and help prevent migraine headaches. Valproate may increase drug levels of phenytoin, phenobarbital, diazepam, carbamazepine, clonazepam and ethosuximide.[39,40]

Ethosuximide (Zarontin)

Ethosuximide is used to treat absence seizures. Doses range from 20 to 40 mg/kg/day divided twice daily with therapeutic serum drug levels between 40 and 100 μg/mL. Side effects include hiccups, headache, nausea and vomiting. Rarely, a lupus-like syndrome, erythema multiforme and Stevens-Johnson syndrome can occur.[39,40]

Clonazepam (Klonopin)

Clonazepam may be useful therapy for absence, myoclonic and atonic seizures. Doses between 0.05 and 0.3 mg/kg/day divided two to four times daily should be used to obtain therapeutic serum levels of 0.02 to 0.08 μg/mL. Its use may cause ataxia, drowsiness and drooling.[39]

Lamotrigine (Lamictal)

Lamotrigine may be useful as monotherapy in generalized tonic-clonic and partial seizures,[40] but it is primarily indicated as adjunctive therapy in partial, atonic, tonic, and myoclonic seizures and Lennox-Gastaut syndrome. Doses range between 5 and 15 mg/kg/day given once or twice daily, but doses may need to be adjusted due to interactions with other antiepileptic medications. Lamotrigine's mood stabilizing effects make it useful in patients with comorbid bipolar disorder or depression, but it may cause headache, diplopia, dizziness, insomnia and gastrointestinal upset.[8,28,39–42]

Felbamate (Felbatol)

Felbamate is useful in refractory seizure therapy and especially in Lennox-Gastaut syndrome. The therapeutic dose ranges between 15 and 45 mg/kg/day divided three to four times daily. The initial dose should be at the low end of the therapeutic range with increases every 1 to 2 weeks, as tolerated. Felbamate increases serum levels of phenytoin and valproate, but decreases serum levels of carbamazepine. Felbamate is often used as monotherapy because its side effects are increased when used concurrently with other medications. These effects include anorexia, vomiting, insomnia and somnolence. More serious side effects, including aplastic anemia and hepatic failure, necessitate frequent monitoring of liver function and blood counts in children on this medication.[8,28,39,41]

Gabapentin (Neurontin)

Gabapentin is used as adjunctive therapy in refractory partial and secondarily tonic-clonic seizures. Its dose ranges between 20 and 70 mg/kg/day divided into three or four doses, and the dose can be titrated up rapidly, as needed. Gabapentin does not interact with other antiepileptic drugs. Side effects include weight gain, dizziness, ataxia, diarrhea and fatigue.[8,39–41]

Vigabatrin (Sabril)

Vigabatrin is effective in the treatment of refractory partial seizures and infantile spasms. Vigabatrin may convert infantile spasms to partial seizures, which is considered by most to be an improvement in this refractory syndrome. Vigabatrin has been shown to be as useful as adrenocorticotropic hormone in patients with infantile spasms associated with tuberous sclerosis. The initial dose of 50 mg/kg/day divided once to twice daily can be increased to 75 to 150 mg/kg/day if improvement is seen with the initial dose. If no response or worsening of symptoms occurs, the patient is considered to be resistant to the drug. Side effects include weight gain, behavioral changes, rash, sedation, ataxia and visual field constriction.[8,39]

Zonisamide (Zonegran)

Zonisamide is useful as adjunctive therapy in children older than 16 years of age who have partial seizures. It is effective in infantile spasms; Lennox-Gastaut syndrome; and generalized tonic-clonic, myoclonic and atonic seizures. It also may be useful as monotherapy for many seizure types including absence seizures.[43,44] The initial dose of 2 to 4 mg/kg/day should be titrated up to obtain maintenance dosing of 4 to 8 mg/kg/day divided once to twice daily. Side effects include fatigue, ataxia, rash and nausea; vomiting and anorexia and are more common early in therapy.[8,41]

Oxcarbazepine (Trileptal)

Oxcarbazepine may be used as monotherapy for partial seizures and adjunctive therapy in many other seizure types. Dosing begins at 5 mg/kg/day and is increased to a maintenance dose of 45 mg/kg divided twice daily. Its use may cause increased serum drug levels of phenobarbital and phenytoin. Twenty-five percent of children allergic to carbamazepine are also allergic to oxcarbazepine. Side effects include nausea, diplopia, ataxia, somnolence and hypersensitivity reactions. Asymptomatic hyponatremia has been reported in adults but has not been seen in children. Oxcarbazepine may aid in mood stabilization.[5,8,40]

Levetiracetam (Keppra)

Levetiracetam is effective as adjunctive therapy in partial seizure treatment. Maintenance dosing ranges between 10 and 60 mg/kg/day. Headache, anorexia, somnolence, infection (rhinitis, pharyngitis, otitis media) and behavioral problems have been reported with its use. Leukopenia has been reported in adults, but this has not been seen in children.[8,40,41,45] IV levetiracetam may be a reasonable alternative in patients who are temporarily unable to take the drug orally, as well as a useful alternative in nonconvulsive status epilepticus.[46,47]

Tiagabine (Gabitril)

Tiagabine is also an adjunctive therapy in partial seizures. Dosing begins at 0.1 mg/kg/day and is titrated up to between 0.5 and 1 mg/kg/day. Multidrug therapy increases the incidence of side effects including fatigue, dizziness, headache, mood disturbances and an inability to concentrate.[8,39,41]

Topiramate (Topamax)

Topiramate is used as an adjunct in the treatment of many seizure types, including partial or generalized tonic-clonic seizures, refractory complex partial seizures, Lennox-Gastaut syndrome and infantile spasms. Initial dosing begins at 1 mg/kg/day and is titrated up to a maintenance dose of 3 to 9 mg/kg divided twice daily. Anorexia, weight loss, kidney stones, fatigue, diplopia, headache and metabolic acidosis may occur with use. Side effects also may include sleep problems and behavioral and cognitive disturbances.[8,39,41] Topiramate use has been associated with hypohidrosis and hyperthermia, as well. These effects resolve once the medication is discontinued.[28,48] Topiramate may have a beneficial effect in patients who suffer from migraine headaches.[28]

KETOGENIC DIET

Patients with many refractory seizure types have been treated with some success using a ketogenic diet. The diet has been used in patients with tonic-clonic, myoclonic, atonic and atypical absence seizures, as well as in patients with infantile spasms and Lennox-Gastaut syndrome. In some studies, this therapy has reported a 50% to 70%

seizure reduction rate.[8,12] The diet works especially well when instituted early in seizure therapy.[49] The low carbohydrate, low protein, high fat diet induces a ketogenic state and leads to a reduction in seizure frequency. The diet is initiated with a 48-hour fasting phase, during which vomiting, dehydration and hypoglycemia can occur. Hospital admission is required during this initial phase to monitor for these side effects and to provide the patient and family with education regarding the diet. Patients on the ketogenic diet are at risk for multiple long-term side effects. These include constipation, weight loss, growth retardation, hyponatremia, hyperlipidemia, renal tubular acidosis, nephrolithiasis and elevation of hepatic and pancreatic enzymes. Patients also may experience increased susceptibility to infection and prolongation of their QT intervals. Before beginning this therapy, a thorough metabolic evaluation and an EKG must be performed. Children must undergo frequent laboratory monitoring and must consume sufficient vitamin supplementation throughout the duration of the diet.[5,8,50] The Atkins' diet, with fewer dietary restrictions and no initial hospital admission, may be better tolerated and as effective as the traditional ketogenic diet.[50]

Other nonmedicinal therapies for refractory seizures are useful in certain patients. These therapies include anterior temporal lobectomy, corpus callosotomy and vagal nerve stimulation therapy. The considerable risks and side effects of these therapies make them appropriate for only a small group of carefully selected patients.[28]

Certain lifestyle modifications, including decreased alcohol consumption and maintenance of regular sleep-wake cycles and circadian rhythms, may lead to a decrease in seizure occurrence. Patients, specifically adolescents, should be educated regarding these adjustments.[28]

DISPOSITION

An asymptomatic, well appearing child can be safely discharged home following a first-time afebrile seizure, provided that sufficient follow-up is ensured. Further workup, including EEG and any required neuroimaging, can be performed safely on an outpatient basis.[5] Patients requiring further inpatient evaluation include those with prolonged seizure activity, those with prolonged postictal state, very young infants or those who required anticonvulsant medications to stop the seizure activity.

PITFALLS

- Failure to treat rapidly reversible causes of seizure activity (i.e., hypoglycemia, opioid intoxication, isoniazid ingestion)
- Failure to check serum drug levels in patients receiving antiepileptic drugs as low levels are a frequent cause of seizures and elevated levels may result in side effects
- Failure to know the definition of a true simple febrile seizure
- Failure to recognize the autonomic signs of seizure activity in newborns such as apnea, bradycardia and hypoxia

REFERENCES

1. Friedman M, Sharieff G. Seizures in children. *Pediatr Clin North Am.* 2006;53:257–277.
2. Gorelick M, Blackwell C. Neurologic emergencies. In: Fleisher G, Ludwig S, Henretig F, et al, eds. *Textbook of Pediatric Emergency Medicine*, 5th ed. Philadelphia, PA: Lippincott Williams & Wilkins; 2006:759–779.
3. McAbee GN, Wark JE. A practical approach to uncomplicated seizures in children. *Am Fam Physician.* 2000;62(5):1109–1116.
4. Roth H, Drislane F. Seizures. *Neurol Clin.* 1998;16:257–284.
5. Shneker BF, Fountain NB. Epilepsy. *Dis Mon.* 2003;49:426–478.
6. Reuter D, Brownstein D. Common emergent pediatric neurologic problems. *Emerg Med Clin North Am.* 2002;20(1):155–176.
7. Tang-Wai R, Oskoui M, Webster R, et al. Outcomes in pediatric epilepsy: seeing through the fog. *Pediatr Neurol.* 2005;33:244–250.
8. Jarrar RG, Buchhalter JR. Therapeutics in pediatric epilepsy, part 1: the new antiepileptic drugs and the ketogenic diet. *Mayo Clin Proc.* 2003;78:359–370.
9. Cossette P, Riviello J, Carmant L. ACTH versus vigabatrin therapy in infantile spasms: a retrospective study. *Neurology.* 1999;52(8):1691–1694.
10. Trevathan E. Infantile spasms and Lennox-Gastaut syndrome. *J Child Neurol.* 2002;17(Suppl 2):2S9–2S22.
11. Elterman RD, Shields WD, Mansfield KA, et al. Randomized trial of vigabatrin in patients with infantile spasms. *Neurology.* 2001;57(8):1416–1421.
12. Vining EP, Freeman JM, Ballaban-Gil K, et al. A multicenter study of the efficacy of the ketogenic diet. *Arch Neurol.* 1998;55(11):1433–1437.
13. Provisional Committee on Quality Improvement, Subcommittee on Febrile Seizures. Practice parameter: the neurodiagnostic evaluation of the child with a first simple febrile seizure. *Pediatrics.* 1996;97:769–772.
14. Gonzalez Del Rey J. Febrile seizures. In: Barkin R, Caputo G, Jaffe D, et al, eds. *Pediatric Emergency Medicine*, 2nd ed. St. Louis, MO: Mosby; 1997:1017–1019.
15. Committee on Quality Improvement, Subcommittee on Febrile Seizures. Practice parameter: long-term treatment of the child with simple febrile seizures. *Pediatrics.* 1999;103:1307–1309.

16. Warden CR, Zibulewsky J, Mace S, et al. Evaluation and management of febrile seizures in the out of hospital and emergency department settings. *Ann Emerg Med.* 2003;41:215–222.

17. Teng D, Dayan P, Tyler S, et al. Risk of intracranial pathologic conditions requiring emergency intervention after a first complex febrile seizure episode among children. *Pediatrics.* 2006;117:304–308.

18. Chiu SS, Tse CYC, Lau YL, et al. Influenza A infection is an important cause of febrile seizures. *Pediatrics.* 2001;108:e63.

19. Trainor JL, Hampers LC, Krug SE, et al. Children with first-time simple febrile seizures are at low risk of serious bacterial illness. *Acad Emerg Med.* 2001;8:781–787.

20. Wirrell E. Neonatal seizures: to treat or not to treat? *Semin Pediatr Neurol.* 2005;12:97–105.

21. Rennie JM, Boylan GB. Neonatal seizures and their treatment. *Curr Opin Neurol.* 2003;16:177–181.

22. Zupance ML. Neonatal seizures. *Pediatr Clin North Am.* 2004;51:961–978.

23. Evans D, Levene M. Neonatal seizures. *Arch Dis Child Fetal Neonatal Ed.* 1998;78:F70–F75.

24. Ng E, Klinger G, Shah V, et al. Safety of benzodiazepines in newborns. *Ann Pharmacother.* 2002;36:1150–1155.

25. Barron T. The child with spells. *Pediatr Clin North Am.* 1991;38(3):711–724.

26. Hirtz D, Ashwal S, Berg A, et al. Practice parameter: evaluating a first nonfebrile seizure in children. *Neurology.* 2000;55:616–623.

27. Arunkumar G, Morris H. Epilepsy update: new medical and surgical treatment options. *Cleve Clin J Med.* 1998;65:527–537.

28. Nadkarni S, LaJoie J, Devinsky O. Current treatments of epilepsy. *Neurology.* 2005;64:S2–S11.

29. Scarfone RJ, Pond K, Thompson K, et al. Utility of laboratory testing for infants with seizures. *Pediatr Emerg Care.* 2000;16:309–312.

30. Sharma S, Riviello JJ, Harper MB, et al. The role of emergent neuroimaging in children with new-onset afebrile seizures. *Pediatrics.* 2003;111:1–6.

31. Shinnar S, Berg AT, Moshe SL, et al. The risk of seizure recurrence after a first unprovoked afebrile seizure in childhood: an extended follow-up. *Pediatrics.* 1996;98:216–225.

32. Prasad A, Seshia S. Status epilepticus in pediatric practice: neonate to adolescent. *Adv Neurol.* 2006;97:229–243.

33. Haafiz A, Kissoon N. Status epilepticus: current concepts. *Pediatr Emerg Care.* 1999;15:119–129.

34. Fitzgerald BJ, Okos AJ, Miller JW. Treatment of out of hospital status epilepticus with diazepam rectal gel. *Seizure.* 2003;12:52–55.

35. Scott RC, Besag FM, Neville BG. Buccal midazolam and rectal diazepam for treatment of prolonged seizures in childhood and adolescence: a randomized trial. *Lancet.* 1999;353:623–626.

36. Wolfe T, Macfarlane T. Intranasal midazolam therapy for pediatric status epilepticus. *Am J Emerg Med.* 2006;24:343–346.

37. Chamberlain JM, Altiere MA, Futterman C, et al. A prospective, randomized study comparing intramuscular midazolam with intravenous diazepam for the treatment of seizures in children. *Pediatr Emerg Care.* 1997;13:92–94.

38. Vilke GM, Sharieff GQ, Marino A, et al. Midazolam for the treatment of out of hospital pediatric seizures. *Prehosp Emerg Care.* 2002;6:215–217.

39. Russell RJ, Parks B. Anticonvulsant medications. *Pediatr Ann.* 1999;28:238–245.

40. Sullivan J, Dlugos D. Antiepileptic drug monotherapy: pediatric concerns. *Semin Pediatr Neurol.* 2005;12:88–96.

41. Bergin AM. Pharmacotherapy of pediatric epilepsy. *Expert Opin Pharmacother.* 2003;4:421–431.

42. Verdru P. Epilepsy in children: the evidence for new antiepileptic drugs. *Acta Neurol Scand.* 2005;112:17–20.

43. Wilfong A. Zonisamide monotherapy for epilepsy in children and young adults. *Pediatr Neurol.* 2005;32:77–80.

44. Wilfong A, Schultz R. Zonisamide for absence seizures. *Epilepsy Res.* 2005;64:31–34.

45. Glauser TA, Ayala R, Elterman R, et al. Double-blind placebo-controlled trial of adjunctive levetiracetam in pediatric partial seizures. *Neurology.* 2006;66:1654–1660.

46. Baulac M, Brodie M, Elger C, et al. Levetiracetam intravenous infusion as an alternative to oral dosing in patients with partial onset seizures. *Epilepsia.* 2007;48(3):589–592.

47. Rupprect S, Franke K, Fitzek S, et al. Levetiracetam as a treatment option in non-convulsive status epilepticus. *Epilepsy Res.* 2007;73(3):238–244.

48. Cerminara C, Seri S, Bombardieri R, et al. Hypohydrosis during topiramate: a rare and reversible side effect. *Pediatr Neurol.* 2006;34:392–394.

49. Rubenstein J, Kossoff E, Pyzik P, et al. Experience in the use of the ketogenic diet as early therapy. *J Child Neurol.* 2005;20:31–34.

50. Kossoff E, McGrogan J, Bluml R, et al. A modified Atkins diet is effective for the treatment of intractable pediatric epilepsy. *Epilepsia.* 2006;47(2):421–424.

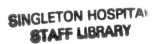

PART III

SPECIFIC SYSTEMS

Linton Yee

INTRODUCTION

Cardiac disease in the infant will always present diagnostic and procedural challenges. Airway management and vascular access require urgent attention in the distressed or obtunded infant with cyanosis or pallor. Decisions must be made expeditiously, and accurate diagnosis will help guide the care of a potentially complicated patient. Much of the history and physical exam may be nonspecific, thus diagnosis can be difficult. By creating a strategy for dealing with cardiac disease, managing these patients can be completed in a timely and efficient manner.

The most critical presentations in the infant with cardiac disease include cyanotic episodes, congestive heart failure (CHF), cardiogenic shock or cardiovascular collapse and arrhythmias. These challenging scenarios may be the initial presentation of the disease or a complication of an already diagnosed lesion.

Cardiac disease in the infant can be the result of structural aberrations, conduction abnormalities and acquired illnesses. Understanding that some of the cardiac lesions are a combination of defects, structural congenital heart disease (CHD) can be divided into cyanotic and acyanotic classifications. The cyanotic group can be further subdivided into increased or decreased pulmonary blood flow. The acyanotic group can be subdivided into categories based on the presence of left to right shunting and left ventricle (LV) outflow obstruction. Disorders in conduction are either congenital or are newly acquired illness. The dysrhythmias commonly seen in early infancy such as supraventricular tachycardia are reviewed in Chapter 5. Cardiomyopathies, myocarditis, pericarditis, endocarditis and Kawasaki's disease are some of the more prominent acquired heart diseases.

The overall color of the infant often gives a clue as to the underlying CHD. The new presentation of cyanosis in a patient strongly suggests the presence of cyanotic CHD with right to left shunting. The appearance of an ashen, mottled or gray infant is most likely the result of cardiogenic shock or collapse from outflow obstruction and pump failure. Color may appear normal in a patient with left to right shunting and CHF.[1–7]

This chapter discusses the interpretation of pediatric electrocardiograms (ECGs) and chest x-rays and the evaluation and management of cyanotic heart disease, acyanotic heart disease, carditis and cardiomyopathies.

CHEST RADIOGRAPHS AND ELECTROCARDIOGRAM INTERPRETATION

The chest x-ray and ECG often offer clues as to the congenital heart lesion in question. Remember, the superior mediastinum is enlarged in the young infant's anteroposterior (AP) chest x-ray due to a normally enlarged thymus. The thymus can take on a variety of shapes and sizes. It can mimic cardiac enlargement, lobar collapse, pulmonary infiltrates and mediastinal masses. The thymus appears "wavy" because it insinuates itself between anterior ribs. It does not push other mediastinal structures. The thymus can protrude to the side, producing a "sail sign" that may be misinterpreted as a pulmonary infiltrate (Figure 15.1).

On the lateral chest x-ray, the space anterior and superior to the heart, just behind the sternum, should be filled with a tissue density (thymus). In older children and adults, this space is air filled. The cardiac width-to-thoracic ratio is not as reliable in young infants. The AP view is affected by inspiration and the thymus. The lateral view can often be more helpful. On the lateral view, if the posterior aspect of the cardiac silhouette extends over the vertebral bodies, then cardiomegaly is present. The anterior tracheal line on the lateral view can be useful. This line, drawn parallel to the anterior tracheal wall inferior

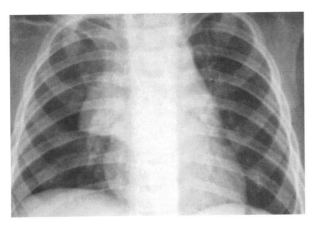

Figure 15.1. Normal infant chest x-ray.

Table 15.1. Pediatric ECG normal intervals

Age	Heart rate	PR interval (seconds)	QRS interval (seconds)
1st week	90–160	0.08–0.15	0.03–0.08
1–3 weeks	100–180	0.08–0.15	0.03–0.08
1–2 months	120–180	0.08–0.15	0.03–0.08
3–5 months	105–185	0.08–0.15	0.03–0.08
6–11 months	110–170	0.07–0.16	0.03–0.08
1–2 years	90–165	0.08–0.16	0.03–0.08
3–4 years	70–140	0.09–0.17	0.04–0.08
5–7 years	65–140	0.09–0.17	0.04–0.08
8–11 years	60–130	0.09–0.17	0.04–0.09
12–15 years	65–130	0.09–0.18	0.04–0.09
>16 years	50–120	0.12–0.20	0.05–0.10

Courtesy of Ra'id Abdullah, MD, University of Chicago, Chicago, IL.

to the diaphragm, should not intersect the heart. It should not be "pushed backward" to intersect the spine above the diaphragm. If it is pushed backward, cardiomegaly exists (Figure 15.2).

The pediatric ECG is often viewed with anxiety, especially in the emergency department (ED) where rapid diagnosis is essential. There are many nuances to the pediatric ECG that relate to age-specific changes as myocardium and conduction tissue mature. It is the variability of "normal" ECGs in children that can sometimes delay interpretation in the ED. We suggest the use of a systemic approach to ECG interpretation with special attention to rate, rhythm, axis, ventricular and atrial hypertrophy and the presence of any ischemia or

repolarization abnormalities.[8,9] Normal pediatric ECG values are listed in Table 15.1.

Heart Rate

The first variable is the heart rate. In children, cardiac output is mostly determined by heart rate and not stroke volume. Hence, age and activity-appropriate heart rates must be recognized. Average resting heart rate varies with age; newborn heart rates can range from 90 to 160 beats per minute (bpm) and adolescent heart rates can range from 50 to 120 bpm. Heart rates grossly outside the normal range for age should be scrutinized closely for arrhythmias (Figure 15.3).

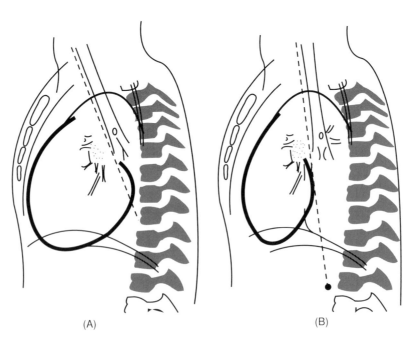

(A)   (B)

Figure 15.2. Anterior tracheal line.

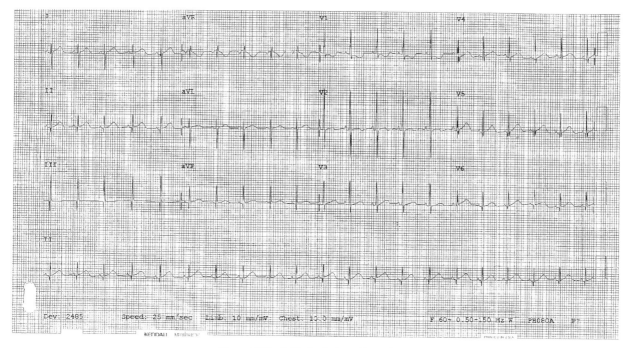

Figure 15.3. EKG of a 5-day-old newborn.

Axis

In the neonate, it is the right ventricle (RV) that is the dominant chamber. In utero, blood is shunted away from the lungs by the patent ductus arteriosus (PDA) and the RV provides most of the systemic blood flow. As a result of this, in the neonate and infant (up to 2 months), the ECG will show RV dominance, and the majority of the QRS will be comprised of RV mass. As the physiology matures, the LV becomes increasingly dominant until it is the ventricle that makes up the bulk of the QRS.

QRS Duration

The QRS duration varies with age. In neonates, it measures 30 to 60 milliseconds (ms), and in adolescents, from 50 to 100 ms. A QRS duration exceeding 100 to 120 ms is referred to as *bundle branch block*. This will result in two distinct spikes in the QRS, which reflect repolarization of the ventricle separately. If it is seen in lead V1, then it is a *right bundle branch block* (RBBB). If it is seen in lead V6, then it is referred to as a *left bundle branch block* (LBBB).

Intervals

The *PR interval* (measured as the time from the onset of the P to the onset of the QRS) also varies with age as the

heart matures. In neonates, it ranges from 80 to 150 ms and in adolescents, from 120 to 200 ms. It is because of wide variability in heart rates that the *QT interval* (measured as the time from the beginning of the QRS complex to the end of the T wave) must be corrected for heart rate. This is done using Bazett's formula:

$$QTc = QT/\sqrt{RR\ interval}$$

T Waves

In the adult population, there is much written about T wave morphology and its assessment for cardiac ischemia. In the pediatric population, however, T wave changes tend to be nonspecific and are often a source of controversy. What is agreed upon is that flat, inverted T waves are normal in the newborn. Upright T waves in V1 after 3 days of age are a sign of RVH.

Chamber Size

Once normal intervals are evaluated, the ECG can be scrutinized for chamber size. If the P wave is taller than two small boxes (1 small box = 1mm in height) in infants and three small boxes in adolescents, then the criteria for right atrial enlargement are met. If the P wave is wider than 2 small boxes in infants or 3 small boxes in adolescents, then the criteria for left atrial enlargement is met. Right ventricular hypertrophy (RVH) is best seen in leads V1 and V2 with an rSR', QR (no S) or pure R (no Q or S). Left ventricular hypertrophy (LVH) is noted in V6 with tall R waves. Biventricular hypertrophy is seen when ECG criteria for enlargement of both ventricles is seen.

These simple rules can be applied quickly in the ED to assess whether an ECG is within acceptable limits for age. Abnormal ECGs can then be referred to a pediatric cardiologist for review.

CYANOTIC HEART DISEASE PATHOPHYSIOLOGY

The transition from fetus to newborn induces a number of changes in the cardiovascular system. The placenta works as the pulmonary system for the fetus, and oxygenated blood travels via the umbilical vein from the placenta to the fetus.

The transition from fetal circulation to newborn circulation creates a number of changes. Blood is oxygenated through the newly created lower resistance pulmonary system, and the shunts that existed between the pulmonary and systemic circulations (the foramen ovale, ductus arteriosus and ductus venosus) close. The patency of the ductus arteriosus becomes important when discussing ductal-dependent cardiac lesions. The ductus arteriosus connects the pulmonary artery to the aorta and shunts blood away from the pulmonary tree during fetal life.

After birth, dilation of the pulmonary vasculature results from the expansion of the lungs and the elimination of fluid from the lungs. This, in turn, decreases pulmonary resistance and increases pulmonary blood flow. Closure of the umbilical vessels, the ductus arteriosus and the ductus venosus is induced when the blood is oxygenated through the pulmonary system. Pulmonary artery resistance decreases and systemic resistance increases, changing blood flow through the atria, with left atrial pressure now greater than the right. This effectively closes the foramen ovale (Figure 15.4).[10,11]

Cyanosis is evident when there is desaturated blood in the capillary beds. Deoxygenated hemoglobin is blue. When cyanosis is present, this corresponds to 3 to 5 mg/dL of deoxyhemoglobin in the blood, which is approximately the same as a room air oxygen saturation of 70% to 80%.[12,13] Oxygen carrying capacity is directly related to the amount of hemoglobin *available* to carry oxygen. This means that a polycythemic and cyanotic infant can still

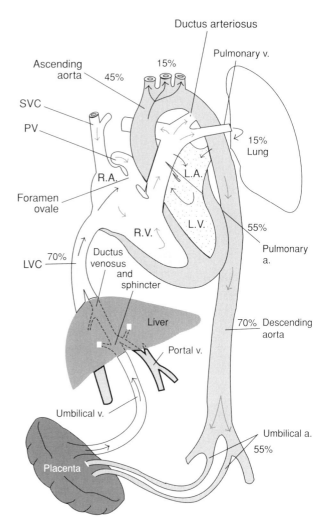

Figure 15.4. Fetal circulation.

deliver oxygen to tissues, in contrast to the anemic infant, who does not appear cyanotic and cannot deliver oxygen to tissues.

The differentiation of central and peripheral cyanosis is important in the evaluation and treatment of the cardiac patient, as management is based on the underlying cause. There are a number of etiologies for central cyanosis. These include pulmonary and cardiac origins as well as central nervous system depression. Sepsis, metabolic disease and toxic ingestions are also included. Peripheral cyanosis can be attributed to acrocyanosis, cold exposure and decreased peripheral perfusion. A method of determining central cyanosis in children is to assess the mucous membranes and tongue. These areas are pink in well-oxygenated children.

The assessment of cyanosis is based on the arterial oxygen saturation, the oxygen-binding capacity (hemoglobin) and the arteriovenous oxygen difference.[12]

Table 15.2. Cyanotic congenital cardiac lesions and typical chest X-ray findings

Cardiac lesion	Chest X-ray findings
Tetralogy of Fallot	Boot-shaped heart, normal-sized heart, decreased pulmonary vascular markings
Transposition of the great arteries	Egg-shaped heart, narrow mediastinum,cardiomegaly, increased pulmonary vascular markings
Total anomalous pulmonary venous return	Snowman sign, significant cardiomegaly, increased pulmonary vascular markings
Tricuspid atresia	Normal to slight increase in cardiac size, decreased pulmonary vascular markings
Truncus arteriosus	Cardiomegaly, increased pulmonary vascular markings

Table 15.3. Cyanotic congenital cardiac lesions and typical ECG findings

Cardiac lesion	ECG findings
Tetralogy of Fallot	RAD, RVH
Transposition of the great arteries	RAD, RVH
Total anomalous pulmonary venous return	RAD, RVH, RAE
Tricuspid atresia	Superior QRS axis with RAH, LAH, LVH
Truncus arteriosus	Biventricular hypertrophy

LAH, left atrial hypertrophy; LVH, left ventricular hypertrophy; RAD, right axis deviation; RAE, right atrial enlargement; RVH, right ventricular hypertrophy.

The presentation of cardiac disease is dependent on the age of the patient and the etiology of the underlying disease. Cyanosis, CHF and cardiogenic shock are the predominant issues in this age group, and all can arise from a number of different scenarios.

In the first couple of weeks of life, cyanosis and shock are the most prevalent. This group is ductal-dependent, and the preservation of ductal patency is essential to patient survival. Many of these patients are diagnosed in the newborn nursery, but with the increasing number of earlier newborn discharges, it is highly probable that these patients will make their initial presentation in the ED when the ductus begins to close.

In general, cyanosis can be seen with any of the cyanotic CHDs commonly referred to as the *Terrible Ts:* tetralogy of Fallot (TOF), transposition of the great arteries (TGA), tricuspid atresia (TA), total anomalous pulmonary venous return (TAPVR) and truncus arteriosus.

During the first 2 weeks of life, cyanosis and shock can be the initial presentation of TA, TGA, TAPVR, truncus arteriosus, hypoplastic right heart syndrome (HRHS), and pulmonary atresia. TOF can present with cyanosis or CHF. Hypoplastic left heart syndrome (HLHS), aortic stenosis and coarctation of the aorta initially present with shock. Tables 15.2 and 15.3 review the common chest x-ray and ECG findings in these patients.

Hypoxemic or worsening cyanotic episodes can occur in infants with known cyanotic CHD, usually TOF. During these episodes, patients present with hyperpnea, irritability and increasing cyanosis as well as a decrease in the intensity of their murmur. The fall in systemic vascular resistance or the rise in resistance to the RV outflow tract increases right to left shunting, leading to hyperpnea, followed by increased systemic venous return. The end result is increased right to left shunting through the ventricular septal defect (VSD), leading to a "tet spell." TOF and pulmonary stenosis patients have critical right heart obstruction and are ductal-dependent. In order to increase their pulmonary blood flow, a decrease in pulmonary vascular resistance will assist in left to right shunting.

Cardiogenic shock is the hallmark of acyanotic lesions that depend on ductal flow. In order to maintain systemic perfusion, cardiac lesions with a critical left heart obstruction (HLHS, aortic stenosis and coarctation of the aorta) are vitally dependent on a patent ductus. A sepsis-like presentation with poor perfusion, diminished pulses and pallor is common when the ductus closes. Supplemental oxygen may lead to no improvement or can make the patient worse, especially if central cyanosis is present. Systemic perfusion is improved by increasing right to left shunting across the ductus arteriosus using potent vasodilators such as prostaglandins.

Tetralogy of Fallot

Representing up to 10% of all CHD, TOF is the most common form of cyanotic CHD in the post infancy period (Figure 15.5).[14-16] There are four major components to TOF: a large VSD, RV outflow obstruction (resulting from pulmonic stenosis), an overriding aorta and RVH. The degree of disease pathophysiology is determined by two of the lesions, as there must be RV outflow obstruction and

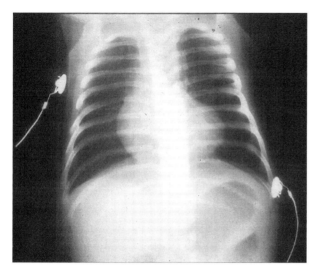

Figure 15.5. Tetralogy of Fallot.

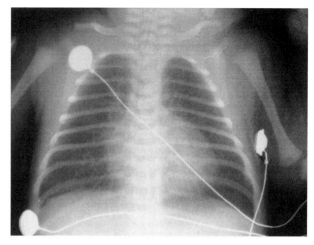

Figure 15.6. Transposition of the great vessels.

the VSD must be large enough to allow for the equalization of pressure in both ventricles.

The level of cyanosis in the patient is determined by the extent of obstruction of the RV outflow tract. The nonrestrictive VSD allows for the balance of systolic pressures in the RV and LV. The degree of RV outflow obstruction determines whether there is a left to right shunt, a bidirectional shunt or a right to left shunt. Severe pulmonic stenosis causes a right to left shunt, which, in turn, causes cyanosis and decreased pulmonary blood flow. An acyanotic TOF is seen when pulmonic stenosis is mild, causing a left to right shunt.

Besides cyanosis, the examination can have a systolic thrill at the lower and middle left sternal border. There is also a loud, single S2, an aortic ejection click, along with a loud grade 3 to 5/6 systolic ejection murmur heard best in the middle to lower left sternal border. The presence of a continuous PDA murmur can also be found.

Transposition of the Great Arteries

The most common cyanotic heart lesion seen in the newborn period is TGA, and it represents around 5% to 8% of all CHD lesions (Figure 15.6).[16] Many variations are seen in TGA. The primary factor is that the aorta originates from the RV and that the main pulmonary artery has LV origins. There are two distinct circulatory systems. The main pulmonary artery has higher oxygen saturation than the aorta, as hyperoxemic blood travels through the pulmonary system and hypoxic blood travels in the systemic

system. The mixing of the circulatory systems is the only way to provide oxygenated blood to the systemic system; therefore, a VSD, an atrial septal defect (ASD) or a PDA becomes essential for survival. A VSD can be found in 20% to 40% of patients. The exam will be remarkable for a loud single S2. When there is a VSD, a systolic murmur will be present.

Total Anomalous Pulmonary Venous Return

TAPVR comprises 1% of CHD (Figure 15.7).[17] Instead of bringing blood from the lungs to the left atrium, the pulmonary veins empty into the right atrium. TAPVR is usually categorized into four groups based on where the pulmonary veins empty. The supracardiac type (50%) has the common pulmonary vein attached to the superior

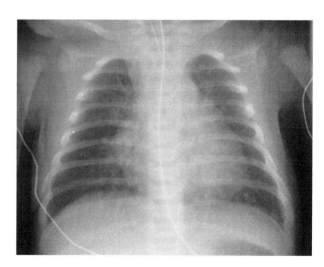

Figure 15.7. Total anomalous pulmonary venous return.

vena cava. The common pulmonary vein empties into the coronary sinus in the cardiac type (20%). The common pulmonary vein drains into the portal vein, ductus venosus, hepatic vein or inferior vena cava in the infracardiac or subdiaphragmatic type (20%). Ten percent of the lesions are of a mixed type, which are a combination of any of the types. Mixing of blood is essential for survival; therefore, ASD or a patent foramen ovale must be present.

Mixing of the pulmonary and systemic circulations occurs when the pulmonary venous return is delivered to the right atrium. Blood then goes through the ASD to the left atrium and also to the RV. Desaturation of the systemic arterial blood results from the mixing of the pulmonary and systemic arterial blood. The extent of desaturation of systemic arterial blood is influenced by pulmonary blood flow. With no obstruction to pulmonary venous return, there is minimal desaturation of the systemic blood. Marked cyanosis will result when there is obstruction to pulmonary venous return. Volume overload (with resultant RV and atrial enlargement) can occur as a result of both pulmonary and venous circulations being pumped by the RV.

Patients with pulmonary venous obstruction may present with a history of frequent pneumonias as well as growth difficulties. CHF is a common presentation, with tachypnea, tachycardia and hepatomegaly in addition to cyanosis. The exam will have a hyperactive RV impulse with a fixed and split S2. A grade 2/6 or 3/6 systolic ejection murmur at the left upper sternal border and a mid-diastolic rumble at the left lower sternal border also are found.

Respiratory distress and cyanosis are seen when there is TAPVR and pulmonary venous obstruction. The cardiac exam typically reveals a loud and single S2 and a gallop rhythm but otherwise will be minimal, frequently with no murmur.

Tricuspid Atresia

TA comprises 1% to 2% of CHD in infancy.[18] No tricuspid valve exists and there is interruption in the development of the RV and pulmonary artery. Pulmonary blood flow is diminished. An ASD, VSD or PDA is necessary for survival because the right atrium needs a right to left shunt to empty as a result of the lack of flow between right atrium and RV. In 30% of cases, the great arteries are transposed, with a VSD and pulmonic stenosis. There is normal artery anatomy in 50% of the cases, with a small VSD and pulmonic stenosis.

As a result of all systemic venous return being shunted from the right atrium to the left atrium, there will be right atrial dilation and hypertrophy. The increased volume of the systemic and pulmonary circulation leads to enlargement of the left atrium and LV. There is an inverse relationship between the degree of cyanosis and the amount of pulmonary blood flow.

Typically, the patient presents with severe cyanosis, tachypnea and poor feeding. The cardiac exam will have a single S2. There is a grade 2 to 3/6 regurgitant systolic murmur from the VSD, heard best at the left lower sternal border. A continuous PDA murmur also may be present. If there is CHF, hepatomegaly will be present.

The ECG is the most outstanding item, with a superior QRS axis with right atrial hypertrophy (RAH), left atrial hypertrophy (LAH) and LVH (Figure 15.8).

Truncus Arteriosus

In truncus arteriosus, all of the pulmonary, systemic and coronary circulations have their origins from a single arterial trunk. Truncus arteriosus represents less than 1% of all CHD.[19] Other abnormalities are associated with truncus arteriosus such as a large VSD, aberrations of the coronary arteries and DiGeorge syndrome (hypocalcemia, hypoparathyroidism, thymus hypoplasia or absence, chromosomal abnormalities). Pulmonary blood flow is dependent on the type of truncus present and can be normal, increased or decreased. The amount of pulmonary blood flow and systemic arterial oxygen saturation are directly related. With decreased pulmonary blood flow there is significant cyanosis, and if there is increased pulmonary blood flow, cyanosis will be minimal. Increased pulmonary blood flow can lead to CHF, as the LV is subject to significant volume overloads.

The patient presents with CHF and cyanosis within the first few weeks of life. A loud regurgitant 2 to 4/6 systolic murmur at the left sternal border is present, and sometimes a high pitched diastolic decrescendo murmur or a diastolic rumble is heard. The S2 is single and prominent.

ACYANOTIC HEART DISEASE

In the first year of life, CHF can have a multitude of etiologies. It can be the result of CHD, and it can be caused by

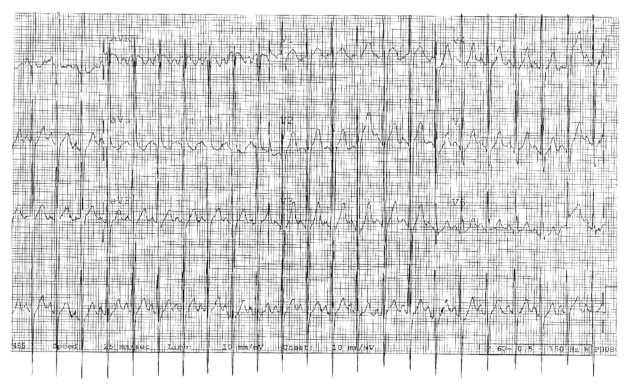

Figure 15.8. EKG of tricuspid atresia.

acquired diseases such as myocarditis, arrhythmias, sepsis, respiratory and metabolic diseases. Factors that contribute to CHF are pressure overload, volume overload, decreased inotropic function, and abnormalities in rhythm. There is a strong CHF association with LV outflow obstruction lesions (coarctation of the aorta and aortic stenosis) and lesions with volume overload (left to right shunts, VSDs, TAPVR). Complete endocardial cushion defects with atrioventricular (AV) valve insufficiency also can present in this manner.

Frequent findings in infants with CHF include difficulty feeding, tachypnea, tachycardia, cardiomegaly, hepatomegaly and rales on pulmonary exam. Feeding can function as a cardiac stress test, and the patient will have prolonged feeding times, less oral intake and diaphoresis. Pulmonary disease can present in a manner similar to cardiac disease, and the administration of supplemental oxygen may not assist in helping with the diagnosis. Echocardiogram is usually the more helpful exam.

The left to right shunt lesions, which comprise approximately 50% of all CHD, are the VSDs, ASDs, PDA and endocardial cushion defects.[20] In left to right shunt lesions, blood is shunted from the systemic system to the pulmonary system. In the neonate, the high pulmonary vascular resistance controls the amount of blood shunted, but when pulmonary vascular resistance starts to decrease in the first few weeks of life, pulmonary blood flow and pressures increase. The magnitude of the lesion is directly related to the extent of the pulmonary vascular blood flow. If there is increased blood flow, this will lead to chamber enlargement, increased pulmonary vascular pressures and CHF. Tables 15.4 and 15.5 review the common radiographic and ECG findings associated with the most common causes of acyanotic heart disease in children.

ATRIAL SEPTAL DEFECTS

ASDs are seen in 10% of CHD.[21] In infancy, about 10% of the patients with an ASD can have complications.[16] With a large defect or associated defects, there can be appreciable left to right shunting and subsequent overloading of the pulmonary circulation. Large defects require surgical intervention, whereas some of the smaller defects close spontaneously. Difficulty with feeding and gaining weight are common complaints.

Ostium secundum defects represent the vast majority of ASDs and are the result of incomplete adhesion of the foramen ovale and septum secundum. Ostium primum

Table 15.4. Acyanotic congenital heart disease lesions and typical chest X-ray findings

Cardiac lesion	Chest X-ray findings
Atrial septal defect	Cardiomegaly with increased vascular markings
Ventricular septal defect	Cardiomegaly with increased vascular markings
Patent ductus arteriosus	Cardiomegaly with increased vascular markings
Endocardial cushion defect	Cardiomegaly with increased vascular markings
Coarctation of the aorta	Cardiomegaly with pulmonary edema
Hypoplastic left heart syndrome	Cardiomegaly
Aortic stenosis	Cardiomegaly
Anomalous origin of the left coronary artery (ALCAPA)	Cardiomegaly

ASDs are caused by the imperfect merging of the septum primum and endocardial cushion and can have abnormalities of the mitral and tricuspid valves. Sinus venosus ASDs occur when the atrium incorrectly merges with the sinus venosus.

The cardiac examination typically reveals a widely split and fixed S2, along with a grade 2 to 3/6 systolic ejection murmur at the left sternal border. A mid-diastolic rumble also may be auscultated.

Table 15.5. Acyanotic congenital heart disease lesions and typical ECG findings

Cardiac lesion	ECG findings
Atrial septal defect	RAD, RVH, RBBB
Ventricular septal defect	LAH, LVH, (RVH in larger VSDs)
Patent ductus arteriosus	LVH, RVH in larger PDAs
Endocardial cushion defect	Superior QRS axis with RVH, RBBB, LVH, prolonged PR interval
Coarctation of the aorta	RVH, RBBB
Hypoplastic left heart syndrome	RAE, RVH, peaked P waves
Aortic stenosis	LVH in severe cases
Anomalous origin of the left coronary artery	Abnormally deep and wide Q waves with ST segment changes in precordial leads

ECG, electrocardiogram; LAH, left atrial hypertrophy; LVH, left ventricular hypertrophy; RAD, right axis deviation; RAE, right atrial enlargement; RBBB, right bundle branch block; RVH, right ventricular hypertrophy.

VENTRICULAR SEPTAL DEFECTS

VSDs are the most prevalent type of CHD and are seen in approximately 25% of all CHD cases.[22] VSDs allow for the mixing of blood in the ventricles. The size of the defect determines the extent of disease, with small defects causing minimal problems and large defects causing pulmonary hypertension and CHF. In large VSDs there is volume and pressure overload in the RV and volume overload in the left atrium and LV.

Poor weight gain and delays in development are common presentations in larger VSDs, and CHF and cyanosis are frequent occurrences.

A grade 2 to 5/6 holosystolic murmur is present and is best heard at the left lower sternal border. A systolic thrill or diastolic rumble, with a narrowly split S2, may also be present.

PATENT DUCTUS ARTERIOSUS

A PDA is seen in 10% of CHD, as the ductus arteriosus remains patent and does not close as it usually would.[20] The magnitude of the shunting depends on the length and diameter of the lesion and pulmonary vascular resistance. Patients are more symptomatic with larger left to right shunts. Generally, in normal patients, the ductus arteriosus closes within 15 hours after birth and then completely seals around 3 weeks of age. It then becomes the ligamentum arteriosum. Prematurity and hypoxia keep the ductus arteriosus patent.

Large PDA defects, as in all left to right shunts, present with CHF.

The cardiac exam typically reveals a grade 1 to 4/6 continuous machinery sounding murmur that is heard best at the left upper sternal border. There can also be a diastolic rumble and bounding peripheral pulses.

ENDOCARDIAL CUSHION DEFECT (COMMON ATRIOVENTRICULAR CANAL)

Defects in the atrial septum, ventricular septum and AV valves will occur when the endocardial cushion does not develop properly. With complete defects, there is involvement of the entire endocardial cushion, and lesions involve the atrial and ventricular septum and the common AV valve. Incomplete or partial defects are seen having atrial involvement with an intact ventricular septum. Also,

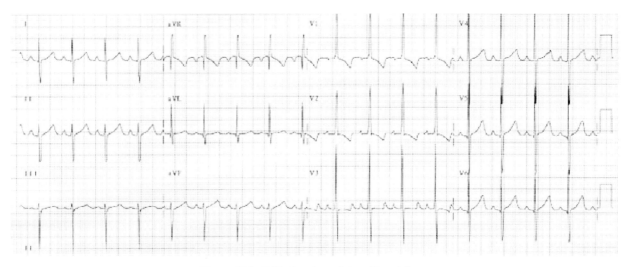

Figure 15.9. EKG of endocardial cushion defect.

variations of complete and incomplete lesions exist. Endocardial cushion defects are seen in about 3% of CHD and about two-thirds are the complete form.[20] A strong association with Down syndrome is seen with the complete form of endocardial cushion defects.

Failure to thrive and a history of multiple respiratory infections are common presentations. Left to right shunting is directly related to the magnitude of the defects, with complete lesions presenting early with CHF from volume overload in the left and RVs.

The exam shows a hyperactive precordium, a systolic thrill, a loud holosystolic regurgitant murmur along with a loud and split S2. The ECG has a superior QRS axis with RVH, RBBB, and LVH as well as a prolonged PR interval (Figure 15.9).

COARCTATION OF THE AORTA

Coarctation of the aorta is seen in 8% to 10% of CHD with a 2:1 male to female ratio.[23] In the region of the ductus arteriosus in the upper thoracic aorta, there is congenital narrowing of the aorta. The degree of narrowing, the length of the narrowing and the presence of other defects determine the magnitude of illness. Infants who become symptomatic early have an RV that supplies the descending aorta via a PDA in fetal life. Other lesions that can be present include a VSD, PDA, aortic hypoplasia and an underdeveloped collateral circulation.

A PDA can temporarily negate the obstructive effects of the coarctation. Also, the PDA can allow for blood flow to areas that are distal to the obstruction. As the PDA closes, pulmonary hypertension will occur, which leads to pulmonary venous congestion and CHF. Blood flow distal to the aortic obstruction is now compromised.

Common presentations include shock, metabolic acidosis, tachypnea, and difficulty feeding. When presenting with CHF, there is a loud gallop and weak pulses. A murmur may or may not be present.

Finding decreased pulses in the lower extremities is a key to diagnosing coarctation. Comparing right upper extremity blood pressures and pulse oximeter readings with the lower extremity help in the diagnosis. However, if the patient is in shock, pulses will be decreased all over.

HYPOPLASTIC LEFT HEART SYNDROME

In HLHS, there is hypoplasia of the LV and hypoplasia of the ascending aorta and aortic arch. Atresia or significant stenosis of the mitral and aortic valves also may be present, as well as underdevelopment of the left atrium. The final result of all of the lesions is minimal LV outflow.[24]

Pulmonary vascular resistance remains higher than systemic vascular resistance in utero. Normal perfusion pressure to the descending aorta and systemic fetal system is maintained by the RV (via the right to left shunt of the ductus arteriosus) and the elevated pulmonary vascular resistance. There is no contribution from the hypoplastic LV. The left atrium is decompressed by an ASD. The entire systemic blood flow depends on the ductus arteriosus. Severe problems occur after birth.

At birth, the fetal pressure system becomes reversed as systemic vascular resistance is now greater than pulmonary vascular resistance. The ductus arteriosus gradually closes. The left side does not function and there is increased systemic vascular resistance; therefore, cardiac output collapses and aortic pressure falls. The end result is circulatory shock and metabolic acidosis. Additionally, increased pulmonary blood flow causes an increase in left atrial pressure, which leads to pulmonary edema.

The patient often presents with a dusky color, tachypnea and listlessness. There is a single heart sound, a systolic ejection murmur and decreased pulses.

AORTIC STENOSIS

Aortic stenosis is found in 6% of CHD, with a 4:1 male to female ratio.[25] Stenosis can occur at the valvular, supravalvular and subvalvular levels and the extent of the obstruction will determine the severity of disease. Patients with severe obstruction (approximately 10%–15%) present in infancy with CHF.[26] Severe stenosis causes LVH. The bicuspid aortic valve is the most common type of aortic stenosis. William syndrome is comprised of supravalvular aortic stenosis, elfin facies, mental retardation, and pulmonary artery stenosis. On examination, there is a systolic thrill at the upper right sternal border, suprasternal notch or carotid arteries. An ejection click may be present. A rough or harsh grade 2 to 4/6 systolic murmur at the right intercostal space or left intercostal space with transmission to the neck also is present.

ANOMALOUS ORIGIN OF THE LEFT CORONARY ARTERY (ALCAPA SYNDROME, BLAND–WHITE–GARLAND SYNDROME)

In the anomalous origin of the left coronary artery syndrome, the left coronary artery originates from the pulmonary artery instead of the aorta. During the second and third months of life, pulmonary artery pressure decreases, and this leads to a fall in perfusion of the LV. The patient becomes distressed and has cardiomegaly and CHF. A murmur consistent with mitral regurgitation also may be present.[27,28] The ECG can show myocardial infarction with abnormally deep and wide Q waves, inverted T waves and ST segment changes in the precordial leads (Figure 15.10).

CARDITIS

Carditis refers to inflammatory disease of the heart and is grouped into myocarditis, pericarditis and endocarditis (with valvulitis).

Myocarditis

Myocarditis is caused by a number of different etiologies such as infectious, autoimmune and toxin mediated.[29,30] The most common etiologies are viral and adenovirus, coxsackievirus, echovirus, mumps and rubella the most frequent causes. Nonviral causes (protozoans) are common outside of the United States. Bacteria, rickettsia, fungal, mycobacteria and other parasites also can be etiologic agents. Myocarditis can be caused by Kawasaki's disease, acute rheumatic fever and collagen vascular disease. Drug ingestion can cause toxic myocarditis.

CHF with tachycardia, tachypnea, a gallop rhythm and decreased heart tones are common presentations as are vomiting, decreased activity and poor feeding. ECG changes are nonspecific. There are tachycardia, low QRS voltages, flattened or inverted T waves with ST-T wave changes and prolongation of the QT interval. Premature contractions also can occur (Figure 15.11).

Pericarditis

Pericarditis is the result of inflammation of the pericardium. In infancy, a viral etiology is the most common cause. Pericarditis frequently is associated with myocarditis, with myocarditis being the more prominent entity. Bacterial etiologies include *Staphylococcus aureus, Streptococcus pneumoniae, Haemophilus influenzae, Neisseria meningitides,* streptococci and tuberculosis. Pericarditis also can be caused by acute rheumatic fever, collagen vascular disease and uremia. Post pericardiomyotomy syndrome can be seen in patients who have had cardiac surgery interrupting the pericardium.

Because the pericardium is a fixed space, the extent of disease is influenced by the rate of accumulation of fluid and by the underlying health of the myocardium. A patient with a healthy myocardium or slow accumulation of fluid will tolerate pericarditis better than a patient with underlying disease and slow collection of fluid or a patient with a rapid collection of fluid. If pericardial tamponade exists, in order to improve hemodynamics, the heart would increase the heart rate (improving cardiac output),

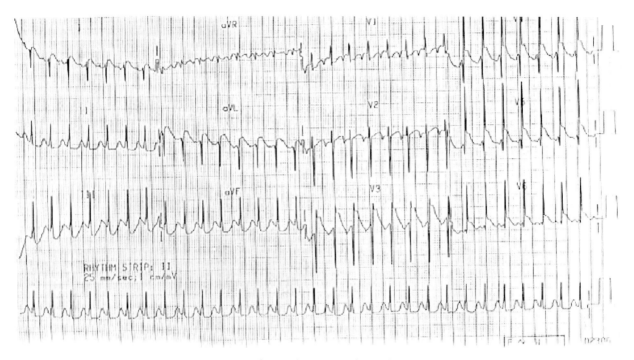

Figure 15.10. EKG of anomalous origin of the left coronary artery.

increase systemic vascular resistance (to compensate for the hypotension), and improve diastolic filling by systemic and pulmonary venous constriction.

The chest x-ray may show cardiomegaly with the heart in a water bottle shape. There is a low voltage QRS complex on ECG. Initially, ST segments are elevated except in V1 and aVR. Later, ST segments normalize and the T waves flatten or invert.

The presence of an effusion is best determined by echocardiogram. Cardiac tamponade can be evaluated also, and, if present, shows collapse of the right atrial wall or RV wall in diastole.

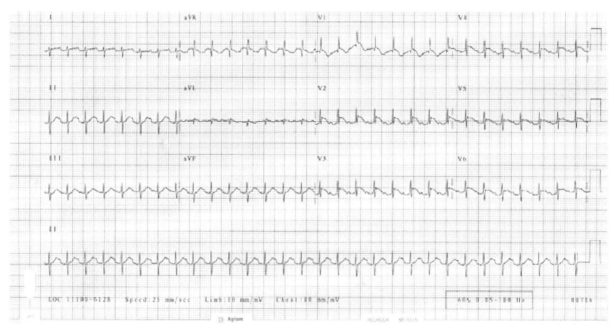

Figure 15.11. EKG of myocarditis.

Cardiac tamponade with associated tachycardia and tachypnea is an immediate concern. Chest x-ray shows cardiomegaly and a pleural effusion. The ECG has ST segment elevation and flat or inverted T waves.

Usually, there is a history of a predisposing illness with an upper respiratory infection. In cases of bacterial pericarditis, pneumonia, empyema, osteomyelitis and pyelonephritis are predisposing factors.

The presence of a pericardial friction rub is diagnostic. The heart is hypodynamic and there may or may not be a murmur.

Endocarditis

Infective endocarditis is frequently linked to CHD. Turbulent flow leads to endothelial damage and thrombus formation, with transient bacteria seeding the damaged areas. The vast majority of CHDs and valvular heart diseases (except the secundum ASD) are predisposed to endocarditis, especially if there is a prosthetic heart valve or graft within the heart. *Streptococcus viridans*, enterococci, *S. aureus* and fungal and bacteria such as *Eikenella* and *Cardiobacterium* are known causes.[31] In infancy, endocarditis is rare and is linked to open heart surgery, presenting with fulminant disease and a septic appearance. There is always fever and a heart murmur.

An echocardiogram, although helpful in finding valvular vegetations, is not 100% sensitive or specific. A negative echocardiogram does not exclude endocarditis. Definitive diagnosis is by obtaining a positive blood culture and isolating a specific microorganism in order to determine specific antibiotic therapy.

The Duke criteria are a combination of diagnostic parameters and echocardiographic findings used to identify infective endocarditis. Clinical diagnosis of definite infective endocarditis requires two major criteria, one major and three minor criteria, or five minor criteria (Table 15.6).

Initial management depends on the patient's presenting condition. Unstable patients require aggressive initial interventions. Maintaining a patent airway, adequate oxygenation and ventilation, and circulatory support are the primary objectives. If a patient presents with signs of embolic phenomena or other complications, therapy should be directed toward those problems until the patient is stabilized. All patients diagnosed with infective

Table 15.6. Duke criteria for infective endocarditis

Major criteria*
1. Isolation of organisms from two blood cultures: Must be typical organisms – *Viridans streptococci, Streptococcus bovis*, HACEK group, or *Staphylococcus aureus* or enterococci in absence of primary focus
2. Persistently positive blood culture: Two or more positive blood cultures for the same organism separated by 12 hours, or three or more positive blood cultures for the same organism with 1 hour between first and last culture
3. Positive echocardiogram for oscillating intracardiac mass at sites where vegetations typically occur
4. Intracardiac abscess identified by echocardiogram
5. New partial dehiscence of prosthetic valve as identified by echocardiogram
6. New regurgitant murmur

Minor Criteria
1. Fever higher than 38°C
2. Predisposing heart condition and/or intravenous drug use
3. Vascular phenomena: includes major arterial emboli, mycotic aneurysms, central nervous system hemorrhages, Janeway lesions, conjunctival hemorrhages, peripheral necrotic skin lesions
4. Immunologic phenomena: includes elevated rheumatoid factor, immune complex glomerulonephritis, Osler's nodes
5. Echocardiogram findings consistent with endocarditis but not meeting major criterion: nonoscillating masses, nodular valve thickening

*Clinical diagnosis of definite infective endocarditis requires two major criteria, one major criterion and three minor criteria, or five minor criteria.
HACEK, *Haemophilus* species, *Actinobacillus actinomycetemcomitans, Cardiobacterium hominis, Eikenella corrodens* and *Kingella* species.

endocarditis, or suspected of having infective endocarditis, should be hospitalized.

Standard treatment consists of parenteral antibiotics, generally at least two agents, for 6 weeks. Multiple organisms cause infective endocarditis; therefore, antibiotic therapy needs to be directed by culture results and sensitivities. Antibiotic combinations for more common infecting organisms – such as *S. viridans, Streptococcus bovis* and enterococci – include intravenous (IV) penicillin G 150,000 units/kg/day divided every 4 to 6 hours (maximum 24 million units/day), or ampicillin 200 mg/kg/day divided every 4 hours (maximum 12 g/day), plus either nafcillin or oxacillin 100 to 200 mg/kg/day divided every 6 hours (maximum 12 g /day), and gentamicin 6 to 7.5 mg/kg/day divided every 8 hours. If the patient is allergic to

Table 15.7. Cardiac conditions requiring prophylaxis against endocarditis

Endocarditis prophylaxis recommended
   High-Risk Category
     Presence of prosthetic valves
     Previous bacterial endocarditis
     Complex cyanotic heart disease
     Surgical systemic pulmonary shunts or conduits
   Moderate-Risk Category
     Other congenital heart malformations
     Acquired valve dysfunction
     Hypertrophic cardiomyopathy
Mitral valve prolapse with regurgitation or thickened leaflets
     Endocarditis Prophylaxis Not Recommended
   Negligible-Risk Category
     Isolated secundum atrial septal defect
     Surgically repaired atrial septal defect, ventricular septal defect or patent ductus arteriosus
     History of coronary bypass graft surgery
     Mitral valve prolapse without regurgitation
     Physiologic, functional or innocent murmurs
     History of Kawasaki disease without valve dysfunction
     History of rheumatic fever without valve dysfunction
     Cardiac pacemakers and implanted defibrillators

Table 15.8. Prophylaxis for dental, oral, respiratory tract or esophageal procedures

Situation	Recommended antibiotic	Dosing regimen
Standard prophylaxis	Amoxicillin	50 mg/kg PO 1 h prior to procedure, not to exceed 2 g
Unable to take oral medications	Ampicillin	50 mg/kg IM or IV within 30 minutes prior to procedure, not to exceed 2 g
Allergic to penicillin	Clindamycin	20 mg/kg PO 1 h prior to procedure, not to exceed 600 mg
	Azithromycin or clarithromycin	15 mg/kg PO 1 hour prior to procedure, not to exceed 500 mg
Allergic to penicillin and unable to take oral medications	Clindamycin	20 mg/kg IV within 30 minutes before procedure, not to exceed 600 mg

penicillin, vancomycin in a dose of 30 mg/kg/day divided every 12 hours (maximum 2 g/day) can be substituted in combination with gentamicin. Patients with staphylococcal infection should be started on nafcillin and gentamicin. Patients with methicillin-resistant strains of staphylococcus or with prosthetic heart valves should be started on vancomycin, rifampin and gentamicin.

Surgery may be necessary in some cases. Indications for surgical intervention include heart failure, an obstructed valve, perivalvular abscess, fungal endocarditis and large vegetations greater than 10 mm.

Stratifying patients into high-, moderate- and low-risk categories is helpful in identifying which individuals need endocarditis prophylaxis (Table 15.7). Those in the negligible-risk category have no greater risk of developing infective endocarditis than the general public; therefore, prophylactic antibiotics are not necessary. Tables 15.8 and 15.9 outline the antibiotic choice and dosing schedules recommended for prophylaxis of individuals that fall into high- and moderate-risk categories.[32]

KAWASAKI'S DISEASE

Kawasaki's disease, also known as *mucocutaneous lymph node syndrome,* is a generalized systemic vasculitis of

Table 15.9. Endocarditis prophylaxis for genitourinary and gastrointestinal procedures

Situation	Recommended antibiotic	Dosing regimen
High-risk patients	Ampicillin and Gentamicin	Ampicillin 50 mg/kg IM or IV, not to exceed 2 g, plus gentamicin 1.5 mg/kg IV, not to exceed 120 mg. 6 hours later ampicillin 25 mg/kg IM/IV or amoxicillin 25 mg/kg PO
High-risk patients with penicillin allergy	Vancomycin and Gentamicin	Vancomycin 20 mg/kg IV over 1–2 hours, not to exceed 1 g, plus Gentamicin as above.
Moderate-risk patients	Amoxicillin or Ampicillin	Amoxicillin 50 mg/kg PO 1 hour prior to procedure, not to exceed 2 g, or ampicillin 50 mg/kg IV/IM within 30 minutes of procedure, not to exceed 2 g
Moderate-risk patients with penicillin allergy	Vancomycin	Vancomycin 20 mg/kg IV over 1–2 hours, complete within 30 minutes of procedure, not to exceed 1 g

indeterminate etiology. The hallmarks are fever, bilateral nonexudative conjunctivitis, erythema of the mucous membranes, rash and extremity changes. Along with Henoch-Schönlein purpura, Kawasaki's disease is one of the most common systemic vasculitic illnesses. Primarily affecting infants and young children, Kawasaki's disease can occur in endemic or community-wide epidemic forms.[33]

In 15% to 25% of untreated children with Kawasaki's, coronary artery aneurysms or ectasia have been found.[34] These coronary lesions can lead to myocardial infarction, sudden death or ischemic heart disease.[35–38]

All parts of the heart (pericardium, myocardium, endocardium, valves and coronary arteries) are involved in the acute phase of Kawasaki's. On examination there can be a hyperdynamic precordium, tachycardia, a gallop and a flow or regurgitant pansystolic murmur. Cardiogenic shock will result from depressed myocardial function.

In the younger patient, an incomplete or atypical presentation is more prevalent. The classic presentation is fever for at least 5 days and involvement of the extremities, the skin, the conjunctivae, the lips and mouth and the cervical lymph nodes. Changes to the extremities include erythema to the palms and soles, with induration and desquamation to the fingers and toes. An extensive erythematous rash appears in the form of a nonspecific diffuse maculopapular rash, with occasional early desquamation of the perineal region. Conjunctival injection (bilateral) involving the bulbar conjunctivae can be seen at the time of the fever. In the lips and mouth there can be erythema, peeling, cracking or bleeding, diffuse erythema of the mucosa and oropharynx, and a strawberry tongue. Unilateral cervical lymphadenopathy is present, with one node larger than 1.5 cm in diameter. Thrombocytosis (appearing in week 2, peaking in week 3 of the illness), leukocytosis and anemia are common as well as elevations in C-reactive protein, erythrocyte sedimentation rate and serum transaminases and gamma glutamyl transpeptidase (GGT). Thrombocytopenia, if found during active disease, is a risk factor for coronary aneurysms.

CARDIOMYOPATHIES

Cardiomyopathies are divided into three categories: hypertrophic, dilated or congestive, and restrictive.

Hypertrophic cardiomyopathies have marked ventricular muscle hypertrophy and increased ventricular contractility. These factors limit ventricular filling. There is an autosomal dominant link.[39] Because the LV is stiff, this affects diastolic ventricular filling. On examination, there is a sharp upstroke of the arterial pulse,[40] and there can be a systolic ejection murmur or a holosystolic murmur.

Dilated or congestive cardiomyopathy is associated with ventricular dilation and diminished contractility. It is the most common form of cardiomyopathy and is usually the end result of an infectious or toxic etiology. CHF is a frequent presentation. There is a pronounced S3 on examination.

The least common form of cardiomyopathy is restrictive. This type limits the diastolic filling of the ventricles and results from noncompliant ventricular walls that have been damaged by an infiltrative process such as a glycogen storage disease.

The hypertrophic cardiomyopathy chest x-ray shows a globular heart.

Hypertrophic cardiomyopathy ECG findings have LVH, ST and T wave changes, deep Q waves, and decreased R waves.

MANAGEMENT

Airway management is of primary importance. Stabilization of the airway and mechanical ventilation can prevent respiratory decompensation. Patients with cyanotic heart lesions will ultimately require surgical intervention. Table 15.10 summarizes the most common surgical procedures performed in these patients.

Cyanotic or hypoxemic episodes are usually associated with TOF. To treat these cyanotic or hypoxemic episodes, the patient should be placed in the knee-chest position to increase systemic vascular resistance. Morphine sulfate (0.1–0.2 mg/kg SC/IM/IV) can stop the hyperpnea. Because the goal is to improve pulmonary blood flow, oxygen may or may not be useful. Acidosis can be treated with sodium bicarbonate (1 mEq/kg IV). Propranolol (0.01–0.2 mg/kg IV over 5 minutes) can be helpful. Phenylephrine (0.02 mg/kg IV) will increase systemic vascular resistance. Ketamine (1–3 mg/kg IV) also will help to increase systemic vascular resistance and will provide sedation.

Ductal-dependent lesions require the prompt initiation of IV prostaglandin E1 (PGE1). In order to improve left to right shunting and to increase pulmonary blood flow, there must be a decrease in pulmonary vascular resistance.

Table 15.10. Cardiac procedures

Procedure	Cardiac lesion	Interventions
Rashkind balloon atrial septostomy	Transposition of the great arteries	Palliative procedure done to make an atrial communication in order to allow mixing of oxygenated and deoxygenated blood
Blalock-Taussig shunt, modified Blalock-Taussig shunt (Gore-Tex shunt with less dissection)	Pulmonary stenosis, pulmonary atresia, tetralogy of Fallot	Connects the subclavian artery to the ipsilateral pulmonary artery allowing for improved pulmonary blood flow
Fontan operation	Hypoplastic left heart syndrome, tricuspid atresia, hypoplastic right heart syndrome, single ventricle lesions	Cavocaval baffle to pulmonary artery anastomosis allows for all systemic venous return to be directed to the pulmonary arteries
Arterial switch operation	Transposition of the great arteries	Aortic trunk attached to left ventricle, pulmonic trunk connected to right ventricle
Glenn operation	Hypoplastic left heart syndrome, hypoplastic right heart syndrome	Cavopulmonary shunt connects the superior vena cava to the right pulmonary artery
Norwood operation, Norwood with Sano modification	Hypoplastic left heart syndrome, single ventricle lesions with aortic atresia or hypoplasia	Reconstruct the aortic arch using the main pulmonary artery and ascending aorta, atrial septectomy, modified Blalock-Taussig shunt in order to provide unobstructed systemic blood flow and satisfactory coronary artery perfusion

The initial dose of PGE1 is 0.05 μg/kg/min. Consultation with pediatric cardiology, if available, and with critical care (neonatal or pediatric) is of great help. Airway management is once again paramount because PGE1 can cause hypotension and apnea. Also, sepsis can present in a similar manner, so evaluation and treatment for sepsis must be initiated. An additional side effect of PGE1 is fever. With certain variants of TAPVR, PGE1 can make the patient worse. Supplemental oxygen can promote the closure of the ductus arteriosus, thus, oxygen must be added cautiously.

Acyanotic lesions that are ductal-dependent require prompt airway management. Mechanical ventilation can increase pulmonary vascular resistance.[40] By increasing right to left shunting over the now PDA using PGE1, systemic perfusion will improve. Volume will treat acidosis and fluid deficits. If decreased ventricular function is evident, pressors can be started.

CHF requires inotropic assistance. Adjustment of preload (end diastolic volume is roughly equal to the intravascular volume), afterload, contractility and heart rate must be made. Cardiac output is the result of heart rate multiplied by stroke volume. Heart rate is the primary mechanism used in the patient 1 year and younger to improve cardiac output.

Dopamine and dobutamine are excellent choices for helping in the management of CHF. Dopamine is started as a continuous infusion at 5 to 10 μg/kg/minute. A rapid response to the chronotropic effects usually follows, with increases in heart rate, blood pressure and urine output. Dobutamine also can be used as a continuous infusion at the same rate but should be used with caution in the patient 1 year of age or younger because of potentially excessive tachycardia. There is less of an arrhythmic potential and chronotropic effect than dopamine. Dobutamine reduces afterload because it has a vasodilatory effect. Dobutamine improves cardiac output without increasing blood pressure; if hypotension is present, dobutamine may be a better choice as an adjunct rather than a primary agent.[4,41]

Amrinone (0.5 mg/kg IV over 3 minutes) and milrinone (loading dose of 10–50 μg/kg IV over 10 minutes) are possible aids in treating CHF. They have inotropic and vasodilator properties but they do not increase heart rate.

In a nonacute setting, digoxin is the inotrope of choice. Digoxin improves cardiac contractility, and because of this, it improves cardiac output. Diuretics, such as furosemide, can be used to promote diuresis.

In Kawasaki's disease, the acute phase is managed with aspirin and IV immunoglobulin (IVIG). High-dose aspirin at 80 to 100 mg/kg/day dosed four times a day along with IVIG have an additive anti-inflammatory effect.[33] IVIG has a generalized anti-inflammatory effect and is dosed at 2 g/kg in a single infusion. The best results are seen when IVIG is initiated within the first 7 to 10 days of illness.

INTERVENTIONAL AND SURGICAL REPAIRS (TABLE 15.10)

Surgical repair of congenital heart lesions continues to evolve, with some lesions repaired in the neonatal period and most lesions repaired in the first couple of months of life.

The Rashkind procedure is a balloon atrial septostomy.[42] In this, an atrial communication is made using a balloon catheter. This allows for the mixing of blood at the atrial level in lesions such as TGA in which there are parallel circulations, and mixing of both is the only way to oxygenate systemic arterial blood.

The Blalock-Taussig shunt is used in TOF. The shunt connects the subclavian artery to the ipsilateral pulmonary artery. The modified Blalock-Taussig shunt uses a Gore-Tex shunt and requires less dissection, is not dependent on vessel length, and has less shunt failure (Figure 15.12).[43]

In severe TOF with marked RV outflow tract obstruction and in older patients, the Rastelli procedure is used. A patch closure of the VSD is done and a conduit from the RV to the pulmonary artery is placed.

For TGA, the Mustard and Senning operations were once done. The Mustard operation was an atrial switch with prosthetic material for an intra-atrial baffle, and the Senning operation used native material for the intra-atrial baffle.

These procedures have been discontinued because of atrial dysrhythmias and the inability of the RV to function as a normal LV later in life. The arterial switch has now replaced these operations and corrects the TGA at the great artery level. The aortic trunk is connected to the LV, whereas the pulmonic trunk is connected to the RV.

The Fontan operation is a shunt that is a cavocaval baffle to pulmonary artery anastomosis. Used in HLHS,

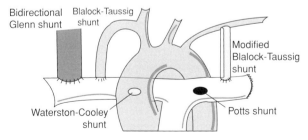

Figure 15.12. Blalock Tausig shunt procedure.

Fontan Operation

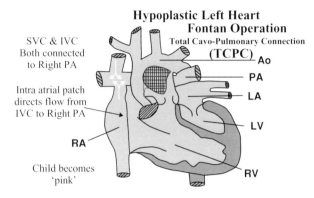

Figure 15.13. Fontan procedure.

TA, and HRHS, the systemic venous return is redirected to the pulmonary artery (Figure 15.13).

In patients with HLHS and HRHS, a bidirectional Glenn (cavopulmonary shunt) or hemi-Fontan operation will anastomose the superior vena cava to the right pulmonary artery. The Glenn operation is done at about 6 months of age and the hemi-Fontan at $1\frac{1}{2}$ years of age.

The Norwood operation is a palliative procedure used in HLHS and is performed in the neonatal period (Figure 15.14).[44] In order to reconstruct the hypoplastic aorta, an aortic or pulmonary allograft is used, the main pulmonary artery is divided, a Gore-Tex shunt is put on the right to establish pulmonary blood flow and the atrial septum is excised to provide interatrial mixing.[45] The Sano modification is done to improve coronary artery perfusion. A small RV to pulmonary artery connection is made in conjunction with a modified Blalock-Taussig shunt, allowing for satisfactory diastolic pressure and improved coronary blood flow.

Stage I-Norwood

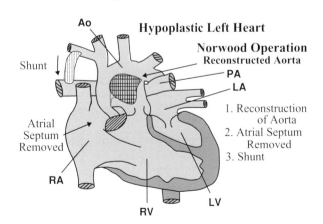

Figure 15.14. Norwood procedure.

Postoperative complications for any of these surgical corrections include dysrhythmias, obstruction of the surgical grafts or conduits, endocarditis, myocardial ischemia or postpericardiotomy syndrome.

PITFALLS

- Failure to recognize that the presentation of cardiac disease in newborns and young infants can mimic pulmonary disease or sepsis
- Failure to realize that preserving ductal patency is paramount to survival in ductal-dependent lesions
- Failure to realize that CHF in young infants can present with nonspecific complaints such as decreased oral intake and poor weight gain
- Failure to consult early with a pediatric cardiologist, a neonatologist, or a pediatric intensivist when CHD is suspected.

REFERENCES

1. Burton DA, Cabalka AK. Cardiac evaluation of infants. The first year of life. *Pediatr Clin N Am.* 1994;41(5):991–1015.
2. Flynn PA, Engle MA, Ehlers KH. Cardiac issues in the pediatric emergency department. *Pediatr Clin N Am.* 1992;39(4):955–968.
3. Woods WA, McCulloch MA. Cardiovascular emergencies in the pediatric patient. *Emerg Med Clin N Am.* 2005;23(5):1233–1249.
4. Gewitz, MH, Woolf PK. Cardiac emergencies. In: Fleisher GR, Ludwig S, eds. *Textbook of Pediatric Emergency Medicine*, 5th ed. Philadelphia, PA: Lippincott Williams & Wilkins; 2006:717–758.
5. Woolridge DP. Congenital heart disease in the pediatric emergency department. Part I: Pathophysiology and clinical characteristics. *Pediatric Emergency Medicine Reports.* 2002;7(7):69–80.
6. Woolridge DP. Congenital heart disease in the pediatric emergency medicine department. Part II: Managing acute and chronic complications. *Pediatric Emergency Medicine Reports.* 2002;7(8):81–92.
7. Hoffman JI, Kaplan S. The incidence of congenital heart disease. *J Am Coll Cardiol.* 2002;39(12):1890–1900.
8. Park MK, Guntheroth WG. *How to Read Pediatric ECGs*, 4th ed. Philadelphia, PA: Mosby; 2006.
9. Park MK. *Pediatric Cardiology for Practitioners*, 5th ed. Philadelphia, PA: Mosby; 2007.
10. Lees MH, King DH. Cyanosis in the newborn. *Pediatr Rev.* 1987;9(2):36–42.
11. Friedman AH, Fahey JT. The transition from fetal to neonatal circulation: normal responses and implications for infants with heart disease. *Semin Perinatol.* 1993;17(2):106–121.
12. Nadas AS, Fyler DC. Hypoxemia. In: Keane JF, Lock JE, Fyler DC, eds: *Nada's Pediatric Cardiology*, 2nd ed. Philadelphia, PA: Saunders; 2006:97–101.
13. Martin L, Khalil H. How much reduced hemoglobin is necessary to generate cyanosis? *Chest.* 1990;97(1):182–185.
14. Waldman JD, Wernly JA. Cyanotic congenital heart disease with decreased pulmonary blood flow in children. *Pediatr Clin N Am.* 1999; 46(2):385–404.
15. Breitbart RE, Fyler DC. Tetralogy of Fallot. In: Keane JF, Lock JE, Fyler DC, eds. *Nada's Pediatric Cardiology*, 2nd ed. Philadelphia, PA: Saunders; 2006:559–579.
16. Studer M, Blackstone E, Kirklin J, et al. Determinants of early and late results of repair of atrioventricular septal (conal) defects. *J Thorac Cardiovasc Surg.* 1982;84(4):523–542.
17. Keane JF, Fyler DC. Total anomalous pulmonary venous return. In: Keane JF, Lock JE, Fyler DC, eds. *Nada's Pediatric Cardiology*, 2nd ed. Philadelphia, PA: Saunders; 2006:773–781.
18. Keane JF, Fyler DC. Tricuspid atresia. In: Keane JF, Lock JE, Fyler DC, eds. *Nada's Pediatric Cardiology*, 2nd ed. Philadelphia, PA: Saunders; 2006:753–759.
19. Williams JM, de Leeuw M, Black MD, et al. Factors associated with outcomes of persistent truncus arteriosus. *J Am Coll Cardiol.* 1999;34(2):545–553.
20. Driscoll DJ. Left to right shunt lesions. *Pediatr Clin N Am.* 1999;46(2):355–368.
21. Mahoney LT, Truesdell SC, Krzmarzick TR, et al. Atrial septal defects that present in infancy. *Am J Dis Child.* 1986;140(11):1115–1118.
22. Kidd L, Driscoll D, Gersony W, et al. Second natural history study of congenital heart defects: Results of treatment of patients with ventricular septal defects. *Circulation.* 1993;87(2 suppl):I38–51.
23. Demircin M, Arsan S, Pasaoglu I, et al. Coarctation of the aorta in infants and neonates: results and assessments of prognostic variables. *J Cardiovasc Surg.* 1995;36(5):459–464.
24. Bailey LL, Gundry SR. Hypoplastic left heart syndrome. *Pediatr Clin N Am.* 1990;37(1):137–150.
25. Fedderly RT. Left ventricular outflow obstruction. *Pediatr Clin N Am.* 1999;46(2):369–384.
26. Bando K, Turrentine MW, Sun K, et al. Surgical management of hypoplastic left heart syndrome. *Ann Thorac Surg.* 1996;62(1):70–77.
27. Chang RKR, Allada V. Electrocardiographic and echocardiographic features that distinguish anomalous origin of the left coronary artery from pulmonary artery from idiopathic dilated cardiomyopathy. *Pediatr Cardiol.* 2001;22(1):3–10.
28. DeWolf D, Vercruysse T, Suys B, et al. Major coronary anomalies in childhood. *Eur J Pediatr.* 2002;161(12):637–642.
29. Towbin JA. Myocarditis. In: Allen HD, Gutgesell HP, Clark FB, et al, eds. *Moss and Adam's Heart Disease in Infants, Children and Adolescents: Including the Fetus and Young Adult*, 6th ed. Baltimore, MD: Lippincott, Williams & Wilkins; 2001:1197–1215.
30. Wheeler DS, Kooy NW. A formidable challenge: the diagnosis and treatment of viral myocarditis in children. *Crit Care Clin.* 2003;19(3):365–391.

31. Danilowicz D. Infective endocarditis. *Pediatr Rev.* 1995;16(4):148–154.

32. Newberger JW, Takahashi M, Gerber MA, et al. Diagnosis, treatment, and long-term management of Kawasaki disease. AHA Scientific Statement. *Circulation.* 2004;110(17):2747–2771.

33. Genizi J, Miron D, Spiegel R, et al. Kawasaki disease in very young infants: high prevalence of atypical presentation and coronary arteritis. *Clin Pediatr.* 2003;42(3):263–267.

34. Dajani AS, Taubert KA, Gerber MA, et al. Diagnosis and therapy of Kawasaki disease in children. *Circulation.* 1993;87(5):1776–1780.

35. Kato K, Koike S, Yokoyama T. Kawasaki disease. Effect of treatment on coronary artery involvement. *Pediatrics.* 1979;63(2):175–179.

36. Rosenfeld EA, Corydon KE, Shulman ST. Kawasaki disease in infants less than one year of age. *J Pediatr.* 1995;126(4):524–529.

37. Baer AZ, Rubin LG, Shapiro CA, et al. Prevalence of coronary artery lesions on the initial echocardiogram in Kawasaki syndrome. *Arch Pediatr Adolesc Med.* 2006;160(7):686–690.

38. Burch M, Blair E. The inheritance of hypertrophic cardiomyopathy. *Pediatr Cardiol.* 1999;20(5):313–316.

39. DeLuca M, Tak T. Hypertrophic cardiomyopathy. Tools for identifying risk and alleviating symptoms. *Postgrad Med.* 2000;107(7):127–140.

40. Atz AM, Feinstein JA, Jonas RA. Preoperative management of pulmonary venous hypertension in hypoplastic left heart syndrome with restrictive atrial septal defect. *Am J Cardiol.* 1999;83(8):224–228.

41. Lee C, Mason LJ. Pediatric cardiac emergencies. *Anesthesiol Clin N Am.* 2001;19(2):287–308.

42. Rashkind WJ, Miller WW. Creation of an atrial septal defect without thoracotomy: a palliative approach to complete transposition of the great arteries. *JAMA.* 1966;196(11):991–992.

43. Ullom RL, Sade RM, Crawford FJ Jr, et al. The Blalock-Taussig shunt in infants: standard versus modified. *Ann Thorac Surg.* 1987;44(5):539–543.

44. Norwood WI, Lang P, Hansen DD. Physiologic repair of aortic atresia with hypoplastic left heart syndrome. *N Engl J Med.* 1983;308(1):23–36.

45. Bove EL, Lloyd TR. Stage reconstruction for hypoplastic left heart syndrome. *Ann Surg.* 1996;224(3):387–394.

46. Wilson W, Taubert KA, Gewitz M, et al. Prevention of infective endocarditis: Guidelines from the American Heart Association: A Guideline From the American Heart Association Rheumatic Fever, Endocarditis, and Kawasaki Disease Committee, Council of Cardiovascular Disease in the Young, and the Council on Clinical Cardiology, Council on Cardiovascular Surgery and Anesthesia, and the Quality of Care and Outcomes Research Interdisciplinary Working Group. *Circulation.* 2007;116;1736–1754.

Dermatology

Maureen McCollough

Skin conditions in young infants can range from the benign, such as birthmarks and neonatal acne, to signs of more serious diseases, such as Kawasaki disease and meningococcemia. Having a solid knowledge of the various conditions that may present is important when caring for young infants in the emergency department (ED). This chapter focuses on dermatological conditions commonly seen in newborns and infants. Other selected important conditions that affect mostly older children also are discussed.

This chapter is organized by grouping skin findings or conditions into several large categories: vesiculobullous (blisters and bullae), vesicular ruptured, pustular, skin-colored, brown or purple-colored, erythematous maculopapular, vascular, papulosquamous and eczematous.

Any newborn or infant who is evaluated for a dermatologic complaint should have a complete history and physical exam performed. Questions include:

When and where on the body did the rash begin?

How has the rash changed?

Are other family members affected?

Are there other associated signs or symptoms such as fever, vomiting, diarrhea, upper respiratory infection (URI) symptoms, itching or pain?

Has there been exposure to a new food or other product such as soap?

What treatment has been tried at home or by other health care practitioners?

The physical exam first should focus on the overall appearance of the infant, well-appearing versus ill or even toxic-appearing. Hydration status and perfusion should be evaluated. A good physical exam is important for diagnoses such as otitis media, oral pathology such as Coxsackie virus, or pneumonia and joint infections. The need

for laboratory studies, radiological studies and management is determined by the age of the infant, the associated signs or symptoms, and the practitioner's confidence in the diagnosis.

Often, when prescribing cream or ointment medication to a child, the question arises, "How many grams do I need to prescribe?" One simplified method is the *fingertip method*.[1] A fingertip unit (FU) is the amount of cream or ointment expressed from the 5-mm diameter end of the medication tube and then applied to the palmar surface of the distal index finger, from the distal interphalangeal joint to the end of the index finger. A measurement of 1 FU can cover the surface equal to two palms of an adult flat hand; 2 FUs equal 1 g of medication (Table 16.1).

VESICULOBULLOUS (BLISTERS AND BULLAE)

Several skins conditions may be present on a newborn's body at birth. *Sucking* or *friction blisters* are solitary, oval, noninflamed blisters or erosions on the skin. Located on the fingers, hands, wrists, forearms or upper lip, these lesions are named appropriately as they are due to the baby's frequent sucking in utero. These lesions will resolve in a few days. *Herpes simplex virus* (HSV) may have similar appearance but exhibits more than one lesion grouped on

Table 16.1. Fingertip unit for measuring prescription amounts

Fingertip unit (FU) = The amount of cream or ointment applied to the palmar surface of the distal index finger, from the distal interphalangeal joint to the end of the finger, using a medication tube with a 5-mm diameter opening

1 FU = An area equivalent to the palms of two adult flat hands

2 FUs = 1 g of medication

an erythematous base. Unroofing of a lesion and subsequent Wright stain can determine the presence of HSV.

Erythema toxicum, a common cause of a vesicular, papular or pustular rash in newborns, is reviewed in the pustular section.

HSV can present in a wide variety of ways in the neonatal and infant age groups. One form seen in infants is *Herpes gingivostomatitis.* Small painful ulcerative lesions occur on the gingiva, mucous membranes, lips, palate and pharynx, and they are associated with fever, dysphagia and subsequent dehydration. Single isolated lesions of the lips or oral mucosa also occur in older children; these lesions traditionally are known as a *herpes labialis* or *cold sores.* Oral HSV can be spread to the fingers in the form of a *herpetic whitlow* via hand-to-mouth transfer. These digital lesions should *not* be incised and drained. Management of the oral form of herpes includes evaluation for signs of dehydration. Infants who are unable to take in adequate fluids due to pain need be admitted to the hospital for intravenous (IV) hydration. Treatment with acyclovir 15 mg/kg, five times per day for 1 week (maximum 200 mg/dose) can shorten the duration of symptoms. Children with oral forms of herpes can shed the virus for 1 to 2 weeks.[2–4]

Corneal involvement requires an ophthalmology consultation (Figure 16.1). Fluorescein staining generally shows a micro-dendritic pattern. A rare complication of neonatal herpes is aseptic meningitis.

Neonatal herpes occurs by contact with an infected genital tract at birth or by exposure to infected oral lesions or secretions. Neonatal herpes is one of the components of the TORCH complex; all these components can mimic neonatal herpes:

T   Toxoplasmosis
O   Other (congenital syphilis and viruses)
R   Rubella
C   Cytomegalovirus
H   HSV

Neonatal herpes presents in three different forms that affect different areas: skin, eyes and mouth; localized central nervous system (CNS); and disseminated.

Skin lesions, including grouped blisters on an erythematous base, are commonly located on the scalp or buttocks, consistent with the portion of the infant presenting through the birth canal. If a fetal scalp electrode was used during labor, this may be an area where lesions coalesce. The lesions develop immediately after birth, with a mean age of onset of 6 days, but they can occur up to 4 weeks of age. The skin lesions present in 50% of infants with neonatal herpes, with most being type 2. Herpes should be considered in any newborn undergoing workup for sepsis who also has elevated liver function tests.

The *CNS form* may be present if the cerebrospinal fluid (CSF) in a febrile infant shows pleocytosis or if the fever is associated with irritability or seizure in the newborn period.[2,3]

The *disseminated form* involves many organs including brain, heart, lungs and liver, and this form also affects the adrenal glands. The infant with the disseminated form of herpes appears septic with poor feeding, dyspnea, hypothermia, jaundice, hepatitis, hepatosplenomegaly, pneumonia, seizures, encephalitis and death.

Diagnosis can be made with Tzanck smear (scrape an intact blister, then treat with Wright or Giemsa stain) showing multinucleated (or single) giant cells with intranuclear inclusions. If herpes is being considered, cultures of the skin, urine, rectum, nasopharynx, eyes and CSF should be obtained. Rapid tests such as direct fluorescent antibody or monoclonal antibodies are 90% accurate. Polymerase chain reactions (PCR) are often used to detect herpes DNA in the CSF.[5] Blood cultures are not usually accurate. Newborns diagnosed with herpes should be admitted to the hospital for IV acyclovir, and antibiotics are usually started concurrently to treat possible bacterial infections. Ophthalmologic herpes should be treated with antiviral agents such as 1% trifluridine, 0.1%

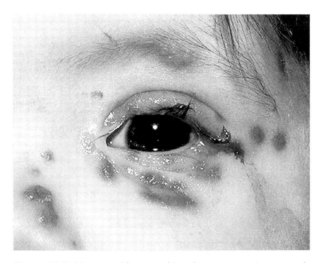

Figure 16.1. Herpes with corneal involvement requires consultation with an ophthalmologist.

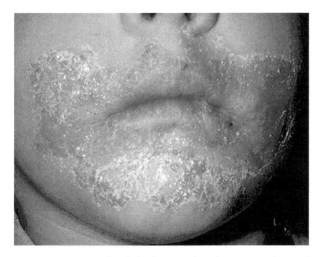

Figure 16.2. Example of the honey-colored crusty exudates of the bacterial infection Impetigo contagiosa.

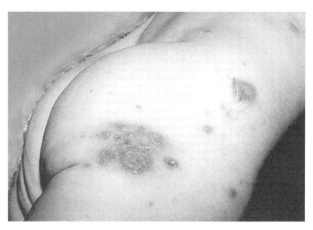

Figure 16.3. Bullous impetigo caused by certain strains of staph present as thin-walled pustules and bullae.

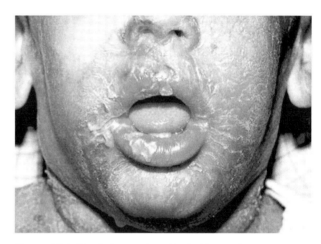

Figure 16.4. Staphylococcal scalded skin syndrome presents with a generalized painful red skin rash, fever and irritability.

iododeoxyuridine or 3% vidarabine.[2,3,6] Topical steroids should be avoided.

Genital herpes, typically a disease of adolescents and adults, is caused by type 2 herpes. Rarely, young children may develop genital herpes because of inoculation with type 1 from an oral lesion. Abuse must be considered in any child with genital herpes. Herpes type 2 in a presexual child supports the diagnosis of abuse; therefore, typing of the lesions is paramount.

Older infants often are plagued by *Impetigo contagiosa*, a bacterial infection causing epidermal vesicles and pustules with honey-colored crusty exudates (Figure 16.2). Caused by *Staphylococcus aureus* and *Streptococcus pyogenes*, the lesions typically start at the nasal area and then spread by self-inoculation. Methicillin-resistant *S. aureus* (MRSA) is implicated more and more.[2] Treatment includes clipping the infant's nails, gently cleansing the area and applying mupirocin cream (Bactroban) three times per day for 7 days. Oral antibiotics to cover staph infection can be used if the lesions are more extensive. Bullous impetigo caused by certain strains of staph present as thin-walled pustules and bullae (Figure 16.3). These lesions rupture, leaving an erythematous base and peeled rim. Bullous impetigo can spread rapidly, especially in newborns. For bullous impetigo, oral antibiotics are used, with coverage to include MRSA in communities with high prevalence. Eradication of colonized staph using a hexachlorophene scrub and intranasal mupirocin cream should be considered.[2]

Staphylococcal scalded skin syndrome (SSSS) is considered by some to be a more extensive version of bullous impetigo. SSSS is caused by staph phage types I, II and III toxins. The pathogen is normally carried in the nose and may begin as a local infection but soon spreads hematogenously. In children younger than 5 years, SSSS presents with a generalized painful red skin rash, fever and irritability.[7] In general, these children are not ill-appearing (Figure 16.4). *Nikolsky's sign* is positive (pressure on the skin causes detachment at the stratum corneum). Bullae often are found in the intertriginous areas, and fissures and crusting are found around the mouth and nose. Large sheets of skin may shear away leaving denuded skin similar to a burn. Mucous membranes are not involved. Cultures of the skin and bullae do not usually reveal the organism. Although the disease is mostly self-limited, treatment includes IV hydration, burn care and IV penicillinase-resistant penicillin. Toxic epidermal necrolysis looks similar but occurs in adults, usually with no fever and usually due to reactions to drugs such as sulfas.

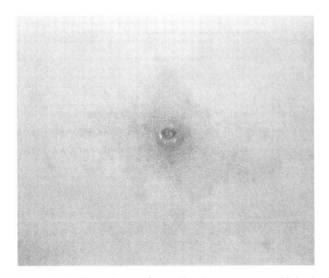

Figure 16.5. Classic lesion of Varicella. This image was published in Color Textbook of Pediatric Dermatology (4th ed.), Weston et al., 2007, copyright Elsevier.

Varicella, or *chicken pox,* is caused by the Varicella-zoster virus (VZV, human herpesvirus [HHV] 3). Varicella has seen a dramatic decrease in incidence since the introduction of the vaccine in 1995, down by 75% to 85%.[8] Varicella becomes clinically apparent after an incubation period of as short as 14 to 16 days or as long as 3 weeks. It is believed to be contagious from 1 to 2 days before the rash begins and remains contagious until all the lesions have crusted, which usually happens 1 week after rash onset. The rash may remain dormant in sensory nerve ganglia, typically of the trunk, and presents as a clinical dermatomal rash called *herpes zoster,* or *shingles.*

The varicella vaccine is administered at ages 12 to 15 months with a booster between 4 and 6 years of age. Because of this, young infants and newborns may be at risk if exposed to an individual with varicella. It is more likely to be maculopapular than vesicular in these young infants.[3] It is also believed to be much less contagious in vaccinated children than in unvaccinated children with standard varicella.

Varicella presents as crops of small macules that become vesicles on erythematous base ("dewdrop" on a rose petal; Figure 16.5). The vesicles soon rupture and crust. Classically, the child presents in various stages of healing. Fever, headache, anorexia, cough, coryza and sore throat are often present concomitant with varicella. Oral or ocular lesions are not uncommon. The lesions are pruritic, and scarring can result.[2,3] Patients with thrombocytopenia may develop hemorrhagic lesions.

The skin should be examined carefully for evidence of secondary cellulitis, the most common complication in varicella, typically caused by group A beta-hemolytic *Streptococcus* or *S. aureus.* Invasive group A *Streptococcus* (GAS) has been shown to cause necrotizing fasciitis and toxic shock in rare cases of varicella.[9] Other complications include acute cerebellar ataxia, encephalitis, post-viral transverse myelitis, Guillain-Barré syndrome, arthritis, nephritis, carditis, myositis, orchitis, hepatitis, thrombocytopenia and Reye syndrome.[10] Varicella rarely causes pneumonia in children but can cause pneumonia in immunosuppressed children, adolescents and adults. Immunocompromised children also may be at risk for hemorrhagic lesions or encephalitis. Severe cases of varicella have been seen in children receiving steroids for asthma or other illnesses.

Congenital varicella syndrome occurs in 2% of infants who are exposed to VZV during the first or second trimester. This syndrome manifests as intrauterine growth restriction (IUGR), microcephaly, cortical atrophy, limb hypoplasia, cataracts, micrognathia, chorioretinitis and skin scarring.[11] Newborn varicella occurs in newborns whose mothers developed varicella lesions within 5 days before birth or within 2 days after birth (no maternal antibodies yet formed that could be passed to the fetus). Mortality in these infants is as high as 30%.[11] Treatment includes acyclovir and Varicella-zoster immune globulin (VZIG). If the mother develops lesions more than 5 days before birth, the resultant varicella is usually less severe in the newborn due to maternal antibodies.

Diagnosis is usually made without any laboratory tests, but for cases that are in doubt, a Tzanck smear can demonstrate multinucleated (or single) giant cells with intranuclear inclusions but are of low sensitivity. Cultures are not timely enough for an ED diagnosis. Direct fluorescent antibody (DFA) tests are rapid and sensitive but less sensitive than PCR testing, but PCR is not available in many health care settings.

Varicella is another self-limiting disease. Lesions usually resolve in 7 to 10 days. Cool compresses, calamine lotion, oatmeal baths or oral antihistamines can be used to help reduce the pruritus. Varicella is transmitted by respiratory droplets and direct contact. Infants diagnosed with varicella should be isolated from newborns, pregnant women and any person who has never had varicella or the vaccine. Treatment includes antipyretics. Ibuprofen is thought to be contraindicated as varicella, at times, can cause thrombocytopenia and hemorrhagic lesions, especially in immunocompromised children. Ibuprofen also has been implicated in the development of necrotizing fasciitis.[12] Aspirin should be avoided as it may be linked to Reye syndrome. Antibiotics for secondary bacterial infections should be aimed toward anti-*Staphylococcal* coverage; these antibiotics include cephalexin, amoxicillin-clavulanate or dicloxacillin. In penicillin-allergic patients, azithromycin or clindamycin could be used.

Antivirals are of limited use in healthy immunocompetent children. Acyclovir is recommended for patients who may be at risk for moderate to severe illness (patients <6 months old, patients >12 years old, patients with chronic skin or pulmonary diseases, patients who use inhaled steroids or chronic salicylates, or patients with ophthalmologic involvement). Immunocompromised patients with acute varicella should be admitted to receive IV acyclovir. VZIG provides passive immunity. Studies have shown the drug will modify or prevent illness in high-risk patients if given within 48 to 72 hours after exposure.[13,14] It is recommended for patients with immunodeficiencies, leukemia or lymphoma; those receiving chemotherapy or immunosuppressive medications; and those with disseminated disease. VZIG is also recommended for newborns whose mothers develop primary varicella either within 5 days before birth or 2 days after delivery or for neonates who develop varicella within 10 days of birth. These infants are at risk for fulminant, disseminated disease.

Zoster is caused by reactivation of the same VZV. Children are affected less often than adults and have milder forms. Those at highest risk are infants who acquired the virus while in utero after 20 weeks gestation or before 18 months of age.[2] Aging and immunosuppression also places patients at high risk. The classic rash is often preceded by painful paresthesias in the dermatome. Children are usually less affected by the neuralgia. The zoster rash appears similar to varicella, grouped vesicles but is only distributed in the area of the affected dermatome. The most common dermatomes affected are the trigeminal and thoracic (thoracic is more common in infants). Involvement of the ophthalmic branch of the trigeminal nerve may involve the cornea, causing keratitis and uveitis. This can lead to permanent corneal damage. Corneal involvement should be suspected when there is a cutaneous lesion on the nose (Hutchinson's sign). Facial nerve palsy and disturbances of hearing and balance constitute Ramsay Hunt syndrome. Fever and lymphadenopathy may also

be present. Although rare, zoster may have complications similar to varicella, such as aseptic meningitis, encephalitis or cerebellar ataxia. Immunocompromised patients may develop more disseminated disease.

Diagnosis of zoster, as with varicella, can be made with a Tzanck smear scraping treated with a Giemsa or Wright stain. DFA can distinguish between herpes and varicella zoster.[15] Management of zoster mandates pain control. Narcotics may be necessary. Steroids may be helpful to decrease post-herpetic neuralgia, but no good studies exist in children.[16] Acyclovir, if started within 72 hours of onset, may shorten the course of the illness and decrease the pain.

Small pox also presents with diffuse blisters of the skin *all at the same stage* and distributed more peripherally. A human case has not been documented in several decades and, if found, needs to be reported to the local health department.

Coxsackie virus is another cause of vesiculobullous rash. Etiology includes the enteroviruses, specifically Coxsackie virus A16 and enterovirus 71, but others have been implicated.[17] Small macules to vesicles to ulcerations are classically seen in the posterior palate ("herpangina"). Small papules or vesicles are often found on the palms, soles of the feet, dorsal surfaces of the hands and feet, and the buttocks, giving this the name *hand-foot-mouth* disease (Figure 16.6). Fever, diarrhea and decreased oral intake are often present. Children generally do not appear ill, but dehydration is a risk. Aseptic meningitis, encephalitis with paralysis, myocarditis, pneumonia or even death can occur due to the same virus but is rare.[18,19] Diagnosis is made most often on clinical findings only. Enteroviruses

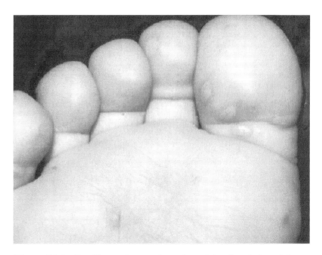

Figure 16.6. Small papules on the soles of the feet in hand-foot-mouth disease.

can be confirmed by culture. PCR is often more rapid and more sensitive than culture.[3] Treatment is symptomatic as the lesions resolve spontaneously within 7 days. Hydration should be encouraged. Popsicles are a fun way for older infants to maintain necessary oral intake during the acute painful phase. Acetaminophen or ibuprofen can be used for fever and pain. A topical suspension of liquid antacids (e.g., Mylanta) with diphenhydramine and viscous lidocaine can be used sparingly (dab suspension onto lesions) to help lessen the pain of the oral lesions. Viscous lidocaine should be used with caution in infants. Patients are contagious from 2 days before the lesions appear to 2 days after onset, but viral shedding continues in feces for 2 weeks.[20]

Contact dermatitis is common in the newborn and infancy period often due to skin irritation from urine or feces. Often appearing as erythematous macules, the dermatitis may include blistering lesions. Contact dermatitis is reviewed in the Erythematous Maculopapular Lesions section.

For any blistering of the skin consistent with a burn either by appearance or history, nonaccidental trauma (child abuse) must be considered if the pattern or history is questionable. Treatment includes pain medication and local wound care. Burn covers such as Biobrane or Vaseline gauze can be cut to the size of the burn, placed on it, then covered with a wrapping such as Kerlix. The Kerlix can be unwrapped daily to check for evidence of infection developing. Every few days, the wound can be soaked to remove the burn cover and then a new cover can be applied, as needed.

VESICULAR ERROSIONS (BURST BLISTERS)

Aphthous stomatitis, also known as *canker sores,* present as 1 to 10 mm erosions with a gray–yellow–pale pink bases appearing on the gums, tongue, palate, lips and buccal mucosa. Burning and tenderness are usually present. Fever is not usually present, and, if present, other diagnoses such as Coxsackie virus or HSV probably should be considered. The aphthous ulcerative lesions generally heal within 7 to 10 days but can recur sporadically or frequently in large numbers. In young infants, URI symptoms may also be present. In older patients, complex aphthosis, Behçet's syndrome or inflammatory bowel disease may also be present. An autoimmune etiology has been suggested. Treatment is symptomatic as these lesions are

self-limited. For young infants, acetaminophen or ibuprofen can be used for pain control. It should be emphasized to parents that infants may find eating too painful but hydration is obviously important. Popsicles, just as with Coxsackie virus, can often be a fun way for older infants to stay hydrated. Severe cases can be treated with a triamcinolone-acetonide base that sticks to the mucosa. Oral prednisone for 3 to 5 days may also be useful for severe cases.[2,3]

PUSTULES

In newborns, one of the most common pustular rashes is *erythema toxicum.* This rash presents as blotchy, erythematous macules, 2 to 3 cm in diameter with 1- to 3-mm papules, vesicles or pustules on this base. The lesions generally appear at 24 to 48 hours old in 50% of newborns. These lesions can continue to develop for the first 10 days. There can be a few scattered lesions to as many as 100 lesions. The erythematous lesions may coalesce, making it more difficult to identify the original lesions. They present on the chest, back, face and proximal extremities; palms and soles are not involved. Eosinophils can be found on Wright stain, and Gram stain is negative. The etiology has not been determined but is thought to be obstruction of the pilosebaceous orifices or possibly a reaction to staph organisms found commonly on the newborn body.[21] Treatment is supportive as these lesions are also self-limited.[2,3]

Transient neonatal pustular melanosis (TNPM) is also seen in newborns with vesicles, either intact or ruptured, or pustules with surrounding scaly edges. The lesions appear on the trunk, extremities and face and can include palms and soles. With time, the lesions will change to hyperpigmented macules. The vesicles and pustules resolve by 1 week but the macules take weeks to months to resolve. TNPM occurs more often in African American newborns. On Wright stain, neutrophils and occasional eosinophils can be seen. Gram stain is negative. The cause is unknown.[3,22]

Neonatal acne, now known as *cephalic pustulosis,* is acne in the neonatal period. Occurring at 2 to 4 weeks, multiple discrete acne-like lesions can be found on the face, chest, back and groin. The papules can become pustules and can persist up to 8 months. These lesions are part of the "miniature puberty of the newborn" including acne, breast enlargement and vaginal bleeding. The causes are hyperplastic sebaceous glands and high hydroxysteroid dehydrogenase activity. Acne as a newborn may indicate more severe acne as a teenager. Treatment is supportive; in severe cases, 2.5% benzoyl peroxide may be used.[4]

Acropustulosis of infancy, also seen soon after birth, can occur in children up to age 3 years old. The lesions appear as discrete erythematous papules or vesicles that become pruritic scaly pustules on distal extremities and are prominent on the palms and soles. Acropustulosis can recur over and over. It can be mistaken for scabies. Treatment can include topical steroids and oral antihistamines for the pruritis.[3,22] (Note: In young infants, "itchiness" may present as irritability; young infants do not have the coordination to scratch.)

Scabies is a pustular rash that brings many infants and young children into the ED. This rash consists of papules and vesicles with excoriated linear or curved burrows (1 mm × 1.5 cm long) in older patients; burrows are less common in children. Scabies in older patients primarily appears in wrists, web spaces, genitals and warm intertriginous areas. Infants have more pustule-like lesions located on the trunk, face, palms, soles and scalp[3] (Figure 16.7). The rash is intensely pruritic, usually worse at night. Scabies is most common in the winter and easily spreads to other family members. The *Sarcoptes scabiei* mite is the culprit; as few as 10 mites per person are common. If unclear, diagnosis can be made by a skin scraping showing mite, ova or feces. The scraping may be negative; if highly

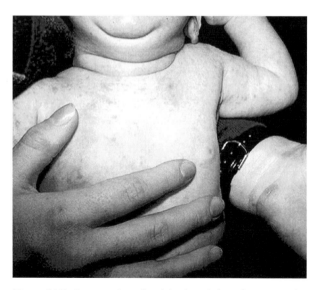

Figure 16.7. Presentation of scabies in an infant shows pustule-like lesions located on the trunk.

suspicious, the recommendation is still to treat. Scabies can be mistaken for eczema from the continuous scratching and secondary infection. Treatment includes washing in hot water all clothes and bedsheets used in the previous 72 hours. If other family members are affected, they also must be treated. Permethrin cream 5% (Elimite) should be massaged into the skin all over below the neck. (Lindane and Kwell should be avoided in infants as it has been linked to seizures and other neurotoxicity).[23] In infants, the head and scalp must also be treated. The itch may still last for days to weeks but no new lesions should develop. A repeat treatment may be needed if new lesions develop. Oral anti-scabies medications are not recommended for infants or children. Antihistamines and topical hydrocortisone can be used for the pruritus. Superinfection should be treated with oral antibiotics. If pruritus persists, undertreatment or reinfection is possible.[2–4] (Note: If a pruritic rash persists for >1 week, consider dry skin, scabies or atopic dermatitis in infants.)

SKIN-COLORED LESIONS

Miliaria rubra, seen in newborns, is due to overheating, and it can consist of skin-colored and erythematous macules. Miliaria rubra are discussed in the Erythematous Maculopapular Lesions section.

Neonatal sebaceous gland hyperplasia is a common neonatal skin condition with multiple 1- to 5-mm yellowish white papules located on nose and cheeks. This is a normal physiological response to maternal androgens stimulating sebaceous glands. These usually resolve in 4 to 6 months.

Milia have similar 1- to 2-mm yellowish white papules located on the face. The lesions are firm and consist of small epithelial-lined cysts arising from hair follicles. They resolve spontaneously.[4]

Molluscum contagiosum, found in infants and children, consists of pearly umbilicated papules appearing on the face, axillae, trunk, and abdomen. Molluscum is caused by a pox virus and is spread by either direct contact or self-inoculation. These lesions are self-limited; reassurance is usually all that is necessary. For bothersome lesions, curettage can be used to remove them.

Pityriasis alba causes flat, hypopigmented lesions and is discussed in the Papulosquamous Lesions section.

Tinea versicolor is discussed in the Papulosquamous Lesions section.

BROWN OR PURPLE LESIONS

Mongolian spots are a very common skin finding in darker-skinned children and can be confused with nonaccidental bruising. Mongolian spots are birthmarks consisting of dark, purplish nonpalpable lesions on back, buttocks and thighs. Mongolian spots will fade over the next several years.[2] Some recent evidence states that Mongolian spots may be more common in infants with certain inborn errors of metabolism such as mucopolysaccharidosis and GM1 gangliosidosis.[24]

ERYTHEMATOUS MACULOPAPULAR LESIONS

Erythematous maculopapular lesions are a very common presentation of a wide variety of infant rashes. One way to think about "red rashes" is those that present *without* fever and those that present *with* fever (Table 16.2).

Those That Present With No Fever

Subcutaneous fat necrosis of the newborn is seen in well-appearing newborns as large firm, erythematous, sharply circumscribed lesions over the cheeks, buttocks, arms and thighs. The lesions first appear at 2 weeks of age and resolve spontaneously over the next several months. Occasionally,

Table 16.2. Erythematous maculopapular rashes

No Fever
  Insect bites
  Drug reaction
  Contact diaper dermatitis
  Candidiasis
  Miliaria rubra or "heat rash"
  Urticaria
  Erythema multiforme
  Stevens-Johnson syndrome
  Erythema nodosum
Fever
  Viral exanthem
  Roseola infantum
  Rubella or German measles
  Rubeola or measles
  Erythema infectiosum or Fifth disease
  Scarlet fever
  Infectious mononucleosis
  Kawasaki disease
  Lyme disease
  Toxic shock

atrophy in the area can occur, leaving a depression in the skin. Calcium levels should be checked periodically as both hyper- and hypocalcemia have been reported.[2]

Insect bites are a common cause of scattered erythematous maculopapular lesions. Areas affected are typically those that are exposed to bed linens, grass or animals. The rash may be pruritic but, in infants who do not have the coordination to scratch, this may come across as irritability. Other family members may be affected by the same rash. Treatment is to stop exposure to the source and antihistamines, either oral or topical, for the pruritus.

Drug reactions in any age group can present as diffuse erythematous maculopapular lesions. In infants, antibiotics are thought to be a common cause of drug-reaction rashes. Unfortunately for many of those infants, a viral source of the febrile condition is probably the true cause of the rash. Treatment for a true allergic reaction rash is to stop the drug in question, and oral antihistamines can be used for significant pruritus. Steroids can be used for severe cases.

Contact diaper dermatitis is a very common condition affecting 7% to 35% of all children younger than 2 years of age.[25] The dermatitis appears as a chaffing maculopapular rash, usually due to urine contact from an infant urinating beyond the diaper capacity, found on the convex surfaces of the buttocks, thighs, and waist. Lesions can become eroded. Contact dermatitis in the perianal region can be due to a diarrheal episode with contact of feces in the area. A diaper area that is already compromised may get secondarily infected with *Candida albicans*. Treatment includes allowing the area to air dry and avoiding plastic pants. Rinsing the urine or feces from the area gently with simple warm water and minimal soap usually suffices. Greasy ointment can be applied to protect the skin from urine and feces. Good old-fashioned petroleum jelly (Vaseline) for protection, followed by cornstarch for absorption, also works well. Cornstarch is no longer implicated in the growth of *Candida albicans*.[26] Talc should probably be avoided because of its affect, when inhaled, on pulmonary tissues. Other emollients found useful include zinc oxide, cod liver oil and lanolin.[27] Hydrocortisone 1% can be used if emollients are not effective but should not be used for more than 2 weeks due to its atrophic affect on skin. Frequent diaper changes are encouraged. Changing the diaper late at night and decreasing fluids right before bed also may encourage healing. On occasion, infants may develop dermatitis from the plastic of disposable diapers.

Switching to cloth diapers should improve the situation. Any diaper dermatitis that does not improve with customary treatment as just described may be infected with *Candida* and should be treated.[2,3]

As stated earlier, any skin in the diaper area that is already compromised by a contact dermatitis from urine is at risk for secondary infection with *Candida albicans*. In infants in whom the diaper dermatitis had been present for more than 3 days, *Candida* was found in up to 80% of the infants.[28] Candidiasis develops in warm, moist areas like the diaper area but will also affect the buccal mucosa (white plaques on an erythematous base called *thrush*) or the angle of the lips (*angular cheilitis*). Candidiasis can also occur in the neck and axillae of young infants due to heat and moisture. Diaper candidiasis will appear as a "beefy" erythematous rash with distinct margins and satellite red plaques. Pustules, vesicles and erosions may be present. Diaper candidiasis can affect the axillae, neck, inguinal and inframammary folds in obese infants. Thumb suckers can also develop a thick disrupted nail surface with cuticle erythema but no tenderness. Potassium hydroxide (KOH) scraping of the lesion will show a single budding yeast. Diaper candidiasis can be treated with a wide variety of antifungal creams including nystatin, ketoconazole, clotrimazole and miconazole.[2,3] Apply the antifungal three times per day for 2 to 3 days. Oral thrush, if present, must also be treated with a nystatin oral solution, 1 cc applied inside both cheeks four times per day for 5 days. If mom is breastfeeding, any nipple changes such as redness or burning should be considered a concurrent yeast infection and treated.

Miliaria rubra, or *heat rash*, is another common erythematous maculopapular rash seen especially in newborns and very young infants. Parents have a tendency to overbundle young infants and this can lead to overheating and sweating. Sweating causes an occlusion of the sweat ducts and the development of a heat rash. Miliaria rubra appears as 2- to 4-mm papules and vesicles surrounded by erythema. They appear on the flexor surfaces such as the neck, axillae, groin, face and upper chest with sweating. Treatment includes avoiding further sweating by not overbundling small infants. These lesions can get secondarily infected with *S. aureus*, which produces pustules.[2–4]

Urticaria can also occur from a variety of causes in infants. Common sources are new fruits introduced into the diet and antibiotic or ibuprofen medications. Any infant who presents with an urticarial rash should also be evaluated for any signs of difficulty breathing or wheezing, as this indicates a more serious allergic reaction. Urticarial rashes in infants, just as in older children, can present with raised maculopapular "wheel-like" erythematous lesions that seem to disappear and then reappear in other areas of the skin. Nikolsky sign is negative. Treatment includes avoiding the food, antibiotic or other source of the allergic reaction. Just as with older patients, oral antihistamines, histamine (H_2) blockers and steroids may all be used.

Erythema multiforme (EM) is a continuation of an allergic process. Symmetrical macular lesions, most targetlike, coalesce to form large geographical patterns. With EM there is no mucosal involvement. If oral or genital lesions are present, this is Stevens-Johnson disease. Etiology for EM or Stevens-Johnson syndrome is viral, drugs or unknown. In children, herpes labialis is a common etiology.[29] Treatment includes stopping the inciting medication or treating the illness, but otherwise is mostly supportive. No studies have been done in children to determine the utility of oral corticosteroids in children with Stevens-Johnson syndrome.[30]

Erythema nodosum is uncommon in children younger than 2 years old but occurs in older children.[2] These lesions consist of tender raised plaques commonly on the anterior tibial area but can affect other areas. Etiology in older patients includes birth control pills, tuberculosis, *Coccidiomycosis,* viral organisms or unknown. In children, however, strep is a common etiology. Treatment includes finding the cause, reassuring the child and parents and providing ibuprofen for pain.

Those That Present With Fever

The other large group of erythematous maculopapular rashes is those that present *with fever*. These rashes can range from the benign viral etiologies to more serious conditions such as Kawasaki disease and measles.

A *viral exanthem* is the most common cause of a diffuse maculopapular erythematous rash in a young infant with a fever. Viral exanthems account for 80% to 90% of all childhood rashes seen in the ED.[3] The original terms for these nonspecific viral rashes were Fourth disease and Duke's disease (Table 16.3). The rash often has a measles-like (morbilliform) appearance. A viral exanthem can also appear as petechial, vesiculobullous, scarlet fever-like or papulonodular. Often caused by enteroviruses or adenovirus, these rashes are usually associated with other viral

Table 16.3. Original classification of pediatric exanthems

First disease: Rubeola, measles
Second disease: Scarlet fever
Third disease: Rubella, German measles
Fourth disease: "Duke's disease," caused by enteroviruses, Echoviruses and coxsackievirus families*
Fifth disease: Erythema infectiosum
Sixth disease: Roseola infantum, exanthem subitum

* One internet resource stated that Fourth disease results from toxin-producing *S. aureus.* Definitions from Wikipedia and Medicine Net.

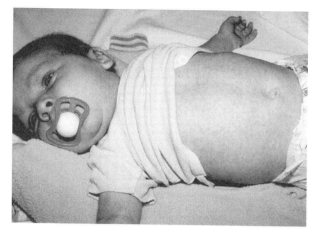

Figure 16.8. A rose-pink maculopapular exanthem appears in Roseola after 3 to 5 days of fever.

symptoms such as upper respiratory symptoms, vomiting or diarrhea.

Echovirus exanthems, of the genus *Enterovirus,* can result in a morbilliform roseola-like pattern or petechial pattern. Echovirus occurs in infants and young children more often than older children. Echovirus 16 is similar to roseola, causing a rash soon after a fever resolves. Lymphadenopathy is often present. Aseptic meningitis can occur but is more often present without the skin rash. Echovirus 9, usually in preschool children, causes a morbilliform rash with petechiae of the extremities. Viral symptoms are usually present including fever, sore throat, abdominal pain and vomiting. Other strains of echoviruses and Coxsackie viruses can cause similar morbilliform rashes.

Infants with viral exanthems are generally well-appearing. As stated previously in the Those That Present With No Fever drug reaction section, what is truly a viral exanthem is often attributed to an allergic reaction to an antibiotic. Differentiating between the two is difficult but parents should be reassured that a viral etiology is more likely the cause of the rash. Treatment for a viral exanthem is supportive with reassurance to the parents.

Roseola infantum, or *Exanthem subitum,* is another common cause of an erythematous maculopapular rash in infants and young children, ages 6 months to 3 years old, with a peak in prevalence at 6 to 7 months. It is the sixth exanthem in the original classification of pediatric exanthems (Table 16.3). Roseola is caused by the HHV 6 and sometimes 7.[20] Roseola begins with a fever for 3 to 5 days; fever often abates before a rose-pink maculopapular exanthem appears (Figure 16.8). Periorbital edema, a bulging anterior fontanel, and posterior cervical lymphadenopathy also may be present. A febrile seizure occurs at the onset of the febrile stage in 25% to 35% of cases.[31] Erythematous papules may be seen on the soft palate or uvula (Nagayama's spots) in up to two thirds of patients.[32] Often, these infants are subjected to workups or fever without a source, such as blood and urine tests, because, before the classic rash develops, the etiology of the higher fever is unknown. Complications are rare but can include seizures, vomiting, cough, hepatitis, thrombocytopenia, disseminated infection or hepatosplenomegaly. Encephalitis can occur.[33] Treatment is supportive.

Rubella, or *German measles,* compared to Rubeola or measles, is mild in most children. Clinical or symptomatic German measles begins with mild headache, low-grade fever, sore throat, anorexia, cough and coryza. A mild lymphadenopathy of the suboccipital and posterior auricular areas develops before the rash. Then a faint, pink macular rash begins on the face and spreads quickly to the trunk and proximal extremities. Petechiae and purpura can also develop. Within 48 hours typically, the face and trunk rash clear and the rash extends to the distal extremities. These children are usually well-appearing with no or low fever in young children. Rubella can usually be cultured from the nasopharynx, blood, urine or CSF, but culture is often unnecessary.

Rubella is mild in infants and young children. Rubella acquired after birth in infants is usually associated with limited prodromal symptoms; up to 50% may be asymptomatic.[34] Rubella acquired during the first trimester of pregnancy can result in congenital rubella in 10% to 20% of patients.[35,36] Earlier transmission results in higher risk. Presentation includes petechiae and purpura from thrombocytopenia, cataracts, glaucoma, sensorineural hearing loss, congenital heart defects such as pulmonary stenosis or patent ductus arteriosus,

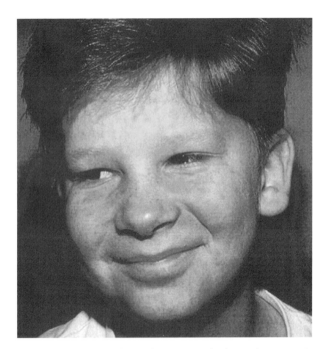

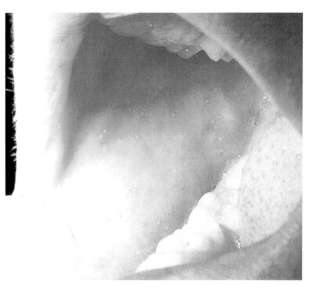

Figure 16.10. Koplik spots also occur in measles. The papules are evident in the mucous membranes of the mouth.

Figure 16.9. The blotchy erythematous rash, that is characteristic of measles.

meningoencephalitis, pneumonia, hepatitis and "blueberry muffin spots."[2] An exposed pregnant woman should be tested for the rubella immunoglobulin G (IgG) antibody at the time of exposure and again 2 to 3 weeks later. If the IgG antibody is present on the first sample, the fetus is protected. If the antibody becomes detectable in the second sample and was not present in the first sample, the fetus is at risk for congenital rubella. If the pregnancy is going to be continued, immunoglobulin 0.55 mL/kg should be administered.[2] For any child with rubella, avoiding pregnant women until 1 week after the rash has appeared is advisable. With the advent of the rubella vaccine, rubella cases have decreased substantially.

Measles, or *Rubeola,* is another febrile illness with an erythematous maculopapular rash that has seen substantial decline since the introduction of its vaccine. Measles has an incubation period of 1 to 2 weeks and begins with the prodrome of high fever, barking cough, rhinitis, conjunctivitis and cervical lymphadenopathy, generally lasting 3 to 5 days. During this prodromal stage and during the exanthem stage, the child can be quite ill-appearing. A blotchy erythematous rash (*morbilliform* means measles-like) appears, comprised of discrete macules and papules, starting on the forehead and face and then spreading to the trunk and extremities (Figure 16.9). The mucous membranes of the mouth may show erythema with 1-mm

white spots called *Koplik's spots* (Figure 16.10). Bacterial otitis media, pneumonia or encephalitis can be sequelae. Other sequelae include myocarditis, pericarditis, thrombocytopenia, hepatitis, glomerulonephritis, and Stevens-Johnson disease.[2] Mortality is 1 per 1000 people, mostly due to pneumonia or encephalitis.[37] No specific treatment combats measles. Vitamin A deficiency has been shown to play a part in the severity of measles; therefore, for children age 1 year older, one oral dose of Vitamin A 200,000 IU is recommended.[2] Measles immunoglobulin (0.25 mL/kg given intramuscularly) may prevent or lessen measles severity if given within 6 days of exposure.[37] Higher dosages (0.5 mL/kg) are recommended for immunosuppressed children. Children with measles are contagious through the third day of the skin lesions. Unimmunized exposed children should receive immunoglobulin 0.25 mg/kg. Higher dosages can be used for immunocompromised or cancer patients. Complications such as the sequelae listed earlier can occur; watch for evidence of recurrent fever, headache, respiratory symptoms and altered mental status.

Erythema infectiosum, or *Fifth's disease,* another febrile exanthem, begins with very erythematous cheeks, so-called slapped cheeks (Figure 16.11). The initial maculopapular erythematous rash then develops on the trunk with a lacy reticular rash on the arms and legs. Parvovirus B19 is the etiology of this rash. (This is not the same strain of parvovirus that affects dogs.) The infant or child is no longer contagious when the rash develops.

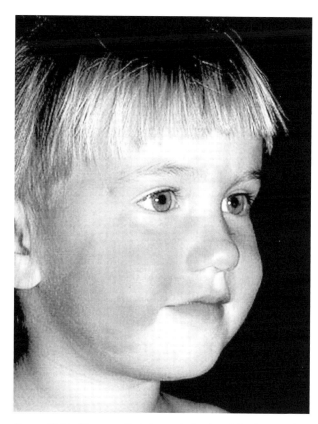

Figure 16.11. The so-called slapped cheeks of *Erythema infectiosum*, or *Fifth's disease*.

Complications include hemolytic anemia and encephalitis. If present in a pregnant woman, parvovirus B19 can cause a small increase in second trimester miscarriage rates. Pregnant women who are exposed to parvovirus B19 should be referred to their obstetrician. Treatment is supportive. IV immunoglobulins (IVIG) may be helpful in immunosuppressed children.[37] The lacy reticular extremity rash may reappear for many months with cold or heat exposure.

Infectious mononucleosis is another infectious disease caused by the HHV 4, 5, 6, and 7 and seen more often in adolescents. Symptoms include fatigue, fever, lymphadenopathy, pharyngitis, headache and splenomegaly. A morbilliform rash can be seen on occasion; a similar appearing drug rash can also be seen when ampicillin or penicillin is given mistakenly for presumed *Streptococcus pharyngitis*.

Scarlet fever, and its subsequent erythematous maculopapular rash and fever, is a relatively uncommon cause of a rash in infants. The etiology is the beta-hemolytic GAS.

Kawasaki disease, or *mucocutaneous lymph node syndrome*, is an uncommon cause of an erythematous maculopapular rash in infants but is important to know about because of its sequelae. Kawasaki disease generally occurs in children less than 5 years old. Male and Asian children are at highest risk. The etiology is unclear but viral organisms and exotoxins have both been suggested as causes.[2] Classically, Kawasaki presents with fever, typically for 5 days, and then four of five criteria are needed for diagnosis:

1. Erythematous maculopapular rash
2. Conjunctival redness
3. Three possible oral changes
   - Red, fissured, crusting lips
   - Erythema of the oropharynx or
   - Strawberry red tongue (Figure 16.12)
4. Cervical nodes
5. Erythema or edema of the palms and soles and desquamation of the fingers

Desquamation of the genitourinary (GU) areas also can occur. These children, as with measles, are usually ill-appearing. Nikolsky sign is negative. Laboratory testing may show elevated platelets, erythrocyte sedimentation rate (ESR) and C-reactive protein (CRP). The most concerning sequelae of Kawasaki disease is the development of coronary artery aneurysms due to a segmental vasculitis. Risks of these aneurysms include myocardial infarction or death, thus early recognition of Kawasaki disease is important for treatment. Kawasaki mimics infantile periarteritis

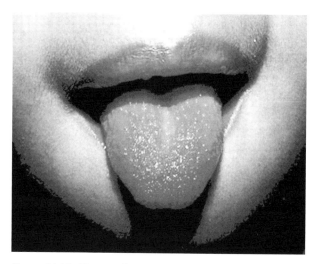

Figure 16.12. The strawberry tongue presentation of Kawasaki disease.

nodosa. Treatment includes aspirin 80 to 100 mg/kg/day for 2 weeks started during the febrile stage. IVIG 2g/kg infused over 12 hours is also recommended to prevent aneurysm formation. Retreatment with IVIG may be needed if the child has persistent fevers. High-dose steroids are contraindicated and may help promote the heart disease. Consulting pediatric cardiology is important as affected children often undergo echocardiogram early looking for evidence of developing aneurysms.[2]

Lyme disease is an uncommon cause of a febrile erythematous rash in young infants. It is often seen in endemic areas in children who have been outside and exposed to tick bites.

Toxic shock is another uncommon cause of a febrile erythematous rash in young infants as there is usually a source for the toxic shock such as tampon or wound. Symptoms generally include fever, a diffuse maculopapular rash, hypotension, and involvement of three organ systems and other areas: gastrointestinal (GI) with vomiting or diarrhea, muscular with severe pain or elevated creatine phosphokinase (CPK) level, mucous membranes with hyperemia, hepatic with elevated liver enzymes, hematologic with thrombocytopenia, renal with elevated blood, urea, nitrogen (BUN) and creatinine levels, or CNS with altered mental status. *S. aureus* is usually the causative organism and treatment should be targeted with beta-lactamase–resistant anti-staphylococcal antibiotics.[2]

VASCULAR LESIONS

Various transient vasomotor conditions appear in the newborn period. *Acrocyanosis of infancy* is seen in newborns and consists of cyanotic hands and feet. This is a benign finding in young infants and is due primarily to the immaturity of vasomotor tone in the distal extremities. Benign acrocyanosis must be distinguished from true central cyanosis by evaluating the face, lips, mucous membranes and tongue. Even in very dark-skinned children, these central areas should be pink in well-oxygenated infants.

Harlequin color change is another benign condition seen more often in low birth weight infants. When the infant is placed on one side, the dependent side develops an erythematous flush. The upper half becomes paler. When the baby is returned to the supine position, the color change will abate but can persist for up to 20 minutes. Again, immaturity of vasomotor tone is believed to be the cause.

Mottling, or *cutis marmorata,* is comprised of a lacy, reticular vascular pattern to the extremities and trunk due to cold, dehydration or sepsis. It can often appear in newborns or young infants who are disrobed for a physical examination in a cold ED exam room. Newborns and young infants have large body surface areas, and with cold exposure they will "clamp down" peripherally in order to retain body heat thus producing the mottling pattern seen. A young infant who is brought to the ED bundled and is found to already have mottling when the baby is disrobed should raise a red flag.

Stork bites or *salmon patches* are capillary malformations seen in most newborns. These patches are located on the back of the neck and in the middle of the forehead. Some experts believe these areas represent remnant fetal vessels, which would explain their regression over time.

Hemangiomas and birthmarks are other very common vascular lesions seen in young infants. Hemangiomas and birthmarks present in a variety of ways including as port-wine stains, isolated hemangiomas, or diffuse hemangiomatosis. Hemangiomas can be present on any part of the body. Often, isolated hemangiomas will grow before shrinking on their own. Because many of these hemangiomas become much smaller after 1 year of age, early treatment is generally not recommended. Any large hemangiomas growing around the neck region may cause airway compromise; early treatment in these cases may be necessary.

Pyogenic granulomas are uncommon causes of vascular lesions in newborns and infants. They usually occur at sites of trauma. *Pyogenic gangrenosum* is a more serious condition resulting often from localized trauma. Beginning as a small papule, the lesion soon progresses to become an inflamed pustule and then an ulcer. The ulcer grows rapidly to greater than 2 cm. The surrounding skin is generally light purple-colored, and there is a loosely epidermal edge to the ulcer.[38] Many causes of the condition have been described but overactive neutrophils are believed to be responsible. It is seen in older children with inflammatory bowel disease, rheumatoid arthritis and myelodysplastic disease.[38] Immunosuppressive drugs have been effective in treating this condition.

Petechiae due to increased thoracic pressure can be seen in infants after pronounced vomiting or coughing. Pertussis pneumonia can cause severe paroxysmal coughing in infants with resultant petechiae, subconjunctival hemorrhages, rectal prolapse, seizures and intracranial

Table 16.4. Purpuric lesions and their etiology

Flat
  Meningococcus
  Rocky Mountain spotted fever
  Measles
  Coagulation disorders
  Vaccine-associated purpura
  EMLA-associated purpura
Palpable
  Sepsis
  Vasculitis
    Henoch-Schönlein purpura
    Hemorrhagic edema of infancy
Neonatal
  Rubella
  Toxoplasmosis
  Herpes
  Syphilis
  Cytomegalovirus
  Coagulation disorders
  Autoimmune disorders, such as systemic lupus
    erythematosus or erythroblastosis fetalis
  Vascular tumors that trap platelets

bleeds. Laboratory studies show normal platelet counts. Petechiae and subconjunctival hemorrhages also commonly are present on a newborn's face and scalp after a prolonged delivery.

Another platelet disorder, *idiopathic thrombocytopenic purpura* (ITP), is a cause of petechiae, generally in older children. *Thrombotic thrombocytopenic purpura* (TTP) is a more serious cause of thrombocytopenia in older patients and is associated with fever, altered mental status and renal insufficiency or failure. Management for both of these conditions can be found in other emergency medicine textbooks.

Purpuric lesions, along with petechiae, mandate evaluation. Purpura can be divided into these categories: neonatal, flat and palpable (Table 16.4). With palpable purpura, both septicemia and a vasculitis can be the etiology. The vasculitis is called a *cutaneous necrotizing venulitis*. IgG or IgA is usually the causative agent and vasculitis of the GI, renal, joint and cerebral vessels can be found.[39]

Henoch-Schönlein purpura (HSP) is an uncommon cause of petechiae in infants. Patients are typically older, 4 to 5 years of age, and more often are male. HSP is a diffuse vasculitis causing palpable petechiae and purpura on the buttocks, arms and legs. IgA deposition seems to be involved in the vast majority of cases.[40] Arthralgias and arthritis (swelling) of the lower extremity joints are common. GI inflammation causes cramping, vomiting and intestinal bleeding. Intussusception can result in 3% to 5% of cases. GU inflammation can cause nephritis with hematuria. Steroids are recommended if the stool is occult blood–positive or the urine shows evidence of hematuria. A recent meta-analysis on the use of steroids for HSP found that steroids are effective in reducing the time to resolution of abdominal pain and in reducing the odds of developing persistent renal disease,[41] although the effect of steroids does remain controversial.[42,43] Prednisone or methylprednisolone pulse therapy is an option for treatment. Therapy for patients with severe renal involvement also includes IVIG, although promising results have also been seen in patients with severe abdominal pain.[44] Other treatment options for patients with severe HSP nephropathy include early treatment with oral immunosuppressants[45] and possibly the use of methylprednisolone and urokinase pulse therapy.[46] A nephrologist should be consulted for patients with renal involvement and follow-up needs to be ensured. Patients can be discharged home if the stool is occult blood–negative and the urinalysis is negative. Treatment is supportive for those patients.

One palpable purpuric condition seen in young infants is *hemorrhagic edema of infancy* (HEI). HEI is a variety of leukocytoclastic vasculitis. Some experts believe this condition is a variant of HSP; others believe this to be a distinct disease.[40] IgA is found in less than one third of the patients with HEI.[40] HEI is uncommon in the United States but is found throughout the world. Large, 10-cm or greater purpuric lesions with associated edema in the area are the hallmark of the condition. They are most frequently seen on the buttocks or genitalia. Associated complaints are similar to HSP, but GI and GU symptoms seem to occur less often. The prognosis is much better. Treatment is supportive if no evidence of GI or GU symptoms exists. Systemic steroids do not seem to alter the course.[40]

Disseminated gonorrhea, with its sparse vascular purple lesions, generally does not occur in newborns and infants.

Endocarditis can occur in infants but is rare. Classic presentation of a patient with endocarditis is a fever and new cardiac murmur with vegetations on a cardiac valve. A purpuric rash can be seen from vegetative emboli. Treatment, after blood cultures are obtained, includes antibiotics until results of cultures are known. Further review of endocarditis can be found in Chapter 15.

Syphilis is an uncommon cause of vascular lesions in infants but is one of the components of the TORCH complex (see Vesiculobullous [Blisters and Bullae] section).

Rocky Mountain spotted fever (RMSF) is another uncommon cause of vascular lesions in infants. RMSF is found in endemic areas and is transmitted by a tick bite. Presentation includes a petechial rash that starts on the distal extremities, headache and arthralgias. Associated findings include hepatosplenomegaly, hyponatremia, myalgias and CNS involvement. Treatment includes doxycycline.

Meningococcemia, although rare, can be a cause of a petechial and purpuric rash in infants with devastating sequelae. Etiology is *Neisseria meningitidis* for which 2% of children and upward of 40% of adults are carriers.[47] Infants up to 6 months old are more immune than older babies due to maternal antibodies. Mortality is high at 5% to 10% with a rate of 90% if disseminated intravascular coagulation (DIC) is present.[47] Presentation begins with symptoms similar to a viral syndrome with URI, headache, vomiting, myalgias and arthralgias. Not all patients appear toxic. Purpura, hypotension, and cardiovascular compromise can suddenly progress. A blood culture showing *Neisseria* is the gold standard. Skin scrapings can also show the *Neisseria* organism on gram staining.[47] Treatment includes intensive care with blood pressure support and broad spectrum antibiotics.

A quadrivalent vaccine exists for meningococcus; however, it is not efficacious in very young children. Thus, the vaccine is recommended for children with terminal complement deficiencies or anatomic or functional asplenia.[47] Prophylaxis with antibiotics is recommended for close contacts including family members, daycare classmates and health care personnel who are exposed to respiratory secretions. Rifampin, ciprofloxacin or ceftriaxone are options.

Disseminated intravascular coagulation (DIC), or *purpura fulminans,* is another devastating cause of a petechial or purpuric rash in infants or children with high morbidity and mortality. The cause, usually sepsis, should be found and treated. Treatment includes fresh frozen plasma and platelet transfusions.

Coin rubbing and cupping are the last of the vascular lesions that can be seen in infants or children. These are caused by cultural healing practices from the Southeast Asian cultures. These are nonabusive attempts by the caretakers to cure the child of various ailments. Coin rubbing involves vigorous rubbing of the trunk with the edge of a coin to treat fever; this leaves a pattern of linear bruising. Cupping involves heating of a cup coated with alcohol; the cup is applied to the skin and as the cup cools, the cup adheres to the skin. When pulled off, the bruised imprint of the cup is left on the skin. Both of these are considered cultural practices and not evidence of abuse.

PAPULOSQUAMOUS LESIONS

Pityriasis rosea does not generally occur in infants, affecting usually older school-age children and young adults. The etiology is probably HHV-7, although debate lingers.[2] Lesions are oval papules or plaques, usually on skin lines, found on the trunk and proximal extremities and can involve the face, arms, and legs. The lesions are classic light scaly collarette appearance. In Caucasians, the lesions are pink; in darker-skinned, patches are darker. A *herald patch,* a single larger patch, is not often seen but if present can be mistaken for tinea corporis. When the more diffuse lesions present, parents can think the "ringworm" is spreading. Treatment includes moisturizing lotion, Aveeno bath, oatmeal bath, and antihistamines for pruritus. Exposure to natural sunlight or sunlamp to the point of minimal redness appears to hasten the disappearance of the lesions.[41] Lesions and pruritus can persist for 8 weeks. Pityriasis rosea is not contagious, but children may need a note to explain to school authorities.

Psoriasis is more common in older children but can manifest itself as persistent diaper dermatitis. Topical steroids are the mainstay of treatment.

Tinea corporis, or *ringworm,* is a common cause of papulosquamous lesions in children but not usually in infants. The causative agents include species of *Microsporum* and *Trichophyton.* The lesions consist of a sharp, scaly, demarcated patch on usually hairless body areas. Diagnosis can be confirmed by scraping the edge with a KOH prep. Treatment includes topical antifungals twice per day until the lesion resolves and then continued once per day for 1 to 2 weeks. Steroids should be avoided.

Tinea versicolor usually affects adolescents and adults with 1- to 3-cm oval, slightly scaly macules on the upper back or chest and proximal upper extremities. Infants can be affected. The etiology is *Pityrosporum ovale (Malassezia furfur).* Mild pruritus may be a complaint. The lesions are usually white, red or light tan in color. The lesions will lighten in sun-exposed areas but darken in sun-protected skin. As tans fade, the lesions will darken. If the infant or child has not bathed, the skin may fluoresce orange. Skin scrapings can be pulled off with tape, KOH applied, and short, curved hyphae with circular spores can be seen ("spaghetti and meatballs"). Topical antifungal treatment usually results in regression. Ketoconazole shampoo (Nizoral 2%) or selenium sulfide 2.5% is also an option. Unresponsive cases may need oral therapy. Pigment changes may take months to clear.

Tinea capitis or *scalp ringworm* has been reported in infants and newborns,[48] but it is more often in African American prepubertal boys. Tinea capitis is more often due to *Trichophyton* species in North America.[2] Lesions of *Trichophyton* appear as an alopecia plaque with broken hair shafts appearing as black dots. *Microsporum canis,* less responsible in North America, appears more as thickened white plaques with broken hairs. Cervical adenopathy may be present. Diagnosis can be made by KOH microscopic evaluation of the scrapings. Fungal cultures may also be taken. Wood's lamp evaluation of the scalp may show yellow-green fluorescence with *Microsporum.*[2] Treatment includes oral antifungals such as griseofulvin orally for 4 to 6 weeks. Liver enzymes should be watched in adolescents but is of less concern in children. During treatment, school attendance is fine with no need to cover the lesion with a hat. One complication of tinea capitis is a kerion, a boggy erythematous tinea capitis lesion. This change is due to a hypersensitivity reaction. Antibiotics are not needed. Severe cases may respond to a steroid taper.

Tinea cruris or *jock itch* is also not seen in infants but is more common in adolescent males. This tinea infection causes sharply demarcated large lesions in the groin area. Treatment includes an antifungal medication twice per day until the lesions are gone and then use the same once per day for 1 to 2 weeks.

Tinea pedis is also not seen in infants and is generally not common before puberty. In children, if feet are dry, cracked, peeling and pruritic, treat them like eczema with moisturizers, topical steroids and clean socks.

Granuloma annulare is also not seen in infants but generally is seen in younger children ages 3 to 7 years. Granuloma annulare has the appearance of tinea corporis lesions but not as scaly. The lesions are generally found on the dorsum of the hands and feet. The etiology is unknown. Most resolve spontaneously. Steroids can be used if the lesions are disfiguring.

Keratosis pilaris is another papulosquamous condition not seen in infants but is seen in older children. Prominent follicular plugs are the etiology. Found on extensor surface of the extremities, buttocks, and cheeks of the face, the skin feels rough and dry. The condition is associated with dry skin and atopic dermatitis, and improves with humid climates. Treatment includes skin lubricants. Extensive cases in older children may need topical keratolytics like lactic acid or topical tretinoin (Retin-A).[3,4]

ECZEMATOUS

Diaper dermatitis is reviewed in the Erythematous Maculopapular Lesions section.

Seborrheic dermatitis is a very common eczematous condition found in newborns, infants and adolescents. This is caused by an overproduction of sebum on the scalp, face, chest and perineum. The scalp is greasy with scales trapped in sebum (seborrhea capitis, "cradle cap"). The scaly lesions are also found in the flexural areas like atopic dermatitis. Adolescents can get erythema and scaling of the nasolabial fold. Treatment includes low potency topical steroids applied twice per day for several days and then occasionally. Keratolytic or antifungal shampoos on the scalp are useful. With shampoo in place, the parent should gently scrub the scalp with a soft brush or toothbrush to remove crusting. Periodic treatment may be necessary, as this condition tends to recur.[2]

Atopic dermatitis or eczema is another common eczematous condition in newborns, infants and older children. The skin appears as dry, pruritic, erythematous, irritated, scaling, papular lesions. Chronic cases appear lichenified and hyperpigmented. Seventy percent have a family history of atopic disease, asthma or

Table 16.5. Topical steroids and potency

Low Potency
Hydrocortisone 1%
Desonide 0.05%
Moderate Potency
Betamethasone valerate 0.1% (Valisone)
Fluocinolone acetonide 0.01% (Synalar)
Hydrocortisone valerate 0.2% (Westcort)
Triamcinolone acetonide 0.025% (Kenalog)
High Potency
Betamethasone dipropionate 0.05% (Diprolene)
Fluocinonide 0.05% (Lidex)

Table 16.6. Exanthems and rashes in pediatric patients

Disease	Season and age group and etiology	Prodromal symptoms	Morphology	Distribution	Associated findings	Complications
Measles (Rubeola)	Winter and Spring 0–20 yo Measles virus	Fever, URI and cough	Erythematous macules and papules, morbilliform, becomes confluent	Face and neck and then spreads to rest of body	Ill-appearing, conjunctivitis, Koplik spots, cough, pneumonia	Common: otitis media, pneumonia Rare:encephalitis, laryngotracheitis
German measles (Rubella)	Spring 5–25 yo Rubella virus	Milder URI symptoms	Maculopapular rash; becomes more pinpoint	Face then spreads quickly to rest of body; recedes rapidly	Tender retroauricular, posterior cervical and occipital lymphadenopathy	Common: arthritis in older patients Rare: encephalitis, orchitis
Roseola (Exanthem subitum)	Spring and Fall 0–3 yo Human herpesvirus 6	High fever for few days Febrile seizure is common	Erythematous to pink macules and papules; "rosette" pattern	Neck, trunk and proximal extremities	Fever subsides and then rash appears	Rare: encephalitis
Erythema infectiosum (Fifth disease)	Winter and Spring 3–12 yo and nonimmune adults Parvovirus B19	Fever and malaise	"Slapped cheeks"; erythematous macular rash then lacy reticular rash	Face then extremities; lacy rash on extensor surfaces of extremities		Rare: arthritis (especially in adults), hemolytic anemia, encephalitis, hydrops fetalis
Chicken pox (Varicella)	Winter and Spring 1–14 yo Varicella-zoster virus	Fever and malaise Headache, abdominal pain and anorexia	Erythematous macules that become serous vesicles	Face, scalp and trunk then spreads peripherally	Lesions on mucous membranes; pruritus	Rare: cellulitis, encephalitis
Kawasaki disease (muco-cutaneous lymph node syndrome)	Winter and Spring <5 yo Unclear etiology – viral?	High fever for several days irritability	Erythematous, maculopapular, morbilliform or vesiculobullous forms	Skin on fingertips and in genital area desquamate after 1 week	Conjunctivitis, strawberry tongue, fissured lips and adenopathy	Risk of coronary artery aneurysms
Henoch-Schönlein purpura	Spring and Fall 6 mo–young adult IgA deposition?	Arthralgias and abdominal pain	Symmetric palpable purpura	Buttocks and extensor surfaces	GI, renal and musculoskeletal	
Meningococcemia	Winter and Spring <2 yo Neisseria meningitidis	Fever, malaise and URI	Petechiae, purpura and bullae	Trunk and extremities, palms and soles	Temperature >40 C, shock and DIC	Loss of distal extremities or digits; death
Rocky Mountain spotted fever	Summer All ages Rickettsia rickettsii	Fever, malaise and headache	Red or rose macules; evolves to petechiae and purpura	Begins peripherally at wrists and ankles, palms and soles involved, spreads centrally	Hepatosplenomegaly, hyponatremia, myalgias, CNS involvement	
Scarlet fever	Winter and Spring 3–12 yrs old Group A beta-hemolytic Streptococcus	Fever, sore throat, vomiting, headache, abdominal pain and tender anterior cervical nodes	Trunk and extremities with "sandpaper" blanching pinpoint red rash most prominent on creases	Flushed face with circumoral pallor Mucosal-pharyngitis, tonsillitis, palatal petechiae and strawberry tongue		Early: otitis media, peritonsillitis and cervical adenitis, sinusitis Late: rheumatic, fever and glomerulonephritis
Staphylococcal scalded skin syndrome	Year round <5 years old or immuno compromised adult S. aureus	Fever and malaise, URI	Bullae formation and desquamation from spread of toxins; Nikolsky sign positive	Skin desquamation; large sheet of skin desquamate		Hypovolemia, hypothermia,, and secondary infection

CNS, central nervous system; GU, genitourinary; URI, upper respiratory infection.

allergic rhinitis.[3,4] Conditions are worse in the winter. In newborns, the condition appears as greasy seborrhea of the scalp with retroauricular erythema and scaling. Infants usually develop erythematous, dry lesions on the cheeks, forehead, scalp, trunk, diaper and extensor areas. The nasal, perioral and periorbital areas are usually not involved. These areas usually resolve by 18 months. Children 2 years to puberty have these atopic lesions on the antecubital, popliteal, neck, buttocks, thighs, and flexural areas of the wrists and ankles. After puberty, hands, flexor surfaces and behind the neck are more common areas.

Atopic dermatitis is commonly known as an "itch with a rash" because of the intense pruritus associated with the condition. The cycle of "itch-then-scratch" is exacerbated by dry skin, irritants, sweating, overheating, secondary infection, and stress. Treatment includes emollients (Eucerin, Aquaphor, Cetaphil or even Crisco) frequently to decrease inflammation and pruritus. Short baths are recommended using simple soaps such as Ivory or Dove. Oil can be added to the bath. Bubble baths should be discontinued, and emollient creams applied generously afterward. Antihistamines for pruritus can be used at night. Anti-sedating versions can be used during the day. Humidifiers in the bedroom at night can help. Placing wet towels around the bedroom at night can also add moisture to the air. Nails should be clean and trimmed. Topical steroids – 1% hydrocortisone for mild cases, low-mid potency for moderate cases – can also be useful (Table 16.5). Ointments are best but greasy; creams and lotions may have an alcohol base. Oral steroids may be necessary for severe cases; prednisone 1 to 2 mg/kg for 4 to 7 days. At times, these atopic lesions may get superinfected. Anti-staph and strep antibiotics are required.

Pityriasis alba is associated with atopic dermatitis. These lesions are 2- to 4-cm hypopigmented, round or oval lesions with vague borders. These lesions do not tan in the sunlight. The etiology is unknown. The lesions usually resolve spontaneously so treatment is not necessary.

Nummular eczema or *little coin* is also not common in infants but appears as 1- to 10-cm, round, symmetrically distributed lesions found on the extremities. Two forms exist – a wet form with oozing and crusting and a dry form with erythema and scaling. These lesions are very pruritic and should be treated with usual atopic dermatitis treatment but may need more potent topical steroids.

Understanding the wide variety of benign and more serious skin conditions that may present in the newborn and early infancy period is important to master as an emergency medicine practitioner. Table 16.6 is a brief summary of some of the more important diseases that have been discussed in this chapter.

PITFALLS

- Failure to recognize other associated symptoms, such as abdominal pain, or signs, such as fever or hypotension, when evaluating a young infant or child with a rash
- Failure to evaluate thoroughly the skin of young febrile children; *Neisseria meningococcemia* can progress rapidly and the first sign may be an early petechial rash
- Failure to educate parents regarding simple treatment of atopic disease such as shortening baths and rehydrating skin with heavy emollient creams
- Failure to start lower potency steroids when beginning steroid treatment for atopic disease, psoriasis or other inflammatory conditions.
- Failure to understand and recognize the sequelae of the more commonly seen pediatric dermatological conditions

REFERENCES

1. Long CC, Mills CM, Finlay AY. A practical guide to topical therapy in children. *Br J Dermatol.* 1998;138(2):293–296.
2. Weston W, Lane A, Morelli J. *Color Textbook of Pediatric Dermatology,* 4th ed. St. Louis, MO: Mosby; 2007.
3. Weinberg S, Prose NS, Kristal L. *Color Atlas of Pediatric Dermatology,* 3rd ed. New York, NY: McGraw-Hill; 1998.
4. Zitelli BJ, Davis HW. *Atlas of Pediatric Physical Diagnosis,* 5th ed. St. Louis, MO: Mosby; 2007.
5. Troendle-Atkins J, Dremmler GJ, Buffone GJ. Rapid diagnosis of herpes simplex encephalitis by using polymerase chain reaction. *J Pediatrics.* 1993;123:376–380.
6. Whitley RJ. Herpes simplex virus infection. *Semin Pediatr Infect Dis.* 2002;186 (Suppl 1):S40–S46.
7. Murono K, Fujita K, Yoshioka H. Microbiologic characteristics of exfoliative toxin-producing staphylococcus aureus. *Pediatr Infect Dis J.* 1988;7:313–317.
8. Decline of annual incidence of varicella – United States, 1990–2001. *Centers for Disease Control and Prevention, Morbidity and Mortality Weekly Report.* 2003;52(37):884–887.
9. Smith EWP, Garson A, Boyleston JA, et al. Varicella gangrenosa due to group A beta-hemolytic streptococcus. *Pediatrics.* 1976;57:306–310.
10. Preblud SR, Orenstein WA, Bart KJ. Varicella: clinical manifestations, epidemiology, and health impact in children. *Pediatr Infect Dis J.* 1984;3:505–509.
11. Derrick CW Jr, Lord L. In utero Varicella-zoster infections in children. *South Med J.* 1998;91:1064–1066.
12. Zerr DM, Alexander ER, Duchin JS, et al. A case-control study of necrotizing fasciitis during primary Varicella. *Pediatrics.* 1999;103:783–790.
13. Arvin AM. Management of varicella-zoster infections in children. *Adv Exp Med Biol.* 1999;458:167–174.

14. Lin F, Hadler JL. Epidemiology of primary varicella and herpes zoster hospitalizations: the pre-varicella vaccine era. *J Infect Dis.* 2000;81:1897–1905.

15. Nahass GT, Goldstein BA, Zhu WY, et al. Comparison of Tzanck smear, viral culture, and DNA diagnostic methods in detection of herpes simplex and Varicella-zoster infection. *JAMA.* 1992;268:2541–2544.

16. Eastern JS. Herpes zoster. eMedicine from WebMD. www.emedicine.com. Accessed December 4, 2007.

17. Lindenbaum JE, Van Dyck PC, Allen RG. Hand, foot, and mouth disease associated with coxsackievirus group B. *Scand J Infect Dis.* 1975;7:161–163.

18. Tindall JP, Callaway JL. Hand-foot-mouth disease. It's more common than you think. *Am J Dis Child.* 1972 Sept; 124(3): 372–375

19. Shimizu H, Utama A, Yoshii K, et al. Enterovirus 71 from fatal and non-fatal cases of hand, foot, and mouth disease epidemics in Malaysia, Japan, and Taiwan in 1997-1998. *Japan J Infect Dis.* 1999;52:12–15.

20. Baren J, Rothrock S, Brennan J, et al, eds. *Pediatric Emergency Medicine,* 1st ed. Philadelphia, PA: Saunders; 2007.

21. Marchini G, Nelson A, Edner J, et al. Erythema toxicum neonatorum is an innate immune response to commensal microbes penetrated into the skin of the newborn infant. *Pediatr Res.* 2005;58(3):613–616.

22. Van Praag MC, Van Rooij RW, Folkers E, et al. Diagnosis and treatment of pustular disorders in the neonate. *Pediatr Dermatol.* 1997;14(2):131–143.

23. Singal A, Thami GP. Lindane neurotoxicity in childhood. *Am J Ther.* 2006;13(3):277–280.

24. Snow TM. Mongolian spots in the newborn: do they mean anything? *Neonatal Netw.* 2005;24(1):31–33.

25. Kazaks EL, Lane AT. Diaper dermatitis. *Pediatr Clin North Am.* 2000;47:909–919.

26. Leyden JJ. Corn starch, *Candida albicans,* and diaper rash. *Pediatr Dermatol.* 1984;1:322–325.

27. Wolf R, Wolf D, Tuzun B, et al. Diaper dermatitis. *Clin Dermatol.* 2001;18:657–670.

28. Hogan P. Irritant napkin dermatitis. *Aust Fam Physician.* 1999;28:385–386.

29. Leute-Labreze C, Lamireau T, Chawki D, et al. Diagnosis, classification, and management of erythema multiforme and Stevens-Johnson syndrome. *Arch Dis Child.* 2000;83:347–352.

30. Yeung AK, Goldman RD. Use of steroids for erythema multiforme in children. *Can Fam Physician.* 2005;51:1481–1483.

31. Barone SR, Kaplan MH, Krilov LR. Human herpesvirus-6 infection in children with first febrile seizures. *J Pediatr.* 1995;127:95–97.

32. Asano Y, Yoshikawa T, Suga S, et al. Clinical features of infants with primary human herpesvirus 6 infection (exanthem subitum, roseola infantum). *Pediatrics.* 1994;93:104–108.

33. Yamanishi K, Okuno T, Shiraki K, et al. Identification of human herpesvirus 6 as a causal agent for exanthem subitum. *Lancet.* 1988;1:1065–1067.

34. Sullivan EM, Burgess MA, Forrest JM. The epidemiology of rubella and congenital rubella in Australia, 1992 to 1997. *Commun Dis Intell.* 1999;23:209–214.

35. Webster WS. Teratogen update: congenital rubella. *Teratology.* 1998;58:13–23.

36. Frey TK. Neurological aspects of rubella infection. *Intervirology.* 1997;40:167–175.

37. Report of the Committee on Infectious Diseases. *Red Book* 2003. Elk Grove, IL: American Academy of Pediatrics; 2003.

38. Bhat RM, Shetty SS, Kamath GH. Pyoderma gangrenosum in childhood. *Int J Dermatol.* 2004;43:205–207.

39. McDougall CM, Ismail SK, Ormerod A. Acute hemorrhagic edema of infancy. *Arch Dis Child.* 2005;90:316.

40. Crowe MA. Acute hemorrhagic edema of infancy. EMedicine from WebMD. www.emedicine.com. Accessed November 20, 2007.

41. Rich SJ, Bello-Quinter CE. Advancements in the treatment of psoriasis: role of biologic agents. *J Manag Care Pharm.* 2004;10:318–325.

42. Huber AM, King J, McLaine P, et al. A randomized, placebo controlled trial of prednisone in early Henoch-Schönlein purpura. *BioMed Central Medicine.* 2004;2:7.

43. Mollica F, Li Volti S, Garozzo R, et al. Effectiveness of early prednisone therapy in preventing the development of nephropathy in anaphylactoid purpura. *Eur J Pediatr.* 1992;151:140–144.

44. Rostoker G, Desvaux-Belghiti D, Pilatte Y, et al: High dose immunoglobulin therapy for severe IGA nephropathy and Henoch-Schönlein purpura. *Ann Intern Med.* 1994;120:476–484.

45. Tanaka H, Suzuki K, Nakahata T, et al. Early treatment with oral immunosuppressants in severe proteinuric purpura nephritis. *Pediatr Nephrol.* 2003;18:347–350.

46. Kawasaki Y, Suzuki J, Nozawa R, et al. Efficacy of methylprednisolone and urokinase pulse therapy for severe Henoch-Schönlein nephritis. *Pediatrics.* 2003;111:785–789.

47. Tanzi EL, Silverberg N. Meningococcemia. eMedicine from WebMD. www.emedicine.com. Accessed December 1, 2007.

48. Gilabarte Y, Rezusata A, Gil J, et al. Tinea capitis in infants in the first year of life. *Br J Dermatol.* 2004:151:886–890.

Jim R. Harley

This chapter discusses two important environmental emergencies: drowning injuries and burns. Information on other injuries is presented in a bullet format in Appendix 4.

SECTION I. NEAR DROWNING

INTRODUCTION

Near drowning or submersion injuries are unusual in children under 1 year of age, but they do occur. Infant deaths are particularly tragic because the majority can be prevented. *Drowning* is defined as death from asphyxia within 24 hours after submersion in a liquid. *Near drowning* is survival beyond 24 hours, regardless of subsequent morbidity or mortality. *Immersion syndrome* is sudden death after contact with very cold water secondary to excessive vagal stimulation from a cardiac dysrhythmia. *Submersion injury* is any submersion that leads to hospitalization or death.

EPIDEMIOLOGY

Drowning is the third most common cause of unintentional death in the United States.[1] Drowning rates peak at 1 to 2 years of age.[2] Whereas drowning rates from 1971 to 1988 have declined for older age children, drowning rates have increased for children younger than 1 year of age.[3] In the United States in 2005, 64 children under 1 year of age and 493 ages 1 to 4 years drowned.[4]

Drowning is the single leading cause of death in children younger than age 5 years. In the 12-year period from 1983 to 1994, 1219 infants drowned in the United States; 85% of these drownings were unintentional.[1] A drowning pyramid of injury has been created to

graphically represent drowning injury and death (Figure 17.I.1). For each fatality, it is estimated that there are 3.65 hospital admissions. For each hospital admission, there are four children seen in the emergency department (ED). For each ED visit, there are 10 near miss submersion events in which a child was in danger but was rescued and did not seek hospitalization.[5,6]

The majority of all infant drowning deaths occur in bathtubs. Typically, a parent or childcare provider leaves the child alone for a brief period of time and then finds that the baby has slipped down with his or her face in the water. There does not have to be much water in the tub. Bathtub seats and rings have been associated with infant drownings. Over a 12-year period, 32 infant drownings in the United States were associated with bathtub ring or seat use. These devices may increase the risk that the child will be left alone in the bathtub or give false reassurance to the caregiver.[7] Almost all cases of infant drowning are secondary to absent adult supervision. Near drowning has been described in water births raising questions to its safety.[8] Other locations that children may

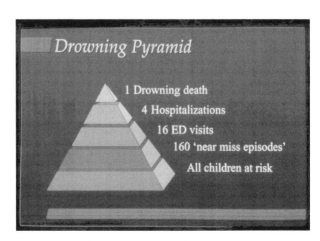

Figure 17.I.1. The Drowning Pyramid.

drown include swimming pools, spas, buckets and natural bodies of water. Residential pools account for the majority of all pool drownings. The child is often left unsupervised for a brief period of time then found unresponsive in the water. A few children drown in small buckets (3–5 gallons) that are holding a small amount of liquid.

Possible abuse should be considered in cases that are atypical for bathtub drownings. The typical bathtub drowning victim is a child age 8 to 24 months who was left alone or with a sibling for a brief period of time. Child abuse victims may have a caregiver with an inconsistent history of how the event occurred, a history of abuse, delayed referral for medical care or other physical signs of abuse such as bruising. A social work consult should be obtained in all cases of bathtub drowning.[9]

PATHOPHYSIOLOGY

The primary damage in a submersion injury is the result of hypoxia. In the majority of drownings, fluid is aspirated in the lungs. In 10% to 20% of drownings, water contact on the vocal cords causes laryngospasm and no water passes into the lungs (dry drownings). Intrapulmonary shunting results from bronchospasm, atelectasis, aspirated water and pulmonary edema. Cerebral edema may develop secondary to asphyxia and hypoxic-ischemic damage. Cardiac arrhythmias are rare but usually the result of hypoxemia and metabolic acidosis. Electrolyte abnormalities occur less than 15% of the time.[10] There is not a significant clinical difference between fresh and salt water drowning.

MANAGEMENT

Prehospital

Initial ED management for a near drowning begins with airway, breathing and circulation (ABCs). Emergency management begins at the site of occurrence. If the victim is not close to shore or a solid surface, mouth to mouth resuscitation should be initiated in the water. The quicker the resuscitation begins, the better the odds of a good outcome. Survivors are much more likely to have received bystander cardiopulmonary resuscitation (CPR) than those who do not survive.[11] Even if the rescuer does not know how to perform CPR, he or she may be instructed on how to do so over the phone by calling 911 and accessing a trained dispatcher.[12] In a Sacramento,

California study, 42% of children who drowned had resuscitation delayed until the arrival of an emergency medical crew.[5] The Heimlich maneuver should not be attempted unless an obstructed airway is suspected that does not clear with airway repositioning.[13]

Emergency medical transportation with aggressive medical care has shown to improve survival.[14] All symptomatic near drowning victims should receive supplemental oxygen. Most drowning victims vomit due to swallowing large amounts of air and water. Providers need to anticipate emesis during resuscitation. The role of prehospital intubation is less clear. In the study by Gausche et al. of prehospital pediatric intubation, there was no improvement in survival and there was a greater risk of esophageal intubation.[15]

EMERGENCY DEPARTMENT

Key elements of patient history are listed:

1. Estimation of submersion time
2. Temperature of the water
3. Condition on removal from the water
4. Time of and response to bystander CPR, if given
5. Time of and response to EMS resuscitation
6. Time to return of pulse and or spontaneous respirations

Other important elements of patient history are whether there may have been a traumatic injury such as a fall, if the patient has a history of seizures, or if there is the possibility of drug ingestion.

Key elements of the physical exam are the body temperature, respiratory rate and oxygen saturation. A special thermometer may be needed to measure low core body temperatures. The physical examination should focus on the patient's respiratory and neurologic status. If the patient's body temperature is low, warming techniques should be used.

ED management should focus on correction of both hypoxemia and metabolic acidosis. The key management question is whether the child needs hospitalization or not. If the child is asymptomatic for a period of at least 4 hours, he or she does not need to be admitted. Children with persistent tachypnea, hypoxia, retractions, abnormal blood gas, abnormal chest radiograph or altered mental status should be admitted to the hospital (Table 17.I.1). Lasix (furosemide) is not recommended as the patient may be volume depleted. Continuous positive airway pressure

Table 17.I.1. Hospital
Admission Criteria

Tachypnea
Hypoxia
Retractions
Abnormal ABG
Abnormal chest radiograph
Neurologic impairment

may be beneficial for patients in mild to moderate distress. Intubation is required for respiratory failure or impending failure. Indications for intubation include severe obtundation, decreasing mental status, an arterial blood gas with a P_{CO_2} greater than 60 or P_{O_2} less than 60 with oxygen administration or a persistent respiratory rate greater than 60 breaths per minute. Early nasogastric tube placement is important to decompress the stomach. A Foley catheter should be placed if the patient is in critical condition in order to monitor urinary output and evaluate perfusion. Antibiotics and steroids are not helpful unless they are given for a specific indication.

Traditional teaching has been that all unconscious drowning victims who may have fallen or struck their head on the bottom of the body of water be kept in cervical spine immobilization. Watson et al.[16] found only 11 of 2244 submersion victims had a cervical spine injury, and none of the victims were younger than age 15 years.[16] A submersion victim less than 5 years of age does not need to be kept in cervical spine immobilization unless either there are obvious signs of trauma or the neck collar is being used to help secure an endotracheal tube.

Barbiturate coma and hypothermia have been used to control the increased intracranial pressure (ICP) that results from hypoxia-induced cerebral edema. However, these methods have not been shown to improve outcome in patients with ICP greater than 20 mm Hg and cerebral perfusion pressure 60 mm Hg or less.[17]

Laboratory and Radiology

If the patient is asymptomatic, no laboratory tests or radiographs are necessary. The patient should be observed for 4 to 6 hours prior to discharge. If the patient is in respiratory distress or is obtunded, a blood gas measurement, complete blood cell count, and electrolyte level should be obtained. A radiograph needs to be obtained if the patient has respiratory symptoms. Electrolyte disturbances are uncommon. Metabolic acidosis is the most common laboratory result. An elevated glucose level is associated with severe hypoxia.

Parent and Caregiver Counseling

The emotional anguish of a parent or caregiver who loses a child to drowning can be extreme. A social worker must be available for immediate counseling. Prehospital care providers may want to consider bringing a child into the hospital even if the child has been pronounced dead in the field so that the family can access immediate counseling services.

Prognosis

The prognosis relates primarily to the length of time the brain is without oxygen and the rapidity of resuscitation. There have been case reports of prolonged submersion in cold water with complete recovery without central nervous system impairment.[18] A child who was submerged for 66 minutes in 5°C water survived after 2 hours of CPR followed by extracorporeal warming.[19] Extracorporeal warming is the most effective way to warm a critically ill hypothermic patient. However, hypothermia is more of a risk factor for near drowning than it is a protective factor. At the sinking of the Titanic in 1912, there were an adequate number of life vests but not enough life boats. Of the 2201 passengers, 1489 died within 2 hours in the 0°C water. The only survivors were in life boats.

Specific historical prognostic factors include length of submersion, presence of respirations, presence of a pulse, papillary response, level of consciousness, blood pH, time to receiving CPR, length of time CPR is given and response to CPR. If a patient has not regained a pulse by the time of arrival to the ER, there is little chance of survival.[20] Elevated blood glucose is a risk factor for a poor prognosis. In one study, 68% of patients with an elevated glucose died or were in a vegetative state.[21] Low initial pH is also a risk factor for poor prognosis.

Brainstem auditory evoked responses (BAERs) can be useful in predicting outcome as abnormal BAERs in the first 6 hours after cardiac arrest are highly correlated with a persistent vegetative state.[22] Serial exams are useful in separating those with a normal neurologic outcome from those who will die or remain in a persistent vegetative state. Bratton found that all intact survivors had spontaneous, purposeful movements at 24 hours with normal brainstem function.[23] For the ED provider, there is no way to accurately predict outcome other than the absence of a pulse on arrival to the ER.

PREVENTION

The majority of all pediatric drownings can be prevented. Parents and caregivers need to be advised that they should never leave their child alone in a bathtub, even for a minute. Bath rings or chairs may give a false sense of security. Whenever infants or small children are near water, there should be a supervising adult at arm's length who is not engaged in other distracting activities. Furthermore, parents should be certain that all caregivers watching their children understand the need for constant supervision.

All residential pools must have a four-sided fence. People with pools need to realize what a risk they are to small children. Physicians need to advocate legislation requiring pool fencing for new and existing residential pools. A walk-on pool cover may provide protection if used properly but has not been tested. Parents and caregivers should learn CPR.[24]

PITFALLS

- Failure to prevent drowning injuries due to inadequate or absent barriers
- Failure to realize that infants should never be left in a bathtub alone
- Failure to recognize that bathtub drownings may not be accidental
- Failure to provide adequate and timely CPR
- Failure to realize that there are not any reliable prognostic indicators for the emergency department physician to use in the initial assessment other than absence of a pulse on arrival

REFERENCES

1. Statistics NCfH. *Compressed Mortality Files: 1983–1994.* Hyattsville, MD: US Department of Health and Human Services; 1995.
2. Gulaid JA Sr. Drownings in the United States, 1978–1984. *MMWR.* 1988;37:27–33.
3. Brenner RA, Overpeck MD. Divergent trends in drowning rates 1971–. *JAMA.* 1994;271:1606–1608.
4. Centers for Disease Control and Prevention, National Center for Injury Prevention and Control. Web-based Injury Statistics Query and Reporting System (WISQARS) [online]. (2008) [cited 2008 June 11]. Available from: URL: www.cdc.gov/ncipc/wisqars.
5. Wintemute GJ, Teret SP, Wright M. Drowning in childhood and adolescence: a population-based study. *Am J Pub Health.* 1987;77:830–832.
6. Spyker DA. Submersion injury: epidemiology, prevention, and management. *Pediatr Clin North Am.* 1985;32:113–125.
7. Rauschschwalge R, Smith GS. The role of bathtub seats and rings in infant drowning deaths. *Pediatrics.* 1997;100(4):e1.
8. Nguyen S, Teele R, Spooner C. Water birth – a near-drowning experience. *Pediatrics.* 2002;110:411–413.
9. Kemp AM, Silbert JR. Accidents and child abuse in bathtub submersions. *Arch Dis Child.* 1994;70(5):435–438.
10. Modell JH. Drowning. *N Engl J Med.* 1993;328:253–256.
11. Kyriacou DN, Arcinue EL, Peek C, et al. Effect of immediate resuscitation on children with submersion injury. *Pediatrics.* 1994;94(2):137–142.
12. Rea TD, Eisenberg MS, Culley LL, et al. Dispatcher-assisted cardiopulmonary resuscitation and survival in cardiac arrest. *Circulation.* 2001;104(21):2513–2516.
13. Rosen P, Harley J. The use of the Heimlich maneuver in near drowning: the Institute of Medicine Report. *J Emerg Med.* 1995;13:397–405.
14. Quan L, Kinder D. Pediatric submersions: prehospital predictors of outcome. *Pediatrics.* 1992;90(6):909–913.
15. Gausche M, Lewis RJ, Stratton SJ, et al. Effect of out-of-hospital pediatric endotracheal intubation on survival and neurological outcome: a controlled clinical trial. *JAMA.* 2000;283(6):783–790.
16. Watson RS, Quan L, Bratton S, et al. Cervical spine injuries among submersion victims. *J Trauma.* 2001;51:658–662.
17. Orlowski JP SD. Drowning: Rescue, Resuscitation, and Reanimation. *Pediatr Clin North Am.* 2001;48:627–646.
18. Sekar TS, MacDonnell KF, Namsirikul P, et al. Survival after prolonged submersion in cold water without neurologic sequelae. Report of two cases. *Arch Intern Med.* 1980;140(6):775–779.
19. Bolte RG, Black PG, Bowers RS, et al. The use of extracorporeal rewarming in a child submerged for 66 minutes. *JAMA.* 1988;260(3):377–379.
20. Peterson B. Morbidity of childhood near-drowning. *Pediatrics.* 1977;59(3):364–370.
21. Ashwal S, Tomasi L, Thompson J. Prognostic implications of hyperglycemia and reduced cerebral blood flow in childhood near-drowning. *Neurology.* 1990;40:820–823.
22. Fisher B PB, Hicks G. Use of brainstem audio-evoked response testing to assess neurologic outcome following near drowning in children. *Crit Care Med.* 1992;20:578–585.
23. Bratton SL, Jardine DS, Morray JP. Serial neurologic examinations after near drowning and outcome. *Arch Pediatr Adolesc Med.* 1994;148(2):167–170.
24. Brenner RA. Prevention of drowning in infants, children, and adolescents. *Pediatrics.* 2003;2003:440–445.

SECTION II. NEONATAL AND INFANT BURNS

INTRODUCTION

Burn injuries are rare in the first year of life, but when they do occur, they are associated with significant morbidity and mortality. The ED is the most common place for burn evaluation and treatment initiation. Severe burns need the expert care that is provided at burn centers. It is vital for the ED physician to be able to assess the child's injury and determine the need for burn center referral. Some pediatric burns are intentional; therefore, it is also of utmost importance for the physician to be able to distinguish intentional and unintentional injuries.

EPIDEMIOLOGY

The majority of burns happen at home. In the first 12 months of life, burns are the eighth most common cause of unintentional death and the fourth most common reason to seek treatment in the ED.[1] Boys sustain more burns than girls. Low income is a significant risk factor for burns. Ten percent of all reported cases of physically abused children involve burns. The majority of patients with burns can be managed in the ED with outpatient follow-up. In one study of ED treatment of burns, only 3% required referral to a burn center.[2]

TYPES OF BURNS

The majority of burns in children are thermal. The most common causes of thermal burns are scalding from hot cooking liquid spills and accidental contact with overheated water. Other types of burns are chemical and electrical.

CLASSIFICATION

Burns used to be classified as first, second, third and fourth degree. Now burns are classified as *superficial* (first degree), *partial thickness* (second degree) and *full thickness* (third degree). The thickness of the burn relates to the amount of energy absorbed, which relates to the time of contact and the temperature of the source.

Superficial burns only involve the epidermal layer. A common cause of superficial burns in small children is inadequate protection from sun exposure. Small children are very susceptible to sunburn. Partial thickness burns extend into the dermal tissue. Blisters are frequently seen. Full thickness burns extend all the way through the dermis. Burns that extend into muscle fascia or bone are fourth degree burns. It is important to realize that there are frequently combinations of superficial and partial thickness burns involved, and it may be very difficult to initially distinguish partial from full thickness burns.

Table 17.II.1. Criteria for Burn Center Referral

1. Partial or full thickness (second or third degree) burns >10% TBSA
2. Partial or full thickness burns involving the face, hands, feet, genitalia, perineum or major joints
3. Full thickness burns >5% TBSA
4. Inhalational injury
5. High voltage electrical injury

TBSA, total body surface area.

INITIAL ASSESSMENT

National guidelines suggest that a burn covering more than 10% of the total body surface area (TBSA) should be considered a critical burn. Children with critical burns must be managed in a burn unit or in a setting in which there are specialists (both physicians and nurses) with expertise in burn treatment. The rule of nines can be used to determine the TBSA of a burn in older children and adults, but this rule does not work well for small children. The Lund and Browder chart can be used to correctly determine the TBSA involved on a small child[3] (Figure 17.II.1). An alternate method is to use the child's palm to represent 1% of the TBSA and to estimate the number of palms it would take to cover the burn. One study revealed that the surface of the palm was only 0.5% TBSA.[4] Superficial burns are not calculated using TBSA. The main job for the ED provider is to determine whether it is a large burn (>10%) or it meets other burn center referral criteria (Table 17.II.1).

TREATMENT

Field Resuscitation

The first treatment is to separate the child from the heat source and apply immediate cooling. The first responders should provide ABCs. Victims of high voltage electrical burns or house fires may require CPR. If the patient has been in enclosed fire, carbon monoxide poisoning is assumed. The patient is given 100% oxygen by nonrebreathing face mask. Pain is assessed and treated appropriately.

The burn should be covered with a clean sheet. Small burns (<3% TBSA) may be covered with dressings soaked in cool water. This will make the patient more comfortable and decrease the extent of injury if applied within less than 1 hour after the injury. Direct cooling for larger

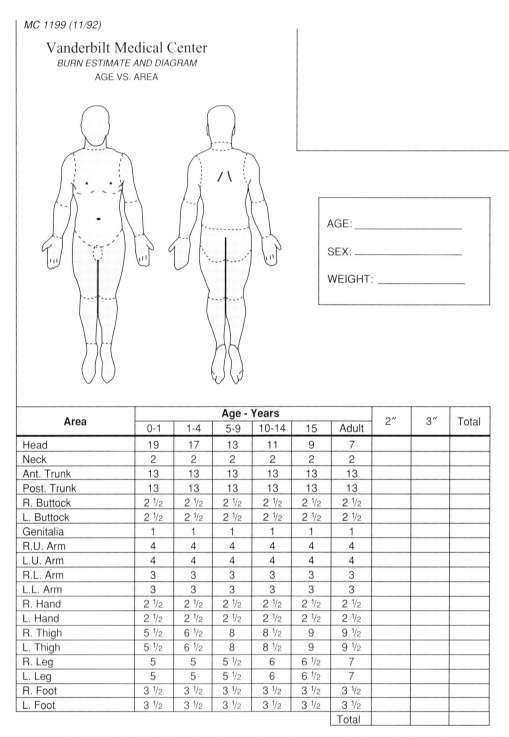

MC 1199 (11/92)

Vanderbilt Medical Center
BURN ESTIMATE AND DIAGRAM
AGE VS. AREA

AGE: _____

SEX: _____

WEIGHT: _____

Area	Age - Years						2″	3″	Total
	0-1	1-4	5-9	10-14	15	Adult			
Head	19	17	13	11	9	7			
Neck	2	2	2	2	2	2			
Ant. Trunk	13	13	13	13	13	13			
Post. Trunk	13	13	13	13	13	13			
R. Buttock	2 ½	2 ½	2 ½	2 ½	2 ½	2 ½			
L. Buttock	2 ½	2 ½	2 ½	2 ½	2 ½	2 ½			
Genitalia	1	1	1	1	1	1			
R.U. Arm	4	4	4	4	4	4			
L.U. Arm	4	4	4	4	4	4			
R.L. Arm	3	3	3	3	3	3			
L.L. Arm	3	3	3	3	3	3			
R. Hand	2 ½	2 ½	2 ½	2 ½	2 ½	2 ½			
L. Hand	2 ½	2 ½	2 ½	2 ½	2 ½	2 ½			
R. Thigh	5 ½	6 ½	8	8 ½	9	9 ½			
L. Thigh	5 ½	6 ½	8	8 ½	9	9 ½			
R. Leg	5	5	5 ½	6	6 ½	7			
L. Leg	5	5	5 ½	6	6 ½	7			
R. Foot	3 ½	3 ½	3 ½	3 ½	3 ½	3 ½			
L. Foot	3 ½	3 ½	3 ½	3 ½	3 ½	3 ½			
						Total			

Figure 17.II.1. The Lund and Browder chart can be used to correctly determine the TBSA involved on a small child.[3]

burns is not recommended as it may lead to hypothermia. Extremities with severe burns should be elevated.

Emergency Department Care

Superficial burns can be treated with a moisturizing lotion and oral analgesics. Most superficial burns will heal within 3 weeks. Partial thickness burns usually have blisters. If the blisters are small (<2 cm) they can be left intact. If they are larger than 2 cm, they should be unroofed, cleaned and covered with an antibiotic ointment. Silver sulfadiazine should be avoided in patients with an allergy to sulfa medications and in premature infants and neonates younger than 1 month of age as it may increase the risk of kernicterus. It is imperative that adequate pain relief be given during wound cleaning. Burns are extremely painful, and the patient may require substantial pain medication.

Airway

Smoke inhalation injuries are uncommon in very small children, but they must be assessed for these injuries. The presence of facial or neck burns should increase suspicion of an inhalational injury; 90% of patients with facial or neck burns have an inhalation injury. Patients may have an inhalation injury without any facial or neck burns, however.[5] Patients with signs of respiratory involvement with wheezing, cough, hoarseness or stridor should be monitored closely. Intubation should be considered early as airway edema may make later intubation difficult. Fiberoptic bronchoscopy is considered the gold standard for the diagnosis and treatment of an inhalational injury. An endotracheal tube can be placed over the scope to insert it in the trachea.

Intravenous access is needed in patients with large burns both for pain medications as well as fluids. Ideally, a large bore catheter is placed through unburned skin. Patients in shock may require an intraosseous line placement followed by a central line.

Fluid Resuscitation

Children with burns of less than 15% TBSA usually do not develop a capillary leak and can be managed with isotonic fluids at 1.5 times their maintenance requirement. Children with more severe burns require more fluids. The recommended resuscitation solution is lactated Ringer's. The Parkland formula estimates fluid requirements as 4 mL/kg per percentage of body surface area burned for the first 24 hours of care.

This formula may underestimate the fluid needs of children who weigh less than 30 kg; in these children, maintenance requirements should be added to the Parkland formula estimate, 100 mL/kg for the first 10 kg and 50 mL/kg for the second 10 kg. For example, a 12-kg child with a 15% TBSA burn should receive 1000 mL for the first 10 kg, 100 mL for the next 2 kg and 720 mL (4 mL/kg x 12 kg x 15%) for the burn, for a total of 1820 mL for the first 24 hours. Of this total, half should be given in the first 8 hours and the second half should be given over the next 16 hours.

Infants under age 6 months pose a more difficult problem due to immature renal function. Young infants retain a larger portion of free water load from fluid resuscitation in burn treatment. Young infants must be carefully monitored for signs of fluid overload. Urine output should be maintained at a minimum of 1 mL/kg/hr. Children who weigh less than 20 kg are at greater risk to develop hypoglycemia. They should receive an IV solution with dextrose to prevent lowering of the blood sugar.[6]

Patients with serious burns should have a nasogastric tube placed to treat adynamic ileus. Decompression of the stomach may improve ventilatory status. A bladder catheter should be placed to monitor urine output. Prophylactic antibiotics and steroids have not been shown to improve the course of burned patients.

LABORATORY

All pediatric patients with severe burns should receive a complete blood cell count, chemistry panel, and urinalysis. The urine should be monitored for myoglobinuria, which is one of the complications of severe burns. A carbon monoxide level should be obtained if the victim was rescued from a house fire.

ELECTRICAL BURNS

Electrical burns are extremely unusual in the first year of life. When children do sustain electrical injuries, they are usually from household current and result from inserting their fingers or metal objects into electrical outlets. These injuries result in superficial burns to the hand and fingers. A serious injury may happen when a child chews through an electrical cord and sustains a burn to the corner of the mouth. These burns can go entirely through the lip and oral mucosa and require plastic surgery repair. Fortunately, the majority of all household electrical current injuries are benign. They do not require hospitalization for cardiac monitoring (see Appendix 4).

INTENTIONAL BURNS

In one study of children presenting to an ED with burns, 20% were suspected to be the victims of abuse or neglect. Suspicion of abuse must arise when there is an unclear history of how the burn occurred, when there are inconsistencies in the history, or when implausible injury patterns with the given history. Scalding to the extremities that involve the entire hand or foot and have a clear demarcated line on injury around the wrist or leg ("glove" or "stocking") should raise suspicion. Another dipping pattern of injury occurs from the child being lowered into a hot liquid while the legs are flexed at the hips with resulting burn of the buttocks, lower back, perineum and lower extremities. This is often done as a punishment for failure at toilet training. Children may sustain thermal burns from intentional forced contact with a hot object such as a clothing or curling iron. Cigarette burns are another form of intentional injury.

Two conditions to be aware of that are mistaken for burns are bullous impetigo and phytophotodermatitis ("lime disease"). Occasionally, children have skin eruptions that simulate a burn after they are in contact with certain chemicals, such as in lime or lemon juice, and then exposed to the sun.[7] A social work consult can be extremely valuable in making the determination of whether or not to suspect abuse. Referral to a burn center or child abuse evaluation center should be made if one is unable to determine whether abuse should be suspected or not.

PREVENTION

The best way to treat pediatric burns is to prevent them from happening. Scald burns are the most common cause of burns in small children. The majority (80%) of these are caused by tap water scalds. Simply decreasing the temperature of the hot water heater to lower than 49°C (140°F) can greatly reduce the risk of an unintentional burn injury.[8] Another measure to prevent pediatric burns is to turn pot handles inward so that toddlers cannot reach up and grab them. Small children need constant supervision, especially when they are near a potential source of heat exposure that might burn the child, such as a boiling pot of water. Irons should be kept away from small children, and parents need to be aware that irons often take a long time to cool off. Parent should cap all unused electrical outlets. It is imperative that families should practice evacuating the house in the event of a fire as is done in school during fire drills.

PITFALLS

- Failure to recognize abusive burns
- Failure to make appropriate referrals to burn centers
- Failure to provide adequate pain relief
- Underestimating fluid requirements in severely burned children

REFERENCES

1. Ten leading causes of injury death by age group. ftp:/ftp.cdc. gov/pub/ncipc/10LC-2003/PDF/101c-unintentional.pdf. 2003. Accessed January 5, 2008.
2. Rawlins J, Khan A, Shenton A, et al. Epidemiology and outcome analysis of 208 children with burns attending an emergency department. *Pediatr Emerg Care.* 2007;23:289–293.
3. Lund C, Browder N. The estimation of areas of burns. *Surg Gynecol Obstet.* 1944;79:352–358.
4. Sheridan R, Retras L, Basha G, et al. Planimetry study of the percent of body surface area represented by the hand and palm: sizing irregular burns is more accurately done with the palm. *J Burn Care Rehab.* 1995;32:605–606.
5. DiVincenti F, Pruitt BJ, Reckler J. Inhalational injuries. *J Trauma.* 1971;11:109.
6. Finkelstein J, Schwartz S, Madden M, et al. Pediatric burns: an overview. *Pediatr Clin North Am.* 1992;39:1145–1163.
7. Richardson A. Cutaneous manifestations of abuse. In: Reece R, ed. *Child Abuse: Medical Diagnosis and Management.* Philadelphia, PA: Lea & Febiger; 1994:167–184.
8. Moritz AR HF. The relative importance of time and surface temperatures in the causation of cutaneous burns. *Am J Pathol.* 1947;23:605–720.

18 Gastrointestinal Emergencies

Christiana R. Rajasingham

INTRODUCTION

In the neonatal and infant periods of life, diagnosing gastrointestinal (GI) emergencies can be especially challenging as the patient population is unable to verbalize or localize their complaints, describe the progression of symptoms or provide a history. Often, the presentation is subtle and nonspecific, with the parent stating that the child "Just doesn't seem quite well" or that the child is feeding poorly. Other symptoms that may lead the clinician to look within the GI tract for a source include vomiting, diarrhea, bleeding, abdominal distention and abdominal pain. It is necessary for the clinician to obtain a very careful and thorough history from the parent and for the clinician to have a very high index of suspicion when evaluating parent's complaints that may seem fairly nonspecific.

Very young children are commonly anxious when separated from their parents and even more so when being examined by a stranger. This anxiety may make examination difficult (and very difficult to interpret), thus it is important to perform much of the physical examination in creative ways. Observing the child in the parent's arms or in a comfortable position prior to approaching him or her may yield important clues as to how uncomfortable movement is for the child. Examining the child while he or she remains with the parent may not be an ideal way to perform a textbook abdominal examination, but it may provide enough information in a nonthreatening setting. In a particularly anxious child, it may even be helpful to have the parent palpate the abdomen while watching for signs of discomfort. The stethoscope can be used as another nonthreatening way to complete an abdominal examination. By pressing more firmly, the examiner may find areas of the abdomen that are tender.

Many of the causes of GI emergencies in the first year of life stem from problems that occur during embryologic development of the GI tract (incomplete rotation of intestines outside of the abdominal cavity leading to malrotation of the intestines), whereas others are acquired or functional in nature (intussusception). This chapter discusses the most common GI reasons that infants present to health care providers.

GASTROINTESTINAL EMERGENCIES IN THE IMMEDIATE NEWBORN PERIOD

Some GI emergencies present so soon after birth that the diagnoses are usually made while the patient is still in the newborn nursery or neonatal intensive care unit (NICU), but as patients are being discharged to home earlier after birth, the emergency department (ED) clinician may be called upon to make some of these diagnoses by him- or herself. As with all of these entities, taking a thorough history and performing a physical examination in addition to having a high index of suspicion are keys to making the diagnosis. Both duodenal atresia and necrotizing enterocolitis (NEC) present relatively early in the postnatal period; in the case of NEC, the presentation may occur later but the child may be either inpatient or at home.

Duodenal atresia is estimated to occur in 1 out of 2500 to 5000 live births in the United States, and infants may have either a complete obstruction of the duodenum or, in the case of other entities such as duodenal stenoses or webs and annular pancreas, an incomplete level of obstruction.[1] Anomalies of the duodenum are usually caused by inadequate proliferation of the endodermal layer or a failure of vacuolization of the epithelial layer of the cord that gives rise to the GI tract; these events normally take place between days 30 and 60 of embryologic development. One third of children with duodenal atresia also have trisomy 21, but children with trisomy 21 do not necessarily have a higher incidence of having duodenal atresia.

Children with duodenal atresia are often diagnosed by prenatal ultrasound,[2] when the ultrasonographer sees evidence of a "double bubble" sign in the fetal abdomen in the setting of polyhydramnios. If the diagnosis is not made prenatally or if the obstruction is incomplete as in duodenal stenosis, neonates will present soon after birth with signs of intestinal obstruction – vomiting within hours of birth that is usually bile-stained, abdominal distention and signs of dehydration and electrolyte abnormalities. When duodenal obstruction is suspected in the postnatal period, plain abdominal x-rays are usually the first studies to be obtained, with a double bubble sign and absent or minimal gas distal to the duodenum being supportive of the diagnosis. Management of this entity is purely surgical; stabilization of the patient with electrolyte replacement and fluid resuscitation must occur simultaneously with plans for the patient to undergo duodenoduodenostomy.

NEC is an entity that is most often seen in the preterm neonate, with the incidence being inversely proportional to gestational age and birthweight. Term infants who develop NEC often have underlying factors that may be contributory, such as birth asphyxia, congenital heart disease and placental insufficiency (from maternal drug use). The etiology of NEC is not known at this time, but it is suspected to be multifactorial. Ischemia and reperfusion insults to the bowel are implicated and, although infection may be a factor, no particular agent has been identified to date. An infant with NEC presents with feeding intolerance, abdominal distention, increased gastric residuals or delayed gastric emptying, ileus, bloody stools, apnea, fever, lethargy, decreased perfusion and, in advanced disease, shock and cardiovascular collapse. In some patients, erythema may be visualized on the abdominal wall.

Laboratory data can be helpful in making the diagnosis of NEC and in helping direct medical therapy. A complete blood cell (CBC) count is valuable as it will show evidence of leukocytosis and anemia (an issue of concern if the patient is experiencing significant hematochezia) as well as thrombocytopenia, which is a hallmark of NEC; a blood culture should be obtained prior to starting antibiotics. Serum electrolytes can show hyponatremia, which is a poor prognostic indicator of capillary fluid leakage in the bowel, as well as signs of acidosis.

The most helpful and readily available radiographic modality in the evaluation for NEC is plain abdominal x-rays. Plain radiography can show abnormal gas patterns

with dilated loops of bowel or scarcity of bowel gas, both of which can be worrisome. Pneumatosis intestinalis is a pathognomonic finding for NEC. Portal gas is also an indicator of NEC but is not considered specific, and free air on an abdominal x-ray warrants urgent consultation with a pediatric surgeon. Medical therapy for NEC depends on the severity of its presentation but always involves bowel rest, nothing by mouth (NPO), antibiotics (the duration of which varies with severity), supportive measures for ventilation and fluid status as needed and surgical involvement for advanced disease.

DISEASE PRESENTATIONS OUTSIDE OF THE IMMEDIATE NEWBORN PERIOD

Pyloric Stenosis

Hypertrophic pyloric stenosis (HPS) occurs more frequently in males than females, and with a rate of 1 out of every 250 births in the United States,[3,4] it is slightly more common in Caucasians and African Americans than in Asian infants. An infant whose parent had HPS has a slightly higher risk of developing HPS when compared with the general population. In HPS, the pyloric canal is narrowed and elongated secondary to hypertrophy of the pylorus muscle; eventually, this hypertrophied muscle acts as an obstruction. The cause for this remains unknown, although some studies have theorized links between *Helicobacter pylori* infection and the development of HPS.

Patients with HPS usually present for evaluation in weeks 2 through 8 of life. The infant usually presents with progressively worsening emesis. The emesis is nonbilious because the obstruction in HPS occurs above the duodenum, and the emesis is initially nonbloody. As the emesis and obstructive symptoms progress, the emesis can become bloody because the mucosa is irritated by the continued vomiting, and secondary gastritis forms, caused by stasis of stomach contents. As time passes, the vomiting progresses to the point at which it occurs predictably with each feed, and the vomiting becomes more forceful to the point at which it is usually described with the classic term *projectile*. The infant with HPS is usually very vigorous and hungry, demanding to be fed soon after each feed as the stomach is emptied with each bout of emesis. As the HPS progresses, the infant begins to show signs of dehydration, malnutrition, electrolyte abnormalities, weight loss and lethargy.

A clinician who is evaluating a child with suspected HPS must first do a very thorough history and physical. Often, the child has been evaluated for vomiting at the primary physician's office or in the ED prior to making the diagnosis, and the family may have been directed to make formula changes initially for the concern of sensitivity to the formula preparations. Also, if the diagnosis is delayed for some time, the family may report a history of constipation in the infant. On physical examination, the enlarged pyloric muscle can often be palpated in the epigastrium or right upper quadrant, and it may feel like an olive in shape and size. It is easier to feel this when the child's stomach is empty and the abdominal musculature is relaxed. If the pylorus is hypertrophied to the point of complete obstruction, the physical exam may reveal peristaltic waves in the upper abdomen and wasting if the child is becoming malnourished.

After the history and physical are obtained, the clinician may want to obtain laboratory and radiographic data to support the suspected diagnosis of HPS. Other entities that need to be considered and excluded include gastroesophageal reflux, gastroenteritis, malrotation, bowel obstruction and inborn errors of metabolism. Classically, electrolytes are obtained and show a metabolic alkalosis with hypochloremia and hypokalemia. These electrolyte derangements are secondary to the fact that the vomiting infant is losing acid and chloride ions in the vomitus and the child's kidneys will try to compensate for the loss of hydrogen ions by exchanging potassium ions, leading to the hypokalemia. The classic electrolyte findings in a child with HPS are hypokalemic, hypochloremic acidosis; however, this is an extremely late finding and may not be present on initial examination. A child with obvious signs of dehydration needs to be fluid resuscitated and may require electrolyte supplementation as well.

To definitively make the diagnosis of HPS, radiologic testing is required. Plain abdominal x-rays may be useful to exclude bowel obstruction as a cause of the infant's vomiting, but they cannot definitively assist in the diagnosis of HPS. An ultrasound in the hands of an experienced operator is very sensitive and specific in making a diagnosis of HPS. The ultrasonographer measures the pyloric muscle thickness and the length of the muscle channel; thickness greater than 3 mm and length greater than 14 mm are considered abnormal (Figure 18.1). An upper GI (UGI) contrast series can show an elongated pyloric muscle with the "string sign" or "double track" where the contrast

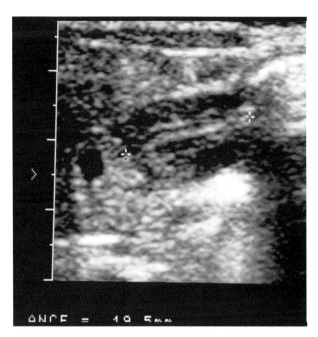

Figure 18.1. Pyloric ultrasound showing an abnormally long pyloric channel measuring 19.5 mm.

is passing through the narrowed pyloric channel (Figure 18.2). In any of these radiographic studies, a false-positive reading can occur if pylorospasm is present.

Once the diagnosis of HPS has been ascertained, the clinician involves a surgeon, as surgical pyloromyotomy is the definitive treatment. If the child is significantly dehydrated, fluid replacement and stabilization should occur prior to surgery. Although surgical correction is the gold standard for treatment of pyloric stenosis, a medical approach has been used in Japan with some success. In this approach, oral atropine for several weeks is used to allow the child to "outgrow" the stenosis, thereby avoiding surgery in some patients.[5]

Biliary Atresia

Biliary atresia occurs in approximately 1 in 10,000 to 15,000 live births in the United States and has a higher incidence in female infants.[6,7] It occurs predominantly in Asian and African American infants almost two times more often than in white infants. Biliary atresia is the most common surgically treatable cause of neonatal cholestasis. Obstruction to bile flow is caused by anomalies within the extrahepatic biliary system, which lead to either discontinuity or blockage of the system. Biliary atresia occurs in two main forms: isolated biliary atresia in 65% to 90% of cases[8] (usually evident in weeks 2–8 of life) and biliary

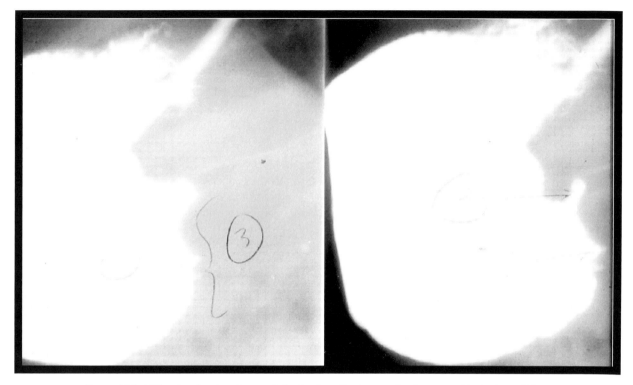

Figure 18.2. UGI series showing abnormal distribution of barium against hypertrophied pylorus ("double track" and "string" signs).

atresia associated with situs inversus and polysplenia or asplenia or other congenital anomalies in 10% to 35% of cases (usually identified by the age of 2 weeks). The more common form is thought to be the result of an inflammatory process that leads to the obliteration of the bile ducts, whereas the more uncommon type is related to problems during fetal development that allow for other anomalies in addition to the abnormal development in the biliary system.[9]

Infants with biliary atresia present with jaundice and a history of dark urine with stools that become lighter, or *acholic*, over the first few weeks of life. Conjugated or direct hyperbilirubinemia is always abnormal, and biliary atresia should be suspected in an infant who presents with direct hyperbilirubinemia or who has prolonged physiologic jaundice (>2 weeks) that turns into a conjugated hyperbilirubinemia. Infants with biliary atresia often present with hepatomegaly, with the liver firm to palpation and midline in the type of biliary atresia associated with splenic and other congenital anomalies. As biliary cirrhosis and portal hypertension develop, the spleen also may be noted to be enlarged on physical exam. Infants with biliary atresia are usually of normal birthweight and, despite their diagnosis, initially may have normal appetites and growth.

It is vital to have a high index of suspicion in making the diagnosis of biliary atresia because early operative intervention (by 2 months of age) is very important in reestablishing bile flow and preventing biliary cirrhosis.

Patients who present with symptoms of neonatal cholestasis need to be evaluated for other entities in addition to biliary atresia. Some other diagnoses to differentiate between include alpha-1-antitrypsin deficiency, choledochal cyst, neonatal hepatitis, viral syndromes including TORCH infections (toxoplasmosis, other infections, rubella, cytomegalovirus, herpes simplex virus), cystic fibrosis and inborn errors of bile acid synthesis. Laboratory data that can help the clinician to establish a diagnosis of biliary atresia include bilirubin levels, alkaline phosphatase (AP), serum transaminases, gamma-glutamyl transpeptidase (GGTP) and serum bile acids.

The infant's total bilirubin is high and, when fractionated, should show a predominant conjugated hyperbilirubinemia. AP is elevated and, if available, the liver-specific fraction of AP 5′-nucleotidase can help differentiate between skeletal and liver sources of AP. GGTP is found in the bile canaliculus and is closely correlated with AP levels; GGTP is elevated in patients with biliary obstruction. The liver transaminases levels do not determine the diagnosis of biliary atresia; however, if the transaminases are markedly elevated, they may help indicate a more likely diagnosis of hepatitis. Making a definitive diagnosis of biliary atresia hinges on other modalities.

Ultrasonography may show some other causes of neonatal cholestasis, such as the presence of a choledochal cyst, but its sensitivity and specificity in diagnosing biliary atresia is less than 80%; it is not a reliable means of making the diagnosis. Hepatobiliary scintiscanning and endoscopic retrograde cholangiopancreatography (ERCP) are other possible means of making the diagnosis of biliary atresia, but the former has significant false-positive and false-negative rates, and the latter is challenging to perform in smaller infants. Percutaneous liver biopsy and intraoperative cholangiography are the two methods that are most likely to provide a definitive diagnosis. Once the diagnosis of biliary atresia is suspected or made, surgical intervention (Kasai procedure or portoenterostomy) is the only option, as there is no established means of medical management.

Malrotation and Volvulus

Malrotation of the intestines is estimated to occur in 1 out every 500 live births in the United States, but studies from autopsy estimate an incidence of malrotation in 0.2% to 1% of the population.[10,11] The actual numbers may be higher, but often malrotation of the intestines is found coincidentally when the patient undergoes laparotomy for some other reason.[12] If a patient with malrotation remains asymptomatic until age 2, the patient may never become symptomatic, but it is believed that a malrotation that is not surgically corrected may result in a volvulus one out of three times over the course of the patient's lifetime. Symptomatic malrotation is most common in children, with 75% to 90% of cases estimated to occur in the first year of life[13]; there is no racial predominance and there is a very slight male predilection in children under 1 year that seems to equilibrate over the entire lifespan.

Malrotation is often associated with other congenital anomalies. During the embryologic development of the GI tract, the intestines undergo a complex set of rotations and movements, and problems that occur with that intricate process are the cause of malrotation. During weeks 5 through 10 of embryologic development, the GI tract (which starts out as a hollow straight tube) undergoes a total of 270 degrees of rotation around a stalk (which includes the superior mesenteric artery) before the intestines become fixed to the posterior abdominal wall. If the rotation does not occur or is incomplete, there will be malposition of some of the abdominal contents and the bowel will not be fixed completely in the abdomen, leaving the intestine at risk of volvulus.

The clinical presentation of malrotation in infants varies with the child's age and level of obstruction. Infants younger than 2 months of age usually present with bilious vomiting and some abdominal distention. In general, the younger the infant at the time of presentation, the more severe the obstruction and the lower the likelihood that the infant will be able to tolerate feeds. Other symptoms in the young infant include loss of appetite, apnea, constipation (from dehydration) and poor growth. Volvulus is an entity that is distinct from malrotation, and although malrotation causes intermittent and partial obstruction of the intestine, volvulus usually causes complete obstruction with disruption of the blood supply to the intestine (either venous congestion or arterial interruption). Ischemia of the bowel caused by volvulus causes significant pain; congestion of blood vessels in the intestine may cause bleeding from the bowel walls (*melena*) and eventually necrosis or gangrene. Infants with complete obstruction and ischemia will become ill quickly and may present in shock.

On initial evaluation of a child with suspected malrotation or volvulus, the clinician may want to obtain some laboratory and radiographic data. Other entities that must be considered in the diagnosis of malrotation and volvulus include duodenal atresia, annular pancreas, gastroesophageal reflux, NEC, pyloric stenosis and inflammatory bowel disease in the older child. A CBC count can yield some valuable information about the child at the time of presentation; the hemoglobin/hematocrit may be decreased if the child is losing blood into the GI tract, and an elevated white blood cell (WBC) count may indicate ischemia. A remarkably high WBC count may indicate the onset of sepsis. A chemistry panel may show signs of dehydration, acidosis and abnormal electrolytes from fluid shifts that occur in the edematous bowel. A positive stool test for occult blood may also provide more evidence that intestinal obstruction is taking place.

Plain abdominal x-rays can be vital in determining if there is complete bowel obstruction. A "double bubble" sign, along with a relative paucity of bowel gas in the lower abdomen, can indicate a high likelihood of obstruction, but normal findings on x-ray do not preclude the

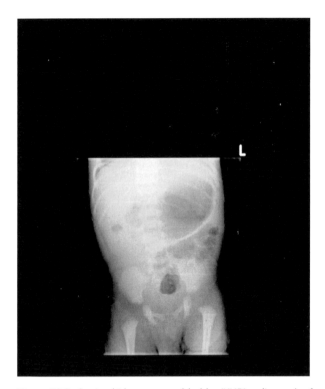

Figure 18.3. Supine kidney, ureter, bladder (KUB) radiograph of 4-day-old infant who presented with bilious vomiting. Note air in the first part of the duodenum but no air in the rest of the right abdomen. This child had malrotation of the intestines with volvulus.

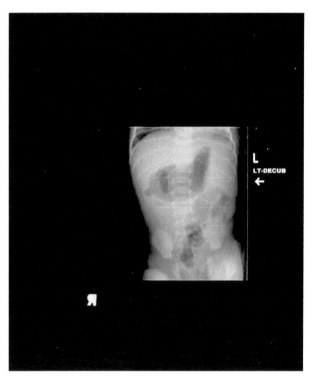

Figure 18.4. Left lateral decubitus radiograph from the same patient in Figure 18.3. The absence of air in the right part of the abdomen is noted again and is suggestive of intestinal obstruction.

diagnoses of malrotation and obstruction in the face of clinical suspicion (Figures 18.3 and 18.4). Definitive radiologic diagnosis comes from a UGI series with contrast follow-through to the small bowel. The *bird-beak sign* (contrast in the dilated proximal duodenum) and the appearance of contrast in a spiral or corkscrew pattern in the duodenum are considered positive signs for malrotation in a UGI exam. A barium or contrast enema also can be helpful in making the diagnosis, but these enemas can be inconclusive and will prevent the clinician from performing a UGI exam to confirm the diagnosis as the contrast from the enema will obscure the data from the UGI contrast. Ultrasonography and abdominal computed tomography (CT) scanning are other radiographic modalities that may help yield the diagnosis of malrotation, but they are considered merely adjuncts to the contrast studies and open laparotomy in making the diagnosis.

Once malrotation or volvulus has been diagnosed, a pediatric surgeon must be emergently consulted as the primary treatment is surgical. It is important to not delay the surgical consultation while awaiting results from the radiologic studies. The infant needs to be stabilized

medically while awaiting surgical correction with the Ladd procedure. In the Ladd procedure, first described in 1932, the surgeon makes an incision in the right upper quadrant, runs the bowel to look for signs of necrosis or infarction, rotates the bowel in a counterclockwise fashion then replaces the bowel in the abdomen in the position that it should have been in embryologically.[14,15] To stabilize the patient, ventilation and oxygenation should be supported; GI decompression with a nasogastric or an orogastric tube is an important initial step. Infants should also be adequately fluid resuscitated and have their electrolytes replaced, if needed. Also, given the propensity of this diagnosis to lead to infection and sepsis, broad-spectrum antibiotics should be started early for prophylaxis, and they should cover both skin and gut flora.

Intussusception

Intussusception is the most common cause of intestinal obstruction in children outside of the neonatal period and younger than 3 years.[16] Approximately two thirds of cases occur in infants younger than 1 year of age.[17] There is a slightly increased proportion of males with intussusception, but there is no reported difference in prevalence among races.[18] Intussusception occurs when a portion of the intestine invaginates into the lumen of the intestine distal to it. This process occurs because the part of the bowel that prolapses (intussusceptum) into the distal bowel (intussuscipiens) acts as a lead point, either because of an effective mass in the bowel wall or because of abnormal peristalsis in that portion of the bowel. Initially, the bowel wall becomes edematous secondary to delay in lymphatic drainage. As time progresses, venous congestion and, eventually, arterial compromise of blood flow ensues. The most common site of intussusception is found at the ileocolic junction.

A child with intussusception traditionally presents with a classic triad of symptoms: vomiting, colicky abdominal pain and bloody, mucoid stools. Most children will not have all three typical symptoms at the time of presentation, however. Another very common presenting symptom is lethargy, although the cause of this symptom is unclear.

Initially, the vomiting is nonbilious in nature but as the bowel obstruction caused by the intussusception progresses, the emesis may become bilious. The abdominal pain is usually episodic and severe, generally lasting minutes, and children draw up their legs and cry during the episodes. Between episodes of pain, the child may seem improved but is usually still somewhat quiet or ill-appearing. On physical exam, occasionally a soft-tissue mass can be palpated in the right side of the abdomen. Rectal exam may reveal guaiac-positive stool or even stool with the pathognomonic "currant jelly" appearance of blood and mucous mixed in with stool, but lower intestinal bleeding is considered a late sign and may not be present at all in the child with intussusception.

After the initial history and physical exam, the clinician will likely need to obtain some laboratory and radiographic data to assist in making the diagnosis of intussusception. The differential diagnosis for intussusception must include colic, gastroenteritis, allergic colitis, appendicitis and, in the patient who presents primarily with lethargy, sepsis. Laboratory data will not provide conclusive information for making the diagnosis, but an elevated WBC count may indicate the onset of gangrene and necrosis and electrolytes may help determine the degree of dehydration and acidosis.

Plain abdominal x-rays may be normal initially and then progress to showing evidence of bowel obstruction,

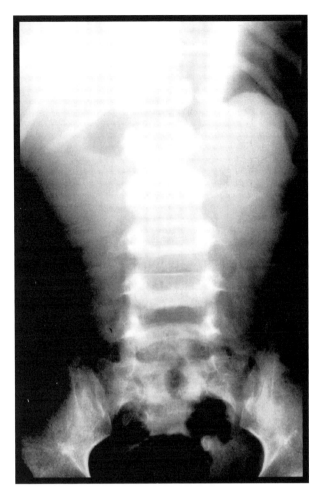

Figure 18.5. Supine radiograph in a child with intussusception. Note the paucity of gas in the right lower quadrant, with the suggestion of a soft tissue mass encroaching into gas-filled bowel in the left upper quadrant ("crescent sign").

such as dilation of small bowel loops and air-fluid levels in the small bowel, later in the course of the intussusception. Paucity of gas in the right abdomen and evidence of a soft-tissue density in the right lower quadrant are findings on plain film that are suggestive of intussusception (Figure 18.5). If air is seen to fill the cecum on x-ray, especially on a left lateral decubitus film, it is unlikely that the child has an ileocolic intussusception.

Ultrasonography may be helpful in making the diagnosis, but results are operator-dependent; it is not always a reliable modality. Abdominal CT scans also may be helpful, but the results are also not consistently reliable, and there are other incurred or implied risks with radiation exposure and use of intravenous (IV) contrast.

The most commonly used and reliable means of both diagnosis and treatment of suspected intussusception is a contrast or air enema. If the intussusception is not reduced with the enema, the procedure may be repeated in accordance with the protocols of the clinician's practice center, but if the repeated attempts are also unsuccessful, the patient needs to undergo surgical release. Most clinical centers advise making a pediatric surgeon aware that there is a patient with likely intussusception prior to doing the enema so that the surgeon can be on standby if the patient requires surgery for release of the intussusception or if the patient has a bowel perforation during the procedure.

Appendicitis

The appendix is a hollow, tubular structure that is attached to the cecum at the ileocecal junction, with the tip pointing into the pelvis, either retrocecally or extraperitoneally. When the lumen of the appendix becomes blocked by stool, food particles or hypertrophied lymph tissue, the appendix becomes inflamed and can progress to becoming infected when bacteria in the intestine multiply. Once the appendix is infected, it may rupture into the peritoneum, or the omentum can wall off the infected structure, leading to formation of an abscess. Appendicitis can occur at any age, but it is rare in infants.[19] The diagnosis of appendicitis in younger children and infants is often made later, once the appendix has perforated.[20–21] Although there does seem to be a family predilection for appendicitis, there is no data to support the presence of a specific gene.[22,23]

The initial presenting symptom of appendicitis is abdominal pain, usually constant, beginning in the periumbilical region and then radiating toward the right lower quadrant of the abdomen within hours. Nausea and vomiting are often present, but, classically, the pain precedes the development of the nausea. Fever, usually low grade, may be present, but it is most common when perforation of the appendix has occurred. In the infant and neonate age group, determining some of these symptoms and their timing is challenging, at best.

Physical examination becomes incredibly important in making the diagnosis in this age group. Young children with appendicitis also show signs of peritoneal irritation; observing the young child's position of comfort and reaction to movement prior to beginning the official physical examination can yield very helpful information. The child likely will minimize his or her own movement to avoid causing more discomfort. Certain physical exam

findings support a diagnosis of appendicitis and peritoneal inflammation or irritation. A positive psoas sign is elicited when the child experiences pain when the right leg is hyperextended while the child is lying on his or her left side, and a positive obturator sign is elicited when the child experiences pain while the right leg is flexed at the hip and internally rotated. Pain experienced in the right lower quadrant when the left side of the abdomen is palpated constitutes a positive Rovsing's sign and also suggests peritoneal irritation. Typically, pain on palpation in McBurney's point in the right lower quadrant is associated with appendicitis; however, the location of maximal tenderness may vary according to where the appendix is located.

Making a diagnosis of appendicitis based solely on history and physical examination in the very young child may be very challenging; laboratory and radiographic evidence can be helpful adjuncts to the clinician's evaluation. Although there is no laboratory result that can specifically prove or disprove a tentative diagnosis of appendicitis, obtaining a CBC count and inflammatory markers may provide information to support a clinical diagnosis. An elevated WBC count, especially when accompanied by a left shift (predominance of neutrophils), is suggestive of inflammation; this finding supports appendicitis as a diagnosis, but neither absence nor presence of this finding is confirmatory. An elevated C-reactive protein level, when available, may also support a diagnosis of appendicitis, but it, too, is a nonspecific inflammatory marker.

Other laboratory data may be helpful in evaluating a patient for other causes of abdominal pain: abnormalities in urinalysis may reveal evidence of urinary tract infection (UTI) or kidney stones, abnormalities of electrolytes on a metabolic panel may reveal evidence of dehydration or metabolic acidosis, and abnormalities of liver and pancreatic enzymes may reveal hepatitis or pancreatitis as causes of abdominal pain.

Various radiographic modalities can be used to assist in the diagnosis of appendicitis as well. Plain x-rays may be obtained to rule out other causes of abdominal pain such as bowel obstruction and stool retention, but they rarely show evidence of an appendicolith to further suggest appendicitis as a cause. The gold standard for radiographic diagnosis of appendicitis is positive visualization of an inflamed or ruptured appendix on ultrasound or CT scan. Ultrasound is a desirable modality as it involves no radiation exposure to the patient; however, its use is limited by availability and the skill or comfort level of the ultrasonographer. CT scanning is a readily available test in most hospital settings, and, when evidence of inflammation surrounding the appendix or an enlarged appendix is found, the diagnosis of appendicitis is easily made. However, performing a CT scan involves exposing the child to radiation, and, in a young child who may be unable to stay still long enough to obtain clear images, sedation may be required to complete the CT scan. Also, the appendix may not always be visualized on CT scan, depending on its position within the abdomen and how early in the disease process the scan is performed.[24]

When a diagnosis of appendicitis is strongly suspected, or confirmed via radiographic tests, urgent consultation with a pediatric surgeon is required. The clinician should be aware of the resources available to him or her; if transfer to another facility is required for access to a pediatric surgeon, telephone consultation and transportation should be arranged as soon as possible. Although treatment includes antibiotics and fluid resuscitation, the primary treatment is surgical; an appendectomy should be performed at the surgeon's discretion. Antibiotic choices vary by institution and surgeon and with the extent of the disease process (e.g., broader coverage of anaerobes is required when the appendix has ruptured). Antibiotics should cover gram-negative flora as well as anaerobic organisms. A second- or third-generation cephalosporin such as cefoxitin or an imipenem such as meropenem are appropriate choices. Another important part of medical therapy is the use of analgesia during the workup phase. Although there has been resistance in the past to giving pain medicine such as morphine to a patient with suspected appendicitis for fear of adversely affecting the physical exam, studies have shown that treating your patient's pain is not only humane but also will not prevent an accurate and prompt diagnosis.[25]

Gastrointestinal Bleeding

There are many causes of both upper and lower GI bleeding in infants; most causes are not serious, but it is important to evaluate each case fully so as not to miss potentially life-threatening etiologies. Table 18.1 lists some of the more commonly found causes of upper and lower GI bleeding in the neonatal and infant age groups. A very careful history of the presenting symptoms and physical exam

Table 18.1. Causes of upper and lower gastrointestinal bleeding

Causes of upper GI bleeds	Causes of lower GI bleeds
Swallowed maternal blood	Allergic colitis (milk protein allergy)
Medication-induced gastritis (indomethacin, NSAIDs, maternal medications such as aspirin, phenobarbital)	Intestinal polyps
Mallory-Weiss tears after emesis	Anal fissures
Erosions of GI mucosa (maternal stress, neonatal peptic ulcer disease)	Meckel's diverticulum
	Intussusception
Hypertrophic pyloric stenosis (from repetitive vomiting)	Infectious diarrhea
	Necrotizing enterocolitis
	Nonbloody entities (food coloring, medications such as iron preparations, bismuth)
	Malrotation and volvulus
	Trauma (consider nonaccidental causes)

GI, gastrointestinal; NSAIDs, nonsteroidal anti-inflammatory drugs.

are tantamount to making a diagnosis and excluding or including serious causes for the bleed. Key elements of the history must include timing and location of bleed (in emesis or in stool); color and quantity of the blood; associated symptoms such as fever, pain, poor feeding, weight loss, abdominal distention, constipation or diarrhea; medications that the child or the breastfeeding mother are taking; recent travel; family history and ill contacts.

Once the history-taking is complete, a thorough physical exam is indicated, including external inspection of the perianal region to look for fissures and a rectal exam to obtain a stool sample for guaiac testing. The guaiac test is important to use in ascertaining whether the red substance in the stool is really blood or a byproduct of food dyes or medication. In the infant who has suspected UGI bleeding because of blood in emesis, an Apt-Downey test can be used to determine if the source of the blood is maternal (swallowed in the birthing process or swallowed from cracked and bleeding maternal nipples in the breastfeeding infant). To perform the Apt-Downey test, 1% sodium hydroxide is mixed with the blood from the emesis and sterile water; if the solution turns yellow-brown, the blood is likely maternal in origin. If the bleeding is minimal or self-limited, further workup may not be warranted; however, if the bleeding continues or the child appears ill, a more extensive evaluation is mandatory.

A CBC count can give the clinician information regarding the possibility of infectious causes if the WBC count is elevated and regarding anemia as an indicator of how severe the blood loss may be. A coagulation panel and electrolytes (including renal and hepatic function testing) also may be helpful in establishing if the child has any evidence of liver dysfunction and the degree of dehydration. Stool studies can be helpful for evaluation of possible infectious causes of lower GI bleeding. Radiographic imaging may be helpful in establishing a diagnosis of GI bleeding secondary to structural anomalies (Meckel's nuclear medicine scan to evaluate for Meckel's diverticulum or ultrasound to evaluate for HPS with frequent emesis leading to Mallory-Weiss tears) or intestinal obstruction (plain x-rays to evaluate for obstruction in malrotation or intussusception), for example.

Meckel's Diverticulum

The vitelline, or omphalomesenteric, duct typically becomes obliterated by gestational week 7, but if it does not completely regress, the remnant is called *Meckel's diverticulum*. Meckel's diverticulum is commonly described by the rule of 2's:

> It typically presents in children younger than 2 years old.[26]
> It is found in approximately 2% of the population.
> Only 2% of people with it are symptomatic.
> It is found in the intestine about 2 feet from the ileocecal junction.
> It is typically 2 inches long.

The Meckel's diverticulum involves all layers of the bowel, and about 60% of the diverticula include some gastric, duodenal, endometrial or pancreatic tissue within them. The typical presentation of a Meckel's diverticulum includes painless bleeding from the rectum, which is a result of the heterotopic gastric tissue secreting gastric enzymes into the diverticulum or the distal ileum. A Meckel's diverticulum may also present with intestinal obstruction (Figures 18.6 and 18.7), intussusception (the diverticulum acts as a lead point), and, in older patients, signs of diverticulitis. There is no definitive laboratory test

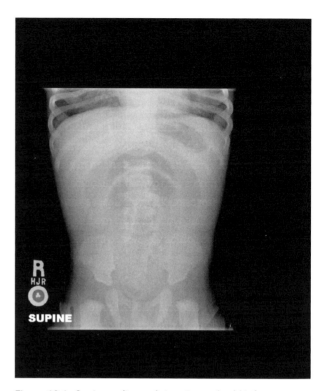

Figure 18.6. Supine radiograph in a 4-month-old infant presenting with abdominal distention and bilious vomiting. Note the paucity of gas in the lower abdomen. This infant had a Meckel's diverticulum that resulted in a small bowel obstruction.

that can make the diagnosis of a Meckel's diverticulum, but a CBC count and metabolic panel may be helpful adjuncts.

Plain radiographs may help establish a diagnosis if the child has a bowel obstruction or bowel perforation. A Meckel's scan, which is a nuclear medicine scan involving technetium-99 tagged red blood cells, may show bleeding from a Meckel's diverticulum with gastric mucosa in 85% of cases,[27] and an arteriogram may show evidence of profuse bleeding from diverticula. When a Meckel's diverticulum is suspected and diagnosed, swift surgical consultation is warranted, emergently if there is evidence of bowel obstruction or perforation or hemodynamic instability.

Management of GI bleeding in the infant depends on the child's clinical appearance, the severity of the bleeding and the underlying cause. The most important priority is to stabilize the patient with fluid resuscitation and hemodynamic support, if indicated. If the child is briskly bleeding from a UGI source, placement of a nasogastric tube can help with diagnosis and help keep the child's stomach decompressed. Endoscopy of the UGI tract and

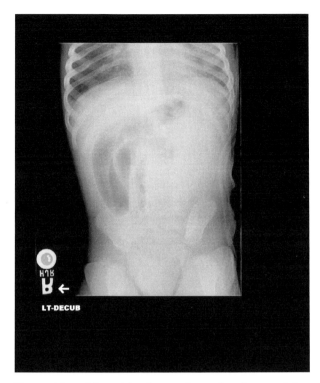

Figure 18.7. Left lateral decubitus radiograph in the same infant pictured in Figure 18.6. Note air-fluid levels suggestive of an obstructive process.

Table 18.2. Common nonsurgical causes of gastrointestinal distress in infants

GI causes	Causes outside the GI tract
Colic	Pneumonia
Gastroesophageal reflux	Urinary tract infection
Constipation	Inborn errors of metabolism
Infectious diarrhea viral (e.g., Rotavirus)	Streptococcal pharyngitis
Bacterial (e.g., Salmonella)	
Hemolytic uremic syndrome	Ingestions (especially iron)
Henoch Schönlein purpura	

GI, gastrointestinal.

colonoscopy can reveal the source of bleeding and even give information about the risk of rebleeding.

COMMON NONSURGICAL CAUSES OF GI COMPLAINTS IN THE INFANT

Parents often bring their infants to the clinician with abdominal pain or distention, vomiting or diarrhea. Table 18.2 lists the common causes of nonsurgical abdominal pain in infants. These are complaints that provoke much anxiety in the caretaker, and the onus is on the physician to evaluate the patient thoroughly to ensure that these symptoms are not caused by a serious or life-threatening disease process. Common causes of vomiting include meningitis, UTIs, otitis media, head injury and inborn errors of metabolism. In addition, pneumonia has been shown to be associated with abdominal discomfort in children. Although ondansetron has been shown to be effective and safe as an antiemetic agent (0.15 mg/kg), the underlying cause of the vomiting should be aggressively sought, particularly in the young infant. Gastroenteritis and constipation are common presenting complaints to the ED and are discussed next in more detail.

Gastroenteritis

Acute gastroenteritis (AGE) is a very common complaint in young children, and it usually has a viral cause. Common viral causes include *Rotavirus* and *Norwalk virus,* and the most common bacterial cause of AGE is *Campylobacter.* The initial presenting symptom is vomiting, and vomiting can precede the onset of diarrhea by hours to 1 or 2 days. Usually, there is no fever or only low-grade temperature elevation in viral AGE. The diarrhea is usually profusely watery or mucoid in viral AGE; consider a bacterial cause of AGE if the diarrhea is bloody, if the child has high fevers or if there is a history of unusual travel or food exposures.

On physical examination, the child may have a minimally tender abdomen and the abdomen may be distended, especially if the child has developed an ileus. Bowel sounds are present and may be somewhat hyperactive. Common causes of acute and chronic diarrhea are listed in Table 18.3.

The risk of developing dehydration is of the highest concern in the young child. Children with frequent vomiting and bouts of diarrhea are at greatest risk. The level of dehydration can be assessed by change in weight from pre-illness levels and clinically by evaluating urine output as well as other indicators. Table 18.4 lists clinical indicators of dehydration.[28]

A particular concern in the young infant is hypoglycemia. Older children have more reserve to deal with low blood sugar, and clinically, an older child is unlikely to be hypoglycemic if he or she appears to be alert and interactive. The clinical exam in an infant is unlikely to provide clues as to blood sugar unless the child is obviously obtunded; therefore, it is advisable to consider obtaining a

Table 18.3. Common causes of acute and chronic diarrheal illness

Common causes of acute diarrheal illness	Causes of chronic diarrheal illness
Bacterial	
Campylobacter	Urinary tract infection
Salmonella	
Shigella	
Yersinia	
Escherichia coli	
Clostridium perfringens	
Clostridium botulinum	
Clostridium difficile	
Cholera	
Staphylococcus aureus	
Aeromonas	
Viral	
Rotavirus	
Norwalk virus	
Adenovirus	
Calicivirus	
Astrovirus	
Torovirus	
Parasitic	
Giardia lamblia	
Cryptosporidium	
Entamoeba histolytica	
Other	
Medication-induced	Postinfectious disaccharide intolerance
Parenteral: Otitis media, upper respiratory infection, urinary tract infection	Irritable bowel syndrome
Food intolerance	Milk or soy protein intolerance
Psychogenic: Anxiety	Food allergy
Necrotizing enterocolitis	Maternal deprivation syndrome
Cystic fibrosis	Cystic fibrosis
Adrenal insufficiency	Celiac disease
Organophosphates	Immunodeficiency disorders
Heavy metals (iron)	Short bowel syndrome (postoperative)
Hirschsprung disease	Inflammatory bowel disease
Intussusception	Tumors (neuroblastoma, carcinoid)
	Stagnant loop syndrome
	Acrodermatitis enteropathica
	Adrenal insufficiency or hyperthyroidism
	Chronic constipation with overflow diarrhea

From Vanderhoof JA. Chronic diarrhea. *Pediatr Rev.* 1998;19:418–422.

Table 18.4. Clinical indicators of dehydration

	5%	5%–10%	>10%
Dehydration	Mild	Moderate	Severe
Skin turgor	Normal	Tenting	No turgor
Fontanelle	Flat	Soft	Sunken
Tears	Present	Decreased	Absent
Mucous membranes	Moist	Sticky/tacky	Dry
Eyes	Normal	Deep-set	Sunken
Heart rate	Normal	Slight tachycardia	Tachycardia
Urine output	Normal	Decreased	Markedly decreased
Mental status	Normal	Irritable	Lethargic

bedside blood sugar check in all children under age 1 with AGE. Rehydration with isotonic fluid and electrolytes is the treatment of choice for children with AGE and dehydration. IV hydration has a role, especially in children with moderate to severe dehydration; however, oral rehydration is also effective in children with milder dehydration, but it is usually more time- and labor-intensive for the parent to perform effectively. Oral rehydration should occur using rehydration a solution such as Pedialyte, which have a sodium and glucose content that approaches the recommendations given by the World Health Organization (60–90 mEq Na$^+$ and 2% dextrose) (Table 18.5). Breast milk is an appropriate means of rehydration if feeds are made shorter and more frequent. Parents should be instructed to rehydrate their children with small amounts of liquid (~5 mL for infants and 15 mL for older children) every 2 to 5 minutes, resting for 10 to 15 minutes if the child vomits before resuming the regimen. Tables 18.6 and 18.7 outline suggested oral rehydration regimens. IV rehydration should include at least 20 to 40 mL/kg of an isotonic solution such as normal saline, with separate supplementation with dextrose, if needed. The child should return to his or her formula or breastfeeding schedule as soon as tolerated in order to allow the child to maintain appropriate nutrition. Some children may experience a transient lactose intolerance following a diarrheal illness, thus some may need to try a lactose-free formula and diet until their intestines fully recover (usually within 1–2 weeks following the illness).

Antidiarrheal medications are not shown to have any proven benefit. Antiemetics can be considered with caution in the older child only, as some have shown increased sedation and risk for dystonic reactions. Ondansetron, an

Table 18.5. Composition of commercial oral rehydration solutions and commonly consumed beverages

Solution	Sodium (mEq/L)	Carbohydrate (g/dL)	Potassium (mEq/L)	Chloride (mEq/L)	mOsm/kg H_2o
World Health Organization	90	2	20	80	310
Pedialyte	45	2.5	20	35	250
Rehydralyte	75	2.5	20	65	250
Gatorade	21	5.9	2.5	1.7	377
Apple juice	0.4	11.9	26	–	700

Data from Colletti JE. Diarrhea. In: Hendey GW, Hendry PL, Linden CH, et al, eds. *Hardwood-Nuss' Clinical Practice of Emergency Medicine*, 4th ed. Philadelphia, PA: Lippincott Williams & Wilkins; 2005:1221.

agent used in treating nausea associated with chemotherapy, has been shown to have some use in older children. As most AGEs have a viral etiology, antibiotics are usually not necessary. If there is suspicion for bacterial AGE (e.g., high fever, bloody stool, significant travel history or known epidemic in daycare), stool cultures should be obtained. *Escherichia coli* O157:H7 should be excluded as a cause before antibiotics are given, so as to prevent the development of hemolytic uremic syndrome. Salmonella infections (nontyphoid) usually do not require antibiotic therapy, except in very young infants or children who are immunocompromised. Shigella infections may be treated with trimethoprim-sulfamethoxazole or erythromycin; *Clostridium difficile* infections are treated with oral metronidazole or vancomycin and Giardia infections can be treated with metronidazole. Table 18.8 lists suggested antibiotic regimens.

Constipation

Although many parents focus on the length of time between bowel movements, a single definition of constipation has not been agreed upon. The North American Society of Pediatric Gastroenterology Hepatology and Nutrition defines *constipation* as a delay or difficulty in defecation present for 2 or more weeks sufficient to cause significant distress to the patient. A determination of normal should encompass stool consistency and the ease with which the stool is passed. The epidemiology and clinical scenarios commonly associated with constipation vary with age. In infants and toddlers, constipation occurs equally in boys and girls. In older, prepubertal children, constipation is more common in boys, with a male-to-female ratio of 3:1. During adolescence, this ratio reverses, with constipation being three times more common in girls.

The major causes of constipation in children can be divided into two broad categories: functional and organic (Table 18.9). *Functional constipation* is defined as constipation without objective evidence of a pathological condition and is truly a diagnosis of exclusion. Although organic causes are responsible for fewer than 5% of cases, failing to diagnose these may result in serious consequences. Anatomic malformations and congenital intestinal disorders are more likely to present in infancy than at a later

Table 18.6. Emergency department management of acute diarrhea with mild to moderate dehydration

- Estimate daily fluid requirements and degree of dehydration.
- Maintenance: 100 mL/kg for first 10 kg body weight, 50 mL/kg for each additional kg over 11–20 kg, and 20 mL/kg for each kg over 20 kg.
- Deficit requirement for 5% dehydration is 50 mL/kg.
- While patient is being monitored in the ED, give 50–100 mL/kg ORS over 4 hours. ORS is best tolerated in small, frequent volumes rather than larger boluses. If vomiting occurs, give 1–2 teaspoons of the solution every 5–10 min.
- Replace ongoing losses:
  <10 kg body weight: 60–120 cc ORS for each diarrheal stool or episode of emesis
  >10 kg body weight: 120–240 cc ORS for each diarrheal stool or episode of emesis
- If stable and retaining fluids, the child may be discharged after deficit fluid is replaced, with phone contact 4–6 hours later.
- After initial hydration, continue breastfeeding or resume an age-appropriate diet.

ORS, oral rehydration salts.

Table 18.7. Suggested oral replacement therapy dosing based on weight and age

Age	Weight	Initial dosing	Volume/hr	First advance	Next advance
0–6 mo	8 kg	5 cc every 5 min	60 cc (10 cc/kg)	15 cc every 15 min	30 cc every $^1/_2$ hr
6–12 mo	10 kg	10 cc every 5 min	120 cc (10 cc/kg)	30 cc every 15 min	60 cc every $^1/_2$ hr
12–18 mo	12 kg	10 cc every 5 min	120 cc (10 cc/kg)	30 cc every 15 min	60 cc every $^1/_2$ hr
18–24 mo	13 kg	10 cc every 5 min	120 cc (10 cc/kg)	30 cc every 15 min	60 cc every $^1/_2$ hr
2–3 yrs	15 kg	10 cc every 5 min	120 cc (10 cc/kg)	30 cc every 15 min	60 cc every $^1/_2$ hr
3–5 yrs	20 kg	15 cc every 5 min	180 cc (10 cc/kg)	45 cc every 15 min	90 cc every $^1/_2$ hr
5–8 yrs	25 kg	15 cc every 5 min	180 cc (10 cc/kg)	60 cc every 15 min	90 cc every $^1/_2$ hr
8–10 yrs	35 kg	15 cc every 2 min	450 cc (10 cc/kg)	90 cc every 15 min	120 cc every $^1/_2$ hr
10–12 yrs	40 kg	15 cc every 2 min	450 cc (10 cc/kg)	90 cc every 15 min	120 cc every $^1/_2$ hr
12–15 yrs	50 kg	15 cc every 2 min	450 cc (10 cc/kg)	90 cc every 15 min	120 cc every $^1/_2$ hr

Courtesy of Mark Hostetler, MD, University of Chicago, Chicago, Illinois.

Table 18.8. Antibiotic therapy based on etiology

Organism	Indications	Therapy
Shigella	Majority are self-limited and do not require antimicrobial agents. Antibiotics are recommended for: Severe disease Dysentery Immunocompromised	77% of *Shigella* are resistant to ampicillin and 37% resistant to trimethoprim-sulfamethoxazole (TMP/SMX) Management depends on susceptibility *Shigella* susceptible strains: TMP/SMX: 8 mg/kg/d divided bid based on the TMP component Resistant stain or unknown susceptibility: Ceftriaxone: 50–75 mg/kg/d IV divided bid for 5 days Azithromycin: 12 mg/kg/d PO for 5 days
Salmonella	Overall: Antibiotics should be avoided Antibiotics and hospital admission are recommended for: Infants <3 months old Immunocompromised Hemoglobinopathies	Ampicillin 200 mg/kg/d IV divided bid for 7–10 days and gentamicin 6–7.5 mg/kg/d IV divided tid
Campylobacter jejuni		Resistant to TMP/SMX, and should be treated with erythromycin: 30–50 mg/kg/d divided tid PO for 5–7 days Azithromycin for 12 mg/kg/d PO for 5–7 days
Giardia	Presence of Giardia on stool testing	Metronidazole: 15 mg/kg/d divided tid for 5–7 days Metronidazole has a cure rate of 80%–95% Tinidazole: 50 mg/kg once with maximum dose of 2 g
Clostridium difficile	*C. difficile* cytotoxin found in stool	Discontinue any current antibiotics In the presence of severe diarrhea or diarrhea that persists despite discontinuation of antibiotics: Metronidazole: 30 mg/kg/d divided qid Vancomycin: 40 mg/kg/d divided qid for 10 days maximum dose of 500 mg is indicated for cases that do not respond to metronidazole. Vancomycin administration is discouraged secondary to promotion of vancomycin resistant organisms.

From American Academy of Pediatrics; Pickering LK, eds. *2006 Red Book: Report of the Committee on Infectious Diseases*, 27th ed. Elk Grove Village, Illinois: American Academy of Pediatrics; 2006.

Table 18.9. Differential diagnosis of constipation

Functional
Developmental: Cognitive handicaps, attention-deficit disorders
Situational: Coercive toilet training, school bathroom avoidance, sexual abuse
Reduced stool volume and dryness: Low fiber diet, dehydration, malnutrition
Organic
Anatomical: Imperforate anus, anal stenosis, anal stricture, anteriorly displaced anus, pelvic mass, rectal abscess
Metabolic/endocrine: Hypothyroidism, hypercalcemia, hypokalemia, cystic fibrosis, diabetes mellitus, gluten enteropathy
Neurologic: Hirschsprung disease, spinal cord abnormalities, neuronal dysgenesis, tethered cord, neurofibromatosis, cerebral palsy
Muscular: Prune belly, gastroschisis, myopathy
Connective tissue disorders: Scleroderma, lupus, Ehlers Danlos syndrome
Drugs: Opiates, phenobarbital, sucralfate, antacids, anticholinergics, antidepressants
Other: Cow's milk intolerance, botulism, lead toxicity, vitamin D intoxication

Courtesy of Le N. Lu, MD, and Dewesh Agrawal

age, but nonorganic causes of constipation predominate at all ages. Botulism is a rare but potentially life-threatening neuroparalytic syndrome from the action of the neurotoxin produced by *Clostridium botulinum.* Although the disease presentation and severity varies, the initial presentation may simply involve constipation, shortly followed by weakness, feeding difficulties, descending paralysis, drooling, anorexia, and a weak cry.

The clinical manifestations of lead poisoning vary with lead level, age of the exposed individual, and acuity of poisoning. Lead colic includes sporadic vomiting and intermittent abdominal pain. Constipation may occur with blood lead levels greater than 60 μg/dL (2.9 μmol/L).

Table 18.10. Oral therapy for constipation

Mineral oil*: 1–4 mL/kg/day divided daily or bid
Milk of Magnesia: 1–3 mL/kg/day divided daily or bid
Lactulose: 1–3 mL/kg/day divided daily or bid
MiraLax: 1 g/kg/day divided daily or bid (maximum 17 g/day; prepared by placing 1 capful of powder into 8 oz of liquid)
Sorbitol: 1–3 mL/kg/day divided bid (70% solution)
Senna: 2–6 years old, 2.5–7.5 mL daily; 6–12 years old, 5–15 mL daily (syrup)
Bisacodyl: 5–10 mg daily

* Contraindicated in infants and children at risk for aspiration; bid, twice daily.

Exhaustive laboratory and radiographic investigation is not usually required in the ED. A test for occult blood in the stool is recommended to be performed in all infants with constipation, as well as in any child who also has abdominal pain, failure to thrive, intermittent diarrhea, or a family history of colon cancer or colonic polyps. If the history is chronic, a urine culture should be taken to avoid missing an occult UTI. An abdominal radiograph is not indicated to establish the presence of fecal impaction if the rectal exam reveals the presence of large amounts of stool. A plain abdominal radiograph may be helpful in confirming the diagnosis when the history or physical examination is confusing or inconclusive.

If fecal impaction is present, disimpaction is necessary prior to initiation of maintenance therapy. Disimpaction can be accomplished by using oral medications (Table 18.10), rectal medications or a combination of the two. Education of the caregiver is paramount, and the treatment for each individual patient should be discussed with the family. Cathartics, suppositories (other than small glycerin suppositories) and especially enemas should generally be avoided in infants. The use of soap suds, tap water and magnesium enemas is not recommended due to potential toxicity. Tap water enemas have been associated with acute hyponatremia, seizures and death.

PITFALLS

- Failure to perform a rectal examination in patients with vomiting, no diarrhea and absent to low-grade fever
- Failure to check for fetal blood in newborns who present with UGI bleeding
- Failure to arrange close follow-up for patients with abdominal pain
- Failure to fully evaluate complaints of progressive or truly bilious vomiting
- Failure to recognize and treat clinical dehydration with oral or IV rehydration
- Failure to examine the genitalia of a child with abdominal complaints

REFERENCES

1. Escobar MA, Ladd AP, Grosfeld JL, et al. Duodenal atresia and stenosis: long-term follow-up over 30 years. *J Pediatr Surg.* 2004;39(6):867–871; discussion 867–871.
2. Hancock BJ, Wiseman NE. Congenital duodenal obstruction: the impact of an antenatal diagnosis. *J Pediatr Surg.* 1989;24(10):1027–1031.
3. Allan C. Determinants of good outcome in pyloric stenosis. *J Paediatr Child Health.* 2006;42(3):86–88.

4. Nazer H, Nazer D. Pyloric stenosis, hypertrophic. http://www.emedicine.com/ped/topic1103.htmeMedicine. Accessed on August 3, 2007.

5. Kawahara H, Takama Y, Yoshida H, et al. Medical treatment of infantile hypertrophic pyloric stenosis: should we always slice the "olive"? *J Pediatr Surg.* 2005;40(12):1848–1851.

6. Bates MD, Bucuvalas JC, Alonso MH, et al. Biliary atresia: pathogenesis and treatment. *Semin Liver Dis.* 1998;18(3):281–293.

7. Schwartz, Steven M. Biliary atresia. http://www.emedicine.com/ped/TOPIC237.htm. Accessed on August 10, 2007.

8. Balistreri WF, Grand R, Hoofnagle JH, et al. Biliary atresia: current concepts and research directions. Summary of a symposium. *Hepatology.* 1996;23(6):1682–1692.

9. Yoon PW, Bresee JS, Olney RS, et al. Epidemiology of biliary atresia: a population-based study. *Pediatrics.* 1997;99(3):376–382.

10. Ford EG, Senac MO Jr, Srikanth MS. Malrotation of the intestine in children. *Ann Surg.* 1992;215(2):172–178.

11. Sing RF, Blasko EC, Kefalides PT. Management of anomalous rotation in adults. *Am Surg.* 1994;60(12):938–941.

12. Hebra A, Miller M. Intestinal volvulus. http://www.emedicine.com/ped/topic1205.htm. Accessed on July 31, 2007.

13. Powell DM, Othersen HB, Smith CD. Malrotation of the intestines in children: the effect of age on presentation and therapy. *J Pediatr Surg.* 1989;24(8):777–780.

14. Ladd WE. Congenital duodenal obstruction. *Surgery.* 1937;1:878–885.

15. Bailey PV, Tracy TF Jr, Connors RH. Congenital duodenal obstruction: a 32-year review. *J Pediatr Surg.* 1993;28(1):92–95.

16. West KW, Stephens B, Vane DW, et al. Intussusception: current management in infants and children. *Surgery.* 1987;102(4):704–710.

17. Stringer MD, Pablot SM, Brereton RJ. Paediatric intussusception. *Br J Surg.* 1992;79(9):867–876.

18. Chahine A. Intussusception. http://www.emedicine.com/ped/topic1208.htm. Accessed on August 5, 2007.

19. Naradzay JFX, Tucker J. Pediatrics, appendicitis. November 15, 2006. http://www.emedicine.com/emerg/topic361.htm. Accessed on September 5, 2007.

20. Brender JD, Marcuse EK, Weiss NS. Is childhood appendicitis familial? *Am J Dis Child.* 1985;139(4):338–340.

21. Nance ML, Adamson WT, Hedrick HL. Appendicitis in the young child: a continuing diagnostic challenge. *Pediatr Emerg Care.* 2000;16(3):160–162.

22. Nwomeh BC, Chisolm DJ, Caniano DA. Racial and socioeconomic disparity in perforated appendicitis among children: where is the problem? Pediatrics. 2006;117(3):870–875.

23. Gauderer MW, Crane MM, Green JA. Acute appendicitis in children: the importance of family history. *J Pediatr Surg.* 2001;36(8):1214–1217.

24. Brender JD, Marcuse EK, Weiss NS. Is childhood appendicitis familial? *Am J Dis Child.* 1985;139(4):338–340.

25. Taylor GA, Callahan MJ, Rodriguez D. CT for suspected appendicitis in children: an analysis of diagnostic errors. *Pediatr Radiol.* 2006;36(4):331–337.

26. Kim MK, Strait RT, Sato TT. A randomized clinical trial of analgesia in children with acute abdominal pain. *Acad Emerg Med.* 2002;9(4):281–287.

27. Brown CK, Olshaker JS. Meckel's diverticulum. *Am J Emerg Med.* 1988;6(2):157–164.

28. Wilton G, Froelich JW. The "false-negative" Meckel's scan. *Clin Nucl Med.* 1982;7(10):441–443.

19 Genitourinary Emergencies

Christy A. Meade and John T. Kanegaye

Genitourinary (GU) complaints are common throughout childhood. Although the diagnoses overlap those of the adult population, a unique range of pathology occurs in infants and younger children. Many GU problems are benign and simply need observation or symptomatic care. Others require rapid evaluation and treatment to avoid long-term morbidity. This chapter discusses the most common male and female GU complaints that may present to the emergency department (ED).

PENILE DISORDERS

Phimosis

Phimosis refers to foreskin that cannot be retracted over the glans. Most cases are physiologic; only 4% of newborn, 25% of 6-month-old, 50% of 1-year-old and 90% of 4-year-old males have a fully retractable foreskin.[1] Pathologic phimosis results from scarring and constriction due to forceful foreskin retraction, recurrent infection, diaper dermatitis, chemical irritation, poor hygiene and congenital abnormalities or as a complication of circumcision.

Most patients with phimosis need no diagnostic evaluation, and parents only need instruction on proper hygiene and counsel against forcefully retracting the foreskin. With severe constriction, a diminished urinary stream with ballooning of foreskin during voiding, pain and hematuria can result. If there is severe obstruction, a dorsal slit procedure may be necessary.[2] Patients with recurrent balanoposthitis and infection may require circumcision or preputioplasty.[3] Short courses of topical corticosteroid (betamethasone valerate 0.6% cream applied twice daily for 2 weeks) in conjunction with preputial stretching may improve the condition and avert the need for surgery.[4]

Paraphimosis

Paraphimosis is an entrapment of the foreskin proximal to the glans, which can lead to progressive venous congestion and edema (Figure 19.1). The foreskin lies retracted and everted as an edematous ring proximal to the glans. The penis is otherwise flaccid with a narrow constriction proximal to the foreskin. Infection, masturbation, trauma, hair or clothing tourniquets may cause paraphimosis.

Maneuvers to reduce edema prior to reduction include cold compresses, circumferential compression, infiltration with a lidocaine-hyaluronidase mixture, or multiple needle punctures.[5,6] During reduction, index and long fingers exert traction on the foreskin while the thumbs apply pressure on the glans to slip it under the constricting ring (Figure 19.2). If all attempts fail, then circumcision or a dorsal slit procedure may be necessary. Patients may be discharged after reduction if they are able to void spontaneously. Patients with cellulitis or necrosis should be admitted for urologic evaluation and intravenous (IV) antibiotics.

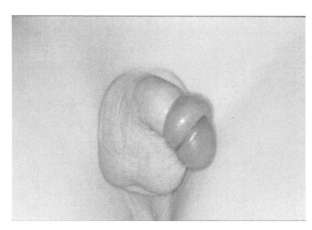

Figure 19.1. Paraphimosis with entrapment of the foreskin proximal to the glans.

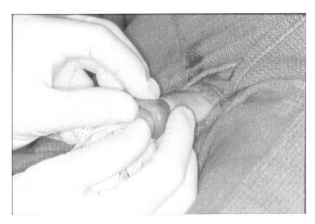

Figure 19.2. Reduction of a paraphimosis using index and long fingers to exert traction on the foreskin while the thumbs maneuver the glans under the constricting ring.

Balanitis and Balanoposthitis

Balanitis is inflammation of the glans, whereas *balanoposthitis* is inflammation of the glans and foreskin. These conditions occur in up to 6% of uncircumcised males.[7] The most common cause of balanoposthitis is infection, typically due to local flora. *Streptococcus pyogenes* has been reported to cause balanitis.[8] Candidal infection may occur, and recurrent cases should raise the suspicion of diabetes mellitus. In addition, sexually transmitted infections should be considered in adolescents. Balanoposthitis may also be caused by chemical irritation, trauma, fixed drug eruption or contact dermatitis.

Physical examination reveals erythema, edema and, at times, discharge (Figure 19.3). Systemic symptoms are rare. Management emphasizing hygiene with gentle retraction may be adequate, depending on the presentation. Discharge may be cultured to guide therapy, but

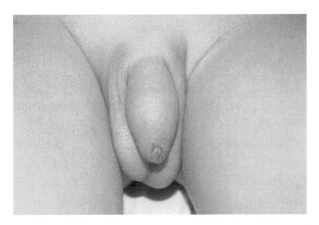

Figure 19.3. Balanoposthitis with erythema, edema and discharge.

empiric treatment directed against *Staphylococcus aureus* and *S. pyogenes* (e.g., a first generation cephalosporin) is appropriate.[9] In adolescents, the discharge should be cultured for *Neisseria gonorrhoeae* and *Chlamydia trachomatis*. Circumcision may be required for recurrent disease.

Priapism

Priapism is engorgement of the dorsal corpora cavernosa in the absence of sexual stimulation, resulting in dorsal penile erection with glans and ventral penile flaccidity. Low-flow priapism is most common and is secondary to decreased venous outflow. The concomitant ischemia causes prolonged, painful erection. Sickle cell disease (SCD) is the most common cause in children (66% of cases); up to 6% of prepubertal boys with SCD will have at least one episode of priapism. Other causes include leukemia (11% of cases), spinal trauma, immunosuppressive disorders and anticoagulation.[10] Prescription drugs such as phenothiazines, sedative-hypnotics, selective serotonin reuptake inhibitors, anti-hypertensive and anticoagulant drugs of abuse such as cocaine, alcohol and marijuana also may be contributory. High-flow priapism is typically associated with penile arterial laceration and excessive inflow of arterial blood without ischemia, resulting in painless corporal engorgement.

If prolonged engorgement of the corpora cavernosa occurs, urinary retention may ensue. Stagnant, hypoxic blood results in thrombosis and ischemia if treatment is not promptly initiated. Complications of priapism include penile fibrosis, impotence and acute urinary retention.

Priapism due to spinal cord injury involves the ventral penis and glans in addition to the dorsal corpora cavernosa. Management centers around hydration, pain control, relief of urinary obstruction and treatment of underlying conditions. Nerve block using local anesthetics without epinephrine may be beneficial as can infiltration of hyaluronidase. In patients with SCD, transfusion may be necessary. The application of hot compresses or sitz baths increases penile blood flow and may be helpful in cases of low-flow priapism.

Cavernosal aspiration and irrigation is effective in patients with low-flow priapism and acidosis. However, in order to be effective, aspiration must be performed within the first few hours of symptom onset, and it is rarely beneficial after 48 hours. Intracorporeal injection or irrigation with a dilute solution of alpha adrenergic agonist (phenylephrine or epinephrine) is a useful adjunct to corporal aspiration. Systemic vasodilators such as papaverine, hydralazine or terbutaline have also been used with varying degrees of success.[11] High-flow priapism can be treated effectively by arterial embolization. If nonsurgical approaches are unsuccessful, a shunt procedure should be considered and is most effective when performed within 24 hours of symptom onset.

Patients with persistent priapism or serious underlying disorders such as SCD or leukemia should be admitted to the hospital. A pediatric urologist should be consulted as soon as possible to determine the best management approach. If the priapism is treated successfully with noninvasive measures without recurrence during observation, the patient may be discharged with close urologic follow-up.

Complications of Circumcision

Existing scientific evidence demonstrates potential medical benefits of newborn male circumcision; however, these data are not sufficient to recommend routine neonatal circumcision.[12] Circumcision may be warranted in the treatment of phimosis, paraphimosis, recurrent balanoposthitis, recurrent urinary tract infections and penile cancer. The main techniques of circumcision are Plastibell or Gomco clamp, excision, or dorsal slit procedure. Hemorrhage, the most common complication, is generally minor and can be managed by direct pressure, silver nitrate application, topical epinephrine or suture placement. Severe hemorrhage is fortunately rare, except in patients with underlying bleeding disorders. Patients with severe bleeding typically require emergent urologic consultation and hospitalization. Hypothermia in a neonate is an important sign of shock; therefore, sequential hemoglobin and hematocrit measurements should be obtained and the patient should be admitted for continued observation.

Immediately after circumcision, pain, edema and urinary retention may occur. Pain usually resolves within 12 to 24 hours. Occlusive dressings can contribute to urinary retention and edema, and should not be used. Infection can rarely occur locally, systemically or in the urinary tract. Typical pathogens include *S. aureus*, *S. epidermidis*, *Escherichia coli*, *Klebsiella pneumoniae*, group D streptococcus, Salmonella spp. and *Proteus mirabilis*. Although quite uncommon, Fournier's gangrene may develop.

With the Plastibell method of circumcision, a small plastic ring is left at the base of the glans. This ring generally falls off in 10 to 14 days. In rare instances, the ring can move proximally or distally and can result in a tourniquet-type effect. The ring can be removed using techniques similar to those employed in a paraphimosis reduction. The lubricated tip of a blunt instrument (the loop of a bent Calgi swab) may be inserted between the retained ring and the glans to allow distal movement of the ring.

Meatal stenosis may occur in circumcised males. Prolonged exposure to the ammoniacal compounds in urine leads to sloughing of the epithelial surface of the meatus and results in a narrowed meatus. Application of an undersized plastibell may also lead to meatal stenosis with a reported incidence of 8% to 31%.[13] Symptoms of meatal stenosis include pain with urination; bloody discharge due to the inflamed meatus; high-velocity, dorsally deflected stream and the need to sit while voiding.

Phimosis may result after circumcision if excessive foreskin remains. Scar formation leads to narrowing of the foreskin opening, with the foreskin slipping over the glans penis. If the constriction is significant, urinary obstruction can occur, mandating dilation of the stenosis; this can be performed with a hemostat. If dilation is unsuccessful, a dorsal slit procedure should be performed, and, ultimately, surgical revision of the circumcision is necessary.[14]

Entrapment Injuries

Zipper entrapment of the foreskin (or the skin of the penile shaft or scrotum) typically occurs in 2- to 6-year-old boys (Figure 19.4). The zipper can be dismantled by

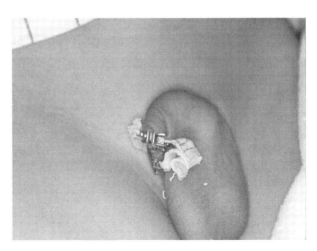

Figure 19.4. Penile zipper entrapment.

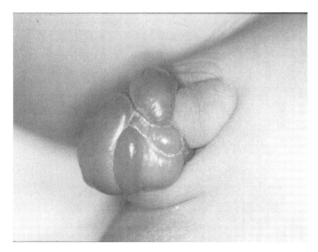

Figure 19.5. Extensive penile hair tourniquet.

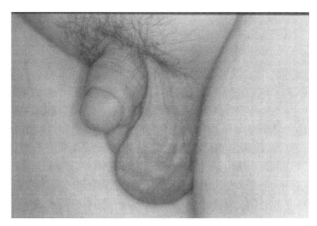

Figure 19.6. Varicocele.

cutting its median bar with bone or metal cutters. The zipper falls apart and the skin is freed. Local anesthesia is not always needed but may be useful if traction on the entrapped skin causes discomfort. There also is reported success with soaking of the entrapped skin in mineral oil prior to zipper removal.[15]

String, wire and human hair can produce a tourniquet, resulting in penile venous and arterial obstruction as well as occlusion of the dorsal nerve supply. The patient presents with swelling of the glans, and the tourniquet may be difficult to visualize due to edema (Figure 19.5). However, the tourniquet fibers may be exposed and divided when the adjacent skin is depressed with a blunt instrument such as a hemostat. Urethral function and penile blood flow should be evaluated prior to discharging the patient.

TESTICULAR AND SCROTAL DISORDERS

Varicocele

Varicoceles, caused by enlargement of the intrascrotal plexus of spermatic veins, are rare in boys younger than 10 years of age,[16] but they occur in 13.7% to 16.2% of adolescents.[17] Because of its sharp angle of drainage into the renal vein, the left spermatic vein is relatively incompetent, and 85% to 95% of cases are left-sided.[18] Vena caval obstruction (due to thrombosis or compression by tumor) should be considered for prepubertal patients, right-sided varicoceles, acute onset or lack of change in the supine position.[19]

A varicocele is best palpated in the upright patient as a "bag of worms" superior and posterior to the testis (Figure 19.6). Patients with uncomplicated varicoceles usually have no symptoms but should receive urologic referral. Ligation may be required for patients with pain, testicular atrophy or large or bilateral varicoceles.[20]

Hydrocele

A *hydrocele* occurs when fluid accumulates within the tunica vaginalis. This may be a simple, benign phenomenon or the result of testicular torsion, epididymitis, trauma or tumor. With communicating hydroceles, the processus vaginalis remains patent between the peritoneum and the scrotum. A communicating hydrocele will change size, often with crying or exertion. Most hydroceles are right-sided. They may be present at birth, are usually painless and may spontaneously resolve by 18 months of age. Examination reveals a transilluminating enlargement of the scrotum. If the hydrocele is secondary to another process, the patient may present with a tender mass, abnormal testicle or changes in the scrotal skin.

Asymptomatic patients may be discharged with pediatric or urologic follow-up. If the patient presents with an acute or symptomatic hydrocele, a Doppler ultrasound should be performed to evaluate for underlying pathology.

Idiopathic Scrotal Edema

Idiopathic scrotal edema is painless erythema and induration of the scrotal skin, unilateral in two thirds of cases. This disorder is rare but typically occurs in prepubertal patients.[21] Its origin is unknown but may be a form of angioneurotic edema. Edema and erythema may extend to the phallus, groin and abdomen wall with minimal tenderness. The testes are nontender and normal in size. Patients are afebrile. If there is no other acute pathology, patients can be managed as outpatients. No treatment is required for idiopathic scrotal edema, which generally resolves spontaneously within 1 to 4 days. Recurrence rates have been reported to be as high as 21%.[10] Purpuric lesions of the scrotum and penis should prompt consideration of Henoch-Schönlein purpura, especially if the characteristic lower extremity eruption is present.

Epididymitis

Epididymitis is inflammation of the epididymis. The most common cause is bacterial infection. Adolescents should be evaluated for possible sexually transmitted infections, such as *N. gonorrhoeae* and *C. trachomatis*. In prepubertal patients, epididymitis is frequently associated with a urinary tract infection or an underlying urologic anomaly.[22] Chemical irritation due to sterile reflux of urine into the vas deferens causes a noninfectious epididymitis.

Patients present with an enlarged, edematous scrotum, with tenderness over the epididymis. A urethral discharge may be present, especially when caused by sexually transmitted infections. Other symptoms can include fever, nausea and lower abdominal pain. Epididymitis can be difficult to distinguish from testicular torsion. Prehn's sign, the relief of pain with scrotal elevation, is unreliable in distinguishing the two.

Evaluation includes a urinalysis and culture. However, half of patients will not have pyuria. Urethral discharge, if present, should be cultured. Doppler ultrasound reveals a normal testis with normal or increased vascular flow on the affected side.[23,24] Treatment includes antibiotics (directed at typical urinary pathogens), pain control with scrotal elevation, ice packs and nonsteroidal anti-inflammatory agents. If urethral discharge is present, a patient should be treated for *N. gonorrhoeae* and *C. trachomatis*. In the prepubertal patient without discharge or pyuria, a reasonable alternative strategy is to withhold antibiotics while awaiting culture results or to discontinue empiric antibiotic therapy if the urine culture is negative.

Patients with systemic symptoms and toxicity should be admitted for IV antibiotics (generally a third-generation cephalosporin). Prepubertal patients may require voiding cystourethrography and renal ultrasound to evaluate for urologic abnormalities.

Orchitis

Orchitis is inflammation of the testis, which is usually the result of an infection. Adjacent epididymitis also can result in orchitis. Orchitis is more common in adolescents and is more likely due to mumps and other viruses (Epstein-Barr virus, arboviruses, enteroviruses) than to bacterial infection. Bacterial orchitis is usually secondary to *E. coli*, *K. pneumoniae*, *Pseudomonas aeruginosa*, staphylococci or streptococci. Granulomatous orchitis may occur with syphilis, fungal infections or mycobacterial disease.

Orchitis usually develops after the first week during a course of mumps and presents with edema and tenderness of the testis with discoloration of the scrotum. Although usually unilateral, bilateral orchitis can develop. Urethral discharge may occur if epididymitis coexists. Bacterial orchitis, although rare, can lead to scrotal abscess formation. Fertility is usually maintained because orchitis is mostly unilateral, although testicular atrophy may occur in up to 50% of patients.[10]

A complete blood cell count may demonstrate a left shift if there is bacterial involvement or a depressed white blood cell count in some cases of viral orchitis. A heterophile antibody test or serologies may be indicated. Doppler ultrasound may be needed in order to exclude torsion. Orchitis usually is self-limiting and treatment is aimed at pain control (scrotal elevation, nonsteroidal anti-inflammatory agents, narcotic agents). Antibiotics should be administered for patients with concurrent epididymitis. Admission for IV antibiotics is warranted for patients who appear toxic, have a scrotal abscess or fail to improve with oral antibiotics.

Testicular Torsion

Testicular torsion or twisting of the spermatic cord is a common cause of an acutely painful scrotum (Figure 19.7). Delayed treatment can result in infertility and in some cases complete infarction of the testis. The incidence of testicular torsion is 1 in 4000 males, with a peak incidence at age 13 years.[21]

The tunica vaginalis normally adheres to the posterior wall of the scrotum and superior pole of the testis. In fetal and early neonatal life, the parietal surface of the tunica is incompletely fixed to the scrotal wall, leading to

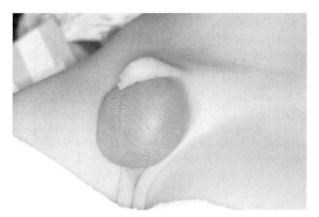

Figure 19.7. Acute painful scrotum.

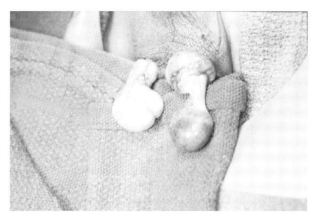

Figure 19.8. Scrotal exploration revealing ischemic left testis shortly following detorsion and normal right testis.

risk for extravaginal torsion. Extravaginal torsion is usually less symptomatic and occurs when the testis and both layers of the tunica undergo rotation. Intravaginal torsion occurs more commonly in the peripubertal period when the unfixed testis rotates within the tunica vaginalis with compromise of arterial flow. Presentation includes acute scrotal pain and swelling, a testicular elevation and absence of the cremasteric reflex.[25] Fever, nausea and vomiting may also develop. In the patient with an undescended testicle who presents with abdominal pain, torsion must be considered.[26] Doppler ultrasound has a reported sensitivity of 82% to 86%, and specificity of almost 100%.[27,28] However, surgical exploration should not be delayed for diagnostic studies, especially in patients who present with less than 12 hours of symptoms.[29] Urgency should be heightened in the presence of thickening or pitting of scrotal skin, a high-riding testis and a horizontal lie.

Testicular salvage depends on time from symptom onset, with a 96% success rate if detorsion occurs in fewer than 4 hours and a less than 10% success rate if longer than 24 hours.[30] Manual detorsion by external rotation is an option for the experienced provider when a surgeon is not available.[31] However, knowledge of this procedure should not delay surgical consultation and intervention. Approximately 40% of patients have improper fixation of the contralateral testis, and contralateral orchiopexy is usually performed during surgery for detorsion (Figure 19.8).

Torsion of Testicular Appendage

There are several vestigial embryologic remnants attached to the testis. The appendix testis (remnant of the mullerian duct) located superiorly and laterally is the testicular appendage involved in 92% of cases of torsion of

testicular appendage (Figure 19.9). Patients typically present with acute onset of moderate to severe unilateral scrotal pain. Fever, dysuria and abdominal pain are rare. In the absence of surrounding inflammation or hydrocele, a tender nodule may be palpable or even visible ("blue dot" sign, present in 14%–22% of cases) beneath the scrotal skin overlying the superolateral pole of the testis.[32] Urinalysis is usually normal. Ultrasound should be performed if there is any doubt in the diagnosis and demonstrates increased flow to the affected side. Treatment is supportive and consists of analgesics and scrotal support. The pain usually subsides within 1 week as the appendage resorbs.

Inguinal Hernia

Inguinal hernias are most common in males younger than 1 year of age and older than 40 years of age. Premature infants are also at increased risk. An indirect inguinal hernia occurs through a patent processus vaginalis and is the most common pediatric hernia. Most hernias are

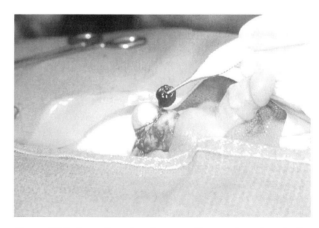

Figure 19.9. Scrotal exploration revealing torsion of testicular appendage.

asymptomatic and detected on routine examination, by patient self-discovery or by parent discovery. Entrapment of adipose tissue, bowel or intraperitoneal organs can occur, especially with smaller hernia defects. If incarceration occurs and persists, venous congestion results in edema and eventually can lead to strangulation or infarction of the entrapped tissue.

Incarceration may present with pain and/or edema over the inguinal canal extending to the scrotum. Low grade fever, nausea and vomiting may be seen. Hernias do not transilluminate unless a reactive hydrocele is also present. A hernia can be diagnosed on examination if an inguinal mass can be palpated and distinguished from the testis. However, ultrasound may be necessary to evaluate for other scrotal pathology.

An inguinal hernia should be reduced if the symptoms are acute. Slow gentle pressure should be applied to reduce the hernia. Pressure at the neck of the hernia helps to return the proximal portion through the inguinal ring. Trendelenburg position, ice packs on the groin to reduce swelling and sedation may facilitate the reduction attempt. If the hernia cannot be reduced or the child appears toxic, fluid resuscitation, broad-spectrum antibiotics and an emergent surgical consultation are warranted. If the hernia is successfully reduced in the ED, close surgical follow-up is warranted for elective repair.[33] Patients with asymptomatic hernias should also be referred for surgical repair because there is an increased risk of incarceration in the first year of life.

Testicular Mass

Testicular cancer accounts for 1% of solid tumors in children. There is an increased incidence in males with a history of cryptorchidism. Patients present with a long-standing and painless unilateral mass. Leukemic infiltration may cause unilateral or bilateral swelling in 2% to 5% of boys with new onset disease. A reactive hydrocele may be seen in 7% to 25% of patients and can result in misdiagnosis and delayed treatment.[10] Evaluation includes ultrasound and referral to a pediatric oncologist and urologic surgeon for staging and management.

Trauma

Scrotal trauma is common in active males and usually results from blunt injury. Although the mobility of male genitalia may reduce the severity of injury, trauma can result in a scrotal hematoma, hematocele, testicular rupture or testicular torsion. Unless the testis is clearly normal on examination, ultrasound should be performed. Surgical exploration is needed for torsion, large hematoceles and testicular rupture.

Scrotal lacerations infrequently accompany blunt injury. ED repair using absorbable suture (or wound adhesive, depending on the size of the wound) is appropriate for superficial wounds. Penetration through the scrotal wall and injury to or exposure of scrotal contents warrant surgical consultation.

FEMALE GENITOURINARY DISORDERS

Genital Examination

A well-prepared and carefully conducted genital examination is neither painful nor threatening. A female chaperone should accompany a male examiner. An assistant may provide instruction and reassurance to the patient as well as organize culture materials and supply skin traction when needed. Frog-leg and knee-chest examinations (Figure 19.10) are complimentary.[34] The supine frog-leg position is the easiest and least threatening and is appropriate for obtaining cultures. Gentle traction of the labia majora in an outward, upward direction provides exposure of the vaginal orifice. To allay patient anxiety, the patient may lie on her parent's lap. The knee-chest position is difficult for fearful patients but allows excellent visualization of the vaginal vault and draws out hymeneal edge for detailed inspection. The patient starts on hands and knees, then rests her head on a pillow and relaxes the abdomen to assume a swayback position. Upward and outward pressure on the buttocks adjacent to the vaginal orifice provides exposure.

The nonestrogenized introitus and hymen are very sensitive; therefore, some texts recommend aspiration by a variety of techniques including small droppers, feeding tubes and the more complex combinations of catheters. However, swabs that only contact the vaginal mucosa appear to be well tolerated and more convenient in the ED setting. A moistened calcium alginate or polyester tip wire swab is suitable for this purpose.

Genital Bleeding

Although possibly physiologic in newborn and pubertal patients, bleeding in prepubertal patients warrants

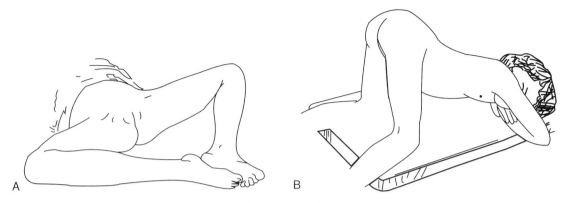

Figure 19.10. Frog-leg and knee-chest positions for the female genital examination.

investigation into the many possible causes. Accidental trauma is common and is usually blunt, affecting external structures only. However, hymeneal or vaginal injuries in the absence of a plausible explanation should raise concern for abuse. Foreign bodies cause 18% of prepubertal bleeding and up to 50% of bleeding without discharge.[35] Local conditions such as vaginitis, lichen sclerosus et atrophicus, and vulvar Crohn's disease may present with genital bleeding.

Anatomic causes include vaginal masses (polyps, hemangiomas, papillomas and malignancies) and nonvaginal lesions such as urethral prolapse, rectal polyps, and rectal prolapse. In addition to the normal physiologic events of newborn withdrawal bleeding and true puberty, endocrine causes include precocious puberty, hypothyroidism and exogenous exposure. Except in the menstruating patient, coagulopathies are less likely to present as isolated genital bleeding. If the examination is unrevealing and the patient is hemodynamically normal, an elective evaluation may include blood studies for concentrations of estradiol; follicle-stimulating, leutenizing, and thyroid-stimulating hormones; ultrasonography; examination under anesthesia or magnetic resonance imaging.[36]

Urethral Prolapse

Urethral prolapse commonly presents with painless blood staining (a minority have urinary symptoms[37]) and appears as a doughnut-shaped mass completely encircling the urethra (Figure 19.11). African American girls between 2 and 10 years of age are most commonly affected.[38] The

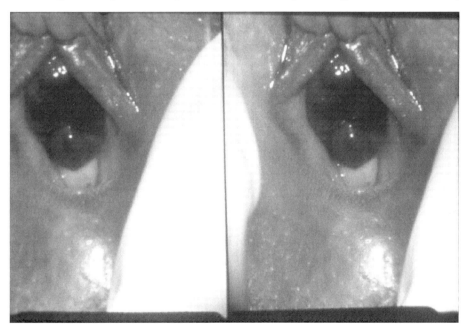

Figure 19.11. Urethral prolapse. (Courtesy of Marilyn Kaufhold, MD.)

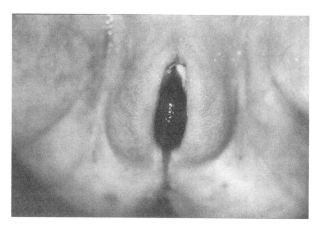

Figure 19.12. Interlabial mass, prolapsed ectopic ureterocele.

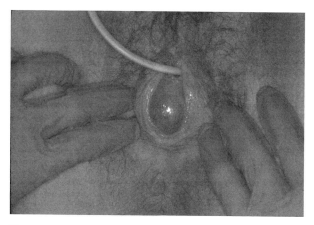

Figure 19.13. Preoperative view of bulging imperforate hymen.

etiology is unknown, but the pathophysiology may involve the presence of redundant mucosa or a cleavage plane between smooth muscle layers.

Because urethral prolapse is the only lesion completely encircling the urethra, visual inspection is sufficient for the diagnosis. If doubt remains, passage of a small urinary catheter through the center of the lesion is diagnostic. Treatment ranges from observation to surgical excision. Small, nonnecrotic prolapses benefit from sitz baths, warm compresses and topical antiseptics. A common recommendation is for topical estrogen daily for 2 weeks,[39] but controlled trials of efficacy are lacking. More complex or necrotic lesions warrant urologic consultation.

Interlabial masses other than urethral prolapse are much rarer.[40] Structural defects include prolapsed ectopic ureterocele (Figure 19.12) arising from a cystic dilation of terminal ureter, prolapsed bladder and hydrometrocolpos associated with imperforate hymen. Acquired masses include urethral or vaginal polyps, hemangiomas, condyloma acuminata, and benign (neurofibromatosis, lipomas, fibromas) and malignant neoplasms (most commonly, sarcoma botryoides). Paraurethral and vaginal wall (Gartner's) cysts usually accompany a normal (or possibly laterally displaced) urethra and introitus and may resolve spontaneously over 1 to 2 months, if not infected.

Imperforate Hymen

If not detected during routine newborn or childhood examinations, imperforate hymen leads to symptomatic outflow obstruction in early infancy or at menarche. The newborn presents with a lower abdominal mass, bulging hymen, hydrocolpos palpable on rectal examination and

mass effect (urinary retention, hydronephrosis, respiratory compromise, lower extremity edema). The pubertal presentation includes amenorrhea, intermittent (not always cyclic) abdominal pain, bulging blue hymeneal membrane and mass effect (urinary retention, constipation, hydronephrosis) (Figure 19.13). Surgical excision is curative. Other variants of vaginal outflow obstruction (transverse vaginal septum, vaginal agenesis) are rarer and often associated with other GU anomalies.

Foreign Bodies

The most common foreign body is toilet paper. A persistent vaginal discharge, especially if brown or bloody,[41] may be the presenting symptom. Vaginal inspection may reveal the foreign body. Techniques for removal include irrigation and vaginoscopy.[41] Rectal examination may assist in location and expression of the foreign body. Recurrence may be due to unchanged behavior, failure to remove all of the foreign body especially if adherent to unestrogenized mucosa, or abuse.

Lichen sclerosus et atrophicus

Lichen sclerosus is most common in postmenopausal women, but 5% to 15% of cases occur in prepubertal girls, occasionally prompting concern for sexual abuse. The history reveals local discomfort (pruritis, pain, dysuria, pain with defecation). The individual lesions are ivory papules that coalesce to form plaques, leaving whitened, parchment-like skin in a figure-eight pattern surrounding the vulva and anus (Figure 19.14). Hemorrhagic lesions and bleeding can occur along with anatomic changes and

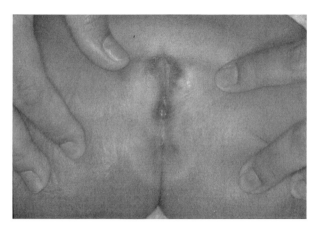

Figure 19.14. Lichen sclerosus with typical figure-eight configuration surrounding vulva and anus with hemorrhagic changes.

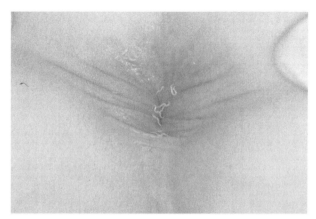

Figure 19.15. Pinworms exposed on anal skin.

scarring in more advanced cases. The etiology is unknown but may be autoimmune. Initial treatment is symptomatic, with removal of local irritant (as with vulvovaginitis), application of bland ointment and night time antipruritics. Persistent or severe cases may require specialty referral for consideration of high potency topical corticosteroids[42] or newer therapies such as calcineurin antagonists.[43]

Vulvovaginitis

Vulvovaginitis, the most common pediatric gynecologic problem, presents as primary vaginitis, primary vulvitis or both. Symptoms of vulvitis include dysuria, pruritis, erythema and secondary excoriation. Vaginitis produces a discharge without external symptoms. In girls younger than 1 month of age and those who have reached puberty, vaginal discharge may represent a physiologic leukorrhea. At other times, the vagina is inactive as a secretory organ, and liquid secretions warrant evaluation.

Important contributors to prepubertal vulvovaginitis include proximity of the vulva and vagina to the anus, increased exposure of the external genitalia due to the absence of hair and paucity of fat in the labia and mons; and lack of estrogen (more alkaline environment with "atrophic" mucosa). Anatomic variants and excess weight predispose to retention of urine, secretions and other irritants (residual soap, detergent, or toilet paper). Modifiable risk factors include poorer hygiene habits; tight-fitting, nonabsorbent garments and prolonged contact with wet swim suits; and external irritants such as soaps, bubble baths and laundry detergents. Discharge can be scant or copious and purulent. Bleeding is often due to denuding

or excoriation and usually a minor component of the complaint. Nonspecific vulvovaginitis accounts for the majority (up to 75%) of cases.[44]

If cultured, predominantly normal flora are present, although overgrowth of subpopulations such as anaerobes, *E. coli*, and Candida may occur. Isolation of a specific pathogen is more likely with a greenish discharge and abrupt onset. Group A streptococcal vaginitis occurs with asymptomatic carriage or scarlet fever and may result from autoinoculation. Intense local erythema and a possibly blood-stained discharge are characteristic. Less commonly, other respiratory organisms may be involved.

Preceding diarrheal illness may predispose to infection with enteric organisms. Shigella vaginitis, particularly *Shigella flexneri*, presents with a mucopurulent to bloody discharge and may require prolonged treatment, even when antibiotics are appropriate to the sensitivities.[45] Although pinworms (*Enterobius vermicularis*) arise from the anus, they can give rise to significant genital symptoms (Figure 19.15). Prepubertal vaginal pH is hostile to yeast; therefore, fungal vaginitis should prompt consideration of diabetes mellitus if the patient is out of diapers and not taking systemic antibiotics or corticosteroids. Although possibly transmitted during birth, sexually transmitted organisms at any other time require an evaluation for sexual abuse.

Because most vulvovaginitis is nonspecific, treatment is primarily symptomatic and includes loose-fitting, absorbent clothing; correct hygiene (wiping front to back, avoiding excess exposure to soaps); and changes in laundry practices (avoiding additives and double-rinsing clothes). During sitz baths, the patient sits with legs abducted in water and uses soap and shampoo in a separate shower.

Vigorous local cleaning is unnecessary, but thorough drying before dressing may hasten resolution. Voiding with legs abducted avoids retention of urine or reflux into the vagina. Antipruritics and bland ointments may be useful, and a low-potency topical corticosteroid can be considered with caution if there is significant irritation. Mebendazole may be given if the history is suggestive of pinworm infestation. Otherwise, the clinician may safely withhold antibiotics unless there is a specific pathogen or long-term failure of local care measures. If follow-up is reliable, the clinician may culture selectively for purulent or bloody discharge, recurrent or persistent symptoms and any suspicion of abuse or sexually transmitted infection.

Other causes of vulvar erythema and vaginal discharge include foreign bodies and other masses; skin conditions such as seborrheic dermatitis, atopic dermatitis and psoriasis; systemic conditions such as toxic shock syndrome, measles, Kawasaki disease and acrodermatitis enteropathica; and urologic anomalies such as ectopic ureter, fistulas and duplicated vagina.

Straddle Injuries

Straddle injuries vary from mild echymoses or shallow lacerations to large hematomas or deep wounds requiring sutures. Such injuries occasionally raise concern over the possibility of abuse. Past literature suggested that anterior injury results from accidental trauma and that posterior injury (posterior fourchette, perineal body) is suspicious for abuse.[46] However, studies of accidental straddle injury demonstrate that, although minor anterior injuries (especially labial) predominate, posterior injuries (Figure 19.16) are common (16%–34%).[47,48] Hymeneal injuries are rare. Findings of concern for abuse include age younger than 9 months; perianal, vaginal and hymeneal injuries without plausible description of an accidental penetrating mechanism; and associated extragenital trauma. Suture repair is rarely necessary, and most wounds heal without sequelae with only local care measures such as sitz baths. At times it is difficult to perform a complete examination in the ED; therefore, a thorough examination in the operating room under anesthesia may be required.

LABIAL ADHESIONS

Labial adhesions are very common and often unrecognized by the parents. Many are asymptomatic, although

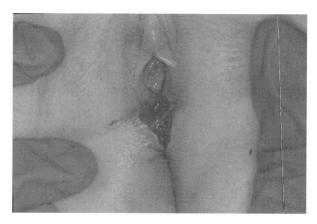

Figure 19.16. Extensive accidental straddle injury requiring repair of posterior fourchette and perineal body.

symptoms suggestive of urinary infection may be present. ED clinicians often encounter them at the time of attempted urethral catheterization for fever evaluation. They range from partial adhesions to near-complete adhesions that leave a mere pinhole for urinary outflow. Examination reveals a thin transparent vertical midline adhesion, although denser adhesions occur (Figure 19.17). Local irritants may cause denuded labial surfaces of nonestrogenized mucosa to come in contact and fuse. The earlier literature suggested abusive etiology,[49] but some degree of adhesion is found in nearly 40% of normal girls.[50] Urine cultures yield bacterial pathogens at a greater rate in asymptomatic[51] and symptomatic[52] patients with adhesions than in patients without adhesions. However, the reliance on clean catch and bag collection methods complicates interpretation of clinical significance.

Although many adhesions readily separate with a mild amount of friction or pressure (e.g., during antiseptic preparation for urethral catheterization), urgent or

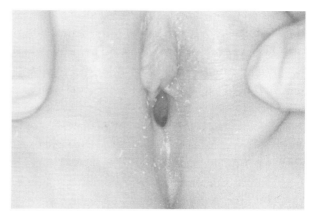

Figure 19.17. Partial labial adhesion (posterior) resulting in false-positive voided urine cultures.

aggressive treatment is rarely necessary. For small adhesions, improved hygiene and application of a bland ointment may suffice. For symptomatic or denser adhesions, sparing topical application of conjugated or synthetic estrogens (conjugated estrogens 0.1% [Premarin] cream or dienestrol .01% cream) to the line of fusion will facilitate separation. Initial application is twice daily for 2 weeks followed by nightly application for 2 to 3 weeks and then continued use of a bland ointment.[53] Careful parent teaching on the proper amount and location of application will prevent local and systemic complications such as telarche, labial pigmentation and the development of downy hairs. Thicker or refractory adhesions may require manual or operative separation.[54] Urethral catheterization, if necessary, is possible by using the catheter to displace (with or without lysis) the opening of the adhesion and then advancing the catheter in the expected location of the urethra.

OVARIAN TORSION

In contrast to testicular torsion, the evaluation of adnexal torsion is complicated by the relatively inaccessible location. Even in adult populations, the presentation is variable and potentially misleading.[55] Pain is typically in the lower abdomen or pelvis and may include sudden onset, colicky nature, radiation to flank, back or groin.

Physical findings include abdominal tenderness (mild in 35%), pelvic tenderness (absent in 29%), and pelvic mass (reported in only 47%). In only half of cases is adnexal torsion the preoperative diagnosis. Clinical information on pediatric torsion is less detailed. Right-sided lesions predominate by a ratio of 1.3:1. Vomiting is present in 73%, and an abdominal mass is palpable in less than 20%. In nearly one third of right-sided lesions, the presumed diagnosis was appendicitis. Operative findings include mature cystic teratoma in 47%; follicular or corpus luteum cyst in 27% (primarily adolescents); otherwise normal ovary in 16%; and other benign and malignant neoplasms in the rest.[56]

Ultrasound is the primary diagnostic modality. Flow abnormalities on Doppler study, although highly specific, may have poor sensitivity (34%–40%) for torsion in adults[57] and children.[58] Adnexal enlargement may be a more reliable sonographic sign[58] and is also evident on computed tomography obtained to evaluate other intra-abdominal conditions. On occasion, plain radiography

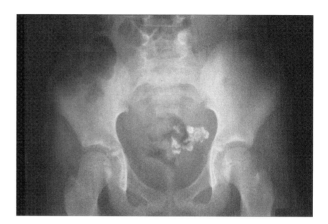

Figure 19.18. Calcified abdominal mass in a young girl presenting with lower abdominal pain. Ultimately, the mass was pathologically demonstrated to be a teratoma.

reveals calcification within a teratoma (Figure 19.18). Surgical intervention with detorsion may lead to ovarian salvage, even if the symptoms are prolonged[59] or the ovary appears to be ischemic at exploration.[60]

PITFALLS

- Failure to perform an adequate genital examination during the evaluation of abdominal, hip or proximal lower extremity pain is an avoidable cause of missed diagnoses of testicular torsion, imperforate hymen, genital trauma and foreign bodies.
- Failure to inspect the perineum of the young girl with dysuria and pyuria may result in unnecessary antibiotic treatment if labial adhesions are the cause of the symptoms.
- Failure to recognize lichen sclerosus may result in the mistaken diagnosis of sexual abuse.
- Failure to treat paraphimosis promptly may result in progressive edema which may impede manual reduction and necessitate a surgical reduction.
- Failure to examine the genitalia of a young female infant or of a premenarchal adolescent female who presents with abdominal mass, abdominal pain, or urinary retention may result in the delayed diagnosis of imperforate hymen.
- After the newborn period and before puberty, vaginal discharge should never be considered normal and should prompt evaluation for underlying pathology.

REFERENCES

1. Van Howe R. Cost-effective treatment of phimosis. *Pediatrics.* 1998;102:1–4.
2. Pontari MA. Phimosis and paraphimosis. In: Seidman EJ, Hanno PM, eds. *Current Urologic Therapy.* Philadelphia, PA: WB Saunders; 1994:392–397.

3. Dewan PA, Tieu HC. Phimosis: Is circumcision necessary? *J Paediatr Child Health*. 1996;32:285–289.

4. Chu C, Chen K, Diau G. Topical steroid treatment of phimosis in boys. *J Urol*. 1999;162:861–863.

5. Kanegaye JT. Reduction of paraphimosis. In: Walsh-Sukys MC, Krug SE, eds. *Procedures in Infants and Children*. Philadelphia, PA: WB Saunders; 1997:386–388.

6. Barone J, Fleisher M. Treatment of paraphimosis using the "puncture" technique. *Pediatr Emerg Care*. 1993;9:298–299.

7. Herzog LW, Alvarez SR. The frequency of foreskin problems in uncircumcised children. *Am J Dis Child*. 1986;140:254–256

8. Orden B, Martin R, Franco A, et al. Balanitis caused by group A beta-hemolytic streptococci. *Pediatr Infect Dis J*. 1996;15:920–921.

9. Chacko MR, Staat MA, Woods CR. Genital infections in childhood and adolescence. In: Feigin RD, Cherry JD, Demmler GJ, et al, eds. *Textbook of Pediatric Infectious Diseases*, 5th ed. Philadelphia, PA: WB Saunders; 2004:562–604.

10. McCollough M, Sharieff G. Renal and genitourinary tract disorders. In: Marx J, Hockberger R, Walls R, eds. *Rosen's Emergency Medicine Concepts and Clinical Practice*, 6th ed. Philadelphia, PA: Mosby; 2006:2635–2656.

11. Mulhall JP, Honig SC. Priapism: diagnosis and management. *Acad Emerg Med*. 1996;3:810–816.

12. American Academy of Pediatrics. Task Force on Circumcision. Circumcision Policy Statement. *Pediatrics*. 1999;103(3):686–693.

13. Persad R, Sharma S, McTavish J, et al. Clinical presentation and pathophysiology of meatal stenosis following circumcision. *Br J Urol*. 1995;75:91–93.

14. Langer J, Coplen D. Circumcision and pediatric disorders of the penis. *Pediatr Clin North Am*. 1998;45:801–812.

15. Kanegaye J. Penile zipper injury: a simple and less threatening approach using mineral oil. *Pediatr Emerg Care*. 1993;9:90–91.

16. Kass E, Reitelman C. Adolescent varicocele. *Urol Clin North Am*. 1995;22:154.

17. Niedzielski J, Paduch D, Racynski P. Assessment of adolescent varicocele. *Pediatr Surg Int*. 1997;12:410–413.

18. Pillai S, Besner G. Pediatric testicular problems. *Ped Clin North Am*. 1998;45:813–830.

19. Bomalaski A, Mills J, Argueso L. Iliac vein compression syndrome: an unusual cause of varicocele. *J Vasc Surg*. 1993;18:1065.

20. Ulker V, Garibyan H, Kurth KH. Comparison of inguinal and laparoscopic approaches in the treatment of varicocele. *Int Urol Nephrol*. 1997;29:71–77.

21. Castillo J, Combest F, Dixon E, et al. Urinary and renal disorders. In: Barkin M, ed. *Pediatric Emergency Medicine: Concepts and Clinical Practice*. St. Louis, MO: Mosby; 1997:1127–1174.

22. Neinstein L, Goldenring J, Carpenter S. Nonsexual transmission of sexually transmitted diseases: An infrequent occurrence. *Pediatrics*. 1984;74:67–76.

23. Herberner TE. Ultrasound in the assessment of the acute scrotum. *J Clin Ultrasound*. 1996;24:405–421.

24. Paltiel HJ. Acute scrotal symptoms in boys with an indeterminate clinical presentation: comparison of color Doppler sonography and scintigraphy. *Radiology*. 1998;207:223–231.

25. Kadish H, Bolte R. A retrospective review of pediatric patients with epididymitis, testicular torsion, and torsion of testicular appendages. *Pediatrics*. 1998;102:73–76.

26. Cilento BG, Najjars SS, Atalar A. Cryptorchidism and testicular torsion. *Pediatr Clin North Am*. 1993;40:1133–1149.

27. Al Mufti RA, Ogedegbe AK, Laftery K. The use of Doppler ultrasound in the clinical management of acute testicular pain. *Br J Urol*. 1995;76:625–627.

28. Coley BD, Frush DP, Babcock DS, et al. Acute testicular torsion: comparison of unenhanced power Doppler US, color Doppler US, and radionuclide imaging. *Radiology*. 1996;199:441–446.

29. Granados EA, Caicedo P, Garat JM. Testicular torsion after 12 hours. III. *Arch Esp Urol*. 1998;51:978–981.

30. Knight PJ, Vassy LE. The diagnosis and treatment of the acute scrotum in children and adolescents. *Ann Surg*. 1984;200:664–673.

31. Cornel EB, Karthaus HF. Manual derotation of the twisted spermatic cord. *Br J Urol*. 1999;83:672–674.

32. Schul M, Keating M. The acute pediatric scrotum. *J Emerg Med*. 1993;11:566–577.

33. Gahukamble DE, Khamage AS. Early versus delayed repair of reduced incarcerated inguinal hernias in the pediatric population. *J Pediatr Surg*. 1996;31:1218.

34. McCann J, Voris J, Simon M, Wells R. Comparison of genital examination techniques in prepubertal girls. *Pediatrics*. 1990;85:182–187.

35. Paradise JE, Willis ED. Probability of vaginal foreign body in girls with genital complaints. *Am J Dis Child*. 1985;139:472–476.

36. Perlman SE. Management quandary. Premenarchal vaginal bleeding. *J Pediatr Adolesc Gynecol*. 2001;14:135–136.

37. Richardson DA, Hajj SN, Herbst AL. Medical treatment of urethral prolapse in children. *Obstet Gynecol*. 1982;59:69–74.

38. Anveden-Hertzberg L, Gauderer MW, Elder JS. Urethral prolapse: an often misdiagnosed cause of urogenital bleeding in girls. *Pediatr Emerg Care*. 1995;11:212–214.

39. Mercer LJ, Mueller CM, Hajj SN. Medical treatment of urethral prolapse in the premenarchal female. *Adolesc Pediatr Gynecol*. 1988;1:181–184.

40. Klee LW, Rink RC, Gleason PE, et al. Urethral polyp presenting as interlabial mass in young girls. *Urology*. 1993;41:132–133.

41. Smith YR, Berman DR, Quint EH. Premenarchal vaginal discharge: findings of procedures to rule out foreign bodies. *J Pediatr Adolesc Gynecol*. 2002;15:22–230.

42. Smith YR, Quint EH. Clobetasol propionate in the treatment of premenarchal vulvar lichen sclerosus. *Obstet Gynecol*. 2001;98:588–591.

43. Strittmatter HJ, Hengge UR, Blecken SR. Calcineurin antagonists in vulvar lichen sclerosus. *Arch Gynecol Obstet*. 2006;274:266–270.

44. Emans SJ. Vulvovaginal problems in the prepubertal child. In: Emans SJ, Laufer MR, Goldstein DP, eds. *Pediatric and*

Adolescent Gynecology, 5th ed. Philadelphia, PA: Lippincott Williams & Wilkins; 2005:83–119.

45. Baiulescu M, Hannon PR, Marcinak JF, et al. Chronic vulvovaginitis caused by antibiotic-resistant *Shigella flexneri* in a prepubertal child. *Pediatr Infect Dis J.* 2002;21:170–172.

46. McCann J, Voris J, Simon M. Labial adhesions and posterior fourchette injuries in childhood sexual abuse. *Am J Dis Child.* 1988;142:659–663.

47. Dowd MD, Fitzmaurice L, Knapp JF, et al. The interpretation of urogenital findings in children with straddle injuries. *J Pediatr Surg.* 1994;29:7–10.

48. Bond GR, Dowd MD, Landsman I, et al. Unintentional perineal injury in prepubescent girls: a multicenter, prospective report of 56 girls. *Pediatrics.* 1995;95:628–631.

49. Berkowitz CD, Elvik SL, Logan MK. Labial fusion in prepubescent girls: a marker for sexual abuse? *Am J Obstet Gynecol.* 1987;156:16–20.

50. McCann J, Wells R, Simon M, et al. Genital findings in prepubertal girls selected for nonabuse: a descriptive study. *Pediatrics.* 1990;86:428–439.

51. Leung AK, Robson WL. Labial fusion and asymptomatic bacteriuria. *Eur J Pediatr.* 1993;152:250–251.

52. Leung AK, Robson WL. Labial fusion and urinary tract infection. *Child Nephrol Urol.* 1992;12:62–64.

53. Leung AKC, Robson WLM, Kao CP, et al. Treatment of labial fusion with topical estrogen therapy. *Clin Pediatr (Phila).* 2005;44:245–247.

54. Muram D. Treatment of prepubertal girls with labial adhesions. *J Pediatr Adolesc Gynecol.* 1999;12:67–70.

55. Houry D, Abbott JT. Ovarian torsion: a fifteen-year review. *Ann Emerg Med.* 2001;38:156–159.

56. Kokoska ER, Keller MS, Weber TR. Acute ovarian torsion in children. *Am J Surg.* 2000;180:462–465.

57. Pena JE, Ufberg D, Cooney N, et al. Usefulness of Doppler sonography in the diagnosis of ovarian torsion. *Fertil Steril.* 2000;73:1047–1050.

58. Servaes S, Zurakowski D, Laufer MR, et al. Sonographic findings of ovarian torsion in children. *Pediatr Radiol.* 2007;37:446–451.

59. Anders JF, Powell EC. Urgency of evaluation and outcome of acute ovarian torsion in pediatric patients. *Arch Pediatr Adolesc Med.* 2005;159:532–535.

60. Pansky M, Abargil A, Dreazen E, et al. Conservative management of adnexal torsion in premenarchal girls. *J Am Assoc Gynecol Laparosc.* 2000;7:121–124.

In this chapter, two important conditions with which infants may present during the first year of life are discussed. Section I reviews sickle cell disease and Section II reviews inherited bleeding disorders. The reader is referred to standard textbooks for a discussion of oncologic disease.

SECTION I. SICKLE CELL EMERGENCIES

Nadeem Qureshi, Stephen Gletsu and Mohammed Al-Mogbil

Sickle cell disease (SCD) represents a group of inherited hemoglobinopathies that are characterized by dysmorphic red blood cells (RBCs), impaired homeostatic balance involving the vascular endothelium, nitric oxide build up leading to microvascular occlusion and resultant multiorgan ischemia-reperfusion injury. The molecular basis of the disease is the substitution of glutamine for valine in the sixth position of the globin beta chain, which permits crystallization of the hemoglobin molecules in conditions of relative hypoxia.

The sickle cell trait is found in 8% to 10% of African Americans. Sickle cell anemia occurs in 1 in 400 to 600 newborns. The disease is seen less commonly in the Hispanic, southern European, and Middle Eastern populations.[1]

Hemoglobin electrophoresis provides rapid and accurate diagnosis of hemoglobinopathies. However, the sickle cell prep (Sickledex) can produce false-negative results before 4 to 6 months of age due to the presence of normal maternal hemoglobin. Today, state mandated newborn screening programs allow for early diagnosis of these disorders. However, unexplained anemia in African American children should raise the suspicion of a hemoglobinopathy. The presence of any sickle forms on a peripheral blood smear is presumptive evidence of sickle cell anemia.

Patients with SCD may present with signs and symptoms involving any organ; however, the majority of emergency department (ED) visits are due to recurrent vaso-occlusive crisis (VOC), invasive infections, acute chest syndrome (ACS), stroke and priapism. The management of priapism is discussed in detail in Chapter 19. The severity of clinical manifestations of these syndromes depends on the specific type of hemoglobinopathy present (Table 20.I.1).

The ED evaluation depends on the patient's presentation. Clinical symptoms may begin as early as 3 to 4 months of age, when significant amounts of hemoglobin S become present. Early recognition and aggressive ED management can improve morbidity and mortality associated with these disorders. Optimal long-term care is best provided through improved parent education and by physicians familiar with the disease and its complications.

CLINICAL PRESENTATIONS AND MANAGEMENT

Sepsis

Sepsis is the leading cause of morbidity and mortality in patients with SCD,[2] even with current vaccination and prophylactic antibiotic regimens. These patients suffer from functional asplenia (5 months–5 years) due to autoinfarction resulting in deficient antibody production and impaired phagocytosis. This leaves the host susceptible to various life-threatening infections (Table 20.I.2).

Streptococcus pneumoniae is the most common cause of sepsis and meningitis in children (<3 years), and it has a mortality rate of 20% to 50%. Bacterial meningitis and septicemia are more than 600 times more common in children with sickle cell anemia than in children without this

Table 20.I.1. Sickle cell syndromes: specific hemoglobinopathy and associated findings

Hemoglobinopathy	Clinical presentations	Hb (g/dL)	Hb S (%)	Hb A (%)	Hb A$_2$ (%)	Hb F (%)
Sickle cell trait (carrier)	Asymptomatic	Normal	40	60	<3.5	0
Sickle Cell Disease (Different Variants)						
Hb SS (sickle cell anemia)	Severe	6–8	>90	0	<3.5	<10
Hb S beta° (thalassemia)	Moderate–severe	7–9	>80	0	>3.5	<20
Hb S beta (thalassemia)	Mild–moderate	9–12	>60	10–30	>3.5	<20
Hb SC	Mild–moderate	10–15	50	0	‡	0

‡, Hb C 50%

Table 20.I.2. Various microorganisms causing lethal infections in patients with sickle cell disease

Microorganism	Infection	Remarks
Bacterial Organisms		
Streptococcus pneumoniae	Septicemia	Common despite prophylaxis and vaccine
	Meningitis	Low frequency compared with pre-vaccine era
	Pneumonia	Rare except in children
	Septic arthritis	Uncommon
Haemophilus influenza type B	Septicemia	
	Meningitis	
	Pneumonia	Low frequency compared with pre-vaccine era
Salmonella species	Osteomyelitis	Most common cause of bone and joint infection
	Septicemia	
Escherichia coli and other gram-negative enteric pathogens	Septicemia	Urinary tract infection
Staphylococcus aureus	Osteomyelitis	Uncommon
Mycoplasma pneumoniae	Pneumonia	Pleural effusions; multilobar involvement
Chlamydia pneumoniae	Pneumonia	
Viral Organisms		
Parvovirus B19	Aplastic crisis	Marked bone marrow suppression
Hepatitis viruses (A, B and C)	Hepatitis	Hyperbilirubinemia

disease.[3] Pneumococcal sepsis, seen in adults, is equally devastating. Table 20.I.3 lists the ED management of sepsis in patients with SCD. Early recognition of a febrile episode and prompt administration of intravenous (IV) antibiotics can lower the risk of severe pneumococcal sepsis. However, resistant strains of pneumococcus have emerged, necessitating an alternative antibiotics (vancomycin) regimen.

Vaccination and daily penicillin prophylaxis starting at 2 months of age has been shown to reduce the incidence of pneumococcal sepsis.[4] The effectiveness of the 23-valent pneumococcal polysaccharide vaccine among children with SCD is 80% to 90%.[5] Penicillin prophylaxis in children younger than 3 years is 125 mg orally twice daily,[6,7] and the prophylaxis dosage is 250 mg orally twice daily for children ages 3 to 5 years. It is imperative that parents are educated about the signs and symptoms of sepsis.

Table 20.I.3. Management of sepsis in patients with sickle cell disease

Evaluation
History: Immunization and penicillin prophylaxis
Laboratory studies: CBC count, electrolytes, Hb S levels,
Cultures (blood, urine, throat, CSF) as indicated
CXR

Treatment
IV Ceftriaxone 75 mg/kg
Add vancomycin 15 mg/kg if meningitis is suspected
Hydration
Analgesia: Morphine 0.1 mg/kg IV (pain relief)
Simple blood transfusion to increase Hb to 9–10g/dL (reduce
    secondary organ damage)

Admission Criteria
Children <1 year of age
High risk: Fever > 40°C , toxic appearing, infiltrate on CXR,
    low Hb

CBC, complete blood cell; CSF, cerebrospinal fluid; CXR, chest x-ray;
Hb, hemoglobin.

Haemophilus influenza type B is the second most common organism responsible for sepsis in these patients. *H. influenza* vaccine given during early infancy provides excellent protection against this organism.

Salmonellosis and osteomyelitis occur more commonly in patients with SCD than in healthy children, probably secondary to infection of the infarcted bone.[8] Osteomyelitis is typically caused by salmonella (twice as common worldwide compared to staphylococcus) and *Staphylococcus aureus*. Infarction is 50 times more common than bacterial osteomyelitis in patients with SCD. Many algorithms have been devised to differentiate between the two etiologies; however, the gold standard for diagnosis remains biopsy and culture.

The ED management for patients with SCD presenting with fever (with or without focus) is to rapidly administer IV ceftriaxone (50–75 mg/kg per dose up to 2 g) after obtaining a complete blood cell count, a reticulocyte count and a blood culture. Based on clinical presentation, patients can be classified as low risk (>1 year of age, well-appearing, white blood cell count between 5000 and 30,000/mm^3, temperature <40°C, absence of pulmonary infiltrates and a reassuring hemoglobin level 8-10gm/dL or patient's usual baseline hematologic parameters) or high risk. High risk patients are admitted for inpatient therapy.[9] Furthermore, children younger than age 1 year who are febrile are typically admitted for appropriate IV antibiotics. Children with a temperature above 103°F should also be strongly considered for hospital admission. Low-risk patients can be managed in an outpatient setting with 24-hour follow-up. However, reliable follow-up must be ensured.

Aplastic Crisis

During normal conditions, the bone marrow erythroid activity is amplified (reticulocytosis >10%) to maintain baseline hemoglobin levels in patients with SCD. This increased erythropoietic activity can be interrupted by various infections, resulting in aplastic crisis. This clinical condition is characterized by a drop in hemoglobin, low or absent reticulocyte count and decreased marrow activity. Parvovirus B19 accounts for 68% of episodes of aplastic crisis followed by *Streptococcus pneumoniae*, salmonellae, and Epstein-Barr virus.

Episodes of erythroid hypoplasia, manifested by progressive anemia with reticulocytopenia (<1%), occur both

sporadically and epidemically in association with the human parvovirus B19.[10] Packed RBC transfusions may be necessary until erythroid production returns, usually within a few weeks. Patients with aplastic crisis require close monitoring as their hematocrit may fall to 10% or lower within a few days. Hydroxyurea has been shown to reduce the occurrence of aplastic crisis.[11]

Acute Splenic Sequestration

Splenic sequestration is a life-threatening condition seen in young children before the onset of autoinfarction of the spleen. Children with Hb SS have an incidence of 30% with a 15% mortality rate. These episodes often occur with viral illness. Over a period of hours, a significant portion of the circulating blood volume is sequestered in the spleen because of vaso-occlusion in the splenic vein. Patients present with hypovolemia, pallor, massive splenomegaly and occasionally, shock and death. Evaluation demonstrates splenomegaly (often massive), anemia and reticulocytosis.

Treatment is aimed at sustaining blood volume until the condition spontaneously reverses, releasing the sequestered blood. Careful monitoring and, often, a transfusion of 10 mL/kg of packed RBCs may be required.[12] Sequestration is recurrent in 50% of cases; therefore, splenectomy is recommended after resolution of acute events. Parents should be educated about how to palpate for an enlarged spleen, especially during viral illness, to detect this complication in early stages.

Acute Painful Vaso-occlusive Crisis

Acute, painful VOC episodes are the most common manifestation of SCD and the most common reason for ED presentation and hospital admission.[13] Pain is the result of tissue ischemia and infarction due to microvascular occlusion and may be severe, unpredictable and relentless. Precipitating factors include infection, dehydration, high altitude and extremes of temperature. Often, however, no precipitating factor is identified.[13]

The average rate of painful crisis per patient is 0.8 episodes per year, although 1% of all patients experience more than six episodes per year and 5% of patients account for 33% of all episodes.[14] The frequency of painful episodes is a marker of disease severity and correlates with increased mortality.[13]

The pain of VOC most often involves the lower back, chest, femoral shafts, hips, knees and abdomen. In children, the hands, feet, fingers and toes are more commonly involved. In individual patients, pain tends to recur in a limited number of sites.[13] Given the propensity of symptoms involving the chest, abdomen and extremities, the ED physician must always consider other diagnoses in SCD patients presenting with acute pain, such as ACS, septic arthritis or acute surgical abdomen. In the absence of complications, physical examination in acute VOC reveals few objective findings.

VOC is a medical emergency. Patients in acute pain presenting to the ED usually have exhausted all home care options and require parenteral opioid analgesia.[15] ED management of painful crises remains inconsistent, and barriers to optimal management persist.[15] The difficulties of treating painful crises in the ED are numerous[13]:

- Patients are treated in episodic encounters in the ED setting by health care providers with whom the patient has no established relationship.
- Patients often report severe pain but lack objective findings.
- Health professionals often fear iatrogenic opioid addiction, and patients with undertreated pain may demonstrate behavior pain that is perceived as drug-seeking in nature.

It has been shown that although patients with SCD who are receiving opioids may develop physiological dependence and tolerance, the rate of addiction in this population is no greater than in the general population.[16]

ED management has traditionally consisted of supplemental oxygen and fluids. There is no evidence that either therapy improves outcome in the nonhypoxic, euvolemic patient, and the chronic anemia and renal impairment that occurs in many patients with this condition put them at risk of pulmonary edema if they are vigorously resuscitated with isotonic fluid.[17]

The mainstay of ED management is parenteral opioid analgesia.[18] Attempts should be made to objectify the severity of the patient's pain using a pain scale. The IV route is preferred, although the subcutaneous route can be used if venous access is difficult. The intramuscular route is not appropriate as this is painful and drug absorption is unpredictable. Morphine and hydromorphone are effective. Meperidine is not recommended due to the cerebral

Table 20.I.4. Suggested approach to emergency department pain control in patients with vaso-occlusive crisis

1. Initial bolus: Morphine 0.1–0.15 mg/kg IV
2. Additional $1/4 - 1/2$ of bolus dose q15–30 minutes until pain is relieved
3. Morphine bolus q2 hours to maintain pain relief
4. If pain relief is maintained, discharge patient with oral analgesics and arrange for outpatient follow-up.
5. If pain relief is not maintained, admit patient.

nervous system toxicity of its renally eliminated metabolite normeperidine.[18]

Effective pain management requires some form of titration to ensure pain relief. One approach involves an initial bolus dose of morphine (Table 20.I.4) followed by repeated small boluses at intervals of 15 to 30 minutes until pain is relieved.[18] Patients should be carefully observed for respiratory depression and hypotension. Pain relief is then maintained with bolus doses on a fixed schedule. If pain relief is maintained, the patient is discharged on an equianalgesic dose of an oral opioid until outpatient reassessment. If pain relief is not maintained following two to three bolus doses, hospital admission is required. Adjunctive medications such as antihistamines and antinauseants may be necessary due to opioid side effects. Parenteral ketorolac cannot be routinely recommended as it does not consistently relieve pain in these patients and is limited by its potential for renal toxicity.[17]

Finally, the ED physician must be aware of the role of hydroxyurea in VOC. Although not indicated in the management of the acute painful event, hydroxyurea has been shown to decrease the incidence of VOC by 44% and is indicated in patients experiencing more than three episodes per year.[19]

Dactylitis (Hand–Foot Syndrome)

The *hand–foot syndrome* represents the symptomatic microinfarcts in the phalanges and metatarsal bones. This syndrome commonly presents between 6 and 24 months of age in children with SCD. These children present with low-grade fever and painful swelling of the hands and/or feet. Hematologic values are usually unchanged. Radiographs at the outset show only soft tissue swelling, but osteolytic and periosteal changes become evident 2 to 3

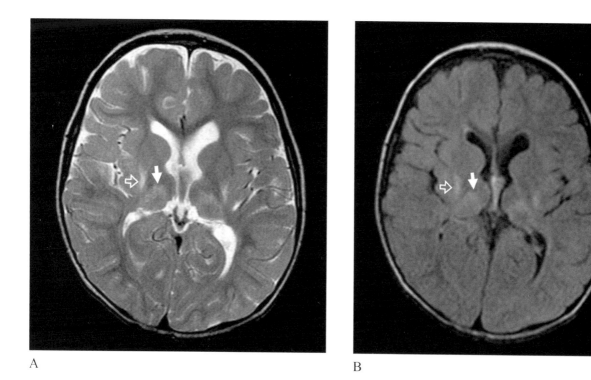

Figure 20.I.1. MRI of a 5-year-old with SCI. Ischemic lesions exist in the thalamus (*white arrows*) and posterior aspect of putamen and globus pallidus (*open arrows*).

weeks after the onset of symptoms. This classical presentation must be differentiated from osteomyelitis (either unifocal or multifocal) and trauma. Therapy consists of hydration at 150% to 200% maintenance (oral or IV fluids) and analgesia. Pain and swelling commonly resolve in 2 to 5 days. Recurrence is uncommon and usually not seen after age 2 years as collateral vascular supplies to these bones develop. Having dactylitis in infancy is a strong predictor of the possibility of severe SCD later in life.[20]

Cerebrovascular Accident

Patients with SCD suffer from neurologic injury with a spectrum that ranges from silent cerebral infarcts (SCIs) to overt strokes (Figure 20.I.1). SCIs are the most common form of neuronal damage in toddlers (<4 years old) and the cumulative incidence increases until 14 years of age. Kinney et al., in the Cooperative Study of the Sickle Cell Disease, identified 266 infants with SCD and followed them for 14 years with a minimum of one MRI at 6 years or older and showed an incidence of 22% SCI in patients without overt stroke.[21] These SCIs result in progressive neuronal damage in school age children, which

leads to lower intelligence quotient and other neurocognitive defects.

Low pain event rate, history of seizure, leukocyte count greater than 11.8×10^9 and SEN globin gene haplotype are associated with increased risk of SCI. SCI is diagnosed on abnormal MRI (focal 3-mm or larger area of abnormal signal intensity) with a normal neurological exam without a history and physical findings associated with an overt stroke. No therapy has been established for the treatment of SCI. Preliminary data from the Stroke Prevention Trial in Sickle Cell Anemia STOP trial demonstrated that blood transfusion therapy showed a 100% relative risk reduction in patients with SCI and elevated transcranial Doppler (TCD) ultrasound velocity measurement of greater than 200 cm/sec[22] (Table 20.I.5). Currently, a large National Institutes of Health funded (Silent Cerebral Infarct Transfusion SIT) trial is looking at the benefit of blood transfusion therapy in patients with SCI and normal TCD measurements.

The most catastrophic neurological event in SCD is stroke. Children with SCD are 200 to 400 times more likely to suffer a stroke, compared to children without SCD. The Cooperative Study of Sickle Cell Disease (CSSCD),[23] a large prospective study, confirmed that stroke is a constant

Table 20.I.5. Management of stroke in patients with sickle cell disease

Evaluation
• CBC count, electrolytes, Hb S levels, sample for RBC antigens
• Urgent CT or MRI (identify thrombotic versus hemorrhagic infarction, cerebral aneurysm and intracranial bleed)
• Arteriography is not indicated as it can precipitate sickling crisis
Treatment
• $1^1/_2$–2 volume exchange transfusion to reduce Hb S <30%
• ICU admission
• Neurology and hematology consultations

CBC, complete blood cell; CT, computed tomography; ICU, intensive care unit; MRI, magnetic resonance imaging; RBC, red blood cell.

threat after age 2, but the incidence is highest in the middle of a child's first 10 years of life. About 11% of all children with homozygous SCD will develop stroke by 20 years of age. In the younger child, the event is usually thrombotic; in the adolescent or adult, it may be hemorrhagic. Patients at increased risk of stroke include those with these traits: familial (genetic polymorphism), parvovirus infection, prior stroke (silent SCI) and TCD more than 200 cm/sec. Children with elevated velocities (>200 cm/sec) have a high rate of stroke (10,000:100,000 patient years). Silent stroke is the strongest risk factor for overt stroke. In the ED, any untoward neurologic event in a patient with SCD is considered a cerebrovascular accident until proven otherwise.

Early recognition and aggressive treatment results in improved outcomes. Long-term treatment necessitates hypertransfusion for several years to reduce the 66% chance of a recurrent cerebrovascular accident.[12,24] Hydroxyurea therapy also has been shown to be effective for prevention of recurrent stroke in patients with SCD.[24,25]

The Acute Chest Syndrome

ACS in SCD is a clinical syndrome with multiple etiologies that share a common pathophysiologic endpoint of acute lung injury.[26,27] ACS is defined by the presence of a new segmental pulmonary infiltrate on chest radiograph accompanied by at least one of the following clinical symptoms or signs[26]:

1. Temperature greater than 38.5°C
2. Chest pain
3. Cough
4. Wheezing
5. Tachypnea

The pathophysiology of acute lung injury in SCD is multifactorial with a final common pathway of pulmonary microvascular obstruction, tissue hypoxia, ischemia and infarction.[26] Recurrent episodes of acute lung injury may lead to chronic restrictive lung disease.[26,27] A large multicenter trial found the most common causes of ACS to be related to fat embolism from infarcted bone marrow, respiratory infections and isolated lung infarction. The most common pathogens identified in this study were Chlamydia, Mycoplasma and respiratory viruses. The rate of fibrin thromboembolism is no greater in patients with SCD compared with the general population, and thromboembolism is very difficult to distinguish from sickle vaso-occlusion on chest CT scan or radionuclide perfusion scanning.[26]

ACS is the leading cause of death among patients with SCD and the second leading cause of hospitalization.[26] One half of all patients with SCD will have one episode of ACS and some patients will experience multiple events. One half of all cases of ACS occur following hospitalization for an acute pain crisis. The peak incidence occurs between the ages of 2 and 4 years.[26] There is a higher incidence of ACS in those with HbSS disease and in patients with higher baseline white blood cell counts. Patients with higher HbF levels have a lower incidence of ACS, which may account for the lower incidence in patients younger than 2 years of age and in patients taking hydroxyurea.[19]

The clinical presentation of ACS in the ED is variable and may mimic that of other chest syndromes in the general population, in particular bacterial pneumonia. It is important for the ED physician to be aware that the clinical course of ACS in a patient with SCD differs from that of the general population presenting with similar findings. SCD patients with ACS may present with a transient benign illness or may present in respiratory failure requiring intubation and mechanical ventilation. In one study, the average length of hospital admission was 10.5 days and 13% of patients required mechanical ventilation.[26] During hospitalization, 11% experienced neurological symptoms and 9% of patients over the age of 20 years died. Factors predictive of a more severe course are age older than 20 years, pain in the arms and legs on presentation, platelet count less than 200,000/μL and multilobar involvement or pleural effusion on chest radiograph.

Table 20.I.6. Emergency department management of acute chest syndrome in children

1. O_2 to keep Sao_2 >92%
2. IV D5: $1/4$ normal saline at 1.5 × maintenance
3. Antibiotics: Ceftriaxone 50-75mg/kg IV and azithromycin 10mg/kg (max 500mg)
   (plus Vancomycin if resistant *S. Pneumoniae* is suspected)
4. Morphine IV titrated to pain relief
5. Salbutamol 2.5–5 mg q1–4 hr
6. Incentive spirometry
7. Simple or exchange transfusion
8. Admission

Clinical findings in ACS appear to be age-dependent. Although fever is the most common presenting finding in all patients, children younger than 10 years of age are more likely to present with cough and wheezing, whereas adolescents and adults more commonly present with chest and extremity pain. Bacteremia is more common in children with ACS, and *S. pneumoniae* is the most common isolate. Initial chest radiographs may be negative in nearly half of cases. In children, upper and middle lobe infiltrates are more common, whereas adults are more likely to have isolated lower lobe involvement and pleural effusions.[26]

The management of ACS is essentially supportive and aims to maintain alveolar ventilation and gas exchange and to prevent further pulmonary injury (Table 20.I.6). Patients should receive supplemental oxygen to maintain oxygen saturation above 92%.[26,27] Fluid deficits should be corrected with normal saline infusion then changed to hypotonic fluid (e.g., 5% dextrose in $1/4$ normal saline at 1.5× maintenance requirement). Overaggressive hydration must be avoided to prevent pulmonary edema. Patients should receive prompt antibiotic therapy to cover the most common organisms identified in this syndrome with consideration given to local sensitivity patterns. A respiratory quinolone by itself or a third or fourth generation cephalosporin in combination with a macrolide should provide adequate coverage.[26,27] Patients should be given bronchodilators as all patients have been demonstrated to have some degree of airflow obstruction, even in the absence of wheezing.[26,27] Ventilation may be compromised by pain secondary to ischemia or infarction of ribs or thoracic vertebrae. Pain should be managed aggressively with parenteral opioids while closely monitoring for respiratory depression associated with these agents. All patients should perform incentive spirometry to prevent atelectasis.

The role of transfusion therapy in the ED management of patients with ACS is not clearly defined; however, RBC transfusion early in the course of ACS is the only therapy that has been shown to acutely stabilize sickle acute lung injury.[26] Simple transfusion is indicated when there is a need to increase oxygen carrying capacity with the objective of decreasing cardiac workload and improving patient comfort. Exchange transfusion should be considered on an urgent basis early in patients with poor prognostic factors who are at risk for respiratory failure; exchange transfusion may produce rapid resolution of ACS.[26,27]

Due to the potential for a rapidly deteriorating clinical course, patients with ACS should be admitted.

HEMOLYTIC TRANSFUSION REACTIONS

Sickle cell hemolytic transfusion reaction (HTR) is a life-threatening emergency seen in patients with SCD after a blood transfusion. Patients with or without alloantibodies develop severe hemolysis following blood transfusion. This results in marked reticulocytopenia and development of a more severe anemia than was present prior to transfusion.[28] Subsequent transfusions may further exacerbate the anemia, which can ultimately be fatal. Serologic studies may not provide an explanation for the hemolytic transfusion reaction.

Corticosteroids are the mainstay of therapy. Recovery from this crisis is manifested by reticulocytosis and gradual improvement in hemoglobin after withholding further transfusion.

PITFALLS

- Failure to recognize that patients may present as early as age 3 to 4 months
- Failure to recognize that the sickle prep is inaccurate before 4 to 6 months of age
- Failure to consider a cerebrovascular accident when evaluating any acute neurological event
- Failure to promptly administer antibiotics in febrile patients with SCD
- Failure to consider aplastic crisis and acute splenic sequestration in the acutely anemic patient with SCD
- Failure to appreciate and adequately treat the severity of pain in acute VOC
- Failure to appreciate the potential for rapid deterioration associated with ACS

REFERENCES

1. Bachman D, Barkin R, Breenan S. Hematologic and oncologic disorders. In: Barkin RM, Caputo G, eds. *Pediatric Emergency Medicine: Concepts and Clinical Practice*, 2nd ed. St. Louis, MO: Mosby; 1997:897–912.

2. Zarkowsky HS, Gallagher D, Gill FM, et al. The Cooperative Study of Sickle Cell Disease: bacteremia in sickle hemoglobinopathies. *J Pediatr.* 1986;109:579.

3. West DC, Andrada E, Azari R, et al. Predictors of bacteremia in febrile children with sickle cell disease. *J Pediatr Hematol Oncol.* 2003;24:279.

4. Dagan R, Melamed R, Zamir O, et al. Safety and immunogenicity of tetravalent pneumococcal vaccines containing 6B, 14, 19F and 23F polysaccharides conjugated to either tetanus toxoid or diphtheria toxoid in young infants and their boosterability by native polysaccharide antigens. *Pediatr Infect Dis J.* 1997;16:1053.

5. Adamkiewicz TV, Sarnaik S, Buchanan GR, et al. Invasive pneumococccal infections in children with sickle cell disease in the era of penicillin prophylaxis, antibiotic resistance, and 23-valent pneumococcal polysaccharide vaccination. *J Pediatr.* 2003;143:438.

6. Hord J, Byrd R, Stowe L, Windsor B, et al. *Streptococcus pneumoniae* sepsis and meningitis during the penicillin prophylaxis era in children with sickle cell disease. *J Pediatr Hematol Oncol.* 2002;24:470–472.

7. Teach SJ, Lillis KA, Grossi M. Compliance with penicillin prophylaxis in patients with sickle cell disease. *Arch Pediatr Adoles Med.* 1998;152:274.

8. Burnett AL, Bivalacqua TJ. Priapism: current principles and practice. *Urol Clin North Am.* 2007;34(4):631–642.

9. Wilimas J, Flynn P, Harris S, et al. Randomized study of outpatient treatment with ceftriaxone for selected febrile children with sickle cell disease. *N Engl J Med.* 1993;329:472–476.

10. Serjeant GR, Serjeant BE, Thomas PW, et al. Human parvovirus infection in homozygous sickle cell disease. *Lancet.* 1993;15:1237.

11. Zimmerman SA, Schultz WH, Davis JS. Sustained long-term hematologic efficacy of hydroxyurea at maximum tolerated dose in children with sickle cell disease. *Blood.* 2004;15:2039.

12. Wanko SO, Telen MJ. Transfusion management in sickle cell disease. *Hematol Oncol Clin North Am.* 19(5):803–826.

13. Yaster M, Kost-Byerly S, Maxwell LG. The management of pain in sickle cell disease. *Pediatr Clin North Am.* 2000;47(3):699–710.

14. Platt OS, Thorington BD, Brambilla DJ, et al. Pain in sickle cell disease. Rates and risk factors. *N Engl J Med.* 1991;325(1):11–16.

15. Silbergleit R. Management of sickle cell pain crisis in the emergency department at teaching hospitals. *J Emerg Med.* 1999;17(4):625–630.

16. Ballas, SK. Current issues in sickle cell pain and its management. *Hematology.* 2007;1:97–105.

17. Linklater DR, Pemberton L, Taylor S, et al. Painful dilemmas: an evidence-based look at challenging clinical scenarios. *Emerg Med Clin North Am.* 2005;23(2):367–392.

18. National Institutes of Health. The *Management of Sickle Cell Disease*, 4th ed. Washington, DC: NIH; 2002.

19. Charache SC, Terrin ML, Moore RD, et al. Effect of hydroxyurea on the frequency of painful crises in sickle cell anemia. *N Engl J Med.* 1995;332(20):1317–1322.

20. Milner PF, Sleeper LA, Pegelow CH, et al. Prediction of adverse outcomes in children with sickle cell disease. *N Engl J Med.* 2000;342:83–89.

21. Kinney TR, Sleeper LA, Wang WC, et al. Silent cerebral infarcts in sickle cell anemia: a risk factor analysis. The Cooperative Study of the Sickle Cell Disease. *Pediatrics.* 1999;103:640–645.

22. Pegelow CH, Wang W, Granger S, et al. Silent infarcts in children with sickle cell anemia and abnormal cerebral artery velocity. *Arch Neurol.* 2001;58:2017–2021.

23. Adams RJ. Stroke prevention and treatment in sickle cell disease. *Arch Neurol.* 2001;58:565.

24. Ware R, Zimmerman S, Schultz W. Hydroxyurea as an alternative to blood transfusions for the prevention of recurrent stroke in children with sickle cell disease. *Blood.* 1999;94:3022–3026.

25. Steinberg MH, Barton F, Castro O, et al. Effect of hydroxyurea on mortality and morbidity in adult sickle cell anemia: risks and benefits up to 9 years of treatment. *JAMA.* 2003;289:1645–1651.

26. Johnson C. The acute chest syndrome. *Hematol Oncol Clin North Am.* 2005;19(5):857–879.

27. Melton CW, Haynes J. Sickle acute lung injury: role of prevention and early aggressive intervention strategies on outcome. *Clin Chest Med.* 2006:27(3):487–502.

28. King KE, Shirley RS, Lankiewicz MW, et al. Delayed hemolytic transfusion reactions in sickle cell disease: simultaneous destruction of recipients' red cells. *Transfusion.* 1997;37:376–381.

SECTION II. INHERITED BLEEDING DISORDERS IN INFANTS

Emily Rose

INTRODUCTION

Rare inherited bleeding disorders command greater respect than their frequency indicates. The clinician caring for infants and neonates must be prepared to care for the time-sensitive emergencies that arise in these vulnerable infants. Infants with bleeding disorders may have a life- or limb-threatening intracranial hemorrhage, hemarthrosis or compartment syndrome from a muscle hematoma. These children often present with lacerations, fractures and other medical disorders that require surgery. With the ability to replace factors and even treat patients prophylactically, children with bleeding disorders are more active than they have been historically. The ED physician

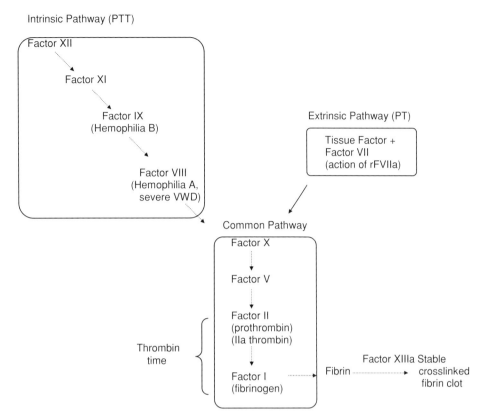

Figure 20.II.1. Simplified coagulation cascade.

must understand the treatment options and requirements of this special patient population.

The most common congenital bleeding disorders are von Willebrand's disease (VWD), hemophilia A and hemophilia B. Multiple other factor-specific and congenital disorders of platelet function also exist, but these disorders are much more rare and will be mentioned only briefly in this chapter.

HEMOPHILIA

Hemophilia A is an inherited deficiency of the clotting factor VIII and occurs in approximately 1 in 5000 male births. *Hemophilia B,* a deficiency of factor IX, is less common, occurring in approximately 1 in 30,000 male births. Both hemophilia A and B are X-linked recessive disorders. There is no geographical or racial predilection for hemophilia inheritance. Hemophilia is a disease of our ancestors as history has documented cases of male siblings afflicted with bleeding diatheses since 200 AD.[1,2]

Hemophilia A and B occur almost exclusively in males but may rarely be seen in females in such cases as a patient with homozygous X chromosomes for hemophilia or in a patient with a diminished or inactivated X chromosome or an absent secondary X chromosome in cases such as Turner syndrome. Approximately 30% of hemophiliacs have no family history of bleeding and so are presumed new, spontaneous mutations.[1,3–5]

The goal of normal hemostasis is to produce a platelet and fibrin plug to seal an injury site. Primary hemostasis involves the formation of a platelet plug, and this occurs normally in hemophilia. Bleeding occurs secondary to a failure of secondary hemostasis. It is the process of stabilizing this platelet plug by fibrin that is defective because inadequate amounts of thrombin are generated. Both factors VIII and IX are central to the generation of thrombin (Figure 20.II.1). After an injury, the complex of tissue factor and factor VII mediate the generation of factor Xa. This production is amplified by factor VIII and IX.[1,6–8]

Disease severity varies based on the plasma activity of the patient's factor VIII or factor IX activity level:

Severe disease: Males with less than 1% factor activity and early onset of symptoms such as joint and muscle bleeding

Moderate disease: 1% to 5% factor activity

Mild disease: Greater than 5% (but <30%) factor activity

Approximately 60% of hemophilia A patients and 50% of hemophilia B patients have severe disease. Typically, patients with hemophilia A present earlier than those with hemophilia B and usually present within the first year of life. Females who are hemophilia carriers typically have factor activity levels ranging from 30% to 70%.[1,9]

Co-inheritance of procoagulant states such as a factor V Leiden mutation may occur in some patients with hemophilia, which may lead to a less severe clinical course despite low specific factor activity.[4,5]

Both factors VIII and IX are synthesized in the liver. Factor VIII is a small multimer that is vulnerable to destruction in circulation and thus is linked to von Willebrand factor (VWF) in order to prevent its degradation once released from the liver.

Multiple mutations have been responsible for the clinical presentations of both hemophilia A and B, which helps explain the significant variance of clinical presentation and disease phenotype.[10]

VON WILLEBRAND'S DISEASE

VWD is the most common inherited bleeding disorder. VWD is typically autosomal dominant, but some forms are autosomal recessive. There are also multiple genetic mutations that lead to clinical disease. Similar to hemophilia, this compound heterogenicity contributes to phenotypic variability. The true incidence of VWD is unknown, and estimates vary from 0.2% to 2.0% with no gender or racial predilection. Less than 5% of individuals who meet criteria for VWD by laboratory screening are symptomatic.[11]

Three main types of VWD exist, as well as numerous subtypes. *Type 1* is the most common form and accounts for 70% to 80% of cases. It is autosomal dominantly inherited. In type 1 there is a partial quantitative deficiency of VWF. *Type 2* can be inherited in either an autosomal dominant or recessive pattern. Type 2 has qualitative abnormalities of VWF and is divided into four subtypes based on the functional abnormality of VWF. *Type 2A* has decreased active multimers of VWF, *type 2B* has increased binding of abnormal VWF to platelets inducing thrombocytopenia, *type 2M* has nonfunctioning VWF multimers and *type 2N*

has a mutation in the factor VIII binding site and is often misdiagnosed as hemophilia secondary to decreased factor VIII activity. Both Types 1 and 2 typically have mild to moderate severity of bleeding. *Type 3* is a rare (1 in 250,000 individuals) autosomal recessive disorder and is usually a severe disease with extremely low or undetectable levels of VWF. Patients present with severe bleeding involving the skin and mucous membranes (secondary to decreased VWF) and soft tissues and joints (due to the low concentrations of factor VIII).[11-13]

VWF is synthesized in endothelial cells and megakaryocytes and serves two important functions in the process of hemostasis. It functions as a mediator of platelet adhesion to damaged endothelium, and it acts as a carrier protein for factor VIII. At the time of vascular injury, VWF binds to subendothelial matrix ligands and promotes adhesion of platelets. Platelets are then activated, de-granulate and recruit additional platelets to the site to form a platelet plug. The platelet surface itself is where coagulation factors are activated to generate a clot. VWF contributes to fibrin clot formation by acting as a carrier protein for factor VIII, thereby prolonging factor VIII's half-life and increasing its plasma concentration. Because factor VIII depends on VWF for its survival in the circulation, lack of VWF, as in severe VWD, results in a secondary deficiency of factor VIII and a clinical presentation similar to hemophilia A.[11,13]

OTHER BLEEDING DISORDERS

Other clotting factor deficiencies are typically autosomal recessive in inheritance and include homozygous forms of factor II, V (also known as *parahemophilia*), VII, X, XI, XIII, and fibrinogen. These factor deficiencies typically do not bleed as frequently as the X-linked recessive forms. Factor X deficiency can be a rare autosomal dominant disorder that results in mild bleeding. Factor X deficiency in an autosomal recessive form tends to occur in populations with consanguineous marriages and has clinically severe bleeding. Combined deficiencies also may occur, such as combined factor V and VIII or factor XII deficiency with VWD (known as *von Willebrand San Diego*).[14-17]

Factor XI deficiency is known as *hemophilia C* and is an autosomal recessive disorder associated with mild to moderate bleeding symptoms. Many ethnic groups are affected, but this disease is most commonly seen in Ashkenazi Jews. The disease phenotype is highly variable.[9]

Table 20.II.1. Clinical characteristics of von Willebrand disease and the hemophilias

Disease type	Hemophilia	von Willebrand disease
Typical bleeding episode	Deep in soft tissues (e.g., joints, muscle hematomas)	Skin, mucous membranes (gingiva, nares, GI and GU tracts)
Ecchymoses	Large, palpable	small, superficial
Minor lacerations	Delayed bleeding/prolonged oozing	Immediate bleeding
Bleeding after surgery	Delayed, severe	Immediate, mild

GI, gastrointestinal; GU, genitourinary.

Vitamin K deficiency in the newborn, previously known as *hemorrhagic disease of the newborn,* is caused by a decrease in factors II, VII, IX, and X that occurs 48 to 72 hours after birth, with a gradual return to normal values by 7 to 10 days of age. This decrease is probably due to a lack of free vitamin K in the mother and therefore poor vitamin K stores in the infant, poor placental transfer, low levels of vitamin K in breast milk, and the absence of bacterial intestinal flora in the newborn that is usually responsible for synthesis of vitamin K.

Onset can occur in the first 24 hours of life and is usually due to maternal medications that interfere with vitamin K such as antibiotics, anticonvulsants and anticoagulants. A common and classic presentation occurs in breastfed newborns, usually at 2 to 7 days of age. Late onset occurs after 2 weeks of age in newborns with diarrhea, hepatitis or other rarer diseases such as celiac disease or cystic fibrosis or simply due to lack of administration of vitamin K prophylaxis at birth.[18]

Other bleeding disorders that involve platelets include inherited thrombocytopenias, homozygous-inherited Bernard-Soulier, and Glanzmann's thrombasthenia.[19–21]

PRESENTATION

Hemophilia

Neither factor VIII nor factor IX cross the placenta; therefore, bleeding symptoms may occur in the fetus or be present from birth.[5] However, the majority of newborns with even severe hemophilia remain undetected during delivery and the first few months of life. Less than one third of patients with hemophilia A and B and 10% of those with other coagulation disorders have hemorrhagic events during the first week of life.[7] Approximately 5% of neonates with hemophilia will have an intracranial hemorrhage.[10] The risk of intracranial hemorrhage

increases with difficult delivery and with the use of birth adjuncts such as forceps or vacuum assistance. Increased irritability in an infant often heralds the onset of a bleed.

Typically, patients with lower factor levels and more severe disease present earlier and often with spontaneous bleeding. Mild disease typically requires trauma or a procedure to induce bleeding. Infants are often diagnosed with hemophilia when they have prolonged or delayed bleeding after blood draws, immunizations, circumcisions or bleeding from the umbilical stump. Multiple sources have demonstrated that only 30% to 50% of hemophiliacs have prolonged bleeding with circumcision.[5,10]

The classic type of bleeding in hemophilia is in the deep soft tissue and joints (Table 20.II.1). Bleeding becomes more frequent as infants become more active and are first crawling or walking and putting more strain on joints and limbs with frequent falls. Excessive bruising into the deep soft tissue, muscle hematomas, intracranial hemorrhage, hemarthrosis and delayed or prolonged bleeding after lacerations are common presentations of infants with hemophilia.

SITES OF BLEEDING

Central Nervous System

Central nervous system (CNS) bleeding is the main cause of death in hemophiliac patients and is responsible for 75% of neurological sequelae among survivors. Infants younger than 2 years of age represent 30% of all hemophiliac patients with intracranial hemorrhages; 90% of these patients have factor levels less than 1%.[22] Intracranial hemorrhages may have a subtle presentation in the infant. Hemorrhage into the spinal cord also can occur and the physician must be vigilant and perform a complete neurological exam after trauma.

Intra-abdominal

Patients with hemophilia are at increased risk for bleeding consequences of blunt trauma. As in patients without hemophilia, the liver and spleen are the most common sources of bleeding after trauma.[23]

Hemarthrosis

In hemarthrosis, bleeding originates from the synovial vessels and can quickly fill the joint cavity. Clinical manifestations in infants are irritability and decreased use of the affected limb. Weight-bearing joints are most commonly affected with the ankles being the most common site of bleeding in children when they are first learning to walk. Knees and elbows are also frequently involved.

Hemarthrosis of the hip joint or acetabulum hemorrhages may result in increased intraarticular pressure and osteonecrosis of the femoral head. Hip involvement in infants is typically clinically apparent by external rotation and abduction with limited and painful range of motion. The infant often refuses to crawl or bear weight. The shoulder is also at risk for avascular necrosis.[7,9,23] Persistent joint swelling associated with fever may indicate a septic joint.

Skeletal Muscle

Hematoma formation can occur, most often affecting the quadriceps, iliopsoas and forearm. Compartment syndrome can occur when a muscle hemorrhages in a closed compartment. Common sites include upper arm, forearm, wrist, volar hand and anterior or posterior tibial compartments. Iliopsoas hemorrhage may be severe and life-threatening, especially if a delay in diagnosis occurs. Presentation often mimics appendicitis.[23]

Head and Neck

Even trivial trauma in a severe hemophiliac may produce life-threatening airway compromise. Coughing or vomiting can produce bleeding into the posterior pharynx which can also lead to airway compromise or obstruction. Epistaxis can be severe.

Gastrointestinal Tract

Gastrointestinal lesions can cause severe bleeding; hematomas of the bowel wall may develop and produce obstruction or intussusception.

Genitourinary Tract

Hematuria frequently occurs, and although it often requires factor replacement, it is not associated with progressive loss of renal function.[13]

Posttraumatic Bleeding

Delayed bleeding is common and can be significant or continuous oozing for weeks.[23]

von Willebrand Disease

Symptoms of VWD can begin at any age and vary based on the genetic mutation and subtype. The classic type of bleeding in VWD is mucosal and cutaneous such as epistaxis, gingival bleeding and bullous hemorrhages on the buccal mucosa (see Table 20.II.1).

As stated previously, patients with type 1 VWD typically present with mild to moderate bleeding and type 2 has multiple subtypes and a range of clinical presentations. Type 3 is the most severe as patients typically have extremely low or undetectable levels of VWF. Severe bleeding occurs involving the skin and mucous membranes (secondary to decreased VWF) and soft tissues and joints (due to low concentrations of factor VIII). Rarely, patients with severe type 3 VWD have joint hemorrhages or spontaneous CNS hemorrhages.[13]

OTHER BLEEDING DISORDERS

Other bleeding disorders beyond hemophilia or VWD should be considered in the undiagnosed spontaneously bleeding patient. Other factor deficiencies have a range of presentation and may present in a manner similar to the hemophilias or VWD (Table 20.II.2).

Common presentations of vitamin K deficiency are bleeding of the mucous membranes, GI tract, umbilicus and circumcision site. Cephalohematomas with bruising are common. Intracranial bleeds can occur and are the main cause of morbidity and mortality.

Severe factor VII deficiency is rare but frequently presents in the neonate as an intracranial hemorrhage.

LABORATORY

General screening tests of a patient with abnormal bleeding include platelet count, bleeding time, prothrombin

Table 20.II.2. Other bleeding disorders (differential diagnosis of hemophilia and von Willebrand disease)

Other factor deficiencies (e.g., factor II, V, VII, XI, and XIII; fibrinogen)

Vitamin K deficiency (*see text*)

Other disorders that prolong the PTT but not the PT include acquired inhibitors to factor VIII and IX, factor XII deficiency or deficiency of prekallikrein or high molecular weight kininogen. Factor XII deficiency, prekallikrein and high molecular weight kininogen do not cause clinically significant bleeding.

Disorders of platelets and platelet function:

    Thrombocytopenia: Most common cause of bleeding diathesis in infants

    Bernard-Soulier syndrome and Glanzmann's thrombasthenia are autosomal recessive disorders and both present with mucocutaneous bleeding in infancy or childhood. Bernard-Soulier syndrome is characterized by a defect in the Ib/IX/V complex resulting in giant platelets and significant bleeding despite relatively mild thrombocytopenia. Glanzmann thrombasthenia has a defect in the GP IIb/IIIa complex with a normal platelet count and morphology but defective platelet aggregation.

    Wiskott-Aldrich syndrome: X-linked recessive disorder associated with thrombocytopenia

    Hermansky-Pudlak syndrome: Oculocutaneous albinism with platelet dysfunction

Ehlers-Danlos syndrome: Easy bruising secondary to vascular defects

Vitamin C deficiency: Easy bruising and petechiae

Data from Drews 2007,[23] Johnson 2005.[35]

time (PT), activated partial thromboplastin time (APTT) and thrombin time (TT)[24] (Table 20.II.3).

A platelet count is important as thrombocytopenia is the most common acquired cause of a bleeding diathesis in children.

Bleeding time assesses the function of platelets and their interaction with the vascular wall. Standardization with a regulated incision length and blood pressure cuff occurs, but the test has significant interlaboratory variation. Platelet function analyzers more accurately measure collagen binding, VWF-mediated adhesion and platelet function.

PT measures the extrinsic clotting system after the activation of clotting by tissue factor (thromboplastin). It is not prolonged with most clotting factor deficiencies except factor VII deficiency. The PT has been standardized using the International Normalized Ratio so that values can be compared among laboratories.

The activated partial prothrombin time (APTT) measures the interaction between all of the coagulation cascade proteins except factors VII and XIII and is typically prolonged in most common clotting factor abnormalities associated with bleeding diatheses. Defects in factors VII and XIII do not prolong the PTT. The PTT range varies among hospital laboratories secondary to differing reagents used in processing.

TT measures the final step of the clotting cascade in which fibrinogen is converted to fibrin. It is prolonged with reduced or dysfunctional fibrinogen or by substances that interfere with fibrin polymerization such as heparin or fibrin split products.

Table 20.II.3. Coagulation disorders and laboratory values

Disorder	Bleeding time	Platelet count	Prothrombin time	Partial prothrombin time	Thrombin time	Fibrinogen
Hemophilias A and B (factor VIII or IX deficiencies)	Normal	Normal	Normal	Increased	Normal	Normal
von Willebrand disease	Prolonged	Normal	Normal	Normal or increased	Normal	Normal
Vitamin K deficiency	Normal	Normal	Increased	Increased	Normal	Normal
Factor VII deficiency	Normal	Normal	Normal	Increased	Normal	Normal
Common pathway deficiencies, factor II (prothrombin), factor I (fibrinogen), factor V or factor X	Normal	Normal	Increased	Increased	Increased (normal in factor X and V deficiency)	Decreased
Factor XII, prekallikrein, HMW kininogen deficiencies (no clinically significant bleeding)	Normal	Normal	Normal	Increased	Normal	Normal

HMW, high molecular weight.

Clotting factor assays are used to test individual clotting factor deficiencies.

Factor assay results are expressed in percent of activity. One unit of factor per milliliter of plasma is equivalent to 1% activity.[9]

If there is an unexplained prolongation of the PT, PTT or TT, a mixing study can be performed. Normal plasma is adding to patient's plasma in a 1:1 ratio and the tests are repeated. Correction of the PT or PTT suggests a clotting factor deficiency as only a 50% level of factor activity is necessary to produce a normal PT or PTT. If the clotting time is not corrected or only partially improved, typically an inhibitor to a factor is present.[9,25,26]

Testing of a neonate is complicated by the fact that neonatal PTT is often prolonged secondary to decreased vitamin K dependent factor activity and decreased factor XI and XII levels. If one is suspicious of hemophilia, direct factor assays of factor VIII or IX should be obtained.[27]

Also in the newborn, factor VIII levels may be artificially elevated because of the acute phase response elicited by the birth process. Factor IX levels are physiologically low in the newborn.[25,28]

Five tests used to screen for VWD are listed[13]:

1. Plasma VWF antigen (VWF:Ag)
2. Plasma VWF activity (ristocetin cofactor activity, VWF:RCo)
3. Factor VIII activity (FVIII)
4. APTT
5. Platelet function analyzer (PFA) or bleeding time (BT).

VWF assays are used to further distinguish factor VIII deficiency from VWD.

Both plasma VWF and factor VIII are acute phase reactants, and their levels can increase one to three times baseline during exercise, adrenergic stimulation or inflammatory processes. Extragenic factors also play role in VWF levels including ABO blood groups, hormones and inflammatory states.[28] All may cause fluctuations in VWF levels and mask a diagnosis.

The most sensitive laboratory test for the diagnosis of VWD is the ristocetin cofactor assay. Ristocetin is an antibiotic that induces platelet agglutination in the presence of VWF. Patients that are deficient in VWF or in the receptor for VWF (e.g., Bernard-Soulier syndrome) have an abnormal ristocetin response. Ristocetin induces

the binding of VWF to the GP1b receptor on platelets. Decreased VWF:RCo in the presence of normal VWF:Ag is indicative of dysfunctional VWF binding to GP1b (as in multiple types 2 VWD). Proportional decreases in both assays are indicative of a quantitative decrease of a normally functioning VWF molecule (as in type 1 VWD).[13]

There are limited laboratory tests for vitamin K deficiency in newborns. A prolonged PT is usually the first abnormal finding, but there is no laboratory test that can confirm the diagnosis.

RADIOLOGY

Clinical suspicion and physical exam are paramount in the diagnosis of hemorrhagic events. Radiology is often used to support diagnosis but is typically performed after appropriate treatment has begun, especially in life- or limb-threatening events.

Hemarthrosis may reveal widening of joint spaces on plain films and fluid-filled joints on ultrasound. Computed tomography (CT) is indicated emergently (after factor replacement is initiated) for any suspected intracranial hemorrhage. A lower threshold for obtaining a head CT scan should be considered in any infant with a bleeding disorder and even minor head trauma. CT may also aid in the diagnosis of intra-abdominal or iliopsoas hemorrhage.

MANAGEMENT

Less than 5% of patients develop significant subgaleal or intracranial hemorrhage in the perinatal period.[29] However, these acute intracranial hemorrhages have high morbidity and mortality and frequently result in long-term neurological complications, and quick recognition and treatment are essential in the management.[30]

As with any infant presenting to the ED, an assessment to evaluate the overall appearance, work of breathing and circulation is imperative. Altered mental status or an ill appearance warrants immediate intervention. As has been stated earlier in this text, the mnemonic THE MISFITS is one way to remember the list of disorders that can result in altered mental status or ill-appearance in young infants:

T   Trauma, consider nonaccidental trauma
H   Heart, hypoxia, hematologic
E   Endocrine

M   Metabolic disturbances (congenital adrenal hyperplasia)

I   Inborn errors of metabolism

S   Sepsis

F   Formula dilution or overconcentration

I   Intestinal catastrophes

T   Toxins

S   Seizures

If the patient does not have a previously diagnosed bleeding disorder, direct pressure should be applied to the compressible bleeding site and immediate coagulation studies ordered including factor assays. If significant or life-threatening bleeding is occurring, fresh frozen plasma (FFP) may be given while awaiting laboratory screening. Factor-specific replacement is much more ideal, especially for hemophilia, as FFP contains low levels of factors VIII and IX and infants may not be able to tolerate the volume of FFP required to obtain sufficient plasma factor levels.

Factor Treatment Products

FFP is separated from the blood's cellular components and contains small and inconsistent amounts of factor VIII and factor IX.

Cryoprecipitate is FFP that is frozen then thawed at 1°C to 6°C creating a cold-resistant precipitant that is rich in factor VIII. Plasma can be fractionated into individual components such as factors VIII and IX and albumin.[24]

Both factor VIII and IX are available in recombinant or plasma-derived forms with intermediate purity concentrates, high purity and ultrahigh purity forms. Plasma-derived factor concentrates are created from pooled donor plasma. The factors are purified from plasma by chromatographic partitioning and monoclonal antibody affinity purification.[31]

Dosing calculations and regimens are targeted at maintaining plasma factor levels based on the patient's bleeding severity and the location of the bleeding. Factor VIII has a shorter half-life than factor IX and should be infused every 8 to 12 hours for an acute bleed while factor IX requires infusion every 12 to 24 hours. Mild muscle and soft tissue bleeds require a minimum of 30% plasma factor level for 1 to 2 days. Plasma factor levels of 90% to 100% are required with major hemorrhage, surgeries or bleeds within the gastrointestinal system or CNS. Major

surgeries and severe bleeds often require continuous factor infusions.[9,32]

Calculations for Targeted Levels
Factor VIII infusions:

Number of units required per dose = [weight (kg)] × [% factor level desired] × [0.5]

Factor IX infusions

Number of units required per dose = [weight (kg)] × [% factor level desired] × [1 (1.2 − 1.4 for recombinant forms)]

Plasma levels are monitored at 1-hour post infusion to guide dose adjustments.

Recombinant VWF replacements is also available in varying purity. See von Willebrand Management section and Tables 20.II.4 and 20.II.5 for dosing.

Prevention of vitamin K deficiency in the newborn involves prophylaxis with vitamin K administration at birth. A single dose can prevent the classic deficiency. Any infant in whom this deficiency is suspected should receive vitamin K subcutaneously. Intramuscular administration may cause a hematoma and intravascular has been associated with anaphylaxis. FFP may be considered for moderate-to-severe bleeding. Classic vitamin K deficiency bleeding is usually not life-threatening; therefore, vitamin K administration is usually sufficient to reverse the condition and return PT values back to normal.[18]

Additional Products

Desmopressin (DDAVP, 1-deamino-8-D-argine vasopressin) is a synthetic formulation of the hormone vasopressin that lacks pressor activity. DDAVP causes release of factor VIII from storage site granules. Successful treatment requires a threefold increase of factor VIII levels in a patient with mild hemophilia A. As much as a four- to sixfold increase of serum factor VIII levels can occur. Typically, DDAVP is only used in mild bleeding episodes as severe bleeding often requires exogenous factor replacement. Serum factor VIII levels increase approximately 30 to 60 minutes after infusion and persist for

Table 20.II.4. Factor replacement guidelines

Bleeding type	% Correction	Hemophilia A (Factor VIII)	Hemophilia B (Factor IX)	von Willebrand (ristocetin cofactor:VWF)
Minor bleeds and procedures (e.g., hemarthrosis, hematoma, minor laceration, fracture)	40–50	DDAVP 0.3 μg/kg or 20–40 U/kg every 12–24 hours for 1–3 doses	30–60 U/kg q24 hours for 1–3 doses	Local measures or DDAVP 0.3 μg/kg; Rarely, VWF:ristocetin cofactor 15–25 U/kg is required
Major bleeds (e.g., ICH, pre-operative, iliopsoas, hip, compartment syndrome)	80–100	40–60 U/kg every 8–12 hours	60–100 U/kg every 12–24 hours	40–80 U/kg (type 1 40–60 U/kg, type 3 60–80 U/kg) load and then 40–60 U/kg q8–12 hours
	Continuous infusion	Load with bolus as above, then 2–5 U/kg/hour	Load with bolus then 5–10 U/kg/hour	May decrease total dose requirements

6 to 12 hours. Side effects include hyponatremia secondary to increased water retention and seizures have been described. Fluid restriction is often encouraged with the use of DDAVP.[1,33–35]

Antifibrinolytic therapy such as aminocaproic acid (Amicar) and tranexamic acid are used to prevent dissolution of a hemostatic plug. Commonly, they are used in mucous membrane bleeding such as in dental procedures. Antifibrinolytic therapy is not useful in obtaining initial hemostasis but prevents rapid clot lysis after hemostasis has been achieved by other means such as desmopressin, replacement therapy or local measures.[1,13]

Table 20.II.5. Treatment of bleeding episodes

Fresh frozen plasma	10–15 mL/kg IV
Cryoprecipitate	1 bag per 10 kg every 8–12 hours
Aminocaproic acid (Amicar)	50–100 mg/kg orally or IV, then 50 mg/kg every 6 hours
Recombinant factor VIII	0.5 × wt (kg) × % correction = number of units
Recombinant factor IX	1.2–1.4 × wt (kg) × % correction = number of units
VWF concentrate	20–30 U/kg (mild bleeding) 50–60 U/kg (severe bleeding)
DDAVP	0.3 μg/kg IV (in 30 mL of normal saline) 0.3 μg/kg SC (in 1.5 mL saline) 150 μg nasal spray 1 puff
Fibrin sealants	Apply to bleeding surface in spray or dual syringe
Topical thrombin	Apply to surface as powder or solution
Microfibrillar collagen	Apply to surface or use strips for packing

Local Hemostatic Blood Products

Topical agents are useful adjuncts to IV management of the hemophilias and VWD. Factor requirements are lower with the use of local hemostatic agents. Examples include fibrin sealant, thrombin powder and microfibrillar collagen.

Fibrin sealant is formed by mixing two plasma-derived protein fractions. One syringe is filled with a fibrinogen-rich concentrate and the other with a thrombin concentrate. Factor XIII (also known as *fibrin stabilizing factor*) is a component of fibrin sealant and plays a role in stabilizing the clot formed by the solution. When the syringes are mixed, the last step of the coagulation cascade is mimicked and a fibrin clot is formed. The components of the sealants can be prepared from either large pools of plasma (commercial preparations) or from single plasma donations (blood bank preparations). This topical therapy can be used via endoscopes, laparoscopes and bronchoscopes for treatment of bleeding.[36,37]

Thrombin powder acts to catalyze the conversion of fibrinogen to fibrin and may be applied as a powder or a reconstituted solution. It is most effective when the thrombin mixes freely with blood as it appears. Rarely, bovine thrombin antibodies develop, which can cross-react with human factor V and cause a factor V deficiency. Human thrombin formulations are available. Gelfoam or Surgicel also may be soaked in thrombin solution and applied to local areas of bleeding.[35]

Microfibrillar collagen is made from purified bovine collagen that is shredded into fibrils; this attracts platelets and triggers platelet activation and aggregation. It is applied topically and is available in strips for packing wounds.

TREATMENT OF SPECIFIC ENTITIES

Hemarthrosis

Hemarthrosis is treated with a goal factor level of 40% to 50%. Typically, only one dose is required. When a single joint undergoes repeated hemorrhage it is labeled a *target joint,* and it may benefit from a short course of corticosteroids to reduce pain and swelling associated with synovial inflammation. Synovectomy may be necessary in older children to decrease hemorrhage and edema. Treatment should be initiated in any suspected joint bleed, even if the diagnosis is unable to be confirmed. Factor dosing may need to be repeated.[1,23]

Suspicion of a septic joint requires antibiotics, arthrocentesis and pre-procedural factor replacement.

Hemarthrosis of the hip or acetabulum requires a minimum factor level of 20%; treatment generally is required for at least 3 days. Joint immobilization with a rigid posterior splint for 24 to 48 hours may be helpful to minimize ongoing trauma.

Hematomas

Intramuscular hemorrhage should have factor correction to levels of 50%. Suspicion of neurovascular compromise requires aggressive treatment with 70% to 100% correction. Aggressive medical therapy with factor correction should always precede surgical intervention.

Iliopsoas hemorrhage requires 100% factor replacement with 3 days of daily infusions and followed by every other day replacement for 10 days.[1,5,9,23,29]

Head and Neck

Epistaxis should have packing and pressure applied. Antifibrinolytic therapy is a useful adjunct in epistaxis and oral bleeding. Topical applications are useful when applicable. Gelfoam or Surgicel can be soaked in topical thrombin and applied locally to the bleeding site.

Hemorrhage involving the neck and surrounding soft tissues requires aggressive management with 80% to 100% factor replacement and protection of airway patency.[1,9,23]

Gastrointestinal

Endoscopy with cauterization is recommended. Antifibrinolytic therapy may be useful.

Hematuria

Manage hematuria with maintenance fluids, factor replacement of 20 to 40 U/kg, and occasionally with steroids. Avoid antifibrinolytic therapy as clotting and obstruction have been described with these products.[1,5]

Wound Management

Correction of clotting factor activity to greater than 50% is required prior to suturing and at the time of suture removal. Hematomas may develop below lacerations and complicate healing. Topical hemostatic agents are useful adjuncts in wound management. Staples should be avoided.[23]

Fractures

Fractures may be associated with intramuscular hemorrhages. A factor level of at least 50% is recommended after cast removal to prevent joint hemorrhages in the rehabilitating limb.[23]

Major Bleeding

Severe episodes such as intracranial or intraabdominal hemorrhage or facial, neck or hip bleeding require 80% to 100% factor level until the hemorrhage has stopped. Continuous infusion is often necessary. Late bleeding after head trauma is common. Seizure prophylaxis is often recommended.[1,9,29]

Severe hemorrhage or head trauma requires aggressive factor replacement and may require patient transfer if a hospital's factor availability is limited.

Management of subdural hematomas in neonates is controversial. Surgical evacuation is commonly necessary (30%–50% of cases). Peyre et al. proposed that an alternative to surgical intervention is medical therapy in conjunction with transcoronal puncture. Two patients were treated in this manner successfully with good neurological outcome.[21]

Table 20.II.6. Treatment of patients with inhibitors

Alternative therapy	Dose	Comments
High purity factor VIII concentrates	100–150 U/kg bolus, then continuous infusion 15–20 U/kg/hour for 3–4 days	Plasmapheresis typically performed prior to treatment to remove inhibitors
Porcine factor VIII concentrates	100–150 U/kg	Risk of hypersensitivity or anaphylaxis. Monitor anti-porcine factor VIII antibodies
Prothrombin complex concentrates (PCC) or activated PCC (aPCC)	100–150 U/kg (PCC) 50–75 U/kg (aPCC)	Difficult to regulate effect, prothrombotic side effects, only used in minor bleeds
Recombinant human factor VIIa	90 μg/kg every 2–3 hours until hemostasis achieved	Promotes coagulation only at local level, therefore no systemic procoagulant effect

Surgery

From 80% to 100% factor levels are maintained for orthopedic surgery with a minimum of 30% factor levels in the ensuing days. Dental surgeries require factor levels of 50%.[2,29]

OTHER MANAGEMENT

Routine immunizations may be given via the usual route or in the deep subcutaneous tissue with the smallest gauge needle available. Pressure and ice should be applied to the site for 3 to 5 minutes after injection. Hepatitis B vaccine is an important vaccination for infants with hemophilia as they will be receiving transfusions from donor plasma. Fibrin glue is helpful for circumcisions if families feel strongly that a baby with known hemophilia should be circumcised.[23,29,36]

Medications affecting platelet function such as aspirin or nonsteroidal anti-inflammatory medications should be avoided.[5]

Safety of Blood Products

Historically, contaminated blood products have been a serious and often lethal consequence of blood transfusion requirements in bleeding disorders. Most people who received factor concentrates prior to 1985 are infected with human immunodeficiency virus (HIV).

Significant advancements have been made to improve the safety of blood derivatives. Factor concentrates have been treated since 1985 to eliminate HIV and since 1988 to eliminate hepatitis C virus. Plasma-derived factors go through a series of viral attenuation steps. Solvent detergents are used to inactivate lipid-enveloped viruses such as HIV, hepatitis B and C. Immunoaffinity and ion-exchange chromatography remove non–lipid-enveloped viruses such as parvovirus and hepatitis A. *Lyophilization* (freeze drying) removes hepatitis A. Advances have also been made in recombinant factors that have little or no human and animal proteins. Prion-born diseases such as Creutzfeldt-Jakob disease may still be transmitted as long as even small quantities of human or animal proteins are present.[31,32,38]

Complications of Treatment

Antibodies to replacement factors can develop and cause difficulty in treatment in patients with severe disease. Immunoglobulin G4 antibodies are inhibitory and neutralize factor VIII or factor IX. These antibodies occur in approximately 30% of hemophilia A and 3% to 5% of hemophilia B patients during the first 15 to 30 infusions and are more common in patients with larger genetic mutations.[1] The presence of inhibitors should be suspected when adequate hemostasis is not achieved with routine replacement therapy. The Bethesda assay is used to measure inhibitors. One Bethesda Unit (BU) is the level of antibody that decreases the plasma factor level by 50% and is expressed in logarithmic fashion. Inhibitors can be transient, low (<5 BU) or high titer (>5 BU). Inhibitor antibodies are more common with factor VIII and in those with more severe disease.[1,5,9]

Inhibitors also can change the phenotype of a patient with hemophilia. A mild to moderately affected individual could be converted to severe disease secondary to inhibitors attacking the native factor and reducing levels to below 1%.[39] See Table 20.II.6 for alternative therapies for patients with inhibitors.[9,39,40]

Vitamin K–dependent factors (e.g., recombinant factor VIIa) can be used as bypassing agents that activate factor

Xa directly, therefore bypassing the need for factor VIII and IX in the coagulation cascade.

The mechanism of action of factor VIIa is twofold. First, recombinant factor VIIa binds to tissue factor, which activates factor X, which initiates a cascade leading to the formation of a hemostatic fibrin plug. Second, recombinant factor VIIa binds to the surface of activated platelets, which also leads to an accelerated clot formation.[27,41,42]

Recombinant factor VIIa dosage is higher in children because they have faster clearance and therefore require higher doses than in adults to maintain plasma levels.[40,42,43]

Long-term management of patients with inhibitors frequently involves immune tolerance induction. Immune tolerance therapy is often used to attempt to eradicate the inhibitor by recurrent exposure to regular infusions of factors VIII or IX.

Factor IX inhibitors carry increased risk of anaphylaxis and nephrotic syndrome when exposed to the antigenic factor; therefore, immune tolerance therapy is typically not performed in patients with hemophilia B with inhibitors.[1,39]

PREVENTION AND PROPHYLAXIS

Preventive measures are important to prevent the onset of chronic sequelae associated with bleeds. Progressive hemophilic arthropathy is associated with significant morbidity. The accumulation of iron within synovial cells triggers an inflammatory response that ultimately causes destruction of cartilage and boney structures. The resultant damaged joint becomes even more susceptible to subsequent bleeding and joint damage.

Prophylactic factor infusion continues to be studied and modified. The goal is to prevent bleeding episodes and the consequent morbidity associated with bleeding. The consequences of prophylaxis include increasing factor requirements (secondary to factor antibodies) and, commonly, indwelling catheter requirements (infection and thrombosis risks). Plasma factor levels should be maintained around 1% to 2% for effective prophylaxis.[1,29]

VON WILLEBRAND MANAGEMENT

Desmopressin is effective in almost all patients with mild or moderate type 1 disease. Type 2 has variable effect with desmopressin and certain types, such as type 2B, can

actually worsen secondary to increased binding of abnormal VWF to the platelets. Treatment for VWD type 2 should occur in consultation with a hematologist. Desmopressin is not effective in patients with type 3 VWD.[44]

Patients with types 2 and 3 VWD often require IV factor concentrate replacements containing VWF. Dosing for recombinant VWF is calculated based on the VWF activity expressed as ristocetin cofactor (vWf:RCoF) units. Multiple products are available containing varying ratios of VWF and factor VIII concentrate. In minor procedures or bleeding, 40 to 50 IU/kg every 8 to 12 hours for one to two doses is typically sufficient. Major surgeries and bleeds require a loading dose of 60 to 80 IU/kg and then 40 to 60 IU/kg every 8 to 12 hours for a minimum of 5 to 10 days in order to keep the vWf:RCoF more than 50%. Any suspected intracranial bleed should receive this higher dosing of recombinant factor.[13,33,45]

Platelet transfusion may be necessary in certain types of VWD such as type 2B, which binds platelets and can cause thrombocytopenia.[33]

In addition to measuring ristocetin cofactor activity, physicians may use the platelet function analyzer (PFA-100) to follow VWF activity after replacement therapy. However, no laboratory test adequately predicts hemostatic effects, and management is often based on clinical response.[33]

Topical agents are frequently used in VWD as oral and nasal bleeds are common.

Recombinant factor VIIa can be used in patients with type 3 VWD with alloantibodies to VWF after replacement therapy.[13]

Gene therapy is the treatment of the future for both VWD and the hemophilias.[46]

OTHER BLEEDING DISORDER MANAGEMENT

Recombinant factor VII is available for treatment of severe factor VII deficiency. Other factor deficiencies require the use of FFP or cryoprecipitate. Vitamin K may be a useful adjuvant treatment with rare combined factor deficiencies.

PITFALLS

- Failure to recognize bleeding early and begin factor replacement prior to further study
- Failure to begin factor replacement with mild symptoms in patients with severe hemophilia
- Failure to recognize inhibitors and treat appropriately

- Failure to recognize how underlying coagulation disorders complicate management of common injuries
- Failure to consult hematology and involve pharmacy during complicated replacements

REFERENCES

1. Dunn AL, Abshire TC. Recent advances in the management of the child who has hemophilia. *Hematol Oncol Clin North Am.* 2004;18:1249–1276.
2. DiMichele D, Neufeld EJ. Hemophilia: a new approach to an old disease. *Hematol Oncol Clin North Am.* 1998;12:16.
3. Bolton-Maggs PHB, Pasi KJ. Haemophilias A and B. *Lancet.* 2003;361:1801–1809.
4. Hoots WK, Shapiro AD. Genetics of the hemophilias. UpToDate serial online. www.uptodate.com. Accessed on May 18, 2008.
5. Montgomery RR, Scott JP. Hemorrhagic and thrombotic diseases. In: Behrman, ed. *Nelson Textbook of Pediatrics*, 17th ed. Philadelphia, PA: Saunders; 2004.
6. Aird WC. Coagulation. *Crit Care Med.* 2005;33.12;S485–467.
7. Greer JP, Forester J, Lukens JN, et al. Clinical features of inherited bleeding disorders. *Wintrobe's Clinical Hematology*, 11th ed. Philadelphia, PA: Lippincott Williams & Wilkins; 2004.
8. Hoffman M, Monroe DM. Coagulation 2006: a modern view of hemostasis. *Hematol Oncol Clin North Am.* 2007;21:1–11.
9. Wong, WY. Hemophilia and related disorders. In: Rakel RE, ed. *Conn's Current Therapy 2007*, 59th ed. Philadelphia, PA: Saunders; 2007.
10. Hoots WK, Shapiro AD. Clinical Manifestations and Diagnosis of Hemophilia. UpToDate serial online. www.uptodate.com. Accessed on May 18, 2008.
11. Rick ME. Clinical Presentation and Diagnosis of von Willebrand Disease. UpToDate serial online. www.uptodate.com. Accessed on May 18, 2008.
12. Michiels JJ, Gadisseur A, Budde U, et al. Characterization, classification and treatment of von Willebrand diseases: a critical appraisal of the literature and personal experiences. *Semin Thromb Hemost.* 2005;31(5):577–601.
13. Gill JC. Diagnosis and treatment of von Willebrand disease. *Hematol Oncol Clin North Am.* 2004;18:1277–1299.
14. Al-Sharif FZ, Aljurf MD, Al-Momen AM, et al. Clinical and laboratory features of congenital factor XIII deficiency. *Saudi Med J.* 2002;5:552–554. [abstract]
15. Anwar M, Hamdani SN, Ayyub M, et al. Factor X deficiency in North Pakistan. *J Ayub Med Coll Abbottabad.* 2004;16(3):1–4.
16. Bolton-Maggs PH, Patterson DA, Wensley RT, et al. Definition of the bleeding tendency in factor XI-deficient kindreds – a clinical and laboratory study. *Thromb Haemost.* 1995;73(2):194–202.
17. Casonato A, Pontara E, Sartorell F, et al. Combined hemophilia A and type 2N von Willebrand's disease: defect of both factor VIII level and factor VIII binding capacity of von Willebrand factor. *Haematologica.* 2001;86:1110–1111.
18. St. John ED. Hemorrhagic disease of the newborn. eMedicine serial. www.emedicine.com; accessed on December 5, 2007.
19. Sood S, Abrams CS. Platelet-mediated bleeding disorders. In: Rakel RE, ed. *Conn's Current Therapy*, 59th ed. Philadelphia, PA: Saunders; 2007.
20. Blanchette VS, Sparling C, Turner C. Inherited bleeding disorders. *Baillieres Clin Haematol.* 1991;4(2):291–332.
21. Neunert CE, Journeycake JM. Congenital platelet disorders. *Hemotol Oncol Clin North Am.* 2007;21(4):663–684.
22. Peyre M, Di Rocco F, Meyer P, et al. Successful conservative treatment of traumatic subacute subdural haematomas in neonates with haemophilia A. *Childs Nerv Syst.* 2008;24(6):679-683.
23. Hampers LC, Manco-Johnson M. Emergency department management of musculoskeletal injuries in children with inherited bleeding disorders. *Clin Pediatr Emerg Med.* 2002;3(2):138–144.
24. Drews RE. Approach to the Patient With a Bleeding Diathesis. UpToDate serial online. www.uptodate.com. Accessed May 18, 2008.
25. Greer JP, Foerster J, Lukens JN, et al. Laboratory methods for study of hemostasis and blood coagulation. *Wintrobe's Clinical Hematology*, 11th ed. Philadelphia, PA: Lippincott Williams & Wilkins; 2004.
26. Sosothikul D, Seksarn P, Lusher JM. Pediatric reference values for molecular markers in hemostasis. *J Pediatr Hematol Oncol.* 2007;29(1):19–22.
27. Brady KM, Easley RB, Tobias JD. Recombinant activated factor VII (rFVIIa) treatment in infants with hemorrhage. *Pediatr Anesth.* 2006;16:1042–1046.
28. Ziv O, Ragni MV. Bleeding manifestations in males with von Willebrand disease. *Haemophilia.* 2004;10:162–168.
29. Hoots WK, Shapiro AD. Treatment of Hemophilia. UpToDate serial online. www.uptodate.com. Accessed on May 18, 2008.
30. Stieltjes N, Calvez T, Demiguel V, et al. Intracranial haemorrhages in French haemophilia patients (1991–2001): clinical presentation, management and prognosis factors for death. *Haemophilia.* 2005;11(5):452–458.
31. Radosevich M. Safety of recombinant and plasma-derived medicinal for the treatment of coagulopathies. *Hematol Oncol Clin North Am.* 2000;14(2):459–470.
32. Shord SS, Lindley CM. Coagulation products and their uses. *Am J Health Syst Pharm.* 2000;57(15):1403–1420.
33. Rick ME. Treatment of von Willebrand Disease. UpToDate serial online. www.uptodate.com. Accessed on May 18, 2008.
34. Nolan B, White B, Smith J, et al. Desmopressin: therapeutic limitations in children and adults with inherited coagulation disorders. *Br J Haematol.* 2000;109:865–869.
35. Johnson LH, Gittelman M. Management of bleeding diasthesis: a case-based approach. *Clin Pediatr Emerg Med.* 2005;05:149–155
36. Burnouf T, Radosevich M, Goubran HA. Local hemostatic blood products: fibrin sealant and platelet gel. *Treatment of Hemophilia.* 2004;36:1–7.
37. Silvergleid AJ. Fibrin Sealant. UpToDate serial online. www.uptodate.com. Accessed on May 18, 2008.

38. Strauss RG. Risks of blood component transfusions. In: Behrman, ed. *Nelson Textbook of Pediatrics*, 17th ed. 2004.

39. Hoots WK, Shapiro AD. Factor VIII and factor IX inhibitors in patients with hemophilia. UpToDate serial online. www.uptodate.com. Accessed on May 18, 2008.

40. Mitsiakos G, Papaioannou G, Giougi E, et al. Is the use of rFVIIa safe and effective in bleeding neonates? A retrospective series of 8 cases. *J Pediatr Hematol Oncol.* 2007;29(3):145–150.

41. Levi M, Peters M, Büller HR. Efficacy and safety of recombinant factor VIIa for treatment of severe bleeding: a systematic review. *Crit Care Med.* 2005:33(4):883–890.

42. Mathew R, Young G. Recombinant factor VIIa in paediatric bleeding disorders – a 2006 review. *Haemophilia.* 2006;12:457–472.

43. Veldman A, Josef J, Rischer D, et al. A prospective pilot study of prophylactic treatment of preterm neonates with recombinant activated factor VII during the first 72 hours of life. *Pediatr Crit Care Med.* 2006;7(1):34–39.

44. Michiels JJ, van de Velde A, van Vliet HHDM, et al. Response of von Willebrand factor parameters to desmopressin in patients with type 1 and type 2 congenital von Willebrand disease: diagnostic and therapeutic implications. *Semin Thromb Hemost.* 2002;28(2):111–132.

45. Federici AB, Castaman G, Franchini M, et al. Clinical use of Haemate P in inherited von Willebrand's disease: a cohort study on 100 Italian patients. *Haematologica.* 2007;92(7): 944–951.

46. High KA. Update on progress and hurdles in novel genetic therapies for hemophilia. *Hematology Am Soc Hematol Educ Program.* 2007:466–472.

21

Metabolic/Endocrine Emergencies

Kenneth T. Kwon and Virginia W. Tsai

INTRODUCTION

Metabolic and endocrine disorders, either acquired or congenital, comprise a variety of entities that cause derangement in normal physiology and metabolism. These may include diseases related to inborn errors of metabolism (IEM), electrolyte imbalances or endocrine dysfunction. Children with metabolic disturbances frequently present with symptoms similar to those with other emergencies, particularly in the newborn period and early infancy. Initial consideration of a metabolic or endocrine disease in the differential diagnosis is important, especially in previously healthy neonates with acute deterioration.

These diseases can vary as much in clinical presentation as they can in classification. Because the symptomatology of these disorders is also associated with a variety of nonmetabolic diseases, many metabolic and endocrine conditions are missed in the emergency department (ED). Differences in presentation can be subtle, especially in the neonatal period. Vomiting, alterations in neurologic status and feeding difficulties are perhaps the most prominent features of metabolic and endocrine diseases. Characteristic clinical manifestations of specific disorders are discussed individually in the following text. Definitive diagnosis is frequently not possible or necessary during the ED course, but proper initial management based on probable diagnosis can be life-saving or reduce neurologic sequelae. Those disorders that are responsive to ED treatment are highlighted.

GENERAL EMERGENCY MANAGEMENT CONSIDERATIONS

Initial ED management for a suspected metabolic or endocrine disorder should begin with the standard ABCs (airway, breathing, circulation) approach. Poorly perfusing or hypotensive infants require standard intravenous (IV) fluid replacement, and antibiotics should be administered promptly when suspecting sepsis. If diabetic ketoacidosis (DKA) is suspected or confirmed, aggressive fluid resuscitation should be avoided in normotensive infants due to its association with cerebral edema.

Careful history may reveal important clues suggestive of metabolic disease. Questions about prenatal care and maternal medications may elucidate an endocrine disorder. Newborn screening test results are important inquiries when considering an IEM, as is a history of consanguinity or sudden infant death in the immediate family. Feeding difficulties, weight loss or association of symptoms with dietary intake or particular types of food are important inquiries, especially in newborns. Vomiting is a prominent feature in most metabolic disorders, both as a primary symptom as well as a compensatory mechanism by which excess body acid is eliminated via the gastrointestinal (GI) tract.

Physical examination should focus on the patient's neurologic and circulatory status. Alterations in consciousness can range from mild lethargy to seizures and coma. Hypotonia with poor suck and Moro reflexes are frequently seen. Dehydration with tachycardia, poor perfusion or hypotension should be recognized early and treated aggressively. Tachypnea is a characteristic sign in acidotic infants, and the degree of tachypnea frequently correlates with the severity of acidosis. A fruity breath can be seen in DKA or other ketotic diseases, whereas other unusual or peculiar body fluid odors suggest IEMs. Hepatomegaly and jaundice may be prominent, especially in glycogen storage diseases and galactosemia.

Emergent diagnostic testing should begin with bedside glucose testing, which should be verified by standard laboratory testing. Electrolytes with calculation of anion gap are important for diagnostic classification. Acid-base status can be more precisely measured with an arterial blood gas, although in the absence of hypoxia or poor perfusion, a venous or capillary measurement may be adequate and less invasive in infants. Concurrent with these studies should be standard investigations for infection, including a complete blood cell (CBC) count, cerebrospinal fluid studies and body fluid cultures, when indicated. Serum calcium, magnesium and liver function tests should also be obtained. Further diagnostic tests to consider are discussed under the specific entities.

Most symptomatic infants with a known or suspected metabolic disorder will require hospitalization, usually in an intensive care setting, for frequent monitoring of metabolic parameters and neurologic status. Prompt consultation should be initiated with a pediatric endocrinologist or metabolic specialist. If appropriate resources are unavailable, transfer should be arranged with a pediatric center skilled in managing metabolic disorders. This should be done expeditiously after resuscitation and empiric treatment for likely causes have been started.

INBORN ERRORS OF METABOLISM

This diverse group of hereditary disorders involves gene mutations, usually of a single enzyme or transport system, causing significant blocks in metabolic pathways and accumulation or deficiency of a particular metabolite. Due to the large number and complexity of IEMs, the reported incidence of these disorders varies greatly, ranging from 1 in 1400 to 200,000 live births.[1,2] It is now possible to screen for many of these defects in the newborn as well as prenatal periods. Some IEMs manifest clinically in the newborn period or shortly thereafter, and failure of early diagnosis may lead to permanent neurologic sequelae and death if specific treatment is not initiated. Although collectively numerous, IEMs that are amenable to specific emergency medications are limited. However, the majority of them should respond to removal of the offending metabolite from the diet. The most common emergent clinical manifestations in the neonatal period include vomiting, neurologic abnormalities, metabolic acidosis and hypoglycemia.[3,4] These nonspecific findings can mimic other disorders, such as sepsis or adrenal crisis, but an IEM should be considered in a previously normal neonate with acute clinical deterioration. Conversely, the presence of infection does not exclude the possibility of IEMs,

as these infants frequently deteriorate and become septic quickly. Standard laboratory values, particularly blood ammonia, electrolytes and urinalysis, can be helpful in further classifying the IEM and tailoring treatment in the ED (Figure 21.1).

Presentation

IEMs can be divided into disorders of amino acid metabolism (phenylketonuria, nonketotic hyperglycinemia), fatty acid oxidation/metabolism (medium-chain acyl-CoA dehydrogenase deficiency, primary carnitine deficiency), energy metabolism (primary lactic acidemias) and carbohydrate metabolism (glycogen storage diseases, galactosemia). Organic acidemias and acidurias (methylmalonic, propionic and isovaleric acidemias; maple syrup urine disease) refer to a specific group of disorders of amino and fatty acid metabolism in which high levels of nonamino organic acids accumulate in serum and urine.

Many patients with IEMs exhibit symptoms as newborns after feedings have been initiated, but a minority may go undetected into infancy or childhood with only psychomotor delay until a stressor causes acute deterioration. Recurrent vomiting, dehydration and acute metabolic encephalopathy are common clinical manifestations. Neurologic symptoms can range from hypotonia to seizures to frank coma. Intractable seizures are characteristic of nonketotic hyperglycinemia and pyridoxine-dependent seizures. Hepatomegaly is a common physical exam finding and can be pronounced in glycogen storage diseases and galactosemia, although it tends to be less evident in infancy. Risk of infection, particularly *Escherichia coli* sepsis, and liver failure are also increased in patients with galactosemia. A peculiar odor in body fluids can be associated with specific disorders and may offer an invaluable aid to diagnosis when present. Maple syrup urine disease is named for its characteristic sweet sugar odor, isovaleric acidemia is associated with a "sweaty feet" scent and methylmalonic and propionic acidemias can exude a fruity ketotic odor similar to that of DKA. Metabolic acidosis with an increased anion gap is very common in many IEMs and can aid in further classification. Hypoglycemia is also common and can be pronounced, particularly in glycogen storage diseases and defects of fatty acid oxidation.[5] Hyperammonemia is most commonly seen in organic acidemias and urea cycle defects.

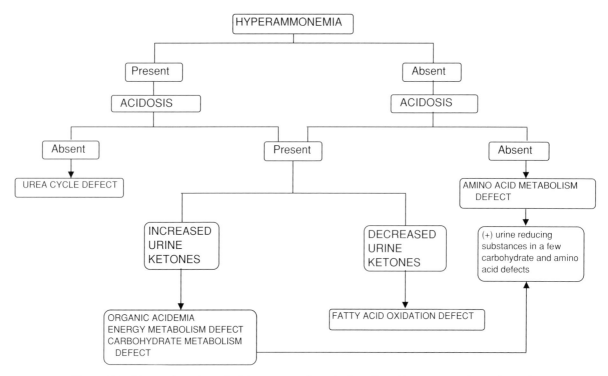

Figure 21.1. Diagnostic pathway for inborn errors of metabolism. Note: Exceptions to this pathway do exist. (Modified from Brousseau T, Sharieff G. The critically ill newborn. *Critical Decisions in Emergency Medicine*. 2003;18:1–7.)

Urea cycle defects are a specific classification of IEMs, which lead to hyperammonemia due to the inability to detoxify ammonia to urea. Common disorders include ornithine transcarbamylase (OTC) deficiency, arginase deficiency (argininemia), and argininosuccinic acid synthetase deficiency (citrullinemia). Clinical manifestations parallel those seen in other IEMs. Neonates frequently present after a few days of protein feeding of either breast milk or formula. Symptoms include vomiting, poor feeding and post-prandial neurologic alterations. Older infants may present with recurrent vomiting, ataxia or developmental delay. Tachypnea is common due to stimulation of the respiratory center by ammonia. The level of hyperammonemia tends to be higher than that seen in organic acidemias. Serum ammonia is usually above 200 μmol/L (normal is <35–50 μmol/L), with some complete enzyme defects reaching levels greater than 500 to 1000 μmol/L.[6,7] Although sicker infants tend to have higher ammonia levels, no strict correlation exists between ammonia levels and clinical findings. The degree of neurologic impairment is thought to be related more to the duration of hyperammonemia than to the level itself. Blood urea nitrogen (BUN) is usually low, but a normal BUN does not exclude a urea cycle defect. Metabolic acidosis

does not occur with these disorders unless they are associated with a concurrent dehydrating illness. Thus the lack of acidosis is helpful in differentiating urea cycle defects from many of the other IEMs.

Differential Diagnosis

When considering an IEM, ammonia levels and acid-base status can help classify a particular disorder (see Figure 21.1). Other entities to consider include adrenal insufficiency, hyperthyroidism, infection or sepsis, gastroenteritis, seizure disorder, dehydration, DKA, hypoglycemia, hyponatremia and metabolic acidosis.

Lab and Radiology

Standard ED testing for metabolic abnormalities and infection should be undertaken. Additionally, serum ammonia level should be obtained in any altered infant in whom an IEM is suspected. Testing for ammonia levels need to be completed within 30 minutes of the blood draw to avoid falsely elevated levels. Ammonia is significantly elevated in urea cycle defects and many of the organic acidemias. Of note is that mild transient elevation of ammonia is common in asymptomatic neonates, especially premature infants. Lactate and pyruvate levels can be of use. Although both acids can be elevated in sepsis and IEMs, the lactate-to-pyruvate ratio tends to be increased in sepsis ($>10{:}1$), whereas in some IEMs, such as primary lactic acidosis, the ratio is usually normal.

Urinalysis will reveal the presence or absence of ketones, which can help to differentiate particular IEMs; the lack of an appropriate ketonuric response to metabolic acidosis is indicative of a fatty acid oxidation defect. The pH of urine is normally less than 5 in organic acidemias, whereas the most common urea cycle defect, ornithine transcarbamylase deficiency, may contain urinary orotic acid crystals. Urine-reducing substances in the absence of glucosuria are indicative of galactosuria and presumptive galactosemia. Urine-reducing substances can also be seen in a few select disorders of amino acid metabolism, such as tyrosinemia.

Additional archival body fluid samples should be appropriately collected and stored if an undiagnosed metabolic disease is considered in the ED and preferably prior to initiation of any therapy. For organic acidemias and other defects in amino acid and fatty acid metabolism, quantitative blood amino acids and urinary amino and organic acids will aid in definitive diagnosis. Although these tests are nonemergent, the ED physician may, on occasion, be requested to order these studies by a consultant.

Management

Treatment for IEMs consists of general measures as well as specific medications if a probable type of IEM is suspected. Unless the infant has a known IEM and is already on a special formula, all dietary intake should be withheld and feedings only re-introduced after consultation with a specialist. IV fluid containing dextrose may be indicated, particularly if a urea cycle defect is suspected, as stimulating endogenous insulin will minimize protein catabolism and ammonia production. After appropriate fluid boluses of normal saline to correct shock, most IEMs can be managed with a standard IV fluid consisting of 10% dextrose in $\frac{1}{4}$ normal saline at 1.5 times maintenance. Metabolic acidosis unresponsive to IV fluids should be treated with sodium bicarbonate boluses of 1 to 2 mEq/kg. Although controversial for other diseases, bicarbonate use for IEMs is indicated, but standard calculations of

Table 21.1. Specific therapies for inborn errors of metabolism

Drug	Dose	Indication
Arginine HCL 10%	210–600 mg/kg IV	Urea cycle defects
Biotin	10 mg IV or PO	Organic acidemias
Carnitine	50–400 mg/kg IV or PO	Fatty acid defects, organic acidemias
Pyridoxine	100 mg IV	Pyridoxine-dependent seizures
Sodium benzoate* and/or phenylacetate*	250 mg/kg IV	Urea cycle defects
Thiamine	25–100 mg IV	MSUD, primary lactic acidosis

* Can infuse over 1–2 hours in dextrose-containing solution.
MSUD, maple syrup urine disease.
Data from Burton,[6] de Baulny,[10] Ozand,[5] and Weiner.[2]

bicarbonate requirements will underestimate actual needs due to ongoing production of acidic metabolites.[6,8] Correction of severe acidosis will often require large doses of bicarbonate, up to 20 mEq/kg in some organic acidemias.[9] Liberal use of bicarbonate, however, should be done in consultation with a metabolic specialist. The rapid removal of toxins may be life-saving in some cases, particularly with severe hyperammonemia. An ammonia level greater than 120 μmol/mL in a newborn is considered neurotoxic. Hemodialysis to remove excessive ammonia is more effective than peritoneal or other extracorporeal routes.[6,10] Temporizing empiric therapy with arginine, with or without sodium benzoate/phenylacetate, can reduce ammonia levels acutely in most urea cycle defects. Table 21.1 lists specific therapies to consider when suspecting particular IEMs.

In the event of a failed resuscitation or imminent death in an infant with a suspected IEM, permission for autopsy and specimen testing should be thoughtfully discussed with parents. Perimortem samples to consider obtaining include frozen blood, plasma and urine specimens; skin biopsy and needle liver biopsy.[6,9] These studies will allow for appropriate genetic counseling for current family members and future siblings.

ADRENAL INSUFFICIENCY

Adrenal insufficiency is due to primary adrenal disease or secondary to pituitary suppression and can be inherited or acquired. Congenital adrenal hyperplasia (CAH) is an important cause of primary adrenal insufficiency in the newborn period, whereas Addison's disease is a more common etiology in infants and older children. Secondary adrenal insufficiency is uncommon in newborns and almost always involves exogenous steroid use for a chronic disease with subsequent discontinuation. Acute adrenal insufficiency or crisis occurs when the adrenal glands fail to produce adequate glucocorticoid and mineralocorticoid in response to stress.

CAH refers to a group of inherited autosomal recessive disorders with defects in adrenal biosynthesis of the glucocorticoid cortisol. The low cortisol production stimulates pituitary production of adrenocorticotropic hormone (ACTH), which causes the characteristic hyperplasia of the adrenal cortex. Depending on the affected enzyme, the synthesis of other steroids such as mineralocorticoids (aldosterone) and androgens may also be affected, and clinical expression will vary depending on the accumulated biosynthetic precursors. Deficiency of 21-hydroxylase (21-OH) accounts for up to 95% of CAH cases, and discussion here is limited to this particular form of CAH. This disorder occurs in 1 in 10,000 to 15,000 live births worldwide.[11] Up to 75% of affected newborns have the classic salt-losing virilizing variant, which is associated with aldosterone deficiency and androgen overproduction (17-hydroxyprogesterone); up to 25% have the non–salt-losing simple virilizing type. The degree of virilization and other clinical signs are usually more pronounced and seen earlier in life in the salt-losing variant.

Many states now screen newborns for CAH. However, these results may not be available for several weeks, allowing for an acute adrenal crisis to occur during this time. Males are particularly prone to missed diagnosis, as their genitalia may appear normal at birth; females will usually exhibit some degree of ambiguous genitalia, such as clitoral enlargement or fusion of labial folds. Another physical examination sign is hyperpigmentation. Although uncommon in newborns, it may be present in the axilla and scrotal or labial areas and is due to the accumulation of a corticotropin precursor, which stimulates melanocytes. With the classic salt-losing type, symptoms may begin 1 to 2 weeks after birth and include weight loss, poor feeding, vomiting, polyuria and dehydration. Progression can occur rapidly, particularly in the setting of infection or trauma, to altered mental status, hypotension or death.

Presentation

The common ED presentation involves a newborn male with an uneventful birth history who presents within the first 2 weeks of life with apparent dehydration or sepsis and circulatory collapse unresponsive to fluid resuscitation. Acute adrenal insufficiency is associated with hyponatremia, hyperkalemia and hypoglycemia. A normal anion gap metabolic acidosis is often seen due to aldosterone deficiency.

Differential Diagnosis

The most important entity to consider in addition to CAH is infection or sepsis. Other diseases to consider include adrenal hypoplasia, hypoglycemia, hyponatremia, hyperkalemia, hypopituitarism, hypothyroidism, congenital heart disease and metabolic acidosis.

Lab and Radiology

Prior to treatment, if possible, blood should be collected for non-emergent testing of specific endocrine hormones and metabolites. For suspected adrenal insufficiency and CAH, additional blood studies to consider include cortisol, ACTH, 17-hydroxyprogesterone, aldosterone, renin, insulin, and growth hormone.

Management

Treatment of acute adrenal insufficiency should be geared toward aggressive fluid resuscitation and rapid stress doses of corticosteroids. Table 21.2 lists various options. Hydrocortisone is the steroid of choice as it has equal glucocorticoid and mineralocorticoid effects; cortisone is an alternative but cannot be given via IV. Stress parenteral dose of hydrocortisone is 25 to 50 mg/m^2 (~2–3 mg/kg), followed by 100 mg/m^2/day in divided doses. The typical dose in a neonate or young infant is 25 mg. Dexamethasone has no mineralocorticoid effect but is advocated by some over hydrocortisone in normotensive patients with an unconfirmed diagnosis due to its noninterference with diagnostic ACTH stimulation testing. An oral mineralocorticoid such as fludrocortisone can be started after initial stabilization with IV fluids and glucocorticoids. Hyperkalemia should correct with fluids and steroid therapy and rarely needs individual correction, as neonates can tolerate elevated potassium levels better than children and adults.

Table 21.2. Corticosteroids for adrenal insufficiency

| Drug | Dose | Potency effect (per mg) | |
		Glucocorticoid	Mineralocorticoid
Glucocorticoid			
Hydrocortisone	25–50 mg/m^2 IV/IM	1	1
	Infant: 25 mg		
	Child: 50 mg		
	Teen: 75 mg		
Cortisone	1 mg/kg IM	0.8	1
Dexamethasone	0.1–0.2 mg/kg IV/IM	40	None
Mineralocorticoid			
Fludrocortisone	0.1 mg PO daily	15	400

IM, intramuscular; IV, intravenous; PO, per os.

THYROID DISORDERS

Neonatal thyrotoxicosis, also called *congenital hyperthyroidism,* is usually due to in utero passage of thyroid-stimulating immunoglobulins from mother to fetus. The incidence is 1 in 4000 to 50,000 live births.[12] By far, most cases are due to maternal Graves' disease, an autoimmune disorder that produces thyroid-stimulating hormone (TSH) receptor antibodies causing increased thyroid hormone release. The prevalence of Graves' disease in pregnant women is 0.1% to 0.4%, with hyperthyroidism seen in 0.6% to 10% of infants born to these mothers.[13] Euthyroid mothers treated for hyperthyroidism are still at risk for having a newborn with thyrotoxicosis.

Hypothyroidism does not occur with acute signs or symptoms and is rarely classified as an emergent condition. Congenital hypothyroidism, however, may occasionally be missed due to laboratory errors in newborn screening, and early ED detection and treatment within the first few weeks of life are important to prevent irreversible brain damage. The incidence is 1 in 4000 live births and is the most common treatable cause of mental retardation. Classic symptoms include prolonged jaundice, poor feeding, hoarse cry, constipation, somnolence and hypothermia. Classic signs include coarse puffy facies, large fontanelles, macroglossia, hypotonia, dry skin, jaundice and distended abdomen with umbilical hernia.

Presentation

Infants with neonatal hyperthyroidism are commonly born preterm with low birthweight, microcephaly and craniosynostosis. They usually present within a few days of life but presentation can sometimes be delayed 10 days or more. Symptoms are transient and usually last fewer than 12 weeks, the duration of which is dependent on the persistence of maternally transmitted immunoglobulins. Symptoms include vomiting, diarrhea, poor feeding and weight loss, sweating and irritability. Most will have a goiter, and many will also have exophthalmos, hyperthermia, tachycardia, hepatomegaly and jaundice. Although transient, neonatal thyrotoxicosis can be life-threatening, with a reported mortality of up to 20%, usually from heart failure.[12] Thyroid storm can occur in infants and consists of extreme signs and symptoms of hyperthyroidism combined with a high fever and altered mental status. It is usually precipitated by infection, trauma or dehydration. Thyroid storm is life-threatening and treatment should be aggressive and similar to adult management.

Hyperthyroidism in older infants and children is almost always due to Graves' disease. Nearly 5% of all patients with hyperthyroidism are younger than 15 years of age, with the majority being adolescents. Unlike adults, children with hyperthyroidism usually have an indolent progression of symptoms over months, although symptoms may occur more abruptly. Personality disturbances or motor hyperactivity may be the earliest symptoms, followed by the classic symptoms of weight loss, heat intolerance, diaphoresis, palpitations, diarrhea and amenorrhea. A goiter is present in nearly 100% of cases, and exophthalmos, tachycardia and hypertension are common.[14]

Differential Diagnosis

Diagnostic considerations include maternal Graves' disease, maternal opioid use and withdrawal, infection or sepsis, congenital heart disease, congestive heart failure and pheochromocytoma.

Lab and Radiology

Emergent thyroid function testing is now available in many laboratories; therefore, these tests should be initiated in the ED when indicated. Although variable studies exist, essential testing should include levels for TSH and free thyroxine (T_4). Normal ranges of T_4 and TSH concentrations are higher in neonates than older infants and children. Also, thyroid function tests may be unreliable in the first few days of life if the mother was taking antithyroid medications before delivery.

Management

Neonatal hyperthyroidism and thyroid storm have many therapeutic options. Beta-adrenergic blockade can be achieved with propranolol 0.01 mg/kg/dose IV and titrated to clinical effect; alternative oral dosing is 2 mg/kg/day in 3 to 4 divided doses. Thyroid hormone synthesis can be blocked using propylthiouracil 5 to 10 mg/kg/day or methimazole 0.5 to 1 mg/kg/day, both in 3 divided oral doses. Iodine can be given in the form of Lugol's solution (8 mg iodine/drop), 1 to 3 drops daily. Iodine should be started at least 1 hour after administering an antithyroid drug, such as propylthiouracil, to avoid increasing thyroid gland stores before the antithyroid effect occurs. Glucocorticoid treatment with hydrocortisone or prednisone may also be helpful in severe cases as it inhibits thyroid hormone release and decreases peripheral conversion of T_4 to T_3.

METABOLIC ACIDOSIS

Metabolic acidosis occurs via three major mechanisms:

1. Loss of bicarbonate from the kidney or GI tract
2. Excess acid from endogenous production or exogenous source
3. Underexcretion of acid by the kidneys

Neonates and infants are more susceptible than older children to develop acidosis due to their lower renal threshold for bicarbonate reabsorption and limited maximum net acid excretion. Thus young infants have a relatively limited compensatory mechanism for an excess acid load.

Presentation

Clinical manifestations of metabolic acidosis are nonspecific and include altered mental status, vomiting, respiratory distress and poor perfusion. An important sign, particularly in neonates, that can alert the ED physician of metabolic acidosis is tachypnea, a compensatory mechanism creating a respiratory alkalotic response. This breathing can range from mild shallow tachypnea to deep Kussmaul respirations of severely acidotic patients.

Differential Diagnosis

The presence of metabolic acidosis has important diagnostic considerations depending on the classification of acidosis as either normal anion gap or increased anion gap. The anion gap is calculated as the difference between serum sodium and the sum of serum chloride and bicarbonate $[Na^+ - (Cl^- + HCO_3^-)]$. A normal anion gap range is somewhat age-dependent but in the pediatric population is 12 ± 4, thus an anion gap of greater than 16 is considered elevated. Causes of metabolic acidosis based on anion gap are listed in Table 21.3. Lactic acidosis is the most common cause of an increased anion gap acidosis in critically ill neonates.[15]

Management

Treatment is focused toward appropriate fluid resuscitation and specific therapy of the underlying cause of the acid-base disturbance. The use of sodium bicarbonate is controversial, but most would only recommend using

Table 21.3. Causes of metabolic acidosis

Normal anion gap
Gastroenteritis/diarrhea
Renal tubular acidosis
Adrenal (mineralocorticoid) insufficiency
Increased Anion Gap
MUDPILES: Methanol, uremia, DKA, paraldehyde, iron or INH, lactic acidosis, ethylene glycol, salicylates
Inborn errors: Carbohydrate, amino acid, or fatty acid metabolism
Starvation
Chronic renal insufficiency

DKA, diabetic ketoacidosis.

it if an inborn error is suspected or if the metabolic acidosis is causing significant arrhythmias or hemodynamic instability. Some advocate its use in DKA with pH lower than 6.9 or significant hyperkalemia or arrhythmias, or in non-DKA metabolic acidosis with pH lower than 7.1 refractory to other treatments. The dose of sodium bicarbonate is 1 to 2 mEq/kg IV. Bicarbonate potentially improves cardiac output and blood pressure, but these benefits are thought to be only transient in neonates.[16] Bicarbonate therapy is potentially harmful as it shifts the oxygen-hemoglobin dissociation curve to the left and can worsen tissue hypoxia, particularly in hypovolemic patients. It can also cause hypernatremia, hypokalemia and paradoxical drop in central nervous system pH leading to decreased consciousness. Albumin 5% infusion in neonates has been shown to be less effective than bicarbonate in correcting metabolic acidosis.[17]

HYPOGLYCEMIA

Hypoglycemia is one of the most commonly encountered metabolic problems, especially in the neonatal period. The definition of *hypoglycemia* is somewhat controversial and age-dependent. In children, infants and term neonates older than 1 to 2 days of life, hypoglycemia is usually defined as a serum glucose concentration less than 40 to 45 mg/dL.[18,19] In term and premature neonates within 1 day of life, levels as low as 30 mg/dL are considered by some to be normal. The laboratory value should be interpreted in the context of the clinical presentation, as symptoms may occur within a continuum of low glucose levels. Thus, glucose levels of 50 to 60 mg/dL combined with symptoms of hypoglycemia may warrant treatment.

Glucose is the main energy substrate for the brain, and its levels represent a balance between exogenous supply and endogenous gluconeogenesis and glycogenolysis. Mobilization and use of glucose is mediated by hormones, primarily insulin. Insulin stimulates glucose uptake in cells and glycogen synthesis, and its actions are opposed by epinephrine, glucagon, cortisol and growth hormone. Hypoglycemia can occur when imbalances exist between exogenous and endogenous substrate supplies, which may involve these hormonal abnormalities.

Early detection of hypoglycemia is critical as permanent brain damage may begin shortly after symptoms develop, particularly in newborns and infants. Bedside glucose testing should be performed on all pediatric patients who appear seriously ill or altered. Hypoglycemia occurring in children requiring resuscitation care is associated with increased mortality.[20]

Presentation

Symptoms of hypoglycemia generally fall into two categories: those associated with activation of the autonomic nervous system (adrenergic), and those associated with decreased cerebral glucose utilization (neuroglycopenic). Adrenergic symptoms are usually seen early with a rapid decline in blood glucose and include tachycardia, tachypnea, vomiting and diaphoresis. Most of these patients are hypoglycemic prior to ED arrival, thus these symptoms are frequently absent. More familiar are the neuroglycopenic symptoms, which are usually associated with slower or prolonged hypoglycemia. These symptoms include poor feeding, altered mental status, lethargy and seizures. These classic symptoms are usually evident in older children and adults, but in infants, the presentation may be subtle and include only hypotonia, hypothermia, jitteriness, exaggerated primitive reflexes or feeding difficulties.

Differential Diagnosis

Causes of hypoglycemia in the pediatric population are listed in Table 21.4. Important etiologies in the ED include infection, adrenal insufficiency, inborn errors and medication-induced emergencies. Hyperinsulinemia, particularly persistent hyperinsulinemic hypoglycemia of infancy, should be considered as a potential cause of intractable hypoglycemia from the newborn period to 6 months of age.

Management

Acute treatment for hypoglycemia begins with IV glucose bolus replacement. The recommended dose ranges from 0.2 to 1 g/kg; thus, a mid-level range of 0.4 to 0.5 g/kg glucose translates to approximately 4 mL/kg of 10% dextrose or 2 mL/kg of 25% dextrose. Some advocate a smaller bolus of 0.2 g/kg (2 mL/kg of 10% dextrose) to minimize hyperglycemia and resultant insulin secretion and possible prolonged hypoglycemia.[21] Generally, 10% solution is used in neonates and infants, whereas 25% solution is used in toddlers and children. More dilute solutions are used in younger patients to minimize vascular injury caused by more concentrated fluids. Continuous glucose

Table 21.4. Causes of hypoglycemia

Decreased production/availability of glucose
Low glycogen stores
Small for gestational age, prematurity
Malnutrition/fasting
Idiopathic ketotic hypoglycemia
Malabsorption/diarrhea

Increased Utilization of Glucose
Hyperinsulinemic states
Infant of diabetic mother
Persistent hyperinsulinemic hypoglycemia of infancy (PHHI)
Nesidioblastosis
Islet cell adenoma/hyperplasia
Beckwith-Wiedemann syndrome
Stress
Infection/sepsis

Combined or Other Mechanism
Inborn errors of metabolism

Hormone deficiency
Adrenal (glucocorticoid) insufficiency
Growth hormone deficiency
Glucagon deficiency

Iatrogenic
Insulin/oral hypoglycemic therapy
Poisoning (ethanol, propranolol, salicylates)
Reye's syndrome

infusion should follow bolus administration to maintain normal glucose homeostasis, especially in neonates. Normal glucose requirement in a neonate is 6 to 10 mg/kg/min, which is roughly equivalent to an infusion of 10% dextrose-containing solution at $1\frac{1}{2}$ times maintenance rate. Glucose levels should be rechecked frequently (every 1–2 hours) and the infusion rate adjusted accordingly.

If hypoglycemia persists despite boluses and infusions, a hyperinsulinemic state should be considered. Glucagon 0.1 to 0.2 mg/kg (up to 1 mg) parenterally can be given to infants for refractory hypoglycemia. Glucagon can be given intramuscularly, thus it can be particularly helpful when IV access is difficult or delayed. Glucagon will not be effective in patients lacking adequate glycogen stores such as those with inherited storage diseases.[22] Hydrocortisone 2 to 3 mg/kg or 25 to 50 mg/m² can also be considered for refractory hypoglycemia.[23]

HYPERGLYCEMIA AND DIABETIC KETOACIDOSIS

Hyperglycemia is typically defined as a glucose concentration of greater than 125 to 150 mg/dL. It is usually seen in critically ill, nondiabetic patients of all ages and can signify increased mortality. Hyperglycemia is frequently seen in the first week of life and is inversely correlated to gestational age, with up to 18 times greater occurrence in neonates with birthweights less than 1000 g.[24,25] It can also be seen in infants who are acutely stressed or septic, are receiving high rates of glucose infusion, or are being treated with corticosteroids or other drugs. In noniatrogenic conditions, hyperglycemia may be a consequence of physiologic stress and higher levels of counter-regulatory hormones including glucagon, catecholamines, cortisol, and growth hormones. Etiologies of hyperglycemia include immaturity in the neonatal period, absolute or relative insulin insufficiency and hepatic and peripheral insulin resistance. Due to their small mass of insulin-dependent tissue, namely muscle and fat, infants have limited glucose utilization compared with larger children and adults.[24,25] The greatest risk of hyperglycemia is dehydration as a consequence of urinary loss of glucose and osmotic diuresis. The hyperosmolarity and osmotic shifts that occur can augment the risk of cerebral bleeding due to brain cell dehydration, dilation of capillaries and inability to autoregulate cerebral blood pressure. Whether infants with stress-induced hyperglycemia are at risk for later development of diabetes mellitus is unknown.[26,27]

Presentation

Insulin-dependent diabetes mellitus (IDDM) diagnosed in the newborn or during the first 6 months of life is exceedingly rare, affecting approximately 1 in 500,000 births.[24,25] More commonly seen is an interim form called *transient neonatal diabetes mellitus*. It resembles permanent diabetes mellitus but resolves within several weeks or months. Patients affected with the transient form during infancy may have reoccurrence of diabetes mellitus later in life.[25] The ultimate cause of neonatal diabetes remains unclear; however, many theories have related to immature metabolic pathways. Most children investigated have low birthweights for their gestational age with some full-term infants weighing less than 1500 g. Other possible associations include short-term maternal enterovirus infection, autoimmune enterocolitis, congenital absence of islet of Langerhans, rare genetic disorders and pancreatic agenesis.[24–26] Interestingly, patients who develop IDDM after the first 180 days of life have genetic profiles and clinical courses similar to other IDDM patients who develop the disease later in life.[25]

Diagnosing IDDM in the young infant can be very difficult for understandable reasons. Polydipsia cannot be communicated by the nonverbal infant, very absorbent diapers may mask polyuria and oral rehydration may obscure acute weight loss. Recurrent cutaneous candidiasis, although common in infants, can be considered an indication for the clinician to check blood glucose levels.[26–28] Infants are often misdiagnosed with pneumonia, asthma or bronchiolitis and undergo treatment with corticosteroids that will only exaggerate the metabolic derangements of IDDM. These difficulties help explain why the younger the patient presents with IDDM, the more likely the patient will present with severe decompensation, including acidosis, obtundation and possibly cerebral edema.[26]

DKA is defined as a glucose level higher than 200 mg/dL with either a bicarbonate less than 15 mEq/L or venous pH lower than 7.3. It is more challenging to recognize and treat in younger patients for several reasons. The higher basal metabolic rate and larger surface area to body mass ratio in infants require exacting amounts of fluid and electrolyte repletion. The smaller patient is also at higher risk to develop cerebral edema due to the immaturity of auto-regulatory mechanisms. Cerebral edema is thought to occur in about 0.5% to 1% of all children with DKA and is the most probable cause of morbidity, with death in 20% to 25% and pituitary insufficiency in 10% to 25% of survivors.[26,28–30] Other causes of mortality in infants with DKA include concomitant pneumonia, sepsis, pulmonary edema and cardiac arrhythmias associated with electrolyte imbalances.

The pathophysiology of DKA can be condensed to a mixture of insulin deficiency and antagonism during physiologic stress with the actions of counter-regulatory hormones. Increased glucose production from glycogenolysis and gluconeogenesis coupled with the inability to use glucose leads to hyperglycemia, osmotic diuresis, loss of electrolytes, hyperosmolarity and dehydration. This fierce cycle occurs concurrently with lipolysis as the body senses a starvation mode and enters oxidative metabolism with resultant ketone (beta-hydroxybutyrate) formation and metabolic acidosis. Lactic acid also adds to the acidosis as tissues undergo anaerobic metabolism with inadequate perfusion. Clinically, the infant will likely present with vomiting, lethargy or frank coma, polyuria, deep

Kussmaul respirations and severe dehydration. DKA can be categorized as *mild,* with a venous pH of 7.2 to 7.3; *moderate,* with a venous pH of 7.1 to 7.2 and *severe,* with venous pH lower than 7.1.

Differential Diagnosis

The differential diagnoses of hyperglycemia and DKA can be endocrine based. IDDM and diabetes insipidus may both present with polyuria, polydipsia and profound dehydration. The metabolic states of pheochromocytoma and hyperthyroidism may lead to hyperglycemia. Toxic etiologies include salicylate toxicity and calcium channel blocker toxicity. Any infection and resulting sepsis may also cause hyperglycemia.

Lab and Radiology

Initial diagnostic tests should include blood draws for serum electrolyte levels, glucose, osmolality (measured and calculated), pH, CBC count, beta-hydroxybutyrate and acetone levels and blood cultures. Blood gases from venous or capillary origin is generally viewed as acceptable in nonintubated and well-perfused infants.[31,32] Catheterized urinalysis and culture should also be performed. Electrocardiogram can be done as a rapid way to assess potassium level. Pseudohyponatremia is usually seen from the dilutional effect of hyperglycemia. Leukocytosis may be from stress response rather than an underlying infection.

Management

Assessment starts with the suspicion of DKA, if the young infant did not previously carry the diagnosis of diabetes. Clinical exam should focus on volume status as well as a search for source of infection, although this may not be the precipitating cause in first time presentations. The patient should be carefully weighed and measured at presentation for accurate fluid therapy calculations. Previously known weights should not be used as the patient may have sustained an unnoticed amount of weight loss. Airway protection with intubation may be necessary in the unresponsive infant or with impending respiratory failure. Care must be taken to set the respiratory rate on the ventilator to match the infant's previous natural rate to compensate the metabolic acidosis. However, aggressive hyperventilation (to P_{CO_2} <22) has poorer neurologic outcomes and is not recommended.[26,28,29]

Initial management should concentrate on rapid expansion of intravascular volume and improvement of acidosis, the two life-threatening circumstances. However, rapid fluid administration to improve glomerular filtration must be carefully followed to avoid excessive hydration and augment the possibility of cerebral edema. Approximately, a 10% fluid deficit in infants with DKA can be assumed. Isotonic solutions of 0.9% saline or Ringer's lactate can be used with a volume of 10 to 20 mL/kg over 1 to 2 hours. If the infant remains severely dehydrated or hypotensive, this volume can be repeated. Once sufficient intravascular volume is obtained, the remaining fluid deficit can be restored over the next 24 to 48 hours, depending on the degree of initial hyperosmolality. The first 4 to 6 hours of replacing fluid deficit can be done with 0.9% normal saline or Ringer's lactate, but ensuing volumes should be replaced with a fluid of tonicity greater than 0.45% saline and added potassium or phosphate. Throughout all this fluid replacement, urinary output must be observed to be adequate.[26]

Insulin therapy is critical to resolving DKA and halting lipolysis and ketone generation. Insulin infusion should begin after the initial fluid bolus, about 1 to 2 hours after the start of resuscitation. Only IV routes should be considered as subcutaneous and intramuscular absorption is irregular or inadequate in the dehydrated patient. Insulin bolus is not recommended in the pediatric population, as widespread evidence shows this may exacerbate the risk of cerebral edema by dropping blood glucose levels too quickly. The dose of insulin should be 0.1 unit/kg/hour (or as low as 0.05 unit/kg/hour in some infants) with the rate of infusion adjusted to achieve a fall in blood glucose of about 50 to 90 mg/dL/hour. Once the blood glucose level falls to about 300 mg/dL, glucose should be added to the IV solution. As long as acidosis persists, insulin infusion should remain with the amount of added glucose adjusted to maintain levels between 150 to 200 mg/dL. Once acidosis has resolved and the patient can tolerate oral intake, subcutaneous insulin can be initiated, usually 1 to 2 hours before insulin infusion is discontinued. The dose for subcutaneous insulin is 0.25 unit/kg.[26,27]

DKA patients generally experience a potassium deficit of about 3 to 6 mEq/kg. Most of the potassium deficit is intracellular as the acidosis, lipolysis, hypertonicity and glycogenolysis promote a general efflux of potassium out of cells. Extracorporeal losses through vomiting and urinary diuresis are also factors to total body potassium deficit. However, at presentation of DKA, the extracellular potassium level that is measured may be decreased, normal or increased. Once insulin therapy is begun and acidosis is improved, potassium is forced back into cells, which may cause a precipitous drop in potassium levels and lead to cardiac arrhythmias. As a general guideline, potassium replacement is necessary in the initial management. If the potassium level is greater than 4 mEq/L, 40 mEq/L of potassium is added to the IV fluids after vascular competency and urine output are restored. If the initial potassium level is less than 4 mEq/L, replacement should be started after the fluid bolus and before insulin therapy. If laboratory values are delayed, the electrocardiogram and cardiac monitor can be used to estimate potassium levels. Potassium phosphate combined with potassium chloride or acetate can be used with the maximum infusion rate of 0.5 mEq/kg/hour. Phosphate depletion, due to osmotic diuresis, can also be expected in DKA patients, but the benefit of phosphate replacement is vague. Although few studies have not demonstrated a clinical benefit to phosphate repletion, severe hypophosphatemia, exhibited by muscle weakness, can be treated through supplementation. However, calcium levels may decline and phosphate infusion should be terminated if hypocalcemia occurs. Potassium phosphate has been shown to be safe for use with close observation of calcium levels.[26]

Bicarbonate therapy in DKA and other acidotic states is discussed in the metabolic acidosis section. Generally, bicarbonate is not recommended, as the acidosis should self-correct during fluid resuscitation and insulin therapy. Some encourage its use in DKA with pH lower than 6.9 or significant hyperkalemia or arrhythmias. The American Diabetic Association recommends consideration of bicarbonate in the pediatric patient if the pH remains less than 7.0 after the first hour of hydration.[33] If given for DKA, bicarbonate can be mixed as an isotonic solution (2 ampules of sodium bicarbonate in 0.45% normal saline) and given over 1 hour.

The treatment guidelines just given were all based on concerns of how to best avoid the development or worsening of cerebral edema. The pathophysiology of cerebral edema is not well described, but DKA itself and its treatment have both been implicated. Perhaps the most universal theory involves fluid entry into the brain due to a brisk drop in serum osmolality concomitant with vigorous fluid resuscitation. It is important to not infuse more than 50 mL/kg over the first 4 hours of treatment as higher volumes have been associated with an increased risk of cerebral edema.[30] Recent studies also suggest a vasogenic, rather than cytotoxic, mechanism of cerebral edema.[26,29,30] Those who present with extreme acidosis, have high levels of blood urea nitrogen and hypocapnia are at greatest risk for cerebral edema. Cerebral edema can be present before the initiation of therapy or anywhere from 4 to 24 hours after treatment.[26,28–30] Radiographic imaging can be normal early on with later signs of focal or diffuse edema, hemorrhage or infarction. Cerebral edema should be considered in infants with persistent vomiting, bradycardia, hypertension, labile oxygen saturation, irritability or lethargy, or in the presence of neurologic findings. Treating cerebral edema has been attempted with mannitol (0.25–1.0 g/kg) or hypertonic saline (3%) at 5 to 10 mL/kg over a period of 30 minutes. Hyperventilation in intubated patients should not be beyond the patient's physiologic tendency.

HYPONATREMIA

Although not as common as hypoglycemia in the ED, hyponatremia is reported as one of the most common electrolyte abnormalities in hospitalized children.[34] *Hyponatremia* is typically defined as a serum sodium level less than 125 to 130 mEq/L, although clinical symptoms are not usually seen until serum sodium falls below 120 mEq/L.

Presentation

Manifestations include altered mental status, lethargy, vomiting, diarrhea, seizures and circulatory collapse. Vomiting can be both a cause and manifestation of hyponatremia. The presence of symptoms is dependent, in part, on the rate of change in serum sodium. Gradual or chronic progression of hyponatremia may not become clinically evident even at levels below 110 mEq/L. Conversely, less severe hyponatremia may be symptomatic if the decline in serum sodium is rapid.

Differential Diagnosis

Hyponatremia can be caused by salt-losing states, such as vomiting or diarrhea, diuretic excess, and adrenal insufficiency, or by excess total body water states, such as infection-induced syndrome of inappropriate antidiuretic hormone (SIADH), nephrotic syndrome and cirrhosis. Factitious, or pseudo-, hyponatremia can occur with hyperglycemia, hyperlipidemia or hyperproteinemia. In infants, hyponatremia is commonly due to excess GI loss from prolonged vomiting or diarrhea, or from inappropriately diluted formulas. Pyridoxine-dependent seizures are a rare cause of intractable seizures in neonates.

Lab and Radiology

In addition to blood electrolytes, urine electrolytes and serum osmolality can help better classify a hyponatremic disorder.

Management

Treatment should be geared toward the underlying cause, and aggressive treatment with 3% hypertonic saline (514 mL/kg) should be initiated only if significant symptoms are present, such as seizures or coma. A dose of 5 mL/kg over 10 to 15 minutes should raise the sodium level by approximately 5 mEq/L; smaller additional doses of 2 to 3 mL/kg can be considered if no clinical improvement. The exact sodium deficit can be calculated as follows:

$$mEq\ Na^+\ needed = 0.6 \times weight\ (kg)$$
$$\times (Na^+\ desired - Na^+\ measured)$$

Acute correction to 125 mEq/L should alleviate symptoms in most cases. After acute correction for symptoms, the goal is to raise the sodium level slowly at a rate of 0.5 mEq/L/hour (maximum 12 mEq/L/day) by using 0.9% normal saline infusion. If SIADH is suspected, consider fluid restriction to two thirds maintenance and administration of furosemide 1 to 2 mg/kg. Pyridoxine 100 mg IV should be considered for neonates with intractable seizures of unclear etiology.[35]

Central pontine myelinolysis is a potential complication of hypertonic saline use, although it has been less well described in children than adults.[34] This may reflect the fact that hyponatremia in the pediatric population tends to occur acutely rather than chronically, and most cases of central pontine myelinolysis after rapid rise of sodium are described in a setting of chronic hyponatremia. Infants can apparently tolerate rapid and large increases in sodium levels without sequelae.

PITFALLS

- Failure to perform rapid bedside glucose testing in any infant with suspected metabolic disease
- Failure to recognize acute adrenal insufficiency in an infant with refractory hypotension
- Failure to recognize that aggressive use of insulin, fluids and bicarbonate in infants with DKA can be detrimental to the patient
- Failure to consider sodium bicarbonate if severe refractory metabolic acidosis is present and an inborn error of metabolism is suspected
- Failure to consider a metabolic disorder in the differential diagnosis in a previously healthy neonate with acute clinical deterioration.

REFERENCES

1. Greene CL, Goodman SI. Catastrophic metabolic encephalopathies in the newborn period. *Clin Perinatol.* 1997;24:773–786.
2. Weiner DL. Metabolic emergencies. In: Fleisher GR, Ludwig S, Henretig FM, et al, eds. *Textbook of Pediatric Emergency Medicine.* Philadelphia, PA: Lippincott Williams & Wilkins; 2006:1193–1206.
3. Calvo M, Artuch R, Macia E, et al. Diagnostic approach to inborn errors of metabolism in an emergency unit. *Pediatr Emerg Care.* 2000;16:405–408.
4. Henriquez H, el Din A, Ozand PT, et al. Emergency presentations of patients with methylmalonic acidemia, propionic acidemia and branched chain amino acidemia (MSUD). *Brain Dev.* 1994;16:S86–893.
5. Ozand PT. Hypoglycemia in association with various organic and amino acid disorders. *Semin Perinatol.* 2000;24:172–193.
6. Burton BK. Inborn error of metabolism in infancy: a guide to diagnosis. *Pediatrics.* 1998;102:e69.
7. Leonard JV, Morris AA. Inborn errors of metabolism around time of birth. *Lancet.* 2000;12:583–587.
8. Hazard PB, Griffin JP. Calculation of sodium bicarbonate requirement in metabolic acidosis. *Am J Med Sci.* 1982;283:18–22.
9. Chakrapani A, Cleary MA, Wraith JE. Detection of inborn errors of metabolism in the newborn. *Arch Dis Child Fetal Neonatal Ed.* 2001;84:F205–210.
10. de Baulny HO. Management and emergency treatments of neonates with a suspicion of inborn errors of metabolism. *Semin Neonatol.* 2002;7:17–26.
11. Merke D, Kabbani M. Congenital adrenal hyperplasia: epidemiology, management and practical drug treatment. *Pediatr Drugs.* 2001;3:599–611.
12. Ogilvy-Stuart AL. Neonatal thyroid disorders. *Arch Dis Child Fetal Neonatal Ed.* 2002;87:F165–171.
13. Zimmerman D. Fetal and neonatal hyperthyroidism. *Thyroid.* 1999;9:727–733.
14. Saladino RA. Endocrine and metabolic disorders. In: Barkin RM, Caputo GL, Jaffe DM, et al, eds. *Pediatric Emergency Medicine: Concepts and Clinical Practice.* St. Louis, MO: Mosby–Year Book; 1997:755–773.
15. Lorenz JM, Kleinman LI, Markarian K, et al. Serum anion gap in the differential diagnosis of metabolic acidosis in critically ill newborns. *J Pediatr.* 1999;135:751–755.
16. Fanconi S, Burger R, Ghelfi D, et al. Hemodynamic effects of sodium bicarbonate in critically ill neonates. *Intensive Care Med.* 1993;19:65–69.
17. Dixon H, Hawkins K, Stephenson T. Comparison of albumin versus bicarbonate treatment for neonatal metabolic acidosis. *Eur J Pediatr.* 1999;158:414–415.
18. Cornblath M, Hawdon JM, Williams AF, et al. Controversies regarding definition of neonatal hypoglycemia: suggested operational thresholds. *Pediatrics.* 2000;105:1141–1145.
19. Cowett R, Loughead J. Neonatal glucose metabolism: differential diagnoses, evaluation, and treatment of hypoglycemia. *Neonatal Netw.* 2002;21:9–19.
20. Losek JD. Hypoglycemia and the ABC's (sugar) of pediatric resuscitation. *Ann Emerg Med.* 2000;35:43–46.
21. Lilien LD, Pildes RS, Srinivasan G, et al. Treatment of neonatal hypoglycemia with minibolus and intravenous glucose infusion. *J Pediatr.* 1980;97:295–298.
22. Pollack CV Jr. Utility of glucagon in the emergency department. *J Emerg Med.* 1993;11:195–205.
23. Kappy MS, Bajaj L. Recognition and treatment of endocrine/metabolic emergencies in children: part 1. *Adv Pediatr.* 2002;49:245–272.
24. von Muhlendahl KE, Herkenhoff H. Long-term course of neonatal diabetes. *N Engl J Med.* 1995;333:704–708.
25. Fosel S. Transient and permanent neonatal diabetes. *Eur J Pediatr.* 1995;154:944–948.
26. Wolfsdorf J, Glaser N, Sperling M. Diabetic ketoacidosis in infants, children, and adolescents: a consensus statement from the American Diabetes Association. *Diabetes Care.* 2006;29:1150–1159.
27. Iafusco D, Stazi MA, Cotichini R, et al. Permanent diabetes mellitus in the first year of life. *Diabetologia.* 2002;45:798–804.
28. Quinn M, Fleishman A, Rosner B, et al. Characteristics at diagnosis of type 1 diabetes in children younger than 6 years. *J Pediatr.* 2006;148;366–371.
29. Shield JPH, Wadsworth EJK, Baum JD. Insulin dependent diabetes in under 5 year olds. *Arch Dis Child.* 1985;60:1144–1148.
30. Glaser N, Barnett P, McCaslin I, et al. Risk factors for cerebral edema in children with diabetic ketoacidosis. *N Engl J Med.* 2001;344:264–269.
31. Harrison AM, Lynch JM, Dean JM, et al. Comparison of simultaneously obtained arterial and capillary blood gas in pediatric intensive care patients. *Crit Care Med.* 1997;25:1904–1908.

32. McGillivray D, DuCharme FM, Charron Y, et al. Clinical decision making based on venous versus capillary blood gas in the well perfused child. *Ann Emerg Med.* 1999;34:58–63.

33. Kitabchi AE, Umpierrez GE, Murphy MD, et al. American Diabetes Association. Hyperglycemic crises in diabetes. *Diabetes Care.* 2004;27(Suppl 1):S94–102.

34. Gruskin AB, Sarnaik A. Hyponatremia: pathophysiology and treatment, a pediatric perspective. *Pediatr Nephrol.* 1992;6:280–286.

35. Gupta VK, Mishra D, Mathur I, et al. Pyridoxine-dependent seizures: a case report and a critical review of the literature. *J Paediatr Child Health.* 2001;37:592–596.

22

Respiratory Emergencies

Seema Shah and Ghazala Q. Sharieff

INTRODUCTION

Neonatal and infant respiratory emergencies account for a large number of emergency department (ED) visits each year. Many of the emergencies may progress rapidly and result in respiratory failure or even death; therefore, they require immediate and aggressive responses. In comparison to adults, infants have a higher frequency of respiratory failure; this may be explained by the differences in anatomy and development of the respiratory system from birth to adulthood.

PATHOPHYSIOLOGY

All infants are obligate nasal breathers until 2 to 6 months of age; any nasal congestion may cause considerable respiratory distress. As compared to adults, infants have smaller airways, have proportionately larger tongues in their oropharynx and have a narrow subglottic area; any obstruction may be clinically significant. Although the differential diagnosis of neonatal and infant respiratory emergencies is broad, here we approach this discussion by dividing the problems into upper and lower airway abnormalities.

UPPER AIRWAY ANOMALIES

Upper airway anomalies frequently present in the newborn period and often present to the ED. In addition to the various infectious causes of upper airway disease, we discuss congenital anomalies and traumatic etiologies of upper airway emergencies. Many upper airway diseases present with symptoms of stridor. Stridor is caused by the oscillation of a narrowed airway, and its presence should be worrisome for obstruction of the larger airways.

Some of the more common upper airway diagnoses are presented next and include anatomic abnormalities such as laryngomalacia, congenital subglottic stenosis and vocal cord paralysis; traumatic injuries that include child abuse, foreign body aspiration and thermal burns; and infectious etiologies that include bacterial tracheitis, croup, epiglottitis and retropharyngeal abscess.

Laryngomalacia

This is the most common upper airway congenital anomaly and the most frequent noninfectious cause of stridor in infants. Unlike other entities, stridor is caused by a collapse of the supraglottic structures during inspiration. Usually, a predisposing illness, such as an upper respiratory infection (URI), exacerbates the symptoms and prompts the parents or caregivers to bring the child to the ED. Laryngomalacia should be suspected in an infant with recurrent episodes of stridor, persistent coughing or wheezing. If symptoms persist or are severe, an otolaryngologist should be consulted to complete the evaluation of these patients with a flexible laryngoscope. A majority of these patients have resolution of symptoms spontaneously; only severely obstructed patients should have surgical intervention. The patients who are more severely affected may have concomitant cor pulmonale, apparent life-threatening events (ALTEs), cyanosis or failure to thrive. Clinicians need to be aware of other associated airway anomalies, including tracheoesophageal fistula.

Congenital Subglottic Stenosis

This is the second most common cause of stridor in infants; however, the stridor is unique in these patients as it is usually biphasic. These patients frequently present to the ED with recurring episodes of croup. Usually a URI is the inciting event that decreases the airway diameter even further. A lateral neck radiograph may depict an airway narrowing, but direct laryngoscopic visualization provides the definitive diagnosis.

Vocal Cord Paralysis

Vocal cord paralysis can occur for various reasons including brainstem compression from a Chiari 1 malformation or vocal cord paralysis from various causes.[1] This is the third most common congenital laryngeal airway anomaly. These infants are often misdiagnosed with wheezing or recurrent stridor, but persistence of symptoms prompts consultation with an otolaryngologist. Diagnosis is made by flexible laryngoscopy in an awake infant. Patients who present in significant respiratory distress occasionally need tracheostomy. Most cases resolve spontaneously in 6 to 12 months.

TRAUMA

Child Abuse

A practitioner should always pay close attention to histories in patients who present with respiratory distress of unclear etiology. Choking, blunt trauma to the neck and oral trauma are examples of child abuse that may present with respiratory distress. A recent case report discusses a series of four infants who had baby wipes pushed into their pharynxes intentionally; all of the patients had other associated findings including fractures, bruises and contusions. The infants presented in various forms of respiratory distress. Three of the four cases resulted in legal outcomes.[2]

Foreign Bodies

Epidemiology/Pathophysiology

Foreign bodies are a significant cause of mortality and morbidity in children. Children under the age of 14 years accounted for 17,537 ED visits for foreign bodies in the year 2000. During that same year, the *Morbidity and Mortality Weekly Report* stated that in that same population there were 160 deaths due to airway obstruction.[3] Foreign bodies are the fifth most common cause of unintentional injury mortality in the United States for children younger

than 1 year of age.[4] Eighty percent occur in children under 3 years of age with a peak incidence of 1 to 2 years.[5] It must be remembered that even very young nonmobile infants are at risk for foreign bodies; sometimes inappropriate toys or food products given by "helpful" siblings result in airway obstruction.

Presentation

A history of a witnessed choking episode has a high sensitivity for the diagnosis of foreign body aspiration.[6] After the aspiration, some patients may have subtle wheezing, persistent cough, inspiratory or expiratory stridor. In severe cases of airway obstruction, patients may present in respiratory distress, potentially with cyanosis. More commonly, infants may have focal examination findings that are suggestive of a foreign body. Although present in only 57% of patients in the Tan et al. study, the triad of cough, wheeze and diminished breath sounds is indicative of an airway foreign body.[7] It must also be remembered that, in infants with very pliable tracheas, a foreign body in the esophagus can cause tracheal compression. The clinical presentation can be very similar to an airway obstruction.

Laboratory and Radiographic Findings

Radiographic findings are often variable, and the absence of findings does not rule out a foreign body aspiration. A majority of the foreign bodies aspirated by infants and toddlers are not radiopaque. If present on chest radiograph, findings may include unilateral hyperinflation, atelectasis and mediastinal shift (Figure 22.1). Some studies demonstrated that imaging studies have a sensitivity of 73% and a specificity of 45%; however, up to 20% of patients will have both negative history and radiographic evaluation.[8] On fluoroscopy, paradoxical movements of the diaphragm may be visualized. Inspiratory and expiratory chest radiographs may assist in the diagnosis as the ball-valve effect from the foreign body partially blocking the bronchus will cause hyperinflation, but this effect is often difficult to visualize on a radiograph in the infant population. A lateral decubitus film can sometimes be used to expose the hyperinflation.

Management

An otolaryngologist should be consulted if the history and clinical examination are suspicious for a foreign body; prompt bronchoscopy should be performed in a controlled setting, such as the operating room (OR). If an

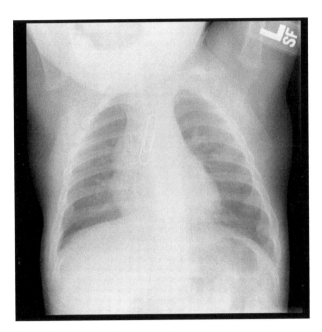

Figure 22.1. Foreign body aspiration.

infant presents with complete airway obstruction, back blows and chest compressions may alleviate the obstruction from either the airway or esophagus.

Removal of the foreign body from the hypopharynx area may be possible with a laryngoscope and pediatric Magill forceps. The patient may need to be intubated to maintain airway patency and ventilation until bronchoscopy. If the foreign body is thought to be occluding the trachea more distally, then forcing the foreign body into the right mainstem using the endotracheal tube (ETT) and stylet with subsequent ventilation of the left lung may be attempted. Other complications that may occur in this complete airway obstruction/foreign body situation are occlusion of the ETT itself with the foreign body (e.g., peanut in the end of the tube) or bilateral pneumothoraces from overzealous bagging.

Thermal Burns

When a patient is being evaluated for burns, facial burns are of particular concern as there may be associated thermal injuries to the airway. Thermal epiglottitis is an entity that closely mimics infectious epiglottitis; however, the patient will be without fever and will have a history of an ingestion, particularly hot beverages. Parents should be educated to not warm bottles in the microwave due to uneven distribution of heat.

INFECTIOUS

Upper Respiratory Infections

A URI or "cold" and its associated symptoms can produce much anxiety on the part of first-time parents. Because young infants are obligate nose breathers, simple URIs can result in decreased oral intake and fussiness. More severe symptoms such as tachypnea and retractions can even result, often improving with simple bulb suctioning or deep nasal suctioning.

Encouraging parents to use good bulb suctioning techniques prior to each feed and prior to sleep should improve oral intake and sleep patterns. Intranasal over-the-counter decongestants such as phenylephrine 0.25% are sold for use in young children. Caution should be applied when using these medications in very young infants. In January 2008, the U.S. Food and Drug Administration (FDA) issued a public health advisory statement that strongly recommends that over-the-counter cough and cold medicines that contain decongestants and antihistamines should not be used for young children under the age of 2.[9] As of the writing of this textbook, most makers of these medications had issued voluntarily recalls. This action was taken for two main reasons: (1) the efficacy of these medications in the pediatric population has not been shown,[10] and (2) a number of deaths in children have been attributed to the overuse of these particular medications.[11] Toxicity and deaths appear to be the result of, in part, the overdosage of these medications in very young children. For now, particularly in children younger than 2 years of age, these cold and cough medications should be used with caution.

Bacterial Tracheitis

Epidemiology/Pathophysiology

Although mentioned in laryngological textbooks in the 1920s through 1950s, it was not until 1979 when Jones et al. better described bacterial tracheitis.[12] *Bacterial tracheitis*, also known as *laryngotracheobronchitis, pseudomembranous croup* or *bacterial croup*, is an uncommon disease; however it may be life-threatening. Similar to viral croup, the peak incidence is in the fall and winter in children between 6 months and 8 years of age.[13] In a recent retrospective case series, bacterial tracheitis was three times more likely to cause respiratory failure than viral croup or epiglottitis.[14]

Marked subglottic edema and thick mucopurulent (membranous) secretions characterize the illness. The organisms most commonly implicated include *Staphylococcus aureus* and *Peptostreptococcus spp.,* and to a lesser extent alpha hemolytic streptococcus, *Haemophilus influenza, Moraxella catarrhalis,* and *Streptococcus pneumoniae.*[15]

Presentation

The clinical presentation of bacterial tracheitis has features of both epiglottitis and viral croup. Typically, the child may have prodromal viral URI symptoms such as low-grade fever, cough and stridor, similar to patients with croup. The patient then develops rapid onset of high fever and respiratory distress and appears toxic. Unlike patients with epiglottitis, these children typically have a cough, are comfortable lying flat and do not drool.[16] Bacterial tracheitis should be considered in any croup patient with high fever who does not respond to standard viral croup therapy.

Laboratory and Radiographic Findings

Radiographs are not definitive or diagnostic as the x-ray is usually normal in appearance. However, on anteroposterior (AP) neck radiographs, bacterial tracheitis can be similar to croup in that marked subglottic narrowing, also known as the *steeple sign,* may be present. Also, a slight irregularity of the proximal tracheal mucosa or clouding of the tracheal lumen may be seen. This irregularity or clouding represents pseudomembranous detachment. This finding varies from 20% to 82% in studies.[13,17]

Routine laboratory data are not indicated; a complete blood cell (CBC) count may show marked leukocytosis; however, Gallagher et al. found that it varied considerably. More common was a left shift.[18] Blood cultures are typically negative.

Diagnosis is made endoscopically by visualizing normal supraglottic structures with prominent subglottic edema, ulcerations and copious purulent secretions. These secretions should be cultured.[16] In several studies, the majority of the patients had a positive Gram stain and culture of the tracheal secretions.[12,17]

Management

Initially, bacterial tracheitis patients are often managed in a manner similar to viral croup patients. The higher fever and lack of significant response to standard croup therapy should alert the practitioner to a possible bacterial component. Patients in severe respiratory distress are best managed in the OR for both the endoscopic diagnosis and intubation.[13,18] However, if ED intubation is required, a tube smaller than the calculated size may be necessary. It is important to note that copious purulent secretions can be suctioned from the ETT. These secretions should be sent for culture. Also, humidification of the inspired air may help prevent mucous plugging.

If endotracheal intubation is unsuccessful, a tracheostomy may be necessary but should be avoided. In the acute setting, a needle cricothyrotomy would be the next emergency intervention. Occasionally, additional endoscopy may need to be performed to remove the pseudomembranous material. Intubation is often required for 3 to 7 days until the patient is afebrile or until there is an air leak present (i.e., passage of air around the ETT), indicating decreased edema and signifying a decrease in the quantity and viscosity of secretions. Antibiotics should be initiated with vancomycin 10 mg/kg every 6 hours in addition to ceftriaxone 50 mg/kg/day. The addition of vancomycin is added for the prevalence of methicillin-resistant *S. aureus* (MRSA).

Complications

Complications of bacterial tracheitis include respiratory failure, post-obstructive pulmonary edema, airway obstruction, pneumothorax, formation of pseudomembranes, and toxic shock syndrome. These patients frequently have concurrent pneumonia.[19]

Croup

Epidemiology and Pathophysiology

Croup, or laryngotracheobronchitis, is the most common cause of infectious airway obstruction in children.[20] Pathophysiology of croup is mucosal inflammation in the subglottic larynx and trachea that is circumferential in nature, with associated involvement and spasm of the vocal cords; however, the epiglottis is not involved. The most commonly affected age group is 6 months to 4 years, with a peak incidence of 60 per 1000 among children 1 to 2 years old.[21] Croup has a peak incidence in early fall and winter, but it may be seen throughout the year. The most frequent causative organism is parainfluenza virus type I; however, other organisms, such as parainfluenza types II and III, *Mycoplasma pneumoniae*, respiratory syncytial

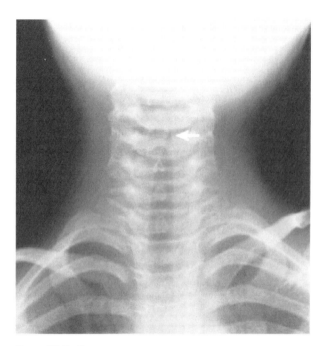

Figure 22.2. Croup.

virus (RSV), influenza A and B and adenovirus have been implicated.

Presentation

Initially, patients have a 1- to 2-day prodrome of nasal congestion, rhinorrhea and cough, but the total duration is less than 1 week with a peak of 1 to 2 days. Often frightening to the caregiver, the patient will have the onset of a harsh, barky cough often described as sounding similar to a seal or a dog bark. The patient may progress to stridor, which is typically inspiratory but may also be biphasic. Crying or aggravation exacerbates the stridor. In addition to nasal flaring, suprasternal and intercostal retractions, tachypnea, hypoxia and the presence of biphasic stridor indicate severe respiratory compromise.[22]

Laboratory and Radiographic Findings

The diagnosis of croup is usually made by history and clinical examination. Laboratory analysis such as CBC counts tends to be normal. Radiographs may be helpful in differentiation of other disease entities such as epiglottitis, retropharyngeal abscess, congenital abnormalities, foreign body or airway hemangioma. The classic radiographic finding in a patient with croup is the steeple sign (Figure 22.2). Distention of the hypopharynx and of the laryngeal ventricle, and haziness or narrowing of subglottic space, may be seen on neck radiograph. However, the absence of these findings does not rule out croup as almost half the patients have normal radiographs.[21]

Management

Although croup is a self-limited disease, treatment options are dependent on the severity of symptoms.[20] A detailed discussion of the adjunctive therapies of croup follows.

Glucocorticoids: Glucocorticoids have proven to be beneficial in severe, moderate and even mild croup. Of the glucocorticoids, dexamethasone is the preferred agent for croup because the half-life of dexamethasone is 36 to 52 hours, and it is not necessary to discharge the patient with additional doses of steroids. Patients with mild croup have also been shown to have faster resolution of symptoms following use of dexamethasone. Although the standard dose of dexamethasone has been accepted to be 0.6 mg/kg, Geelhoed et al.[23, 24] showed similar efficacy in patients with moderate croup using lower doses of 0.15 mg/kg and 0.3 mg/kg.

In comparison with placebo, oral or intramuscular (IM) dexamethasone was found to decrease hospitalization rates. Donaldson et al. found no difference between oral and IM dexamethasone, both at 0.6 mg/kg, for children with moderate to severe croup at 24 hours or at any time in the week after treatment.[25]

Studies by Klassen et al. and Johnson et al. have shown clear improvement in children with severe croup treated with steroids. Both studies also compared dexamethasone to nebulized budesonide dosed at both 2 mg and 4 mg and found similar benefits in treatment of croup as single-dose therapy.[26,27]

Racemic Epinephrine: Racemic epinephrine was introduced in the United States in 1971. It contains a 1:1 mixture of the levo (l)- and dextro (d)- rotatory isomers of epinephrine. Inhaled epinephrine is believed to be effective by reducing airway edema as a result of its α-adrenergic effect on vasculature within the mucosa.

Nebulized epinephrine is considered the mainstay of treatment for moderate to severe croup. Although epinephrine does not alter the natural course of croup, it may reduce the need for emergent airway management. The preferred dose of racemic epinephrine is 0.25 to 0.5 mL of a 2.25% solution diluted in 3 cc of normal saline. Ledwith and Shea recently allayed the concern for the rebound phenomenon. Patients who also received corticosteroids and experienced a sustained response to racemic epinephrine 3 hours after treatment were shown to be safe for discharge.[28] Patients who receive nebulized epinephrine should also receive dexamethasone.

Racemic epinephrine has traditionally been recommended for use in patients with croup, but L-epinephrine, which lacks the inert (d)-isomer, can be used in its place with equal efficacy. Equivalent dosages of L-epinephrine would be 0.5 cc/kg of 1:1000 concentration diluted in 3 cc normal saline with a maximum of dose of 2.5 cc per dose for children younger than 4 years old and 5 cc per dose for children older than 4 years old. The administration of racemic epinephrine is reserved for more ill patients due to the potential for cardiotoxic effects.

Mist Therapy: Theoretically, patients with croup have received humidified air in order to sooth the inflamed mucosa, thereby decreasing the amount of coughing due to mucosal irritation. However, Neto et al. described that mist therapy was not effective in improving clinical symptoms in children presenting to the ED with moderate croup.[29] Furthermore, Scolnik et al. found that 100% humidity was not more effective when compared with mist therapy in the treatment of moderate croup.[30]

Severe Croup: Only a minority of cases of croup result in complete obstruction of the airway. However, if respiratory failure is imminent, management of the airway is essential. Additional therapies such as heliox, a mixture of helium and oxygen, have been shown to mix results in randomized trials in the treatment of croup.[31] Terrigino et al., in a prospective, double-blind study comparing Heliox with humidified oxygen in children with acute viral croup, found no statistically significant difference in croup scores between the two groups.[32] In another prospective, randomized, double-blind trial comparing the additive effect of heliox to racemic epinephrine on a modified croup score in patients with moderate to severe croup, no difference was found between the groups in mean croup score, oxygen saturation, respiratory rate or heart rate, at baseline or at the treatment end period.[33]

In patients who have severe croup that is unresponsive to nebulized epinephrine, corticosteroids and possibly heliox, endotracheal intubation and ventilation may be necessary. If intubation is necessary, then an ETT with a diameter smaller than recommended for age and size should be used.

Complications

Patients who have persistent tachypnea, have hypoxia, are unable to tolerate oral fluids or require more than two treatments of inhaled epinephrine should be admitted to the hospital. Complications include potential airway obstruction, pneumonia and respiratory arrest.

Epiglottitis

Epidemiology/Pathophysiology

First described in 1878 by Michel and labeled *angina epiglottidea anterior, supraglottitis,* better known as *epiglottitis,* is an airway emergency. Epiglottitis not only is an acute bacterial cellulitis of the lingual surface of the epiglottis but also involves the structures surrounding it including the aryepiglottic folds and the arytenoid soft tissue. Obstruction occurs as the edema of the surrounding structures worsens. It is more common in the winter but can occur throughout the year. Peak incidence occurs in children between 2 and 7 years of age, but cases of children younger than 1 year of age have been reported. In 1987, prior to widespread vaccination against *H. influenza* type B (HiB), the incidence of epiglottitis was 41 cases per 100,000 in children younger than 5 years old. This decreased to 1.3 per 100,000 in 1997.[34] Since the widespread use of HiB vaccination, the most commonly identified organisms causing epiglottitis are Group A β-hemolytic *Streptococcus, Streptococcus pneumoniae, Klebsiella, Pseudomonas,* viruses, and *Candida.*

Presentation

Usually abrupt in onset, epiglottitis presents with high fever, irritability, throat pain, airway obstruction, marked anxiety and a toxic appearance. Some patients have a 6- to 24-hour prior duration of illness. On presentation, these children are often found in the sniffing position with the nose pointed superiorly to maintain an adequate airway. The preferred position is a tripod position. As the supraglottic edema worsens, it becomes difficult for the patient to swallow saliva; therefore, drooling is apparent and is a common complaint.[35] Often a "hot potato" muffled voice may be present as well as air hunger. On physical examination, an erythematous epiglottis may be seen protruding at the base of the tongue. A tongue depressor should not be used routinely in any infant suspected of having epiglottitis as manipulation may result in complete obstruction of the airway. A fever as high as 104°F (40.0°C) and tachycardia may also be present. Blackstock et al. described the "4 Ds" of epiglottitis: drooling, dyspnea, dysphonia, and dysphagia.[36] Cyanosis is usually an ominous sign indicating impending airway obstruction.

Laboratory and Radiographic Findings

As this is a true airway emergency, establishment of a definitive airway is the first priority. It is not necessary to obtain routine laboratory data before establishing the airway, especially because phlebotomy may induce agitation of the child and worsen symptoms. Only after a definitive airway has been established should cultures and sensitivities be obtained from both the blood and supraglottic region. Radiographs are helpful if the diagnosis is unclear and the patient has a stable airway. Caution should be exercised when making the decision to send patients with possible airway compromise to radiology. A lateral neck radiograph, especially when done in hyperextension during inspiration, may further distinguish croup, retropharyngeal abscess or foreign body, but treatment should not be delayed to obtain radiographs. The classic finding is the "thumbprint sign," indicative of a round and thick epiglottis (Figure 22.3). However, this finding may be negative in up to 20% of cases.[37]

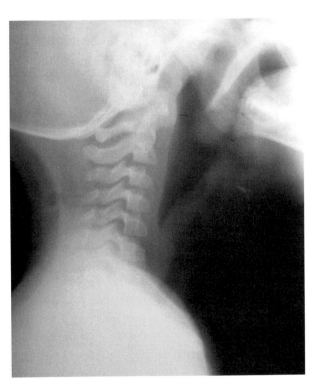

Figure 22.3. Epiglottitis.

Management

When a definitive diagnosis of epiglottitis is established, every effort should be made to avoid any anxiety provoking procedures, including phlebotomy or intraoral examination. It is imperative to allow the patient to sit in the most comfortable position and allow them to be held by their caregivers. The confirmatory diagnosis of epiglottitis is made by direct visualization with a laryngoscope; however, this should be performed in a controlled setting such as an OR.

The supraglottic structures, including the epiglottis, arytenoids and aryepiglottic folds, may appear cherry red and edematous and pooling of secretions may be present as well. Severe airway compromise requires immediate airway management by orotracheal intubation and typically requires a tube size smaller than calculated for age. In cases in which intubation is not successful, a surgical airway is necessary. If time permits, the assistance of an anesthesiologist or ear, nose, throat specialist is helpful.

After securing the airway, the patient is started on broad-spectrum antibiotics such as second or third generation cephalosporins; ceftriaxone (100 mg/kg/day intravenously [IV]) or cefotaxime (200 mg/kg/day in four divided doses) or ampicillin/sulbactam (450 mg/kg/day in four divided doses) as an alternative until cultures return. Patients with mild symptoms may be observed in the intensive care unit. Patients who do not require immediate intervention are ideally taken to the OR for airway control. One advantage of the OR for airway control in the stable patient is the use of inhaled anesthetics for sedation. Steroids are also not routinely indicated in the management of epiglottitis.

Complications

While the patient is bacteremic, other sites may become involved through seeding. Patients who are not vaccinated against HiB may develop meningitis, septic shock, cellulitis or septic arthritis. A majority of the complications associated with this disease are centered on airway obstruction, including pulmonary edema, pneumonia and respiratory arrest.

Retropharyngeal Abscess

Epidemiology

A retropharyngeal abscess is an infection of one of the deep spaces of the neck and another potential life-threatening infection in children. The retropharyngeal space is a potential space located between the anterior border of the cervical vertebrae and the posterior wall of the esophagus; the space contains connective tissues and lymph nodes that receive lymphatic drainage from adjacent structures. There are two potential ways that the space may become infected: (1) through a URI that causes inflammation of the retropharyngeal nodes, and (2) through an infection introduced through penetrating trauma to the oropharynx (e.g., children who fall with an object in their mouths).

Fifty percent of retropharyngeal abscesses occur in patients between 6 months and 12 months of age, and 96% of all cases occur in children younger than 6 years of age, as the nodes of Ruvier that drain the retropharyngeal space typically atrophy after this age.[37] There is also a slight male predominance, in some studies up to 75% of cases.[38] The most common causative organisms are group A streptococcus, anaerobic organisms and *S. aureus*.

Presentation

The clinical picture of retropharyngeal abscess is similar to that of other illnesses such as croup, epiglottitis, tracheitis and peritonsillar abscess. The patients frequently present with symptoms of a URI, fever, dysphagia, odynophagia, trismus, neck stiffness and poor intake. As the purulent material collects, a fluctuant mass may compress the pharynx or trachea. Patients may then present with drooling, stridor, and respiratory distress. On examination, visualization of oropharynx may reveal a mass; however, this is only present in half of all children with retropharyngeal abscess.[39]

Laboratory and Radiographic Findings

In general, the AP diameter of the retropharyngeal space should not exceed that of the contiguous vertebral body. The lateral neck radiograph with attention to the retropharyngeal space is very useful in the initial diagnosis of retropharyngeal abscesses. In children, the normal parameters are that the soft tissue should measure no more than 7 mm at the level of the second cervical vertebrae (or <33% of the AP diameter of the second vertebral body), less than 5 mm anterior to the third and fourth cervical vertebrae (or <40% of the AP diameter of the vertebral body) and 14 mm at the sixth cervical vertebrae (or <100% of the AP diameter of the sixth vertebral body) on a film done with proper neck extension (Figure 22.4). Incorrect positioning of the infant during the lateral radiograph can result in a

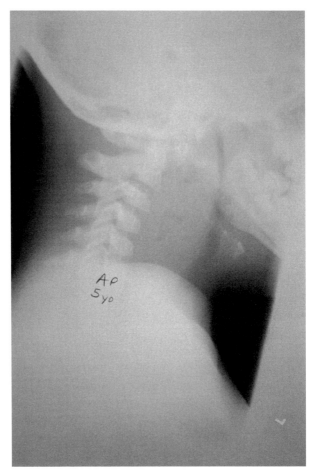

Figure 22.4. Retropharyngeal abscess.

false widening of the soft tissue. Retropharyngeal thickening is seen in 88% to 100% of retropharyngeal abscess cases on the lateral neck radiograph.[38,40,41] In clinically stable patients, a computed tomography (CT) scan of the neck is helpful to delineate whether there is a retropharyngeal cellulitis rather than a true abscess.[42]

Routine laboratory testing is not useful in the diagnosis of a retropharyngeal abscess. Occasionally, there may be a leukocytosis on a peripheral CBC count, but a normal white blood count (WBC) count does not rule out retropharyngeal abscess.

Management

Previously, the standard of care for management of retropharyngeal abscess had been surgical drainage. For patients who are of concern for airway obstruction, endotracheal intubation followed by surgical drainage by a qualified surgeon is still the treatment of choice. In cases of retropharyngeal abscess diagnosed by CT, antibiotics alone successfully treated 37%.[42] Antibiotic therapy is initiated in these patients; clindamycin is an appropriate first choice (30 mg/kg/day IV divided four times a day) and, as an alternative, cefazolin (100 mg/kg/day IV divided four times a day). If endotracheal intubation needs to be undertaken due to airway compromise, caution should be taken when visualizing the airway due to distortion from the mass and the possibility of inducing rupture.

Complications

Retropharyngeal abscess is a life-threatening airway illness; therefore, all patients should be closely monitored and admitted. Complications include airway compromise, abscess rupture leading to asphyxiation or aspiration pneumonia, or spread of infection to adjacent structures in the neck including infection of carotid artery sheath, osteomyelitis of the cervical spine or infection of the structures of the mediastinum. Necrotizing fasciitis is also a complication of the infection itself.

LOWER AIRWAY EMERGENCIES

The lower airway encompasses the bronchi, alveoli, interstitium and pleura. In the lower respiratory tract, the major differences between infants and adults reside in the fact that infants have fewer and smaller alveoli, which is suggestive of a lower surface area where gas exchange occurs. The lower cartilaginous content of the smaller airways and small diameter make an infant easily susceptible to obstruction. This section discusses reactive airway disease (RAD) and various infectious and congenital etiologies of lower respiratory emergencies.

Congenital Diaphragmatic Hernia

Epidemiology and Pathophysiology

Congenital diaphragmatic hernia (CDH) is the presence of intestinal viscera in the chest through a congenital opening in the diaphragm with most presenting on the left. Most herniations occur through the foramen of Bochdalek found at the back of the thoracic cavity; however, some occur through the foramen of Morgagni. The incidence is 1 in 2500 live births worldwide. Despite advances in medical and surgical therapies, mortality continues to be high, ranging from 52% to 66%.[43-45] Although uncommon, blunt abdominal trauma may cause a rupture of the diaphragm and can present in a delayed manner.

Although most patients present in the newborn period, it is postulated that up to 10% of patients present after that time. The high mortality and morbidity was once thought to be the result of mechanical compression of the lung. It is now thought that a combination of pulmonary hypertension, surfactant deficiency and an ongoing cycle of hypoxia, acidosis and intrapulmonary shunting significantly contribute to the mortality and morbidity.[46] However, in late presentation of CDH, infants may also present with bowel obstruction and respiratory distress.

Presentation

On presentation, patients with CDH may be in significant respiratory distress and be cyanotic, or they may be exhibiting symptoms of bowel obstruction. Also present may be a scaphoid abdomen or a barrel-shaped chest. Careful examination may reveal the presence of bowel sounds in the chest. Auscultation of cardiac sounds can be present on the right side of the chest when left-sided defects are present; severe defects may lead to poor perfusion and pneumothorax.

Laboratory and Radiographic Findings

A blood gas evaluation should be completed in a patient presenting in respiratory distress to assess the pH, $Paco_2$ and Pao_2, as acidosis is a frequent complication in conjunction with pulmonary hypertension. In late presenting CDH, radiographs have often been obtained for persistent respiratory distress or other nonspecific symptoms of cough, fever, abdominal pain or vomiting. On chest radiograph, loops of bowel may be visualized (Figure 22.5). If the loops of bowel give the appearance of pneumonia with pneumatocele formation, clarification by passage of a nasogastric tube will be of assistance. More definitively, a barium swallow study or CT of the abdomen will better delineate the diagnosis.

Management

Maintenance of the airway is important, especially in infants presenting with respiratory distress. Intubation should be undertaken early as excessive bag-valve-mask ventilation may further distend the intestine, thereby causing more pulmonary compromise. Definitive management is surgical repair; a pediatric surgeon should be consulted urgently. If there is concern for bowel ischemia, emergent surgical therapy may be required.

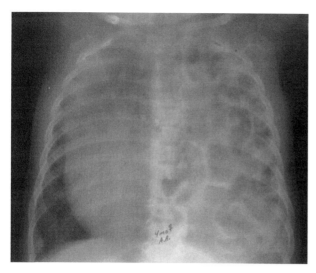

Figure 22.5. Congenital diaphragmatic hernia.

Complications

Most complications arise from pulmonary compromise including pulmonary hypertension, pneumothorax, bowel ischemia, pleural inflammation, chronic lung disease and death. Other congenital anomalies are associated with CDH, such as Cornelia de Lange syndrome.

INFECTIOUS

Bronchiolitis

Epidemiology and Pathophysiology

Bronchiolitis is the most common and potentially life-threatening lower respiratory tract infection in infants. It is characterized by fever, cough, coryza, expiratory wheezing, and respiratory distress.[47] The disease causes marked inflammation, edema and necrosis of the epithelial cells of the smaller airways, increased mucous production and bronchospasm.[48] Although it may occur in all age groups, the larger airways of older children better accommodate the mucosal edema; therefore, severe symptoms are usually seen in children under the age of 2 years. An estimated 120,000 hospitalizations for bronchiolitis occur each year, and bronchiolitis is the main cause of hospital admission for respiratory illnesses.[49]

The most common cause of bronchiolitis is RSV, isolated in 75% of children younger than 2 years of age who were hospitalized for bronchiolitis.[50] Other causes include parainfluenza virus types 1 and 3, influenza B, adenovirus type 1, 2 and 5, *Mycoplasma*, rhinovirus, enterovirus, and

herpes simplex virus. In temperate climates, RSV epidemics occur yearly beginning in winter and continue until late spring, whereas parainfluenza epidemics typically occur in the fall.

History of underlying conditions such as prematurity, cardiac or pulmonary disease, immunodeficiency or previous episodes of wheezing should be identified.[51] The natural course of the illness is about 7 to 10 days but can last several weeks to a month. Unfortunately, re-infection with RSV is common throughout life.[52]

Presentation

Most clinicians recognize bronchiolitis as a constellation of clinical symptoms and signs including a viral URI prodrome followed by increased respiratory effort and wheezing in children younger than 2 years of age. Clinical signs and symptoms of bronchiolitis consist of rhinorrhea, coughing, wheezing, tachypnea and increased respiratory effort manifested as grunting, nasal flaring and intercostal or subcostal retractions.[51]

Respiratory distress in these children manifests as tachypnea, with respiratory rates as high as 80 to 100 breaths per minute, nasal flaring and intercostal and supraclavicular retractions, apnea, grunting and cyanosis. Common caregiver complaints include poor feeding and increased fussiness, usually as a result of difficulty sleeping. Other associated findings are tachycardia and dehydration.

Laboratory and Radiographic Findings

Virologic tests for RSV, if obtained during peak RSV season, demonstrate a high predictive value. However, the knowledge gained from such testing rarely alters management decisions or outcomes for the vast majority of children with clinically diagnosed bronchiolitis.[48] The diagnosis of bronchiolitis should be a clinical one.[53] If necessary, the workup may include a nasopharyngeal swab for a rapid enzyme-linked immunosorbent assay (ELISA) to test for RSV. A chest x-ray often shows hyperinflation, flattening of the diaphragms and peribronchial cuffing (Figure 22.6). Although routine chest x-rays are not necessary, they are helpful in ruling out potential complications such as atelectasis, pneumothorax or pneumonia, especially when patients are not improving at the expected rate or have acute decompensation of unclear etiology.

Infants younger than 3 months of age who have bronchiolitis and fever are frequently studied to determine the

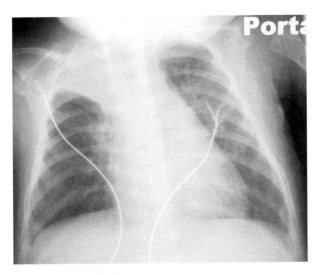

Figure 22.6. Bronchiolitis.

risk of serious bacterial infection. Melendez and Harper showed that the risk of bacteremia or meningitis among infants younger than 90 days with fever and bronchiolitis is low. However, it has been shown that the risk of urinary tract infection in febrile RSV-positive patients younger than 60 days of age may still be significant.[54,55]

Management

The mainstay of treatment of bronchiolitis is supportive care, including ensuring hydration, oxygenation, nasal suction or even endotracheal intubation and ventilation for children with respiratory failure. Many therapies have been studied including epinephrine, β_2-agonist bronchodilators, corticosteroids and ribavirin but little evidence supports a routine role in management.[56]

β_2-**Agonist Bronchodilators:** In actual hospital practice, β_2-agonists have been shown to be used about 53% to 73% of the time in various studies.[57,58] According to the American Academy of Pediatrics (AAP) Subcommittee on Diagnosis and Management of Bronchiolitis, bronchodilators should not be used in routine management of all patients with bronchiolitis; inhaled bronchodilators should be used, however, if there is a documented positive clinical response.[51] Bronchiolitic infants with a family history of RAD seem to show variable clinical response to bronchodilators.[59]

Nebulized Epinephrine: In a 2003 report, the Agency for Healthcare Research and Quality noted that nebulized epinephrine has "some potential for being efficacious."[48]

A meta-analysis of randomized controlled trials evaluating the efficacy of nebulized epinephrine by Hartling et al. showed some favorable short-term benefit.[60] In contrast, a later multi-center controlled trial by Wainwright et al. concluded that epinephrine did not impact the overall course of the illness as measured by hospital length of stay.[61] The AAP Subcommittee also could not find sufficient evidence of the efficacy of inhaled epinephrine for bronchiolitis.[51]

Hypertonic Saline: Nebulized hypertonic saline is theoretically thought to improve mucus transport rates, increase the volume of airway surface liquid and increase rates of mucociliary clearance. Based on that presumption, two studies recently demonstrated improvement in patients and showed decrease in length of stay for hospitalized infants.[62,63] Whether or not it is efficacious in the ED to prevent hospitalization for bronchiolitis remains to be seen.

Steroids: Steroids, such as prednisone and prednisolone, have traditionally been used in the treatment of bronchiolitis, but numerous studies have not been able to show any significant difference in decreasing admission rates or lowering hospital length of stays.[51] Dexamethasone was recently investigated in a large multi-center study and found that a single dose of oral dexamethasone 1 mg/kg did not significantly alter the respiratory status after 4 hours of observation, the rate of hospital admission or other later outcomes.[64]

Adjunctive Therapies: Because lower respiratory tract inflammation and secretions are a significant result of bronchiolitis, deep airway suctioning can be extremely helpful in infants who present with acute distress. These thick secretions compromise the infant's airway, and this simple therapy can provide immediate relief. The clinician should give close attention to the patient's hydration status, especially in children who present with respiratory distress as they are often quite dehydrated due to insensible losses and inability to take adequate oral intake during the preceding hours to days.

Prevention

The subset of infants particularly prone to apnea and respiratory failure are those with underlying conditions such as bronchopulmonary dysplasia, chronic lung disease, congenital heart disease or immunodeficiencies, and close evaluation should be completed, as they are prone to apnea and respiratory failure.

Synagis (palivizumab) has shown to be effective in preventing severe bronchiolitis when given prophylactically in these compromised infants. Synagis is a monoclonal antibody given IM on a monthly basis through the RSV season. The AAP has established guidelines for administration of Synagis, but, in general, it is given to children under the age of 24 months who have comorbidities such as prematurity less than 28 weeks, congenital heart disease, severe immune deficiencies, severe neuromuscular disease or congenital airway abnormalities. Unfortunately, a recent study in an ED demonstrated that only half the infants who met the AAP criteria were receiving Synagis.[65]

Complications of bronchiolitis include apnea, respiratory failure and pneumonia. Sweetmann et al. found an incidence of neurologic complications of 1.2% (0.7% seizures) in a total of 964 patients with RSV bronchiolitis.[66]

Admission Criteria

Patients with persistent hypoxia, respiratory distress, apnea or inability to tolerate fluids or patients in whom close follow-up cannot be ensured should be admitted. The AAP recommends supplemental oxygen when the room air oxygen saturation is less than 90%. Infants with comorbid disease may require supplemental oxygen sooner.[51] Willwerth et al. demonstrated that infants who fall into a high-risk group are at risk for apnea, whereas the low-risk group had an apnea risk of <1%. A child was considered to be at high risk for apnea if he or she met the following criteria:

1. The child was born at full-term and was younger than 1 month of age.
2. The child was born preterm (<37 weeks estimated gestational age) and was younger than 48 weeks post-conception.
3. The child's parents or a clinician had already witnessed an apnea episode with this illness before inpatient admission.[67]

Pneumonia

Epidemiology

Community-acquired pneumonia is one of the most serious infections of childhood, leading to significant mortality and morbidity in the United States. The annual incidence in Europe and North America for children younger than 5 years of age is 34 to 40 cases per 1000.[68-71] There are several definitions for pneumonia; however, McIntosh et al. stated that the most commonly accepted definition is the presence of fever, acute respiratory symptoms or both, plus evidence of parenchymal infiltrates on chest radiograph.[72]

Etiology

The most causative organisms vary by age group (Table 22.1). In the first month of life, Group B streptococcus, gram-negative bacteria and *Chlamydia* are common bacterial pathogens; all occur from vertical transmission from the mother.

From 1 to 3 months, *Streptococcus pneumoniae* is the most common bacterial pathogen. Other potential bacteria include *Mycoplasma pneumoniae*, *H. influenzae*, *S. aureus*, *Moraxella catarrhalis*, *Chlamydia* and *Pertussis*. Beyond 3 months of age, viruses, such as Adenovirus, Parainfluenza and influenza, are the predominant causative organisms.

Presentation

The clinical features of pneumonia depend on various factors, such as the age of the patient, presence of immunosuppression or comorbid diseases and the causative organism. Bacterial pneumonia generally has an abrupt onset with fever and chills, productive cough and chest pain. Frequently, respiratory rate and work of breathing have been studied as predictors of pneumonia; however, a study showed that tachypnea was predictive of only 24% of cases of pneumonia, based on a respiratory rate of greater than 40 breaths per minute.[73] Another study reviewed the predictive factors for the presence of focal infiltrates in children and found that decreased breath sounds, crackles, grunting and retractions were clinically significant.[74] Wheezing is typically associated with viral pneumonias, Mycoplasma or Chlamydial infections.

Bacterial pneumonia may not necessarily always present with obvious respiratory symptoms. Toikka et al. found that 93% of patients with bacterial pneumonia had a high fever (>39.0°C), 28% had no respiratory symptoms (although in this study, cough was not considered a respiratory symptom) and 6% presented with only gastrointestinal symptoms such as vomiting and vague abdominal pain in addition to fever.[75] Upper lobe pneumonias may

Table 22.1. Treatment of pneumonia based on age and type

Age	Birth to 4 Weeks	4 to 8 Weeks	8 Weeks to 3 Years	3 to 12 Years
Organisms	Group B Streptococcus Gram-negative enteric bacteria Cytomegalovirus *Listeria monocytogenes*	*Chlamydia trachomatis* Respiratory syncytial virus Parainfluenza 3 *Streptococcus pneumoniae* *Bordetella pertussis* *Staphylococcus aureus*	Respiratory syncytial virus, parainfluenza viruses, influenza virus, adenovirus, rhinovirus *Streptococcus pneumoniae* *Haemophilus influenza* (non–B type) *Mycoplasma pneumoniae*	*Mycoplasma pneumoniae* *Chlamydia pneumoniae* *Streptococcus pneumoniae* Respiratory syncytial virus, parainfluenza viruses, influenza virus, adenovirus, rhinovirus
Inpatient Therapy	Cefotaxime 50 mg/kg IV q8h and ampicillin 50 mg/kg IV q6h	Ceftriaxone 50 mg/kg IV q24h	Ceftriaxone 50 mg/kg IV q24h. Vancomycin for resistant *Strep* should be considered in critically ill appearing children	Ceftriaxone 50 mg/kg IV q24h. Vancomycin for resistant *Strep* should be considered in critically ill appearing children
Outpatient Therapy	Admit	High dose amoxicillin 90 mg/kg div q8h	High-dose amoxicillin 90 mg/kg div q8h *or* Azithromycin 10 mg/kg day 1 then 5 mg/kg qd for 4 days* *or* Augmentin 40 mg/kg div q8h	Azithromycin[†] 10 mg/kg day 1 then 5 mg/kg qd for 4 days

* Erythromycin or clarithromycin are acceptable alternatives.
[†] Preferred agent.
div, divided.

manifest as suspicion for meningitis as pain may radiate to the neck. The presence of vague abdominal pain and fever should also raise the suspicion for pneumonia.

Laboratory and Radiographic Findings

The decision to obtain a chest radiograph for an infant with clinical signs of pneumonia – productive cough, tachypnea, grunting, retractions, decreased breath sounds, crackles or hypoxia – is easier than making that decision in an asymptomatic febrile infant without a clinical source for the fever. Literature reviews looking at the need for a chest radiograph come to the conclusion that, unless the infant has evidence of lower respiratory tract disease, the utility of a chest radiograph is low.[76] One study by Bachur appeared to show that *occult pneumonia*, defined as definite radiographic evidence of an infiltrate in a child lacking clinical signs of pneumonia, may be present in up to 26% of children with fevers without a source and a WBC count higher than 20,000/mm^3.[77] Limitations of this study include the fact that residents rather than attending physicians performed these exams in the majority of cases, no

interobserver reliability between radiologists was reported and viral and bacterial infiltrates can have similar appearance on chest x-ray. Preliminary data from other studies seem to show similar occult pneumonia results[78–80]; therefore, chest radiographs may be considered in young infants with higher fevers and no source for that fever.

Classic characteristic radiographic findings vary by causative organism such as lobar infiltrates with air bronchograms seen in bacterial pneumonia or perihilar infiltrates seen in atypical pneumonia (Table 22.2). However, many of these radiographic findings may be seen in both bacterial and viral infections.[81] Decubitus chest radiographs are helpful in the evaluation of pleural effusions. It should be noted that children who are dehydrated might not have an infiltrate on initial radiography.

In an uncomplicated patient with lower respiratory tract infection who is otherwise stable, no additional laboratory testing is necessary. A peripheral WBC count as well as a sedimentation rate and C-reactive protein have been shown to not assist in differentiating a viral from a bacterial infection.[82] Another diagnostic test is the *Mycoplasma*

Table 22.2. Radiographic findings of various types of pneumonia

Type of pneumonia	Classic radiographic findings
Viral	Diffuse perihilar infiltrate
Bacterial: Pneumococcal	Round or unilobar infiltrates
Bacterial: Staphylococcal	Pneumatoceles
Bacterial: Nonspecific	Lobar infiltrates with air bronchograms
Atypical: Mycoplasma	Diffuse perihilar infiltrate, occasional pleural effusion
Pneumocystis carinii	Bilateral "fluffy" interstitial infiltrate
Tuberculosis	Upper lobe infiltrate; cavitary lesion

immunoglobulin M (IgM); this can be helpful in children younger than 3 years of age who present with pneumonias that are not responsive to amoxicillin.

Management

Once a diagnosis has been made, management is based on the age of the patient and the presumed causative agent. For either bacterial or viral pneumonia, supportive care should be initiated with hydration, maintenance of oxygenation and continuous cardiorespiratory monitoring for the ill-appearing child. If a virus is suspected, supportive care should be continued.

Children with large pleural effusions who are ill-appearing or immunocompromised should have a thoracentesis as well as chest tube placement in order to relieve respiratory distress and for diagnostic purposes. Bronchodilators and steroids should be considered in patients with wheezing or a history of RAD. An arterial or venous blood gas may be helpful in ill-appearing infants in respiratory distress. Endotracheal intubation followed by mechanical ventilation should be initiated in children with respiratory failure. Empiric antibiotics should be initiated based on the presumptive causative organism (see Table 22.1).

For infants younger than 2 months of age who are diagnosed with pneumonia, the clinician should strongly consider obtaining blood, urine and cerebrospinal fluid (CSF). Caution should be exercised in obtaining CSF from ill-appearing or toxic infants. Pulse oximetry during the lumbar puncture should be used to detect apnea. For older infants, blood cultures are rarely positive in pneumonia.[83] Infants younger than 2 months of age should be

admitted for IV antibiotics due to their high risk for sepsis and meningitis.

Other patients who meet admission criteria include those who have persistent hypoxia, are unable to tolerate fluids, experienced outpatient antibiotic failure or are in a difficult social situation in which appropriate follow-up is difficult.

Complications

Complications of pneumonia include bacteremia, with seeding of infection causing meningitis, pericarditis, epiglottitis and septic arthritis.

Chlamydia

Epidemiology and Pathophysiology

Chlamydia trachomatis infection is the leading cause of sexually transmitted disease in the United States. Neonatal infection is the source of significant mortality and morbidity. Transmission is thought to occur during delivery when the infant is exposed to maternal genital flora. Occasionally, there may be transmembranous transmission, which has been reported in infants born by cesarean section.

After exposure, it is presumed that the infant develops pneumonia after either direct inoculation of the tract or by drainage of the infected conjunctival secretions.[84] Studies have indicated that up to 30% of all newborns who have been exposed to *C. trachomatis* will develop pneumonia. The serotypes that are implicated in neonatal infection are B and D through K.

Presentation

These infants typically present between 4 and 12 weeks of age, but they rarely present earlier than 2 weeks or beyond 4 months of age. Chlamydia pneumonia presents in usually well-appearing infants 1 to 3 months of age with a staccato-like cough and no fever. The infant may have had a history of conjunctivitis (80%) or a mucoid rhinorrhea or nasal congestion (80%).[84]

Laboratory and Radiographic Findings

The typical radiographic findings include hyperinflated lungs with diffuse bilateral interstitial infiltrates. Lobar consolidations or pleural effusions are rarely seen. A CBC count is rarely useful in aiding diagnosis, as it frequently will be normal. For infants with suspected *C. trachomatis* pneumonia, the gold standard for diagnosis is isolation by obtaining cultures from the nasopharynx and, to a lesser extent, the conjunctiva. If the patients are intubated, additional cultures may be obtained from the tracheal aspirates.

Management

The treatment of *C. trachomatis* pneumonia is erythromycin base or ethyl succinate (50 mg/kg/day in four divided doses orally).[84] For infants who are unable to tolerate erythromycin, sulfisoxazole orally (150 mg/kg/day in four divided doses) is an alternative, but it should be used with caution in infants younger than 1 month of age due to the risk of hyperbilirubinemia.

Pertussis

Epidemiology

Pertussis, or *whooping cough,* is an acute infection of the respiratory tract caused by *Bordetella pertussis,* first isolated in 1906. There are other organisms that may cause a similar clinical syndrome, such as *Bordetella parapertussis,* adenovirus, or *Chlamydia.* Following the introduction of immunization in the mid-1940s, pertussis incidence declined more than 99% by 1970 and to an all-time low of 1010 cases by 1976. However, since then, an increase in disease incidence has been documented, with nearly 26,000 cases reported in 2004, 40% of which are present in children younger than 11 years old.[85] The concern regarding the rising number of cases is that an increase in the number of reported deaths from pertussis among very young infants has paralleled the increase in the number of reported cases.[86]

Clinical Features

Pertussis can be divided into three phases. The *catarrhal phase* is usually characterized by mild cough, conjunctivitis and coryza, and may last 1 to 2 weeks. The *paroxysmal phase* involves a worsening cough for 2 to 4 weeks. The classic description of the cough in this phase is after a spasmodic cough, the sudden inflow of air produces a whoop. In infants, the cough is usually staccato and there is an absence of the "whoop." Vomiting frequently occurs after the episodes as well. Generally, there is no fever. In infants younger than 2 months of age, apnea is a worrisome presentation of pertussis. Conjunctival hemorrhages and facial petechiae may be noted due to harsh coughing.

The *convalescent phase* is typified by a chronic cough that may last several weeks.

Laboratory and Radiographic Findings

The gold standard for diagnosis is culture. However, a polymerase chain reaction test of the nasopharyngeal specimens is available. Classically, pertussis is known to cause significant leukocytosis with predominant lymphocytes. The leukocytosis may reach 20,000 to 50,000/mm^3; however, this finding is not often seen in children younger than 6 months of age. According to Heininger et al., 75% of unvaccinated patients with pertussis have a lymphocytosis on CBC count.[87] A poor prognosis in infants is associated with leukocytosis with a lymphocytic predominance and the presence of pulmonary infiltrates.[88] Chest radiographs are usually normal, but they may infrequently show a shaggy right heart border.

Management

Antibiotic therapy is directed at preventing disease dissemination as treatment is of minimum benefit by the time the paroxysmal phase has begun. Prophylaxis is recommended for all close contacts regardless of age and vaccination status. The options are listed in Table 22.3. Erythromycin use has been associated with a risk of pyloric stenosis in infants younger than 1 month of age.[89]

Infants younger than 2 months old diagnosed with pertussis should be admitted because of the risk of apnea. A limited number of studies have demonstrated that most deaths from pertussis occur in infants younger than 3 months of age, most of whom are not vaccinated.[90] A recent study found that infants who have received their first vaccinations at 2 months of age have a protective effect against disease severity.[91]

An admitted patient with pertussis should be placed in respiratory isolation in order to prevent further infections. If the patient is not vaccinated, a series should be initiated. If the patient is younger than 2 months of age and has a known diagnosis of pertussis, then a complete sepsis workup may not be necessary. However, if the patient is ill appearing or is febrile but testing has not yet revealed a suspected diagnosis of pertussis, then consider a sepsis evaluation.

Complications

Major complications of pertussis infection include secondary bacterial pneumonia (20%), encephalopathy and

Table 22.3. Pertussis antibiotic therapy and prophylaxis

First-line antibiotic therapy	Dosing guidelines	Comments
Azithromycin	10 mg/kg on day 1, then 5 mg/kg for 4 days	For <6 months, use 10 mg/kg qd for 5 days
Clarithromycin	15 mg/kg div q12h for 7 days	Not recommended for use in infants <6 months of age
Erythromycin ethylsuccinate	50 mg/kg/day div q6h for 14 days	Linked to infantile hypertrophic pyloric stenosis in infants <1 month
Macrolide Allergy		
Trimethoprim-sulfamethoxazole	8 mg/kg/day div q12h for 14 days	Contraindicated in infants <2 months

div, divided.

seizures (1%), failure to thrive and death (0.3%). Pneumonia accounts for 90% of deaths from pertussis.[88] Other secondary complications as a result of severe coughing and increased intrathoracic pressure are intracranial hemorrhage, diaphragmatic rupture, pneumothorax and rectal prolapse.

Reactive Airway Disease

Epidemiology and Pathophysiology

RAD reflects airway hyperreactivity to various stimuli but encompasses a broad differential diagnosis. The term *asthma* is often used interchangeably with RAD, but not all children who wheeze have asthma and only 30% of infants who wheeze progress to asthma. Frequent precipitants of airway hyperresponsiveness include infection (commonly RSV), tobacco smoke, stress, drugs and various allergens including dust mites, pet dander and cockroaches.[92–93]

Presentation

On examination of the lungs, wheezing should be distinguished from other respiratory findings such as stridor. Stridor is usually an upper airway phenomenon and is present on inspiration, whereas wheezing is accentuated on expiration. During auscultation, the clinician should pay careful attention to the symmetry of the breath sounds as asymmetry may represent an obstructive process. Subtle wheezing may be auscultated by a "squeezing the wheeze" technique, in which the clinician applies manual compression in the AP dimension of the chest.

Patients may present in significant respiratory distress with cyanosis, flushing, nasal flaring, intercostal retractions and an increased inspiratory-to-expiratory ratio. "Abdominal breathing" can also be an indication of increased work of breathing. Infants may also present with poor feeding, diaphoresis and dehydration.

Laboratory and Radiographic Features

In most infants who present with RAD, most laboratory testing is of limited utility. A blood gas analysis has often been suggested as useful in determining impending respiratory failure. But with the addition of continuous pulse oximetry and the ongoing evaluation of the patient's mental status and work of breathing, the need for arterial blood gas analysis has lessened.

A CBC count may demonstrate hypereosinophilia, and an IgE level may be elevated. Routine chest radiography is not recommended unless an infant presents with focal exam findings suggestive of pneumonia, foreign body or fever.[94–95] Hyperinflation, peribronchial thickening and atelectasis may be seen on chest radiograph. Bronchoscopy or a barium swallow should be conducted in an infant who has persistent or recurrent wheezing and in whom other etiologies are being considered, such as gastroesophageal reflux, vascular rings or slings or tracheoesophageal fistulas. The barium swallow should be performed once the child is stable and without respiratory distress as the study does carry a risk of aspiration of the barium.

Management

Most therapies have not been well studied in children younger than 4 years of age. The National Asthma Guidelines were updated in 2007[96]; the expert research panel recommended the following steps be followed during acute exacerbations:

1. Administer supplemental oxygen to correct significant hypoxemia in moderate or severe exacerbations.
2. Administer repetitive or continuous short-acting β-antagonists (SABAs) to rapidly reverse airflow obstruction.

Table 22.4. Quick dosing reference guide

Disease	Initial therapy	Comments
Croup Mild to Moderate	Decadron 0.3 mg/kg PO/IM, maximum 16 mg in 24 hr	If not improved after first nebulizer treatment, repeat
Croup Severe	Decadron 0.6 mg/kg PO/IM, maximum 16 mg in 24 hr	
	Racemic epinephrine 0.25 cc or 0.5 cc in NS nebulized or L-epinephrine 1:1000 0.5 cc/kg/dose (max 2.5 cc for <4 years old and 5 cc for >4 years old)	
Bacterial Tracheitis	Vancomycin 10 mg/kg q6h	Establish airway
	plus	Immediate consultation with otolaryngology
	Ceftriaxone 100 mg/kg/day qd	
Epiglottitis	Ceftriaxone 100 mg/kg/day IV in one dose	Establish airway
	Or	Immediate consultation with otolaryngology
	Cefotaxime 50 mg/kg q6h	
	Or	
	Ampicillin/sulbactam 200-400 mg/kg/day div q 6h	
Retropharyngeal Abscess	Clindamycin 30 mg/kg/day IV in four divided doses	Establish airway
	Or	Immediate consultation with otolaryngology
	Cefazolin 100 mg/kg/day IV in three divided doses	
Reactive Airway Mild	Albuterol 0.5 cc nebulized prn	Admission for persistent distress
Moderate	Albuterol 0.5 cc nebulized for 3 doses	
	Ipratropium 0.25 mg nebulized	
	Prednisone/Prednisolone 1–2 mg/kg for 5 days	
Severe	Continuous albuterol nebulization	Admission
	Magnesium sulfate 25 mg/kg IV	
	Solu Medrol 2 mg/kg IV/IM	
	Systemic beta-agonists – terbutaline, epinephrine SQ, IV	

IM, intramuscular; IV, intravenous; PO, per os; prn, as needed; SQ, subcutaneous.

3. Administer oral systemic corticosteroids to decrease airway inflammation in moderate or severe exacerbations or for patients who fail to respond promptly and completely to SABA treatment.
4. Monitor response to therapy with serial assessments.

Supplemental Oxygen: The National Asthma Guidelines' expert panel recommended that supplemental oxygen be administered to maintain an oxygen saturation of greater than 90%. In infants, an Sao_2 of less than 90% indicated severe distress. The clinician should monitor the patient until clear improvement has been seen with other therapies.

Short-Acting β-Antagonists: The National Heart, Lung and Blood Institute Guidelines have made minimal changes to the recommendation of SABA therapy.

Currently, the recommended doses are 0.15 mg/kg (minimum dose 2.5 mg) every 20 minutes for three doses then 0.15 to 0.3 mg/kg up to 10 mg every 1 to 4 hours as needed, or 0.5 mg/kg/hour by continuous nebulization. The guidelines also added that levalbuterol may also be used as a SABA. Albuterol is a 50:50 mixture of synthetic *R*-albuterol and *S*-albuterol, whereas levalbuterol contains only the active enantiomer, *R*-albuterol. *R*-albuterol is thought to have isolated effects on the smooth muscle of the bronchi. However, levalbuterol has not been shown to be superior to albuterol for the treatment of acute pediatric asthma.[97] Another consideration is that the cost of levalbuterol is significantly more than albuterol.

Anticholinergics: Anticholinergics such as ipratropium bromide have been shown to provide further benefit beyond β-agonists in patients with asthma.[96] They should not be the first-line therapy, however. Ipratropium can be delivered in the same nebulizer as albuterol at a dosage of 0.25 mg for infants (Table 22.4).

Steroids

Steroids are a mainstay of treatment in most cases of RAD seen in the ED. Initial dosing should be started in the ED for patients in moderate to severe distress and then continued as an outpatient at 1 to 2 mg/kg/day in one to two divided doses for 5 days.

Recently, there have been several studies advocating the use of dexamethasone in lieu of prednisone. The most recent study showed no clinical difference in patients treated with a single IM dose of dexamethasone as compared to a 5-day course of oral prednisone for the treatment of moderate asthma exacerbations.[98]

Systemic Therapies

Systemic β-agonists have also been used extensively in both adult and pediatric RAD. No significant improvement of subcutaneous over inhaled epinephrine or terbutaline has been found.[96] There is little literature on the use of IV epinephrine in children for acute RAD. A recent study found a trend toward improvement, but not significant, in hospitalized children with severe asthma who received IV terbutaline.[99]

Theophylline/aminophylline is not recommended because it appears to provide no additional benefit to optimal SABA therapy and increases the frequency of adverse effects.[96]

Magnesium sulfate should be considered in patients in severe exacerbations refractory to conventional therapy. A meta-analysis of the use of magnesium sulfate in asthma exacerbations showed that patients with moderate to severe exacerbations probably benefit from the use of magnesium sulfate.[100] The National Heart, Lung and Blood Institute report recommended 25 to 75 mg/kg up to 2 g in children of magnesium sulfate in these exacerbations.

Complications

Complications include cardiac arrest, pulsus paradoxus, pneumothorax, pneumomediastinum (Figure 22.7), respiratory failure and death.

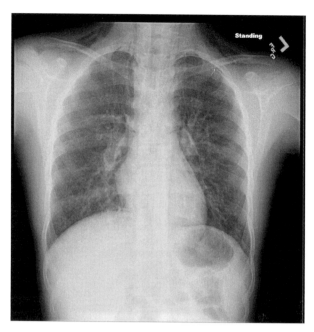

Figure 22.7. Pneumomediastinum.

PITFALLS

- Failure to recognize that infants in respiratory distress are frequently dehydrated due to insensible losses
- Failure to consider anatomical abnormalities in patients with recurrent croup
- Failure to consider bacterial tracheitis in an ill-appearing child with high fever and with croup-like symptoms that are refractory to conventional treatment with epinephrine and corticosteroids
- Failure to correctly position the infant for the lateral neck radiograph may give the false appearance of an enlargement of the retropharyngeal space
- Failure to include pertussis in the differential diagnosis of infants presenting with apnea or cyanosis after episodes of prolonged coughing

REFERENCES

1. Maschka DA, Bauman NM, McCray PB Jr, et al. A classification scheme for paradoxical vocal cord motion. *Laryngoscope.* 1997;107:1429–1435.
2. Krugman SD, Lantz PE, Sinal S, et al. Forced suffocation of infants with baby wipes: a previously undescribed form of child abuse. *Child Abuse Negl.* 2007;31(6):615–621.
3. Centers for Disease Control and Prevention (CDC). Nonfatal choking-related episodes among children – United States, 2001. *MMWR Morb Mortal Wkly Rep.* 2002;51:945–948.
4. WISQARS leading cause of death reports 1999–2001. National Center for Injury Prevention and Control. http://webappa.cdc.gov/sasweb/ncipc/leadcaus10.html. Accessed on May 20, 2008.

5. Burton EM, Brick WG, Hall JD, et al. Tracheobronchial foreign body aspiration in children. *South Med J.* 1996;89(2):195–198.

6. Even L, Heno N, Talmon Y, et al. Diagnostic evaluation of foreign body aspiration in children: a prospective study. *J Pediatr Surg.* 2005;40(7):1122–1127.

7. Tan HK, Brown K, McGill T, et al. Airway foreign bodies (FB): a 10-year review. *Int J Pediatr Otorhinolaryngol.* 2000;56(2):91–99.

8. Freidman EM. Update on the pediatric airway: tracheobronchial foreign bodies. *Otolaryngol Clin North Am.* 2000;33(1):179–185.

9. Food and Drug Administration. *Public Health Advisory. Nonprescription Cough and Cold Medicine Use in Children.* January 17, 2008.

10. Smith MB, Feldman W. Over-the-counter cold medications: a critical review of clinical trials between 1950 and 1991. *JAMA.* 1993;269(17):2258–2263.

11. Centers for Disease Control and Prevention (CDC). Infant deaths associated with cough and cold medications – two states, 2005. *MMWR Morb Mortal Wkly Rep.* 2007;56(1): 1–4.

12. Jones R, Santos JI, Overall JC Jr. Bacterial tracheitis. *JAMA.* 1979;242(8):721–726.

13. Liston SL, Gerhz RC, Siegel LG, et al. Bacterial tracheitis. *Am J Dis Child.* 1983;137(8):764–767.

14. Hopkins A, Lahiri T, Salerno R, et al. Changing epidemiology of life-threatening upper airway infections: the reemergence of bacterial tracheitis. *Pediatrics.* 2006;118(4):1418–1421.

15. Brook I. Aerobic and anaerobic microbiology of bacterial tracheitis in children. *Pediatr Emerg Care.* 1997;13(1): 16–18.

16. Donaldson JD, Mathby CC. Bacterial tracheitis in children. *J Otolaryngol.* 1989;18(3);48:101–104.

17. Bernstein T, Brilli R, Jacobs B. Is bacterial tracheitis changing? A 14-month experience in a pediatric intensive care unit. *Clin Infect Dis.* 1998;27:458–462.

18. Gallagher PG, Myer CM 3d. An approach to the diagnosis and treatment of membranous laryngotracheobronchitis in infants and children. *Pediatr Emerg Care.* 1991;7(6):337–342.

19. Duncan NO, Sprecher RC. Infections of the airway. In: Cummings CW, ed. *Otolaryngology – Head and Neck Surgery,* 3rd ed. St. Louis, MO: Mosby; 1998:388–400.

20. Denny FW, Murphy TF, Clyde WA Jr, et al. Croup: an 11-year study in a pediatric practice. *Pediatrics.* 1983;71(6):871–876.

21. Skolnik NS. Treatment of croup: a critical review. *Am J Dis Child.* 1989;143(9):1045–1049.

22. Shroeder LL, Knapp JF. Recognition and emergency management of infectious causes of upper airway obstruction. *Semin Respir Infect.* 1995;10(1):21–30.

23. Geelhoed GC, Turner J, Macdonald WB. Efficacy of a small single dose of oral dexamethasone for outpatient croup: a double blind placebo controlled clinical trial. *BMJ.* 1996;313(7050):140–142.

24. Geelhoed GC, Macdonald WB. Oral dexamethasone in the treatment of croup: 0.15 mg/kg versus 0.3 mg/kg versus 0.6 mg/kg. *Pediatr Pulmonol.* 1995;20(6):362–368.

25. Donaldson D, Poleski D, Knipple E, et al. Intramuscular versus oral dexamethasone for the treatment of moderate-to-severe croup: a randomized, double blind trial. *Acad Emerg Med.* 2003;10(1):16–21.

26. Klassen TP, Craig WR, Moher D, et al. Nebulized budesonide and oral dexamethasone for treatment of croup: a randomized control trial. *JAMA.* 1998;279(20):1629–1632.

27. Johnson DW, Jacobson S, Edney PC, et al. A comparison of nebulized budesonide, intramuscular dexamethasone, and placebo for moderately severe croup. *N Engl J Med.* 1998;339(8):498–503.

28. Ledwith C, Shea L. The use of nebulized racemic epinephrine in the outpatient treatment of croup. *Pediatr Emerg Care.* 1993;9:318.

29. Neto GM. Kentab O. Klassen TP, et al. A randomized controlled trial of mist in the acute treatment of moderate croup. *Acad Emerg Med.* 2002;9(9):873–879.

30. Scolnik D, Coates AL. Controlled delivery of high vs. low humidity vs. mist therapy for croup in emergency departments: a randomized controlled trial. *JAMA.* 2006;295(11):1274–1280.

31. Gupta VK, Cheifitz IM. Heliox administration in the pediatric intensive care unit: an evidence-based review. *Pediatr Crit Care Med.* 2005;6(2):204–211.

32. Terregino CA, Nairn SJ, Chansky ME, et al. The effect of heliox on croup: a pilot study. *Acad Emerg Med.* 1998;5(11):1130–1133.

33. Weber JE, Chudnofsky CR, Younger JG, et al. A randomized comparison of helium–oxygen mixture (heliox) and racemic epinephrine for the treatment of moderate to severe croup. *Pediatrics.* 2001;107(6):E96.

34. Centers for Disease Control and Prevention. Progress toward eliminating *Haemophilus influenza* type b disease among infants and children – United States, 1987–1997. *MMWR Morb Motal Wkly Rep.* 1998;47(46):993–998.

35. Mauro RD, Poole SR, Lockhart CH. Differentiation of epiglottitis from laryngotracheitis in the child with stridor. *Am J Dis Child.* 1988;142(6):679–682.

36. Blackstock P, Adderhey RJ, Steward DJ. Epiglottitis in young infants. *Anesthesiology.* 1987;67:97–100.

37. Loos GD. Pharyngitis, croup and epiglottitis. *Prim Care.* 1990;17(2):335–345.

38. Yeoh LH, Singh SD, Rogers JH. Retropharyngeal abscesses in a children's hospital. *J Laryngol Otol.* 1985;99:555–556.

39. Broughton RA. Nonsurgical management of deep neck infections in children. *Pediatr Infect Dis J.* 1992;11(1): 14–18.

40. Coulthard M, Isaacs D. Retropharyngeal abscess. *Arch Dis Child.* 1991;66:1227–1230.

41. Morrison JE, Pashley NRT. Retropharyngeal abscesses in children: a 10-year review. *Pediatr Emerg Care.* 1988;4: 9–11.

42. Craig FW, Schunk JE. Retropharyngeal abscess in children: clinical presentation, utility of imaging, and current management. *Pediatrics.* 2003;111:1394–1398.

43. Stege G, Fenton A, Jaffray B. Nihilism in the 1990s: the true mortality of congenital diaphragmatic hernia. *Pediatrics.* 2003;112:532–535.

44. Cannon C, Dildy GA, Ward R, et al. A population-based study of congenital diaphragmatic hernia in Utah: 1988–1994. *Obstet Gynecol.* 1996;87:959–963.

45. Torfs CP, Curry CJ, Bateson TF, et al. A population-based study of congenital diaphragmatic hernia. *Teratology.* 1992;46:555–565.

46. Fleischer GR, Ludwig S. *Textbook of Pediatric Emergency Medicine.* Philadelphia, PA: Lippincott Williams & Wilkins; 2000.

47. Klassen TP. Recent advances in the treatment of bronchiolitis and laryngitis. *Pediatr Clin North Am.* 1997;44:249–261.

48. Agency for Healthcare Research and Quality. Management of Bronchiolitis in Infants and Children. Evidence Report/Technology Assessment No. 69. Rockville, MD: Agency for Healthcare Research and Quality; 2003. AHRQ Publication No. 03-E014.

49. Hall CB. Respiratory syncytial virus and parainfluenza virus. *N Engl J Med.* 2001;344(25):1917–1928.

50. Carlsen KH, Orstavik I, Halvorsen K. Viral infections of the respiratory tract in hospitalized children. A study from Oslo during a 90 months' period. *Acta Paediatr Scand.* 1983;72(1):53–58.

51. American Academy of Pediatrics Subcommittee on Diagnosis and Management of Bronchiolitis. Diagnosis and management of bronchiolitis. *Pediatrics.* 2006;118(4):1774–1793.

52. Shay DK, Holman RC, Roosevelt GE, et al. Bronchiolitis-associated mortality and estimates of respiratory syncytial virus-associated deaths among US children, 1979–1997. *J Infect Dis.* 2001;183:16–22.

53. Bordley WC, Viswanathan M, King VJ, et al. Diagnosis and testing in bronchiolitis: a systematic review. *Arch Pediatr Adolesc Med.* 2004;158(2):119–126.

54. Melendez E, Harper MB. Utility of sepsis evaluation in infants 90 days of age or younger with fever and clinical bronchiolitis. *Pediatr Infect Dis J.* 2003;22(12):1053–1056.

55. Zorc JJ, Levine DA, Platt SL, et al. Multicenter RSV-SBI Study Group of the Pediatric Emergency Medicine Collaborative Research Committee of the American Academy of Pediatrics. *Pediatrics.* 2005;116(3):644–648.

56. King VJ, Viswanathan M, Bordley WC, et al. Pharmacologic treatment of bronchiolitis in infants and children: a systematic review. *Arch Pediatr Adolesc Med.* 2004;158(2):127–137.

57. Mansbach JM, Edmond JA, Camargo CA. Bronchiolitis in US emergency departments 1992 to 2000: epidemiology and practice variation. *Pediatr Emerg Care.* 2005;21:242–247.

58. Plint AC, Johnson DW, Wiebe N. Practice variation among pediatric emergency departments in the treatment of bronchiolitis. *Acad Emerg Med.* 2004;11:353–360.

59. Tepper RS, Rosenberg D, Eigen H, et al. Bronchodilator responsiveness in infants with bronchiolitis. *Pediatr Pulmonol.* 1994;17(2):81–85.

60. Hartling L, Wiebe N, Russell K, et al. A meta-analysis of randomized controlled trials evaluating the efficacy of epinephrine for the treatment of acute viral bronchiolitis. *Arch Pediatr Adolesc Med.* 2003;157(10):957–964.

61. Wainwright C, Altamirano L, Cheney M, et al. A multicenter, randomized, double-blind, controlled trial of nebulized epinephrine in infants with acute bronchiolitis. *N Engl J Med.* 2003;349:27–35.

62. Tal G, Cesar K, Oron A, et al. Hypertonic saline/epinephrine treatment in hospitalized infants with viral bronchiolitis reduces hospitalization stay: 2 years experience. *Isr Med Assoc J.* 2006;8(3):169–173.

63. Kuzik BA, Al-Qadhi SA, Kent S, et al. Nebulized hypertonic saline in the treatment of viral bronchiolitis in infants. *J Pediatr.* 2007;151(3):266–270.

64. Corneli HM, Zorc JJ, Majahan P, et al. A multicenter, randomized, controlled trial of dexamethasone for bronchiolitis. *N Engl J Med.* 2007;357(4):331–339.

65. Mansbach J, Kunz S, Acholonu U, et al. Evaluation of compliance with palivizumab recommendations in a multicenter study of young children presenting to the emergency department with bronchiolitis. *Pediatr Emerg Care.* 2007;23(6):362–367.

66. Sweetman LL, Ng YT, Butler IJ, et al. Neurologic complications associated with respiratory syncytial virus. *Pediatr Neurol.* 2005;32(5):307–310.

67. Willwerth BM, Harper MB, Greenes DS. Identifying hospitalized infants who have bronchiolitis and are at high risk for apnea. *Ann Emerg Med.* 2006;48(4):441–447.

68. Murphy TF, Henderson FW, Clyde WA Jr, et al. Pneumonia: an eleven-year study in a pediatric practice. *Am J Epidemiol.* 1981;113:12–21.

69. Foy HM, Cooney MK, Allan I, et al. Rates of pneumonia during influenza epidemics in Seattle, 1964 to 1975. *JAMA.* 1975;241:253–258.

70. Jokinen C, Heiskanen L, Juvonen H, et al. Incidence of community-acquired pneumonia in the population of four municipalities in eastern Finland. *Am J Epidemiol.* 1993;37:977–988.

71. McConnochie KM, Hall CB, Barker WH. Lower respiratory tract illness in the first two years of life: epidemiologic patterns and costs in a suburban pediatric practice. *Am J Public Health.* 1988;78:34–39.

72. McIntosh K. Community-acquired pneumonia in children. *N Engl J Med.* 2002;346(6):429–437.

73. Rothrock SG, Green SM, Fanella JM, et al. Do published guidelines predict pneumonia in children presenting to an urban ED? *Pediatr Emerg Care.* 2001;17(4):240–243.

74. Lynch T, Platt R, Gouin S, et al. Can we predict which children with clinically suspected pneumonia will have the presence of focal infiltrates on chest radiographs? *Pediatrics.* 2004;113(3 Pt 1):e186–189.

75. Toikka P, Virkki R, Mertsola J, et al. Bacteremic pneumococcal pneumonia in children. *Clin Infect Dis.* 1999;29:568–572.

76. American College of Emergency Physicians Clinical Policy for Children Younger Than Three Years Presenting to the Emergency Department With Fever. *Ann Emerg Med.* 2003;42:530–545.

77. Bachur R, Perry H, Harper MB. Occult pneumonias: empiric chest radiographs in febrile children with leukocytosis. *Ann Emerg Med.* 1999;33(2):166–173.

78. Aaron K, Moro-Sutherland D, Shook JE. Prevalence of occult pneumonia in febrile children with elevated white blood cell count. *Pediatrics.* 1998;102:719. [abstract]

79. Blumenreich R, Ryan JG, Catapano M, et al. Prevalence of abnormal chest radiographs in febrile children from 90 days to 36 months. *Ann Emerg Med*. 1998;32:S18. [abstract]

80. Murphy CG, van de Pol AC, Harper MB, et al. Clinical predictors of occult pneumonia in the febrile child. *Acad Emerg Med*. 2007;14(3):243–249.

81. Korppi M, Kiekara O, Heiskanen-Kosma T, et al. Comparison of radiological findings and microbial aetiology of childhood pneumonia. *Acta Paediatr*. 1993;82:360–363.

82. Nohynek H, Valkeila E, Leinonen M, et al. Erythrocyte sedimentation rate, white blood cell count and serum C-reactive protein in assessing etiologic diagnosis of acute lower respiratory infections in children. *Pediatr Infect Dis J*. 1995;14:484–490.

83. Shah SS, Alpern ER, et al. Risk of bacteremia in young children with pneumonia treated as outpatients. *Arch Pediatr Adolesc Med*. 2003;157(4):389–392.

84. Feigin RD, Cherry J, Demmler GJ, et al. *Textbook of Pediatric Infectious Diseases*, 5th ed. Philadelphia, PA: Saunders; 2004:910–913, 2482–2495.

85. Centers for Disease Control and Prevention (CDC). *Pertussis. Epidemiology and Prevention of Vaccine-Preventable Diseases (The Pink Book) Course Textbook*. Washington, DC: CDC; 2007:79–96.

86. Vitek C, Pascual B, Murphy T. Pertussis deaths in the United States in the 1990s. In *Abstracts of the 40th Interscience Conference on Antimicrobial Agents and Chemotherapy, September 17–20, 2000, Toronto, Ontario, Canada*. Washington, DC: American Society for Microbiology, 2000.

87. Heininger U, Klich K, Stehr K, et al. Clinical findings in Bordetella pertussis infections: results of a prospective multicenter surveillance study. *Pediatrics*. 1997;100(6):E10.

88. Greenberg DP, von Konig CH, Heininger U. Health burden of pertussis in infants and children. *Pediatr Infect Dis J*. 2005;24(5 Supp):S39–43.

89. Cooper WO, Griffin MR, Arbogast P, et al. Very early exposure to erythromycin and infantile hypertrophic pyloric stenosis. *Arch Pediatr Adol Med*. 2002;156(7):647–650.

90. Galanis E, King AS, Varughese P, et al; IMPACT investigators. Changing epidemiology and emerging risk groups for pertussis. *CMAJ*. 2006;174(4):451–452.

91. Briand V, Bonmarin I, Lévy-Bruhl D. Study of the risk factors for severe childhood pertussis based on hospital surveillance data. *Vaccine*. 2007;25(41):7224–7232.

92. Huss K, Adkinson NF Jr, Eggleston PA, et al. House dust mite and cockroach exposure are strong risk factors for positive allergy skin test responses in the Childhood Asthma Management Program. *J Allergy Clin Immunol*. 2001;107(1):48–54.

93. Rosenstreich DL, Eggleston P, Kattan M, et al. The role of cockroach allergy and exposure to cockroach allergen in causing morbidity among inner-city children with asthma. *N Engl J Med*. 1997;336(19):1356–1363.

94. Roback MG, Dreitlein DA. Chest radiograph in the evaluation of first time wheezing episodes: review of current clinical practice and efficacy. *Pediatr Emerg Care*. 1998;14(3):181–184.

95. Mahabee-Gittens EM, Bachman DT, Shapiro ED, et al. Chest radiographs in the pediatric emergency department for children < or = 18 months of age with wheezing. *Clin Pediatr (Phila)*. 1999;38(7):395–399.

96. National Heart, Lung and Blood Institute. Guidelines for the Diagnosis and Management of Asthma (EPR-3). July 2007. www.nhlbi.nih.gov/guidelines/asthma. Accessed on May 20, 2008.

97. Qureshi F, Zaritsky A, Welch C, et al. Clinical efficacy of racemic albuterol versus levalbuterol for the treatment of acute pediatric asthma. *Ann Emerg Med*. 2005;46(1):29–36.

98. Gordon S, Tompkins T, Dayan PS. Randomized trial of single-dose intramuscular dexamethasone compared with prednisolone for children with acute asthma. *Pediatr Emerg Care*. 2007;23(8):521–527.

99. Bogie AL, Towne D, Luckett PM, et al. Comparison of intravenous terbutaline versus normal saline in pediatric patients on continuous high-dose nebulized albuterol for status asthmaticus. *Pediatr Emerg Care*. 2007;23(6):355–361.

100. Cheuk DK, Chau TC, Lee SL. A meta-analysis on intravenous magnesium sulphate for treating acute asthma. *Arch Dis Child*. 2005;90(1):74–77.

23

Toxicologic Emergencies

Raemma P. Luck and Adam Barouh

INTRODUCTION

According to data compiled by the American Association of Poison Control Centers (AAPCC), there were more than 2.4 million incidents of human exposure reported to regional poison centers in 2005 alone.[1] Of the reports made, about 1.2 million, or 51%, were reported in children younger than 6 years of age. The vast majority of these exposures occurred at home, involved a single-agent and was unintentional in nature. Most of these pediatric poisonings were managed by the Poison Control Center at the site of exposure (90%) rather than in a health care facility (10%). About 96% of these exposures had either no effect or only minor effects requiring no follow-up.

Because children are inquisitive by nature and have a strong tendency to put objects in their mouths, ingestion is the most common means of exposure, followed by dermal contact.[1] Cosmetics and personal care products, household cleaning substances, and foreign bodies such as toys, plants and pesticides are the top five nonpharmaceutical poisons to which children younger than 6 years of age are exposed (Table 23.1). Among pharmaceutical products, analgesic agents, topical preparations, cold and cough medications, vitamins and antihistamines are the most frequent substances reported in this age group.

In order to understand the complex interplay among the child, the agent and the environment in toxic exposures, knowledge of the approximate age of key developmental milestones is important. For example, most 7-month-old infants are able to sit without support, reach out and grasp large objects with their hands. At 9 to 10 months, they can pull up to stand, crawl, cruise along furniture, grasp small objects using their thumbs and forefingers (pincer grasp) and consequently put things in their mouths. After 12 months, children can walk alone, start to drink from a cup and feed themselves with their fingers.[2]

Table 23.1. Top ten pediatric poisons in children younger than 6 years old, 2005

	Total No.	Total exposures (%)
No pharmaceuticals		
Cosmetics/personal care products	165,329	13.4
Household cleaning substances	121,498	9.8
Foreign bodies/toys/ miscellaneous	91,422	7.4
Plants	49,410	4.0
Pesticides	49,232	4.0
Pharmaceuticals		
Analgesics	100,595	8.2
Topical preparations	88,859	7.2
Cold and cough preparations	70,398	5.7
Vitamins	48,604	3.9
Antihistamines	35,766	2.9

Data from Lai MW, Lein;Schwartz W, Rodgers GC, et al. 2005 Annual Report of the American Association of Poison Control Centers' national poisoning and exposure database. *Clin Toxicol (Phila)*. 2006; 44:803–932.

The attainment and mastery of these developmental milestones means that children have a wider area of exploration that creates opportunities not only for learning but also for injuries. The increase in mobility and fine motor ability combined with easy access to common household poisons and lapse in supervision by caretakers results in this age group having the highest incidence of toxic ingestions. Children cannot discriminate between safe and unsafe products, are attracted to colored objects and imitate caretakers who take medications. Contrary to popular belief, poisoning occurs in families of all economic strata and educational backgrounds. Caretakers often put household chemicals in familiar containers such as soda bottles or store them in areas that are not locked.[3] Some agents look similar to candy, may be odorless or may even have a pleasant taste. As mentioned previously, a majority

Table 23.2. Top five causes of all fatal poison exposures in the US, 2005

Substance	% of All exposures
Stimulants and street drugs	0.55
Antidepressants	0.32
Cardiovascular drugs	0.30
Sedatives/antipsychotics	0.28
Analgesics	0.25

Data from Lai MW, Lein-Schwartz W, Rodgers GC, et al. 2005 Annual Report of the American Association of Poison Control Centers' national poisoning and exposure database. *Clin Toxicol (Phila)*. 2006; 44:803–932.

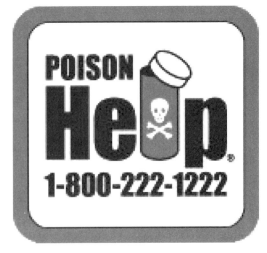

Figure 23.1. The AAPCC's new Poison Help logo showing the national number to call anywhere anytime in the United States for any poisoning related inquiries.

of ingestions in the first few years of life are innocuous, involve small quantities of a known substance and result in favorable outcomes. In contrast, ingestions by adolescents and adults are often intentional in nature, involve multiple and large quantities of drugs and result in worse outcomes.

In the United States in 2004, poisoning was second only to motor vehicle crashes as the most common cause of death from unintentional injury.[4] Most of the poisoning deaths from drugs were due to either abuse of prescription medications or use of illegal drugs.[5] In 2005, there were 1261 fatalities from poisoning recorded in the AAPCC database.[1] The top causes of these fatalities are listed in Table 23.2. Of these fatalities, 56% occurred in the 20- to 49-year-old age group. In contrast, there were 24 deaths (1.9%) in children younger than 6 years of age, the lowest recorded since 1985. Considering that there were 1.2 million reports to the Regional Poison Control Centers in this age group, these fatalities, as a percentage of total reports, are a very small fraction (0.003%), reflecting the benign nature of most pediatric poisonings.

The decrease in morbidity and mortality from poisoning is the result of many interventions from both the private and the public sectors. One effective piece of legislation is the Poison Prevention Packaging Act (PPPA) of 1970.[6,7] The PPPA was created to prevent children younger than 5 years of age from accidentally ingesting hazardous substances. The PPPA restricted children's access to prescription and over-the-counter (OTC) medications by making it difficult for them to open the packages while allowing easy access for adults. The U.S. Consumer Product Safety Commission was charged with the responsibility and authority to carry out the PPPA, and continues to this day to issue requirements regarding child-resistant packaging.

Another intervention that helped decrease childhood morbidity and mortality from poisoning was the creation of Poison Control Centers with the first center starting in Chicago in 1957.[8] Presently, there are 61 centers which have joined together to form the AAPCC in 1999. Staffed by toxicology specialists, these centers can be accessed anywhere in the U.S. by a national telephone number 24 hours a day, 7 days of the week through the Poison Help Hotline (1-800-222-1222) (Figure 23.1). This number will direct the caller to the nearest regional poison control center. The specialists provide free immediate consultation about a potential poison, treatment recommendations as well as poisoning prevention education.

Physician- and pharmacy-based educational intervention programs designed for children and their parents are effective ways to increase awareness of childhood poisonings. Anticipatory guidance provided to parents and children by staff at the physician's office during scheduled well-child visits also can include strategies to decrease childhood poisoning. Repeat poisoning is common; emergency department (ED) physicians should take the opportunity to discuss poisoning prevention with caretakers of every patient who has experienced a toxic exposure.[9]

GENERAL APPROACH TO A TODDLER WITH UNKNOWN EXPOSURE

Occasionally, the ED physician is called upon to manage a symptomatic infant or toddler who has ingested an unknown substance. The goal is to simultaneously initiate treatment, uncover the diagnosis and assess the severity of the exposure within a short but critical period of time.

Primary Survey

The initial phase of management is similar to the primary and secondary surveys advocated by the American College of Surgeons' Advanced Trauma Life Support model.[10,11] In the primary survey, airway, breathing and circulation (ABCs) are assessed expeditiously and supported as needed. Oftentimes, all that is needed to support the airway is the administration of oxygen by a simple face or nonrebreather mask. If there is evidence of airway obstruction or decreased ability to protect the airway, intubation must be initiated immediately using rapid sequence intubation. A child with intact airway reflexes but with altered mental status and possible clinical deterioration should be electively intubated sooner rather than later.

An intravenous (IV) access line, preferably two, needs to be secured while the patient's circulatory status is still stable. While drawing blood specimens for laboratory analysis, a rapid bedside glucose level should be obtained because a number of drugs, such as beta-blockers, ethanol, oral hypoglycemic agents and insulin, can cause hypoglycemia in a toddler.[11,12] Vital signs, such as heart rate, respiratory rate, blood pressure and oxygen saturation (using a pulse oximeter) should be continuously monitored. Abnormalities in vital signs can provide a clue to the class of drugs taken. For example, tachycardia in a child who is hard to arouse may suggest cocaine, heroin, anticholinergic or antihistamine poisoning. Bradycardia is seen in children who ingest beta-blockers, calcium-channel blockers, digoxin, anticholinesterase drugs or clonidine.

In the ABCDs of possible toxicologic overdose, "D" not only stands for Dextrostix but also stands for disability or a mini-neurologic exam, drugs and decontamination. The Glasgow Coma Scale or the simpler alert, verbal stimulus response, painful stimulus response, unresponsive (AVPU) scale often is used to assess level of consciousness.[13] Pupillary size and reactivity also can give clues to the class of substances ingested. Miosis can be observed in children who have ingested clonidine, cholinergics, opiates, organophosphates, phenothiazines and sedative-hypnotics (COPS mnemonic).[14] Mydriasis, on the other hand, is seen in sympathomimetics and anticholinergics.

Unlike in many adult overdose patients, thiamine and naloxone are not routinely used among pediatric patients with ingestions. However, many OTC medications such as cough and cold remedies and antidiarrheal agents contain opioid derivatives. Hence, a trial of naloxone (0.4–2 mg/dose) should be used as a therapeutic and diagnostic maneuver in suspected opioid poisoning or in a toddler with altered mental status and respiratory depression.

The need for emergent decontamination depends on the type and amount of substance exposed, risk for aspiration, approximate time of exposure and presence or absence of life-threatening symptoms. Ocular exposure necessitates immediate and copious saline irrigation after penetrating injury to the eye has been ruled out. Likewise, simple removal of clothes and washing with soap and water works well for many dermal exposures. In most instances, the type of decontamination cannot be determined until further history, a focused physical exam and a firmer suspicion of the type of exposure can be drawn.

Secondary Survey

After the patient has been assessed and stabilized for life-threatening conditions, a more thorough secondary survey can be carried out. During this phase, a brief history about the circumstances and the events leading to the discovery of the symptomatic patient should be obtained. Poisoning in infants younger than 1 year of age is unusual because of their limited motor development. Caretakers should be questioned more closely for inadvertent dosing of another medication, repetitive dosing of the same medication and passive exposure to recreational drugs. *Intentional administration of a substance by a sibling or the caretaker should always be considered.*[15] Any suspicion of possible child abuse or neglect should be explored and reported.[16] Family members should be asked where the child was found, who was taking care of the child, and what the child was doing just prior to the change in behavior. Caretakers may underestimate the amount the child ingested due to lack of knowledge or out of fear of being reported for child neglect or abuse. Other pertinent questions include the timing and progression of symptoms and past medical problems including previous ED visits for poisoning or burns. Also ask for a history of recent trauma and a list of all medications taken by the child or other family members. If the caretaker presents a container with the probable poison, every effort should be made to quantify the dose taken by calculating the possible maximum amount ingested per weight and by sending the material to the laboratory for further analysis. Physicians should also ask emergency medical services personnel to corroborate the caretaker's account regarding the behavior of the patient, condition at the scene and any interventions done.

The physical examination should focus on the central and autonomic nervous systems, cardiovascular and respiratory systems as well as the skin. Toxic overdoses can cause confusion, central nervous system (CNS) depression, psychosis and even coma. Some of the substances that can cause coma include lead, lithium, ethanol, tricyclic antidepressants, oral hypoglycemics, flunitrazepam (Rohypnol), insulin, clonidine and carbon monoxide.[14] Seizures are seen in children who have ingested tricyclic antidepressants, cocaine, amphetamines, anticholinergics, phencyclidine, isoniazid and alcohol. Focal neurologic findings, abnormal posturing or loss of pupillary functions should prompt the clinician to look for a structural intracranial process other than a toxic ingestion.[17]

Cardiovascular system dysfunction, such as tachycardia, bradycardia, hypotension or hypertension, is often the first sign of toxic exposure. Respiratory system stimulation or depression also could be the initial finding. An asymptomatic patient with a possible toxic exposure can become symptomatic or unstable within a short period of time. To prevent serious outcomes, it is important to repeat vital signs and perform serial physical examinations, including neurologic examinations, during the entire ED stay.

Toxidromes

In cases of single-drug ingestions, recognition of distinctive signs and symptoms associated with certain classes of drugs may aid the ED physician in making the diagnosis, anticipating symptoms and providing therapy.[11,14] Common toxidromes seen in the pediatric age group are cholinergic, anticholinergic, sympathomimetic and opioid drugs. Examples of cholinergic agents are organophosphates and carbamates found in insecticides. The toxidrome is often remembered with the mnemonics SLUDGE and DUMBBELLS[11,14]:

S   Salivation
L   Lacrimation/lethargy
U   Urination
D   Diarrhea
G   Gastric cramping
E   Emesis

D   Diarrhea
U   Urination
M   Miosis/muscle weakness
B   Bradycardia
B   Bronchorrhea
E   Emesis
L   Lacrimation
L   Lethargy
S   Salivation/sweating

Examples of anticholinergic agents include antihistamines either alone or in combination with many OTC cough and cold and analgesic medications. The toxidrome consists of delirium, coma or convulsions, tachycardia, hypertension, fever, dilated but sluggish pupils, diminished bowel sounds and flushed, dry skin. It is best remembered by the description "hot as a hare, dry as a bone, red as a beet, blind as a bat and mad as a hatter."[11,14]

Sympathomimetic agents include stimulants and street drugs such as cocaine, amphetamines, phencyclidine and cold and cough preparations containing pseudoephedrine and ephedrine. The toxidrome is similar to that for anticholinergics except for the presence of bowel sounds, diaphoresis and large but reactive pupils.

Opioids are commonly prescribed powerful analgesic agents such as morphine, codeine, hydrocodone, oxycodone or street drugs such as heroin and methadone. The triad of miosis, coma and respiratory depression suggests opioid overdose and thus warrants a trial of naloxone.

Ancillary Evaluation

A majority of exposures in the first 2 years of life are nontoxic or minimally toxic and involve a known substance; therefore, extensive laboratory testing is often not necessary. For symptomatic toddlers with unknown exposures, readily available tests such as bedside glucose level, electrocardiogram (ECG), blood gas, urinalysis and electrolytes provide the largest amount of information. The anion gap (Na - (Cl + HCO_3) and osmolal gap (2Na + Glucose/18 + blood urea nitrogen [BUN]/2.8) are easy to calculate from the electrolytes and may narrow the differential diagnoses.

ED physicians should resist reflex ordering of labor-intensive and expensive comprehensive toxicology screens. Results are often not available or helpful during the critical phase of management.[18–20] Limitations of these "tox screens" include the inability to detect other dangerous drugs. A negative "tox screen" may give a false sense of security to the clinician. A positive "tox screen" may not be the cause of the patient's symptoms, may reveal a drug that is not actually toxic or may show a drug that was taken several days earlier that remains in the urine.[14,21] Instead, selective qualitative screening for drugs that have blood levels predictive of toxicity and guide therapy should be ordered. Acetaminophen levels are particularly important in patients with unknown ingestions because acetaminophen poisoning remains one of the top causes of fatalities among poisoned children.[1,18] Other tests to consider are an abdominal radiograph for possible iron overdoses and a chest radiograph for patients with respiratory distress or hypoxemia.

Gastrointestinal Decontamination

In the struggle to remove poison early, many decontamination techniques have been advocated. However, procedures such as gastric emptying with emesis and lavage have been found to have limited efficacy and are dependent on the time administered and the type of drug ingested. There is no evidence that these procedures have improved clinical outcomes.[22,23] In 2003, the American Academy of Pediatrics (AAP) issued a policy statement stating that ipecac should no longer be used routinely as a poison treatment strategy at home and that remaining ipecac be disposed of safely. It also recommended that the first action a caregiver of a child who has ingested a potentially toxic substance should take is to consult the Poison Control Center.[24] A position statement by the American Academy of Toxicologists in conjunction with the European Association of Poison Centers and Clinical Toxicologists also stated that gastric lavage should not be used routinely, if ever.[23] It may be considered in select patients who have taken a large amount of poison if it can be done safely within 1 hour of ingestion.[25]

Activated charcoal remains the most common method of gastric decontamination and is most effective when used within 1 hour of ingestion.[26] It is recommended for potentially toxic ingestions that can be adsorbed by charcoal. It is not routinely recommended for nontoxic ingestions seen in many pediatric exposures. Similar to gastric emptying techniques, activated charcoal's effectiveness decreases with time, is dependent on the type of drug being adsorbed and has not been shown to improve clinical outcomes. The recommended dose is 1 g/kg. Adding syrup or soda can make it more palatable. Charcoal should only be given to patients with intact airway reflexes because aspiration is a serious complication. Contraindications include patients with decreased level of consciousness and unprotected airway, bowel perforation and obstruction and those with increased risk of aspiration.[26] Cathartics, with or without activated charcoal, have not been recommended as a method of decontamination.[27] They have not been found to reduce the availability of drugs in the body or improve clinical outcomes. A single dose of cathartics such as sorbitol or magnesium citrate is well tolerated and safe for patients older than 1 year of age. Multiple dose activated charcoal can increase the clearance of certain drugs by acting as a "gut dialyzer." It is recommended for use in carbamazepine, phenytoin, phenobarbital, quinine, digoxin and theophylline overdoses.[28] Several substances are not adsorbed by charcoal and can be remembered by the mnemonic SHIELA:

S	Solvents
H	Hydrocarbons
I	Iron and insecticides
E	Electrolytes
L	Lithium
A	Acids, alkali and alcohol

Whole bowel irrigation is also useful for certain drugs such as iron, metals and sustained-release medications but should not be used for unknown ingestions.

Not every patient who presents a few hours after ingestion needs decontamination because most of the drugs would have been absorbed by then.[29] Exceptions are those who ingested sustained-release or enteric-coated medications. These toddlers can be observed in the ED for a few hours and sent home if asymptomatic. The Poison Control Center will often follow-up with these patients. A patient with an unknown ingestion who becomes symptomatic early in the ED course needs to be transferred expeditiously to a pediatric facility where critical care services and toxicology consultation are available.

SPECIFIC TOXINS COMMONLY INGESTED BY TODDLERS

Acetaminophen

Acetaminophen is one of the medications most commonly ingested by children. It is available to the public both as a prescription and as an OTC medication. It is sold under more than 50 brand names and incorporated in even more drug combinations.[30] A favorite among households with children, acetaminophen, when used appropriately and in the correct dosage, provides an antipyretic as well as an analgesic response. When used inappropriately however, the outcomes can be fatal. In 2005, there were 46,167 patients younger than 19 years of age who ingested acetaminophen as reported to the AAPCC with 138 deaths directly related to its ingestion.[1]

After oral ingestion, acetaminophen is rapidly absorbed within 30 minutes for liquid preparations and 45 minutes for immediate-release tablets. Most of it is absorbed within 1 to 2 hours with peak plasma concentration reached at 4 hours.[31] It is metabolized in a complex fashion using three separate metabolic pathways. The majority (95%) of the acetaminophen compound is metabolized via glucuronidation and sulfonation processes with the remainder being handled by the cytochrome P450 system within the liver. N-acetyl-p-benzoquinone-imine (NAPQI) is the byproduct of the cytochrome P450 system that is highly toxic to the liver tissues. In prescribed doses, this compound conjugates with glutathione to form a nontoxic metabolite. However, in overdoses, the body's stores of glutathione are depleted, thus allowing the toxic byproduct to accumulate with resultant liver damage.[11,32] The antidote, N-acetylcysteine (NAC), acts as a glutathione precursor and replenishes glutathione stores, thereby preventing hepatic injury.

The typical prescribed dosage of acetaminophen is weight-based and calculated at 15 mg/kg/dose to be given every 4 to 6 hours as needed for fever and pain relief. The maximum recommended daily dose of acetaminophen is 4 g for adults and 90 mg/kg for children, whereas the toxic single dose is approximately 10 g for adults and 150 mg/kg for children.[33] An infant with mild acetaminophen toxicity presents with nonspecific findings such as anorexia, vomiting, abdominal tenderness, lethargy or pallor that resolves after 24 hours. An infant with severe toxicity will have increasing abdominal tenderness and jaundice with elevated liver enzymes. If left untreated, 2% to 4% will develop hepatic failure and death.[11]

In calculating the dose of an acetaminophen ingestion, the ED physician must take into consideration the weight of the child, the concentration of the preparation, the timing of ingestion and whether it is an acute or chronic overdose or an immediate or extended-release formulation. In cases in which the exact amount cannot be ascertained, the dose for a worst case scenario is often calculated. For example, if there are 10 tablets (325 mg/tablet) remaining in a bottle that originally held 20 tablets and the child's weight is 10 kg, the estimated dose taken is 325 mg/kg. If the child took more than 150 mg/kg, a 4-hour acetaminophen serum level post ingestion (or longer) will give the clinician an estimate of the severity of liver injury when plotted on the acetaminophen nomogram developed by Rumack and Matthew[34] (Figure 23.2). A serum level of 200 μg/mL or higher at 4 hours post ingestion stratifies risk for hepatic toxicity. However, in order to prevent undertreatment, a second line (25%) under the original line at 150 μg/mL was established to guide treatment options.[35] The nomogram should not be used for chronic acetaminophen ingestion.

Activated charcoal can be used if the child presents to the ED within 1 to 2 hours of a toxic ingestion and if the maximum potential dose taken is more than 150 mg/kg.[33] Once toxicity has been established by a 4-hour acetaminophen level and the decision to treat has been made, the recommended therapeutic agent remains NAC. When given within 8 to 10 hours of a toxic acetaminophen ingestion, NAC, in either the oral and IV form, appears to be equally effective in the prevention of hepatic toxicity.[36–38] If the time of ingestion is unknown but the potential dose ingested is greater than 150 mg/kg, the clinician should begin treatment with NAC as soon as possible while awaiting serum acetaminophen levels. If the level is above the lower line of the nomogram, the physician should continue NAC treatment. The patient should be admitted to an inpatient hospital floor and monitored closely while receiving treatment with NAC. The current recommended dosing schedule of oral NAC is a loading dose of 140 mg/kg followed 4 hours later by 70 mg/kg every 4 hours for a total of 17 doses.[11,36] For patients with chronic or repetitive overdosing over several days, treatment is controversial.

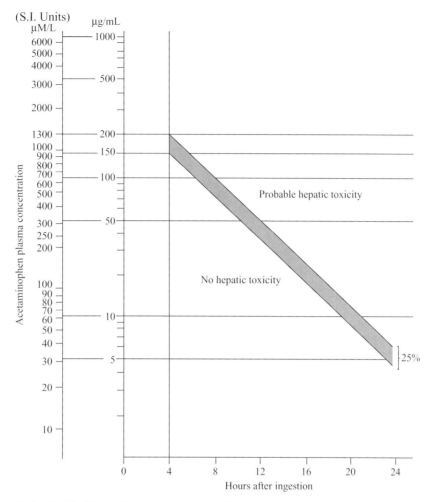

Figure 23.2. Modified Rumack-Matthew acetaminophen nomogram. (From Rumack BH, Matthew H. *Pediatrics*. 1975;55:871–876.)

Early consultation with the Regional Poison Control Center is important.

Salicylate

Salicylate poisoning, both acute and chronic, continues to be a common occurrence in patients who present to the ED.[39] Salicylates are found in a variety of compounds, most commonly in acetylsalicylic acid (aspirin) products, methylsalicylate (oil of wintergreen), keratolytics containing salicylic acid, sunscreens with homo methylsalicylate, antidiarrheals with bismuth subsalicylate and teething gel preparations containing salicylates.[40,41]

Salicylates have analgesic, antipyretic and anti-inflammatory effects. The pharmacologic effects are mediated through the inhibition of cyclooxygenase, which leads to a decreased production of prostaglandins, the mediator of fever and inflammation. With proper dosing, salicylates reach a peak level within 1 to 2 hours for standard preparations and 4 to 6 hours for enteric-coated tablets.[40] In an acute overdose, delays in the peak serum concentration (up to 10–60 hours) can be due to the formation of insoluble concretions, food in the stomach as well as by co-ingestions of substances that reduce gastric emptying time (anticholinergic drugs).

Salicylates exert several effects[11,42,43]:

1. Stimulate the medullary respiratory center causing tachypnea and respiratory alkalosis
2. Uncouple oxidative phosphorylation and inhibit lipid, amino acid and carbohydrate metabolism, producing lactic and ketoacidosis, hyperglycemia, electrolyte disturbances, an increase in metabolic rate and heat

3. Inhibit platelet function and interfere with clotting factors, producing a coagulopathy

4. Induce hepatic injury, leading to elevations in hepatic enzymes

5. Cause local corrosive effects to the gastrointestinal (GI) tract, producing bleeding or bezoars

6. Damage the cochlear hair cells, causing ototoxicity manifesting as tinnitus

Salicylates are metabolized in the liver and eliminated from the body via the kidney. The rate of excretion of free salicylate is variable and largely dependent upon the urine pH. Alkaline urine enhances excretion, whereas acidic urine slows excretion due to reabsorption of the free salicylate by the renal tubules. In children, the therapeutic dose of acetylsalicylic acid is 10 to 20 mg/kg/dose and can be given every 4 to 6 hours, as needed. The therapeutic range is 15 to 30 mg/dL, but above this level, signs and symptoms of toxicity may appear. A single dose greater than 150 mg/kg/dose is considered mildly toxic, whereas serious toxicity is seen with ingestions of 300 to 500 mg/kg/dose.[11,40] Oil of wintergreen (98% methylsalicylate), a common analgesic liniment, deserves special mention because 1 teaspoon contains 7000 mg of salicylate. It can be fatal to a 10 kg toddler who ingests even less than 1 teaspoon.[18]

Depending upon the severity and timing of the ingestion, children may present in a variety of ways. The earliest presenting symptoms include nausea, vomiting, abdominal pain, tachypnea, fever and irritability from tinnitus.[39–41] These nonspecific symptoms are often mistaken for other diagnoses such as viral syndrome, gastroenteritis, iron intoxication and diabetic ketoacidosis. Those with severe toxicity (serum level of 100 mg/dL) progress to altered mental states, seizures, signs of sepsis, pulmonary edema, renal failure, acid-base disorders and electrolyte abnormalities. Cardiopulmonary arrest and death may follow.

Management of a patient with salicylate ingestion begins by performing the primary and secondary surveys, ruling out life-threatening conditions and securing the patient's airway as needed. Important patient history includes amount of salicylate ingested, type of preparation used and whether this is an acute or chronic ingestion. The patient is placed on continuous cardiac, ventilatory and oxygen saturation monitoring. IV fluids should be given to correct electrolyte abnormalities, restore hydration and

enhance elimination. To increase tubular secretion of salicylate, the urine is alkalinized with sodium bicarbonate mixed in a hypotonic solution such as 5% dextrose. Adding sodium bicarbonate to normal saline can create a hyperosmolar solution and should be avoided. Potassium is added to the IV fluids as hypokalemia can be exacerbated by the addition of bicarbonate. Urine output should be maintained at 1 to 2 mL/kg/hour.

Keeping in mind the mechanisms of salicylate toxicity, laboratory testing includes a bedside glucose level, initial salicylate level, arterial blood gas (ABG) measurement, electrolyte panel, liver function tests, complete blood cell count, prothrombin and partial thromboplastin times, urinalysis and an ECG. Peak salicylate concentrations may not be reached until 4 to 6 hours post ingestion and may be delayed in cases of overdose; therefore, the initial salicylate level may not be accurate. Instead, serial salicylate levels, together with blood gas analysis and serum electrolytes, need to be obtained every 2 to 4 hours until the level is decreasing and then followed every 4 to 6 hours until the level is less than 30 mg/dL.[40,44,45]

After careful consideration of the patient's risk for aspiration, activated charcoal may be given to patients with salicylate poisoning, even 6 hours after presentation, because of delayed gastric emptying. Multiple dose activated charcoal may be used every 3 to 4 hours in cases of significant ingestion.[39,40] Hemodialysis is reserved for patients with salicylate concentrations above 100 mg/dL, evidence of end-organ injury, renal failure, refractory acidosis and hypotension, persistent neurologic dysfunction and clinical deterioration despite standard therapy.[39]

Iron

Although iron is still a leading cause of poisoning in children younger than 6 years of age in the United States, significant strides have been made in the past decade to decrease its morbidity and mortality.[1,46,47] A common scenario is a toddler who eats his mother's prenatal iron tablets that look like candy while the mother is preoccupied with the new baby. Each prenatal iron tablet (ferrous sulfate) contains 65 mg of elemental iron and, even when fewer than 10 tablets are ingested by a 10 kg toddler, symptoms of iron overdose are seen.

In the nontoxic state, ferritin stores iron in the intestinal lining and transferrin binds free iron in the serum. During overdose, these molecules are saturated. Free iron causes toxicity due to its corrosive effects in the GI tract and the uncoupling of oxidative phosphorylation leading to the formation of free radicals. The GI tract and liver are the primary sites of injury.[48]

There are five clinical stages of iron toxicity starting from 30 minutes post ingestion and lasting up to 4 to 8 weeks.[48] The clinical *stage 1* of iron intoxication is the GI stage and is characterized by abdominal pain, vomiting, diarrhea, hematemesis and hematochezia leading to volume and blood loss. The onset is usually within 2 hours of a toxic ingestion. Absence of GI complaints, especially vomiting, in the first 6 hours post iron ingestion suggests a nontoxic exposure.[11,48] *Stage 2*, 6 to 24 hours post ingestion, is a relatively stable period during which patients may have minimal GI symptoms but with continued subclinical hypoperfusion and metabolic acidosis. Most iron poisoning deaths occurs during *stage 3* (24–72 hours post ingestion), during which shock, metabolic acidosis and multisystem failure are characteristic. *Stage 4*, seen within 48 to 96 hours of a severe ingestion, is characterized by hepatic necrosis with jaundice and elevated liver enzymes. *Stage 5*, rarely seen, is characterized by bowel obstruction, notably vomiting, resulting from stricture formation 2 to 6 weeks after iron toxicity.

Toxicity from iron ingestion depends on the amount of elemental iron the product ingested contains as different preparations contain varying concentrations. For instance, a chewable multivitamin with iron contains less elemental iron than prenatal iron tablets. One study of adults found that an elemental iron ingestion of 20 mg/kg leads to GI toxicity and elevated serum iron levels.[49] A more recent evidence-based guideline for out-of-hospital management of iron overdoses recommended that an ingestion of 40 mg/kg of elemental iron is significant, and patients with this level of ingestion should be referred for management in a health care facility.[50]

In practice, however, the amount ingested is often not known. If iron ingestion is suspected, the clinician should obtain a serum iron level within 3 to 5 hours. If enteric-coated tablets were ingested, serial levels are indicated. A patient with a serum iron level of less than 350 μg/dL is usually asymptomatic, levels between 350 and 500 μg/dL have mild systemic symptoms, greater than 500 μg/dL have moderate toxicity and greater than 1000 μg/dL have significant morbidity and mortality.[11,48]

Other tests of diagnostic importance include abdominal radiographs (looking for opacities within the GI tract),

ABG measurements (looking for the presence of acidosis), serum electrolyte panel and liver function tests including a coagulation panel.

Total iron binding capacity is no longer useful. A white blood cell count of greater than 15,000/mm^3 and blood glucose levels of greater than 150 mg/dL are sensitive but not specific for iron toxicity.

The initial phase of resuscitation is similar to any overdose; assessment and intervention are performed simultaneously as dictated by the primary and secondary surveys. While serum iron level, blood studies and abdominal films are ordered, decontamination is started.

Activated charcoal has no role in the treatment of iron intoxication, as it will not absorb iron. Whole bowel irrigation using 500 mL/hour of polyethylene glycol electrolyte solution via a nasogastric tube is the decontamination of choice in children.[11] It should be used until the rectal effluent comes out clear and repeat abdominal radiographs are clear of pill fragments. Deferoxamine, a chelating agent, forms a complex with the ferric form of iron that is then easily excreted in the urine. It is infused at a dose of 15 mg/kg/hr when one or more of the following are present: serum iron levels greater than 500 μg/dL, signs and symptoms of toxicity and metabolic acidosis.[11,48]

Lead

Lead is most commonly encountered as a chronic poisoning in children, especially those with pica. It is often asymptomatic and detected by routine lead checks at the primary care physician's office. Repeated exposure to small amounts of lead can lead to serious health problems affecting many organ systems but particularly the child's hematologic, renal and central nervous systems.[11] Lead interferes with calcium-dependent metabolic pathways in the cell and has special affinity for enzymes and structural proteins with sulfhydryl groups. Common sources of lead are listed in Table 23.3.

The symptoms of lead poisoning in children can be mistaken for other diagnoses because they are nonspecific (Table 23.4). Presence of additional risk factors such as age between 1 and 5 years, history of pica, residence in a city, renovation in an older home and iron deficiency anemia should increase one's suspicion of possible lead poisoning.[11] Those with levels between 10 and 50 μg/dL are usually asymptomatic. Patients with mild to moderate lead poisoning (50–70 μg/dL) may present with

Table 23.3. Common sources of lead

House paint before 1978 (peeling or unpeeling)
Painted toys made outside of the United States
Water (lead plumbing)
Soil with lead paint dust, leaded gasoline
Arts and crafts tools (paint sets)
Printing dyes, jewelry fittings, ceramics
Fishing supplies
Battery casings

Data from Osterhoudt et al,[11] Henretig F[51] and Price.[53]

Table 23.5. Sources of methemoglobinemia*

Most Common	Other causative agents
Dapsone	Metoclopramide
Local anesthetics	Naphthalene
● Benzocaine	Nitric oxide
●Prilocaine	Nitroglycerin
●Lidocaine	Nitroprusside
Sulfonamide antibiotics	Phenytoin
Anti-malarial drugs	Rifampin
	Silver nitrate
	Sodium valproate
	Sulfasalazine
	Sulfa-containing compounds

* Data from Price[53] and Cohen and Manno.[54]

abdominal pain, vomiting, constipation, listlessness and irritability. Severe toxicity may present as pallor, persistent vomiting, and loss of developmental milestones, seizures, encephalopathy or coma.[51,52]

The most useful test for lead toxicity remains a venous sample. Normal or acceptable lead level is 10 μg/dL or less; a level higher than 10 μg/dL is defined as *lead poisoning.*[52] A blood smear may show microcytic anemia with basophilic stippling of the erythrocytes. An abdominal radiograph may show evidence of lead flakes or concretions that show up as opacifications throughout the intestinal tract, whereas long bone radiographs may show dense metaphyseal bands (lead lines).[11,51] Erythrocyte protoporphyrin (EP) levels are used during the inpatient course in severe lead poisoning but are not recommended in outpatient management.

Management of children with elevated lead levels includes environmental education such as identifying sources of lead and nutritional counseling. Asymptomatic children with lead levels between 45 and 69 μg/dL can be managed with an oral chelating agent, succimer (dimercaptosuccinic acid [DMSA]) plus environmental investigation. Symptomatic cases, especially those with encephalopathy, require parenteral chelation therapy with 2, 4 dimercaptopropanol (BAL) and edetate calcium disodium (CaEDTA).[51,52]

Table 23.4. Symptoms of lead toxicity

Mild to moderate lead toxicity	Severe lead toxicity
Abdominal pain	Seizures, paresthesias, headache
Vomiting	Loss of developmental milestones
Constipation	Increased intracranial pressure
Weight loss	Encephalopathy
Irritability	Coma
Hyperactivity	

Data from Osterhoudt et al,[11] Henretig F[51] and Price.[53]

Methemoglobin-Inducing Substances

Methemoglobinemia results when the heme iron of the hemoglobin molecule remains in the ferric state and thus is unable to carry oxygen to tissues and cells.[53] Toddlers are often exposed to substances that can cause acquired methemoglobinemia. Examples of these substances include the teething gels containing benzocaine, topical anesthetics such as prilocaine and lidocaine, naphthalene balls, sulfa-containing compounds, antimalarial agents, bladder anesthetic such as phenazopyridine and well water containing nitrates[53,54] (Table 23.5). Acquired causes of methemoglobinemia are also seen in infants younger than 4 months who have immature nicotinamide adenine dinucleotide (NADH)–dependent methemoglobin reductase enzyme systems and in transient in infants with GI illness of unknown cause. The congenital forms of methemoglobinemia are due to *hemoglobin M,* a deficiency of the NADH-dependent methemoglobin reductase enzyme, and characterized by chronic cyanosis.

Symptoms depend on the methemoglobin level and are exacerbated by anemia. Patients with a methemoglobin level between 15% and 20% present with cyanosis that is unresponsive to oxygen therapy. At levels of 20% to 50%, dyspnea, headache, fatigue and dizziness are common. Dysrhythmias, seizures, and coma are seen at methemoglobin levels higher than 50%, and death occurs at levels higher than 70%.[53,54]

Methemoglobinemia should be suspected in an infant who is cyanotic yet has no obvious cardiac or pulmonary disease. The serum will have a chocolate brown appearance unlike normal blood, which is bright red. Measured oxygen saturation by pulse oximetry may be inaccurate because it can only detect wavelengths absorbed by oxyhemoglobin and deoxyhemoglobin. As the methemoglobin levels increase, the pulse oximetry readings decrease, but not proportionately, leading to overestimation of oxygen saturation. An ABG determination by co-oximetry can give more accurate oxygen saturation readings and determine the concentrations of different hemoglobins, such as methemoglobin and carboxyhemoglobin. Other laboratory studies a complete blood cell count to look for evidence of anemia and electrolyte studies to look for acidosis.

Treatment of methemoglobinemia involves removal of the offending agent, supportive care (ABCs), high-flow oxygen and watchful waiting for asymptomatic patients with methemoglobin levels lower than 30%.[53,54] For symptomatic patients at any level, methylene blue at 1 to 2 mg/kg over 5 to 10 minutes hastens the conversion of the abnormal methemoglobin to the physiologic form of the hemoglobin. This may be repeated in 1 hour if symptoms persist. All patients with acquired methemoglobinemia should be admitted for close observation and further evaluation.

Over-the-Counter Cough and Cold Preparations

OTC cough and cold medications consist of varying combinations of analgesics, antihistamines, antitussives, decongestants and expectorants. In 2005, there were more than 95,000 ingestions of various OTC cough and cold preparations by children younger than 19 years of age with over 70,000 of these ingestions by those under the age of 6 years.[1] There were 21 deaths reported as a direct result of ingestions from these medications in all age groups in 2005.[1] Thirty-nine percent of households purchase these products with 95 million packages purchased every year.[55]

The dosing of OTC cough and cold medications was extrapolated from adult studies because of limited studies in children. A critical review of studies done from 1950 to 1991 concluded that these OTC medications are not effective in relieving symptoms in children younger than 6 years of age.[56] Other reviews did not find that these medications had any advantage in relieving symptoms when compared with placebo.[57,58] In 1997, the AAP recommended that pediatricians educate parents about the lack of proven benefit, the potential risks and the adverse effects regarding use of dextromethorphan- and codeine-containing cough medications.[59] In 2007, the

Centers for Disease Control and Prevention reported the deaths of three infants from use of OTC cough and cold medications.[60] The Food and Drug Administration, in response to a citizen petition, held an advisory meeting to discuss the safety of these medications. Subsequently, in late 2007, makers of these products voluntarily withdrew from the market OTC cough and cold products labeled for infants younger than 2 years of age until further evaluation.[61]

Household Cleaning Agents

Household cleaning products are easily accessible to infants and toddlers at home, making them one of the top exposures reported to the poison centers every year. Most of them are classified as either acids or alkalis and include laundry detergents and dishwashing agents, disinfectants, drain and oven cleaners, bleaches and ammonia-containing solutions. As a result of the PPPA, caustics with a concentration of more than 2% need to be packaged in child-resistant containers.[62] However, because these products are often transferred to familiar containers such as soda bottles or empty glasses, curious children mistake them for beverages, leading to injury.

Household cleaning agents are considered caustics or corrosives because they can cause damage on contact with biologic tissues. The degree of damage is determined by the duration of contact, volume ingested, concentration, pH, food in the stomach and amount of material needed to neutralize the caustic. Neutralization by the tissues causes an exothermic reaction, releasing heat and leading to burns.[62] Acids produce damage by coagulation necrosis with superficial involvement of the tissues. Alkalis cause liquefaction necrosis that penetrates deeply into the tissues. Serious injuries can result in perforation and stricture formation. Examples of acids include hydrochloric acids (muriatic acid), sulfuric acids and hydrofluoric acids. Common household alkalis include sodium hydroxide (lye) found in oven cleaners and drain pipe cleaners (e.g., Drano or Easy-Off), laundry and dishwasher detergents and sodium hypochlorite (bleach). Table 23.6 lists the most common exposures to household cleaning substances.

By and large, most exposures are through ingestions, although dermal and respiratory exposures are common. Fortunately, ingestions by toddlers are typically

Table 23.6. Exposures to household cleaning products, 2005

Product	Ingestions age <19 years	Total ingestions all ages	Total treated in health care facilities	Total deaths
Bleaches (all)	26,790	56,183	11,974	8
Drain cleaners (acid)	271	1172	272	2
Drain cleaners (alkali)	836	3677	1201	5
Dishwasher detergents (all)	12,741	14,178	629	0
Ammonia cleaner	753	1882	429	0

Data from Lai MW, Lein-Schwartz W, Rodgers GC, et al. 2005 Annual Report of the American Association of Poison Control Centers' national poisoning and exposure database. *Clin Toxicol (Phila)*. 2006; 44:803–932.

unintentional and usually involve minimal amounts of the substance. Engaging the Poison Control Center early to help determine the nature of the product and its toxicity is important. Decontamination measures such as emesis, lavage or charcoal are contraindicated. Dilution, although intuitive, should not be attempted in the symptomatic patient.

Children who have ingested a caustic agent often complain of pain or a burning sensation in the oral mucosa. Depending on the amount, type and concentration of the caustic agent, other symptoms of laryngeal, esophageal or gastric injury may be seen. Absence of oral burns does not predict absence of esophageal or gastric injury.[63] Presence of stridor, drooling, dysphagia, chest or abdominal pain and vomiting is predictive of a serious injury.[11,62] A symptomatic toddler with unintentional ingestion or a patient with intentional ingestion, regardless of symptoms, requires endoscopy to delineate extent of injury.[64] Admission and early consultation with our otolaryngology colleagues are necessary. Airway protection may be necessary for patients with severe symptoms. Asymptomatic toddlers deemed to have minimal exposures can be observed in the ED for several hours and discharged after a trial of clear fluids.[62]

DEADLY PILLS IN SMALL QUANTITIES

Several medications, taken even in small quantities by a toddler, can result in severe poisoning or even death (Table 23.7).[18,65–68] ED physicians should familiarize themselves with these drugs because parents occasionally bring a small child into the ED alleging that the child took only 1 to 2 doses of the parent's medicine. Table 23.7 lists medications that were responsible for about 40% of fatalities among toddlers from 1990–2000.[66]

Tricyclic Antidepressants

Tricyclic antidepressants (TCAs) are potent inhibitors of norepinephrine reuptake and, to a lesser degree, serotonin reuptake. They also inhibit histamine, dopamine D_2, muscarinic and sympathetic alpha-1 receptors as well as fast sodium channels in the cardiac cells. This leads to serious toxicity affecting the CNS and cardiovascular system. Symptoms of an anticholinergic toxidrome are present. CNS manifestations include altered mental states, hallucinations, seizures and coma. Cardiovascular effects include heart blocks, tachycardia, hypotension and arrhythmias. The ECG may show prolonged QRS intervals and torsades de pointes.

The minimum potentially toxic amount of antidepressants that have resulted in mortality among the small children is 15 mg/kg.[69] The mortality associated with a toxic ingestion is secondary to the cardiotoxic and neurodepressant effects of the drug. Management of TCA ingestions involves supportive care (ABCs) and close monitoring of the patient for cardiovascular and CNS deterioration. Sodium bicarbonate, by overcoming sodium channel blockade of the cardiac membranes, is the mainstay of treatment. It is given as a bolus with an initial dose of 1 to 2 meq/kg.[18,65] Seizures respond well to benzodiazepines. Physostigmine is no longer recommended.

Calcium Channel Blockers

Calcium channel blockers, such as nifedipine, diltiazem and verapamil, can cause serious morbidity and mortality in doses as little as 15 mg/kg.[66] They are commonly used for migraines, hypertension, glaucoma and angina. These medications predominantly exert their effects by blocking calcium entry into cardiac and vascular smooth

Table 23.7. Top ten drugs fatal to a toddler (10 kg) in small doses

Drug	Minimal lethal dose/kg	Dose unit (tablets or teaspoon)
Antiarrhythmics (procainamide)	70 mg/kg	1000 mg/tab
Antimalarials (chloroquine)	<30 mg/kg	500 mg/tab
Antipsychotics (chlorpromazine)	20 mg/kg	200 mg/tab
Calcium channel blockers (verapamil)	<40 mg/kg	240 mg/tab
Camphor	<100 mg/kg	1000 mg/5 mL
Cyclic antidepressants (imipramine)	~20 mg/kg	150 mg/tab
Methyl salicylate	~200 mg/kg	1400 mg/1 mL
Narcotics (codeine)	7–14 mg/kg	30 mg/tab
Oral hypoglycemics (glyburide)	~1 mg/kg	5 mg/tab
Theophylline	~50 mg/kg	500 mg/tab

Data from references 11, 18, 65–68.

muscle cells causing conduction abnormalities, decreased contractility and vasodilation. Symptoms can be apparent within 1 to 5 hours for immediate-release preparations or may take longer to manifest with sustained-release preparations. Patients can present with bradycardia, refractory hypotension and arrhythmias and may require fluid resuscitation, atropine and calcium gluconate or calcium chloride boluses.

Sulfonylureas and Diabetic Agents

Oral hypoglycemic agents are the cornerstone of pharmacologic treatment for type 2 diabetes mellitus, the most common endocrine condition in Western society.[65] Sulfonylureas cause a drop in the serum glucose concentration by directly inhibiting adenosine triphosphate-dependent potassium channels of the pancreatic beta cells, causing depolarization and subsequent release of insulin.[65] Elevated insulin levels prevent glycogenolysis, causing severe, refractory hypoglycemia. Studies have documented that as few as 1 or 2 tablets can cause severe hypoglycemia and death in toddlers.[70–72]

Symptoms associated with hypoglycemia include lethargy, behavior changes, seizures or coma. Previously, children with sulfonylurea ingestions were admitted for a minimum of 24 hours for observation of the development of hypoglycemia.[65] A more recent study recommended an observation period with serial glucose monitoring of at least 8 hours for immediate-release tablets. If a patient does not develop hypoglycemia within this period, he or she can be discharged home with instructions.[72] Patients who ingest extended-release tablets need hospital admission with close monitoring and correction of the

hypoglycemia. Octreotide, by preventing insulin release, has been effective in refractory hypoglycemia caused by oral hypoglycemic agents.

Opioids, Clonidine and Imidazolines

Although opioids are commonly prescribed as analgesic agents, they are also present in many cough-suppressant medications and antidiarrheal agents. Methadone, oxycodone and codeine ingestion are the most common causes of deaths from opioid overdose in children younger than 6 years of age.[18,65,66] Toxicity results in respiratory depression, miosis and CNS depression. Respiratory depression can be observed at doses greater than 5 mg/kg for codeine and 0.5 mg/kg for methadone.[73,74]

Clonidine is a central-acting alpha-2-adrenergic agonist that is used to treat a variety of medical conditions including hypertension, neuropathic pain, opioid detoxification, insomnia and attention-deficit hyperactivity disorder. It is available in oral preparations from 0.1 mg to 0.3 mg per tablet and in transdermal preparations, which deliver 2.5 mg, 5 mg and 7.5 mg per patch of the drug.[18] In overdose, patients present with an opioid toxidrome and have a decreased level of consciousness, bradycardia, hypotension, decreased respiratory drive and miosis. Toxic effects of clonidine in children typically occur within 30 to 90 minutes of ingestion and, because of a long half-life, these effects may persist for 1 to 3 days. Treatment for opioid and clonidine overdose is supportive. Naloxone in doses of 0.1 mg/kg up to a total of 10 mg has been shown to be effective in reversing respiratory and CNS depression.[18,65]

Camphor

Camphor is a common ingredient in many OTC topical anesthetic ointments and liniments such as Vicks VapoRub, Bengay, Tiger Balm, Absorbine Jr. and Campho-Phenique gels. In the United States, OTC products containing camphor are limited to a concentration of 11% or less.[75] Minimal fatal dose is estimated to be 100 mg/kg or less.[11,66] Overdose is primarily from ingestion, which produces a burning sensation in the mouth, GI irritation and vomiting. In toxic ingestions, CNS stimulation manifests as delirium, restlessness is followed later by seizures, coma and respiratory failure. Treatment is primarily supportive because no antidote exists for camphor. Seizures may be managed with benzodiazepines.

PITFALLS

- Failure to use the resources of the Regional Poison Center early in the management of toxic exposures
- Failure to repeat vital signs and perform serial examinations
- Failure to consider child abuse or neglect in poisoned infants younger than 1 year of age
- Failure to consider intracranial pathology other than a toxic ingestion in patients with focal neurological findings, abnormal posturing or loss of pupillary functions
- Failure to recognize that a negative comprehensive drug screen does not mean absence of a toxic exposure
- Failure to recognize that absence of oral burns from caustic ingestions in a symptomatic patient does not predict absence of esophageal or gastric injury
- Failure to provide anticipatory guidance is a missed opportunity in preventing another poisoning

REFERENCES

1. Lai M, Klein-Schwartz W, Rodgers G, et al. 2005 Annual Report of the American Association of Poison Control Centers' national poisoning and exposure database. *Clin Toxicol (Phila)*. 2006;44:803–932.
2. Fergelman S. The first year. In: Behrman RE, Kliegman RM, Jenson HB, et al, eds. *Nelson Textbook of Pediatrics*, 18th ed. Philadelphia, PA: Saunders; 2006.
3. Jacobson BJ, Rock AR, Cohn MS, et al. Accidental ingestions of oral prescription drugs: a multicenter survey. *Am J Public Health*. 1989;79:853–856.
4. Centers for Disease Control and Prevention (CDC). Web-based Injury Statistics Query and Reporting System (WISQARS). http://www.cdc.gov/ncipc/wisqars. Accessed on May 22, 2008.
5. Paulozzi LJ, Ballesteros MF, Stevens JA. Recent trends in mortality from unintentional injury in the United States. *J Safety Res*. 2006;37:277–283.
6. Rodgers GB. The safety effects of child-resistant packaging for oral prescription drugs: two decades of experience. *JAMA*. 1996;275(21):1661–1665.
7. Walton WW. An evaluation of the Poison Prevention Packaging Act. *Pediatrics*. 1982;69:363–370.
8. Miller TR, Lestina DC. Costs of poisoning in the United States and savings from poison control centers: a benefit-cost analysis. *Ann Emerg Med*. 1997;29:239–245.
9. Demorest RA, Posner JC, Osterhoudt KC, et al. Poisoning prevention education during emergency department visits for childhood poisoning. *Pediatr Emerg Care*. 2004;20:281–284.
10. *American College of Surgeons' Advanced Trauma Life Support*, 7th ed. Chicago, IL: ACS.
11. Osterhoudt KC, Ewald MB, Shannon M, et al. Toxicologic emergencies. In: Fleischer GR, Ludwig S, Henretig FM, et al, eds. *Textbook of Pediatric Emergency Medicine*, 5th ed. Philadelphia, PA: Lippincott Williams & Wilkins; 2006:951–1007
12. Michael JB, Sztajnkrycer MD. Deadly pediatric poisons: nine common agents that kill at low doses. *Emerg Med Clin North Am*. 2004;22:1019–1950.
13. Kelly CA, Upex A, Bateman DN. Comparison of consciousness level assessment in the poisoned patient using the alert/verbal/painful/unresponsive scale and the Glasgow coma scale. *Ann Emerg Med*. 2004;44:108–113.
14. Erickson TB, Thompson TM, Lu JJ. The approach to the patient with an unknown overdose. *Emerg Med Clin North Am*. 2007;25:249–281.
15. Meadow R. Munchausen syndrome by proxy. *Arch Dis Child*. 1982;57:92–98.
16. Bays J, Feldman KW. Childhood poisoning by abuse. In: Reese RM, Ludwig S, eds. *Child Abuse: Medical Diagnosis and Management*. Philadelphia, PA: Lippincott, Williams & Wilkins; 2001:405–441.
17. Delaney KA, Kolecki P. Approach to the poisoned patient with central nervous system depression. In: Ford M, Delaney K, Ling L, et al, eds. *Clinical Toxicology*. Philadelphia, PA: Saunders; 2001:137–145.
18. Eldridge DL, Van Eyk J, Kornegay C. Pediatric toxicology. *Emerg Med Clin North Am*. 2007;15:283–308.
19. Belson MG, Simon HK, Sullivan K, et al. The utility of toxicologic analysis in children with suspected ingestions. *Pediatr Emerg Care*. 1999;15:383–387.
20. Belson MG, Simon HK. Utility of comprehensive toxicologic screens in children. *Am J Emerg Med*. 1999;17:221–224.
21. Sugarman JM, Rodgers GC, Paul R. Utility of toxicology screening in a pediatric emergency department. *Pediatr Emerg Care*. 1997;13:194–197.
22. Position paper: ipecac syrup. *J Toxicol Clin Toxicol*. 2004; 42:133–143.
23. Vale JA, Kulig K; Academy of Clinical Toxicology; European Association of Poisons Centres and Clinical Toxicologists. Position paper: gastric lavage. *J Toxicol Clin Toxicol*. 2004; 42:933–943.

24. American Academy of Pediatrics Committee on Injury, Violence and Poison Prevention. Poison treatment in the home. *Pediatrics*. 2003;112:1182–1185.

25. Kulig K, Bar-Or D, Cantrill SV, et al. Management of acutely poisoned patients without gastric emptying. *Ann Emerg Med*. 1985;14:562–567.

26. Chyka PA, Seger D, Krenzelok EP, et al. American Academy of Clinical Toxicology; European Association of Poisons Centres and Clinical Toxicologists. Position paper: single-dose activated charcoal. *Clin Toxicol*. 2005;43:61–87.

27. Position paper: cathartics. *J Toxicol Clin Toxicol*. 2004; 42:243–253.

28. Position statement and practice guidelines on the use of multi-dose activated charcoal in the treatment of acute poisoning. American Academy of Clinical Toxicology; European Association of Poisons Centres and Clinical Toxicologists. *J Toxicol Clin Toxicol*. 1999;37:731–751.

29. Tenenbein M. Recent advancements in pediatric toxicology. *Pediatr Clin North Am*. 1999;46:1179–1188.

30. Smith DH. Managing acute acetaminophen toxicity. *Nurse*. 2007;37:5–63.

31. Ameer B, Divoll M, Abernethy M, et al. Absolute and relative bioavailability of oral acetaminophen preparations. *J Phar Sci*. 1983;72:955–958.

32. Marzullo L. An update of *N*-acetylcysteine treatment for acute acetaminophen toxicity in children. *Curr Opin Pediatr*. 2005;17:239–245.

33. Dart RC, Erdman AR, Olson KR, et al. Acetaminophen poisoning: an evidence-based consensus guideline for out-of-hospital management. *Clin Toxicol (Phila)*. 2006;44:1–18.

34. Rumack BH, Matthew H. Acetaminophen poisoning and toxicity. *Pediatrics*. 1975;55:871–876.

35. Rumack BH, Peterson RC, Koch GG, et al. Acetaminophen overdose: 662 cases with evaluation of oral acetylcysteine treatment. *Arch Intern Med*. 1981;141:380–385.

36. Kanter MZ. Comparison of oral and i.v. acetylcysteine in the treatment of acetaminophen poisoning. *Am J Health System Pharm*. 2006;63:1821–1827.

37. Perry HE, Shannon MW. Efficacy of oral versus intravenous *N*-acetylcysteine in acetaminophen overdose: results of an open-label clinical trial. *J Pediatr*. 1998;132:149–152.

38. Buckley NA, Whyte IM, O'Connell DL, et al. Oral or intravenous *N*-acetylcysteine: which is the treatment of choice for acetaminophen (paracetamol) poisoning? *J Toxicol Clin Toxicol*. 1999;37:759–767.

39. O'Malley GF. Emergency department management of the salicylate-poisoned patient. *Emerg Med Clin North Am*. 2007; 25:333–346.

40. Donovan WJ, Akhtar Jawaid. Salicylates. In: Ford MD, Delaney MK, Ling LJ, Erickson T, eds. *Ford: Clinical Toxicology*, 1st ed. WB Saunders; 2001:275–280.

41. Brubacker JR, Hoffman RS. Salicylism from topical salicylates: a review of the literature. *J Toxicol Clin Toxicol*. 1996; 34:431–436.

42. Krause DS, Wolf BA, Shaw LM. Acute aspirin overdose: mechanisms of toxicity. *Ther Drug Monit*. 1992;14:441–451.

43. Cazals Y. Auditory sensori-neural alterations produced by salicylate. *Prog Neurobiol*. 2000;62:583–631.

44. Dugandzic RM, Tierney MG, Dickinson GE. Evaluation of the validity of the Done nomogram in the management of acute salicylate intoxication. *Ann Emerg Med*. 1989;18:1186–1190.

45. Flomenbaum N. Salicylates. In: Flomenbaum N, Goldfrank L, Hoffman R, et al, eds. *Goldfrank's Toxicologic Emergencies*. New York, NY: McGraw- Hill Medical Publishing; 2006:550–564.

46. Woolf A. Progress in the prevention of childhood iron poisoning. *Arch Pediatr Adolesc Med*. 2005;159:593–595.

47. Tenenbein M. Unit-dose packaging of iron supplements and reduction of iron poisoning in young children. *Arch Pediatr Adolesc Med*. 2005;159:557–560.

48. Madiwale T, Liebelt E. Iron: not a benign therapeutic drug. *Curr Opin Pediatr*. 2006;18:174–179.

49. Burkhark KK, Kulig KW, Hammond KB, et al. The rise in total binding capacity after iron overdose. *Ann Emerg Med*. 1991;20:352–355.

50. Manoguerra AS, Erdman AR, Booze LL, et al. Iron ingestion: an evidence-based guideline for out of hospital management. *Clin Toxicol*. 2005;43:553–570.

51. Henretig F. Lead. In: Flomenbaum N, Goldfrank L, Hoffman R, et al, eds. *Goldfrank's Toxicologic Emergencies*. New York, NY: McGraw-Hill Medical Publishing; 2006:1308–1324.

52. Committee on Environmental Health. Lead exposure in children: prevention, detection, and management. *Pediatrics*. 2005;116(4):1036–1046.

53. Price D. Methemoglobin inducers. In: Flomenbaum N, Goldfrank L, Hoffman R, et al, eds. *Goldfrank's Toxicologic Emergencies*. New York, NY: McGraw-Hill Medical Publishing; 2006:1734–1745.

54. Cohen AR, Manno CS. Hematologic emergencies. In: Fleischer GR, Ludwig S, Henretig FM, et al, eds. *Textbook of Pediatric Emergency Medicine*, 5th ed. Philadelphia, PA: Lippincott Williams & Wilkins; 2006:934–936.

55. Consumer Healthcare Products Association (CHPA). Briefing information for the Food and Drug Administration joint meeting of the Nonprescription Drugs Advisory Committee and the Pediatric Advisory Committee. http://www.fda.gov/ohrms/dockets/ac/07/briefing/2007-4323b1-01-CHPA.pdf. Accessed on December 29, 2007.

56. Smith MB, Feldman W. Over-the-counter cold medications. A critical review of clinical trials between 1950 and 1991. *JAMA*. 1993;269:2258–2263.

57. Schroeder K, Fahey T. Should we advise parents to administer over the counter cough medicines for acute cough? Systematic review of randomised controlled trials. *Arch Dis Child*. 2002;86:170–175.

58. Paul IM, Yoder KE, Crowell KR, et al. Effect of dextromethorphan, diphenhydramine, and placebo on nocturnal cough and sleep quality for coughing children and their parents. *Pediatrics*. 2004;114:e85-90

59. American Academy of Pediatrics, Committee on Drugs. Use of codeine-and dextromethorphan-containing cough remedies in children. *Pediatrics*. 1997;99:918–920.

60. Infant deaths associated with cough and cold medications – two states, 2005. *MMWR Morb Mortal Wkly Rep*. 2007; 56:14.

61. Consumer Healthcare Products (CHPA). Makers of OTC cough medicines announce voluntary withdrawal of oral infant medicines. http://www.chpa-info.org/ChpaPortal/PressRoom/NewsReleases/2007/10_11_07_CCMedicines.htm. Accessed on May 22, 2008.

62. Fulton JR, Rao RB. Caustics. In: Flomenbaum N, Goldfrank L, Hoffman R, et al, eds. *Goldfrank's Toxicologic Emergencies.* New York, NY: McGraw-Hill Medical Publishing; 2006:1405–1416.

63. Previtera C, Guisti F, Guglielmi M. Predictive value of visible lesions (cheeks, lips, and oropharynx) in suspected caustic ingestion: may endoscopy reasonably be omitted in completely negative pediatric patients? *Pediatr Emerg Care.* 1990; 6:176–178.

64. Crain EF, Gershel JC, Mezey AP: Caustic ingestions – symptoms as predictors of esophageal injury. *Am J Dis Child.* 1984;138:863–865.

65. Michael JB, Sztajnkrycer MD. Deadly pediatric poisons: nine common agents that kill at low doses. *Emerg Med Clin North Am.* 2004;22:1019–1050.

66. Bar-Oz B, Levichek Z, Koren G. Medications that can be fatal for a toddler with one tablet or teaspoonful: a 2004 update. *Pediatric Drugs.* 2004;6(2):123–126.

67. Henry K, Harris CR. Deadly ingestions. *Pediatr Clin North Am.* 2006;53:293–315.

68. Leibelt EL, Shannon ML. Small doses, big problems: a selected review of common highly toxic medications. *Pediatr Emerg Care.* 1993;2:292–297.

69. Rosenbaum TG, Kou M. Are one or two dangerous? Tricyclic antidepressant exposure in toddlers. *J Emerg Med.* 2005;28:169–174.

70. Spiller HA, Villalobos D, Krenzelok EP, et al. Prospective multicenter study of sulfonylurea ingestion in children. *J Pediatr.* 1997;131:141–146.

71. Quadrani DA, Spiller HA, Widder P. Five year retrospective evaluation of sulfonylurea ingestion in children. *J Toxicol Clin Toxicol.* 1996;34:267–270.

72. Little GL, Boniface KS. Are one or two dangerous? Sulfonylurea exposure in toddlers. *J Emerg Med.* 2005;28:305–310.

73. Sachdeva DK, Stadnyk JM. Are one or two dangerous? Opioid exposure in toddlers. *J Emerg Med.* 2005;29:77–84.

74. von Muhlendahl KE, Scherf-Rahne B, Krienke EG, et al. Codeine intoxication in childhood. *Lancet.* 1976;2:303–305.

75. United States Food and Drug Administration. Proposed rules: external analgesic drug products for over the counter human use; tentative final monograph. *Fed Reg.* 1983; 48:5852–5869.

24 Trauma

Minor trauma and nonfatal traumatic injuries in children account for more than 10 million emergency department (ED) visits each year. It is essential that each ED be fully prepared to care for and treat these patients. The main causes of nonfatal injuries in children younger than 5 years of age include falls, child abuse, drowning, burns and motor vehicle accidents (MVAs). Head injury, suffocation and drowning are the main causes of fatal injuries.

Some of the anatomic differences between children and adults are listed in Table 24.I.1. Although a complete discussion of trauma care is beyond the scope of this chapter, the authors highlight pertinent trauma issues that occur in the first year of life: child abuse, minor head injury and orthopedic injuries. The reader is referred to advance trauma life support (ATLS) for the current pediatric trauma guidelines.

Table 24.I.1. Anatomic differences in the pediatric patient

- Children have open skull sutures that fuse by 12–18 months of age.
- Cervical injuries occur at the C1-C3 level in infants and children younger than 8 years of age.
- Pseudosubluxation between C2 and C3 is common (see orthopedic chapter).
- Children have a thinner abdominal wall with less musculature. The adult pelvic organs such as the bladder are intra-abdominal.
- Children have a compliant chest wall. It is more likely for children to have pulmonary pathology than to experience rib fractures because it takes significant force for a child to sustain a rib fracture.
- Infants require full diaphragmatic excursion for normal breathing to occur; therefore, gastric distention can result in respiratory compromise.
- Children are more likely to experience a fracture than a sprain.
- Infants have a vascular scalp and can become hypotensive from a scalp laceration.
- Children have poor temperature regulation due to thin skin, higher body surface to mass ratio and smaller fat stores; therefore, they can become hypothermic rapidly.

SECTION I. CHILD ABUSE

Sharon E. Mace

INTRODUCTION

Unfortunately, child abuse, more recently termed *child maltreatment,* is not infrequent. More than 3 million cases of child maltreatment are reported annually in the United States; about 30% of these are confirmed cases[1,2] and about 1500 to 2000 result in death.[1–3] The actual incidence of maltreated children and deaths from maltreatment is undoubtedly higher; the true number of maltreated children is estimated to be two to five times the reported cases[3,4] and deaths are estimated to be at least double the reported cases.[5,6] Only half of the children who died of maltreatment, as determined by a child fatality review committee, had death certificates that listed maltreatment as a cause of death.[6] Another study indicated that child homicides due to abuse were under-recorded by nearly 60%.[5] Underascertainment of deaths from child maltreatment occurs because most estimates of child maltreatment fatalities are derived from the coding (e.g. ICD 9 codes) on death certificates.

Child maltreatment is differentiated into the following categories: neglect (54%), physical abuse (25%), sexual abuse (11%), emotional abuse (3%), and Munchausen's syndrome (factitious disease by proxy).[7] The incidences of the types of maltreatment vary depending on the data sources used and the mandated reporters.[7,8] EDs report child maltreatment rates of physical abuse (55%), physical neglect (30%), and sexual abuse (15%).[8] The

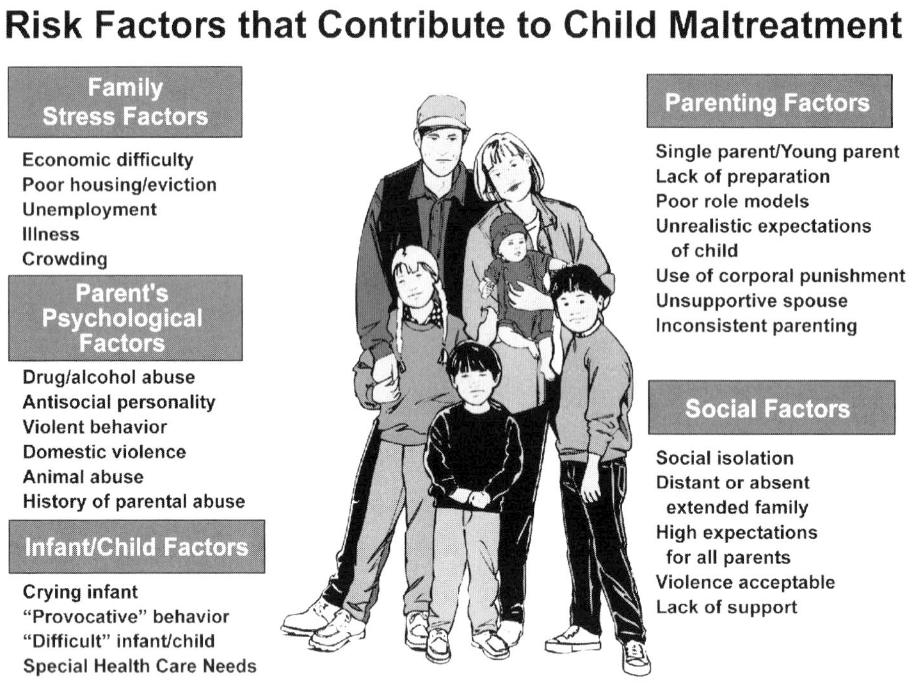

Risk Factors that Contribute to Child Maltreatment

Family Stress Factors

Economic difficulty
Poor housing/eviction
Unemployment
Illness
Crowding

Parent's Psychological Factors

Drug/alcohol abuse
Antisocial personality
Violent behavior
Domestic violence
Animal abuse
History of parental abuse

Infant/Child Factors

Crying infant
"Provocative" behavior
"Difficult" infant/child
Special Health Care Needs

Parenting Factors

Single parent/Young parent
Lack of preparation
Poor role models
Unrealistic expectations
  of child
Use of corporal punishment
Unsupportive spouse
Inconsistent parenting

Social Factors

Social isolation
Distant or absent
  extended family
High expectations
  for all parents
Violence acceptable
Lack of support

Figure 24.I.1. Factors that contribute to child maltreatment. (Courtesy of Sharon E. Mace, MD, and the Center for Medical Art and Photography at the Cleveland Clinic, Dave Schumick, Medical Illustrator.)

striking increase in reported child maltreatment cases in recent decades is probably due to an increased recognition and reporting of child abuse by mandated reporters and others, changing societal notions of what constitutes abuse, as well as to a higher incidence of child maltreatment.[9–11]

AGE AND CHILD MALTREATMENT

Most physically abused children are younger than 4 years old.[3] There are many variables that increase the risk for abuse in infants and toddlers: increased or total dependency on parents and caregivers; limited or no ability to resist, seek help or run away; and increased time at home. Of all children younger than 3 years old who were seen in the ED with trauma, 1 out of 10 (10%) suffered trauma secondary to an inflicted injury.[12] Nearly one third (30%) of all fractures in children younger than 2 years old are nonaccidental.[12] A Child Fatality Review Committee, which reviewed all death certificates of children younger than 17 years, attributed 5% of all pediatric deaths to child maltreatment; only half of the death certificates correctly attributed death to maltreatment.[6] The highest rates of mortality secondary to child maltreatment occur in children younger than 1 year of age.[6] Homicide is the number

one cause of infant injury death in the United States,[13] and the infant homicide rate is increasing to almost one infant homicide per day.[9]

In addition to the mortality, there is a substantial morbidity associated with child maltreatment. Each year in the United States as a consequence of child maltreatment, more than 140,000 children suffer from serious injury, 18,000 incur a lifelong disability[3] and countless others undergo psychological distress, which frequently results in lifelong psychological disorders and dysfunctional behavior.[14–18] Failure to detect child maltreatment has major consequences. Children whose maltreatment is not detected have an up to 50% chance of enduring further abuse and a 10% chance of dying.[19–22]

Child maltreatment occurs in all socioeconomic, racial, ethnic and cultural groups.[23–26] Certain variables, however, are associated with an increased incidence of child maltreatment: domestic violence (history of partner abuse or sibling maltreatment), parental substance (drug or alcohol) abuse, parental mental illness or antisocial personality, social isolation, poverty, animal abuse, and a history of the parent being abused[27–32] (Figure 24.I.1). A background constellation of elements (so-called right parent or caregiver, right family or environment, right child or infant, right day) are usually present with a

Maltreatment: Risk Factors and Sequelae

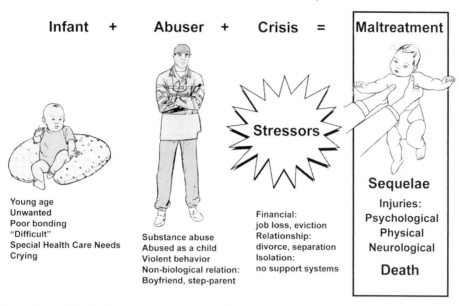

Figure 24.I.2. Child maltreatment: risk factors and sequelae. (Courtesy of Sharon E. Mace, MD, and the Center for Medical Art and Photography at the Cleveland Clinic, Dave Schumick, Medical Illustrator.)

socioeconomic crisis or crises (e.g., job loss, eviction, separation or divorce) triggering the abusive incident[33] (Figure 24.I.2).

Certain characteristics are noted with increased frequency among abused children (*right child or infant*): young age, "unwanted," born from a previous relationship or during a crisis period, poor maternal–child bonding, "difficult" and special health care needs.[27–32] The *right family or environment* refers to social isolation, socioeconomic difficulties (e.g., single parent, financial stress, separation or divorce, unwanted pregnancy).[34] The *right caregiver* has features including substance abuse, violent behavior, aberrant nurture and young age[27–32] (see Figure 24.I.1). One caveat must be remembered. Although these features or characteristics are noted with an increased incidence in maltreated infants or children and their families, not all infants or children with these characteristics are maltreated, and infants or children lacking these features may be victims of abuse.[24]

The majority of child maltreatment is perpetrated by parents or parental figures such as a step-parent or an unrelated male caregiver (e.g., mother's boyfriend).[1,6,34–36] Although child maltreatment can occur at any age, the majority of cases occur in children younger than 3 years of age: about one third of victims are older than age 3 years, one third are between 6 months and 3 years, and one third younger than 6 months.

INFLICTED TRAUMATIC BRAIN INJURY

Trauma is the primary cause of death in children, and traumatic brain injury is the number one cause of death and disability secondary to trauma in children.[37] Nonaccidental head trauma is the number one cause of traumatic death[38] and serious head injuries in infants.[39] The risk of abusive head trauma is greatest in infancy (age <1 year), with the majority of inflicted traumatic brain injury (iTBI) occurring in infants (age <12 months).[40] In about 24% of children younger than 2 years old with a head injury admitted to the ED, the injury was due to nonaccidental trauma.[39] According to one study, excluding uncomplicated skull fractures, 64% of all head injuries and 95% of all life-threatening head injuries in infants (age <1 year) were a result of child abuse.[41] In a study of pediatric abusive head trauma, the perpetrators were father (37%), mother's boyfriend (20.5%), female babysitter (17.3%) and mother (12.6%).[42]

Shaken Baby Syndrome

The association between closed head injury and child abuse was described decades ago when the dyad of chronic subdural hematomas and long bone fractures was described by Caffey.[43] *Shaken baby syndrome* (SBS) describes the occurrence of an intracranial hemorrhage without any apparent external injuries resulting from the vigorous shaking of an infant.[44,45] SBS, also referred to as *whiplash SBS*, is defined by the following triad: severe intracranial injury, retinal hemorrhages and minimal or no external signs of trauma.

The head injury pattern seen in SBS is thought to be caused by shaking followed by an impact. Acceleration and deceleration forces occur from shaking then throwing the infant against a bed or on the floor, causing an impact. Thus, SBS has been renamed *shaken impact syndrome*.[46] More recently, the terms *iTBI, abusive head trauma* (AHT), and *nonaccidental head injury* (NHI) have been used to denote the clinical findings occurring in pediatric victims of abusive head trauma.[47] Shaken impact syndrome generally occurs in children younger than 3 years old with the majority of cases occurring during the first year of life. Infants' weak cervical musculature and relatively large heads make them especially vulnerable to shaking injuries. The increased susceptibility of infants and toddlers to any traumatic brain injury is detailed in Section II on minor head injury.

When diagnosing shaken impact syndrome, the physician should look for the usual history clues and physical examination findings of possible child maltreatment (Tables 24.I.2 and 24.I.3). With shaken impact syndrome, the physical examination may reveal no obvious external signs of trauma. The physician should look for two key findings during the physical examination: (1) small bruises (the size of fingertips) on the chest or upper arms where the infant was held while being shaken and (2) retinal hemorrhages. Yet according to a study of bruising in children with fatal inflicted head injuries, 21% of the victims had no external bruises, but they all had internal, generally intracranial, hemorrhage[48]; the absence of external bruises does not rule out shaken impact syndrome.

Ophthalmic Findings with Shaken Baby Syndrome

Retinal hemorrhages occur in the majority (65%–90%) of shaken infants,[39,45–55] although iTBI can occur without retinal hemorrhages and retinal hemorrhages can occur with severe trauma other than SBS, such as an MVA, and in other conditions and diseases[38,47,56–58] (Tables 24.I.4 and 24.I.5). Thus, controversy surrounds the association between SBS and retinal hemorrhages. However, the characteristics (type, number, location) of the retinal hemorrhages with iTBI can be indicative of SBS.[59–61] Although retinal hemorrhages are the most common ophthalmologic finding with SBS, other ocular findings include vitreous hemorrhage, subretinal hemorrhage, optic nerve sheath hemorrhage, retinal folds, retinal tears, papilledema and retinal detachment.[38,59–61]

Perhaps a better term for the ocular findings of SBS is *intraocular hemorrhages* (instead of just *retinal hemorrhages*) because retinal, vitreous, preretinal and subdural optic nerve sheath hemorrhages can be seen on the funduscopic examination.[38,59–61] These ophthalmologic findings are suggestive of SBS; therefore, it is critical to obtain a pediatric ophthalmology consult when the diagnosis of SBS is being considered, although this consult does not necessarily need to be done while the infant is in the ED and may be obtained after the infant is admitted. Although ED physicians and other nonophthalmologists are fairly accurate (13% false-negative rate) in diagnosing the presence of retinal hemorrhage, they may inadvertently omit critical ophthalmologic forensic information.[62] Consequently, it is mandatory to obtain an ophthalmology consult in cases of suspected nonaccidental pediatric head trauma because forensic information regarding the type, number and location of retinal hemorrhages and other ocular findings must be well documented. The ophthalmology consultant must take retinal photographs to document the ocular involvement.

Given the following facts, the ophthalmic findings indicative of SBS should be considered pathognomonic of SBS and noncontroversial:

1. Birth-related retinal hemorrhages are mild and resolve relatively quickly.
2. Clinical disorders in which retinal hemorrhages occur are rare and can be diagnosed easily.
3. Retinal hemorrhages with nonaccidental trauma are infrequent.
4. The severity, characteristics, and associated ophthalmologic (and other clinical) findings in a given clinical context that are found with iTBI support the diagnosis.

One important caveat to remember is that the absence of intraocular hemorrhages does not rule out SBS.

The outcome of SBS is grim: about two thirds (65%) of children either die or suffer permanent neurological disability. The mortality for pediatric victims of nonaccidental head trauma is estimated to be from 15% to 38%.[40,54,63] The morbidity is also extremely high; neurological or cognitive deficits occur in up to 85% (30%–85%) of the survivors and only 15% to 30% of the survivors have a chance of full recovery.[63,64]

Table 24.I.2. Clues to child maltreatment in the history

Chief complaint
- Multiple presentations: Frequent ED/office/clinic visits may signify that the caregiver/parent is having trouble caring for the child, can't cope and is at risk
- ED visit(s) for nonexistent or trivial complaints. Again, this may indicate the caregiver/parent is having trouble caring for the child, can't cope and is at risk

History of present illness: explanation of injury event
- No history of trauma
- History of low impact trauma
- History of injury attributed to cardiopulmonary resuscitation
- Unexplained history: Caregiver has "no idea" how the child was injured
- Variable history: History changes when recounted at different times by same person
- Discrepant history: Different history given by different individuals (parents, older siblings, grandparents, babysitter, neighbors)
- Implausible history: Injury is not possible given the child's age/developmental level with the mechanism
- Accusatory history: Older child or sibling may name a specific person; anonymous reports and parental accusations against each other (especially in custody cases) should be investigated but be cautious
- History of self-inflicted injury: Does a young child or infant have the skills or physical dexterity to explain the injury? For example, an infant can't turn the knob on the hot water faucet and burn him- or herself
- History of playmate or sibling causing injury: Similarly, does the playmate or sibling have the physical ability or skills? For example, a 2 year old does not have the physical force to fracture a mandible if he or she hits a 1 year old

History of present illness: information to be obtained by physician
- Who, if anyone, was responsible for the injury?
- Who, if anyone, was present when the injury occurred? Was the infant/child left unattended (neglect)?
- What was the cause of the injury? Be specific. If a fall, off what and how high (how many feet) on to what surface? A 2-ft fall off a couch onto a carpeted floor does not cause significant head injury
- When (time of injury): Was there a delay in seeking care?
- Where did the injury occur? At home, school, relative's house, etc?
- Mechanism of injury: Obtain details (how many stairs did the child fall down?)
- Child protective services may need to visit the home and place of injury to document the conditions

Family history
- Parental history: Substance abuse, domestic abuse, violent behavior/criminal record
- Medical illness/disorders: Bleeding, metabolic, or genetic disorders, orthopedic or bone diseases that are in the differential for child abuse
- Any recent stressors or crises at home? Job loss, eviction, financial problems, separation/divorce
- Sibling's history: Illnesses (possible inherited disorders)/injuries (abuse may involve several family members)

Social history
- Members of the household, others (relatives, friends, neighbors) who may have visited household and have access to the child/infant
- Older children: Daycare, school
- Caregivers
- Diet

Past medical history
- Neonatal history
- Developmental history
- What is child capable of?
- Special care needs child?
- Previous surgery/hospitalizations/ED or clinic or office visits
- Previous injuries or illnesses (abuse, neglect, Munchausen's)

The differential diagnosis of SBS is extensive, ranging from gastroenteritis to sepsis. About one third (31.2%) of patients with SBS are misdiagnosed when seen in the ED.[54] The most common misdiagnoses for SBS are listed in Table 24.I.6. The average delay in diagnosis for iTBI was 7 days.[54]

Skull Fractures and Child Abuse

A skeletal survey for child abuse includes frontal and lateral skull radiographs.[65] Significant skull fractures in pediatric patients, especially fractures without a history of major trauma such as an MVA, should raise suspicion of

Table 24.I.3. Physician observations and physical examination*

Observations to Be Documented
- Child/Infant
  - Behavioral/emotional state
    - Older child: Withdrawn, fearful, apprehensive, hyperactive
    - Infant: Listless, lethargic, crying, irritable
  - Developmental level: Motor milestones
    - Infant: Can child sit, stand, walk, run, grasp, transfer objects
    - Toddler: Can child walk up and down stairs, use hands (turn knobs)
  - Older child: Record quotes regarding injury events
- Parent/Caregiver
  - Appearance/demeanor: Ill kept, intoxicated, inappropriate, unstable, abusive, hostile, upset, evasive
- Family Unit
  - Interaction of parents with each other
  - Interaction of child with each parent
  - Caregiving of parent for infant: How well does parent feed the infant, change diapers?
- Growth Parameters
  - Record weight, height or length, head circumference (Is there failure to thrive with weight <10th percentile from neglect? Increased head circumference from traumatic injury?)

* In addition to the usual history and physical examination.

child abuse. Characteristics of skull fractures that are most common with nonaccidental head trauma include multiple, complex configuration (versus simple linear), depressed, wide, growing, bilateral, involvement of two or more cranial bones, location other than parietal bone and associated intracranial injury (including subdural hematoma) (Figure 24.I.3). Features consistent with accidental skull fractures are single, narrow, linear, generally in the parietal bone and with no associated intracranial injury.[24]

PHYSICAL ABUSE

Abdominal and Thoracic Trauma

Abdominal injuries are the second most common cause of death from child abuse.[66,67] Nonaccidental abdominal injuries have a 40% to 50% mortality rate.[67,68] In young children and infants, child abuse ranks second only to MVA as a cause of abdominal trauma. Any abdominal injury in an infant or toddler who has no history of significant trauma such as an MVA should have child abuse in the differential diagnosis.[69]

Table 24.I.4. Causes of retinal hemorrhages in infants*

Central Nervous System Injury
- Shaken impact syndrome
- Increased intracranial pressure[1]
- Subarachnoid hemorrhage[1]
- Accidental trauma

Blood Dyscrasias/Coagulopathies
- Hematologic disorders
- Coagulopathies
- Thrombocytopenia

Ophthalmologic Disorders
- Retinopathy of prematurity
- Retinal dysplasia

Cardiovascular Disease
- Severe hypertension

Vasculitis

Poisonings
- Carbon Monoxide

Birth Trauma[2]
- Secondary to delivery/birth trauma occurs in up to 34% of newborns
  - Highest incidence with vacuum-assisted delivery (75%–78%)
  - Lowest incidence with cesarean section 7%–8%
  - Vast majority of retinal hemorrhages from birth trauma resolve within 1 month (one infant s/p vacuum-assisted delivery retinal hemorrhage lasted 58 days)

Metabolic Disorders
- Galactosemia
- Glutaric aciduria type I: Can have acute subdural hematoma, chronic subdural effusion, retinal hemorrhage

Intrauterine Infections
- Cytomegalovirus

Infections
- Meningitis
- Rickettsia
- Malaria
- Bacterial endocarditis

[1] Subarachnoid hemorrhage and/or increased intracranial pressure can occur with inflicted traumatic brain injury.

[2] Retinal hemorrhages secondary to birth trauma should resolve by 1–2 months of age.

* With all these causes of retinal hemorrhage other than shaken baby syndrome, the retinal hemorrhages are not multiple, not severe and resolve fairly quickly.

[1] Even in patients with a coagulopathy, cardiopulmonary resuscitation does not cause multiple or severe retinal hemorrhages.

Abdominal trauma secondary to child abuse generally involves blunt trauma from blows or kicks to the abdomen. Abdominal injuries of this type can be deceptive and are frequently misdiagnosed not only because there is generally no history of trauma or a history of only minimal trauma but also because there

Table 24.I.5. Characteristics of retinal hemorrhages with shaken baby syndrome versus other causes of retinal hemorrhages

Characteristic	Shaken baby syndrome	All other causes
Number	Multiple	Usually single, few in number
Severity	Severe	Mild
Location	Anterior pole	Posterior pole
Duration	Last months	From birth trauma, resolves within 1 month (rarely lasts 2 months)
Characteristics	Bilateral but can be unilateral Intra-retinal Extended to periphery of retina Involves all layers of retina Pre-retinal hemorrhage present Pre-macular hemorrhage present Retinal detachment/tears/folds	Unilateral
Associated ophthalmologic findings	Retinal detachments/tears/folds Vitreous hemorrhage Papilledema	

is no external evidence of injury because the force is transmitted to the intra-abdominal structures. Abdominal injuries secondary to child abuse include lacerations of the spleen or liver, perforated bowel with secondary peritonitis, intraperitoneal bleeding, mesenteric tears, retroperitoneal hematomas, duodenal hematomas (which can lead to intestinal obstruction) and pancreatitis.[66–70] Pancreatitis secondary to nonaccidental abdominal trauma is the most common cause of non–medication-associated pancreatitis in children.[70] Pediatric victims of inflicted abdominal trauma may present with vomiting, abdominal pain, abdominal distention, obstruction or shock.

The following thoracic injuries have been reported following nonaccidental trauma: rib fractures, hemothorax, pneumothorax, chylothorax, pulmonary contusion, myocardial contusion and cardiac tamponade. Only bilateral multiple rib fractures, especially posterior rib fractures, are pathognomonic for child abuse in the absence of major trauma such as an MVA.

Head, Eyes, Ears, Nose and Throat Trauma

Any abnormalities must be well documented. Bilateral orbital swelling or fractures rarely occur secondary to accidental trauma. The mouth and throat examination may reveal tears of the frenulum from forced feeding or abnormalities of the corners of the mouth secondary to gagging injuries.[24] The ears may have bruises or circular marks from someone grabbing the ears. Broken hairs or alopecia may be secondary to traction from pulling on the hair. Circular marks on the neck may indicate strangulation. Any swelling, skin abnormalities, tenderness or fractures on the face, skull or neck should be noted.

Fractures

Fractures secondary to inflicted trauma should be considered in young children, especially in nonambulatory children and children younger than 2 years old.[71,72] More than half of all fractures (56%) in infants (age $\leq$12 months) are

Table 24.I.6. Differential diagnosis of shaken baby syndrome

Gastrointestinal
- Vomiting
- Diarrhea
- Gastroenteritis
- Feeding difficulties/poor feeding
- Reflux

Neurologic
- Seizure disorder
- Accidental head trauma
- Increasing head size
- Macroencephaly

Infectious
- Rule out sepsis
- Otitis media
- Influenza
- Other
  - Apnea
  - Sudden infant death syndrome

Nonaccidental Manifestation of Abuse: Fractures

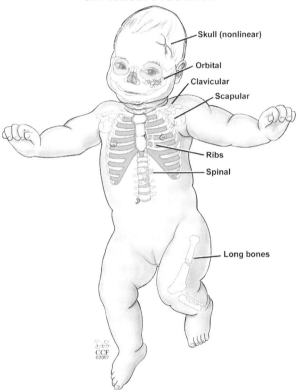

Figure 24.I.3. Nonaccidental manifestation of abuse: fractures. (Courtesy of Sharon E. Mace, MD, and the Center for Medical Art and Photography at the Cleveland Clinic, Dave Schumick, Medical Illustrator.)

Table 24.I.7. Skeletal injuries suspicious for abuse

Fractures of Trunk
- Sternal fracture
- Scapula fracture
- Vertebral fracture
- Rib fractures (especially posterior rib fractures)
- Costosternal separation

Fractures Based on Age
- Fracture in nonmobile infants (<6 months of age)

Long Bone Fractures
- Metaphyseal chip fractures
- Metaphyseal fracture ("corner," "bucket handle" fractures)

Extremity Fractures
- Multiple metacarpal fractures
- Multiple metatarsal fractures
- "Toddler's fracture" in a nonambulatory infant

Multiple Fractures
- Multiple fractures of various ages
- Repeated fractures at the same location

Fractures Based on Mechanism of Injury
- Implausible fracture based on history: Fracture is highly unlikely based on injury (e.g., femur fracture in an infant who rolled off the couch, falling 24 inches onto padded shag carpeted floor)

Skull Fractures
- Anything other than a simple linear skull fracture
- Depressed skull fractures
- Multiple linear skull fractures

from nonaccidental trauma.[73] Fractures are found in over one third (36%) of physically abused children.[74]

Certain fractures are highly specific for inflicted injury. These include fractures in nonmobile infants and rib (especially posterior rib), scapular, spinal and metaphyseal ("bucket handle" or corner) fractures[75–81] (Table 24.I.7; see Figure 24.I.3). A childhood ambulatory spiral tibial (CAST) fracture or "toddler fracture" is a fracture that results from a twisting injury to the tibia as the young child falls on it. This is not from inflicted trauma. However, a spiral tibial fracture in a nonambulatory infant is suspicious for nonaccidental trauma. Remember that any fracture can be the result of abuse.

Falls and Cardiopulmonary Resuscitation as Injury Mechanisms

As with iTBI, minor falls are often cited by the abuser as a mechanism for injury resulting in fractures and

blunt abdominal injuries.[82] Although household falls in infants and children are common, they are generally harmless.[83–85] In one study, nearly one fourth (22%) of all infants younger than 6 months of age were involved in a household fall with less than 1% resulting in any serious injury (either a concussion or fracture).[83] Only one fracture (of a clavicle) occurred in over 1700 falls (1:1700 <1%).[83] Similar findings occurred in hospitalized children younger than 6 years of age who fell from 25 to 54 inches with only 2 fractures (one clavicle, one simple skull fracture) reported out of 207 falls (2:207 <1%).[85] Fractures resulting from falls in infants (age <1 year) were uncommon compared with older children, and child abuse was suspected in half (50%) of all the infants with fractures, according to one report.[84]

Cardiopulmonary resuscitation (CPR) is often mentioned by the abuser as a cause of rib fractures.[82] The evidence suggests otherwise. Studies of children who received CPR indicated that rib fractures are very rarely, if ever, due to CPR.[86–88] No rib fractures were detected on radiographic examination or at autopsy in 91 infants who underwent CPR,[86] which confirms similar findings in earlier studies.[87] Another autopsy study found a 35% incidence of posterior rib fractures in those children who died from abuse versus no posterior rib fractures and only 2% (2:94) anterior rib fractures located in the mid-clavicular line in infants dying of natural causes who underwent CPR.[88]

RADIOGRAPHIC EVALUATION OF CHILD PHYSICAL ABUSE

In any child younger than 2 years and in some children from 2 to 5 years in whom physical abuse is suspected, a skeletal survey is indicated and is the primary radiographic evaluation.[65,69] A so-called babygram x-ray lacks sufficient detail to reveal all fractures and should not substitute for a skeletal survey in these patients.[65] Bone scans are less effective during the acute phase of the injury (<24 hours), are unreliable in detecting linear skull fractures and use radioactive material that is preferentially picked up by rapidly healing bone. Bone scans can identify fractures that occurred more than 24 to 48 hours before the scan but not fractures that occurred more recently. Bone scans should be considered an adjunct to the skeletal survey and are used mainly to evaluate questionable fractures noted on the skeletal survey.[65]

Acute fractures occasionally are not evident on initial plain x-rays; therefore, repeat films in 10 to 14 days are indicated when a fracture is suspected that may show the healing bony callus indicative of a fracture. Rib fractures that have just occurred may be especially difficult to detect on plain radiographs, either chest or rib films. When rib fractures are suspected but are not evident on the initial plain radiographs, oblique views, repeat films in 10 to 14 days,[89] and radionuclide scanning are helpful techniques to use.[90]

BURNS AND BRUISES

When child maltreatment is in the differential diagnosis, the skin must be examined and the findings documented, including appearance, location, size (measured with a ruler), shape, pattern, color (if a bruise), severity (if a burn) and associated findings[24] (Table 24.I.8; Figures 24.I.4A and B and 24.I.5).

Fully undress the infant or young child and note any abrasions, lacerations, bruises, burns, bite marks, hematomas and areas of tenderness, which may suggest an underlying injury. In the past, attempts were made to date bruises based on their color; however, because many factors can affect the color of a bruise, it is better to describe them accurately in detail than to assign a specific age. For any visible injuries, make diagrams and take photographs with a ruler and a color scale in place.[24] Use a ruler to measure the distances between the teeth in a bite mark; this can help differentiate an adult's from a child's bite and a human's from an animal's bite. Take a bite mark sample by wiping a cotton swab moistened with sterile saline over the bite mark, air dry the swab and put it in a sterile vial. Obtain a second control sample from the child's uninvolved skin. Send both samples for forensic testing including DNA, while making sure to maintain the chain of evidence.[24] Circumferential marks on the skin – especially around the wrists, ankles, or neck – may be caused by physical restraints (Table 24.I.8).

SEXUAL ABUSE

The diagnosis of sexual abuse can be very difficult, especially in infants, for many reasons. Older children who have been sexually abused may relate information such as, "Daddy touched me down there." It is not possible to acquire this type of information from preverbal children and infants. Furthermore, physical findings are rarely diagnostic. Reports have indicated that the likelihood of diagnostic findings in prepubertal girls,[91,92] including those who have been penetrated, is less than 5%.[91,92] Factors accounting for the high incidence of normal or nonspecific findings in sexual abuse cases include the wide range of normal, children's and infant's ability to heal rapidly, the fact that sexual abuse (even with penetration) may not show signs of physical damage, and, frequently, the disclosure of sexual abuse occurs long after the actual incidents.[69] In prepubertal children, the transfer of biological material, such as semen or sperm, rarely lasts longer than 24 hours.[93,94] Data also indicate that the greatest recovery of biological transfer material (e.g., semen or sperm) in prepubertal girls (age <10 years) is from clothing or bedding related to the assault and not from body sites.[95] This explains why it is extremely important to forensically collect all underwear, clothing and bedding, even if this process entails sending community resources, such as police or child protective services officers, to obtain it. Data also suggest that even qualified practitioners are

Table 24.I.8. Cutaneous manifestations of inflicted injury: burns and bruises

Parameter	Inflicted	Accidental	Inflicted injury example
Appearance	Uniform Regular Recognizable pattern Shape of an object Symmetric Circumferential Bilateral	Nonuniform Irregular No pattern No recognizable shape Asymmetric Not circumferential Unilateral	Bruise: Belt buckle, rope Burns: Iron, cigarette marks
Location	Nonexposed, protected areas Extensor/posterior surfaces	Exposed areas shins, forehead Peripheral distribution: Lower extremities, arms, forehead Flexor/anterior surfaces	Chest, neck, axilla, ear pinna, buttocks, genitalia, oral mucosa, inner aspect of arm, back of hands, inner thighs, back of knees, small of back, trunk (more central)
Location: Specific Injuries	Strangulation Restrained/tied down Grabbed/shaken (as with shaken baby syndrome) Force feeding Toilet training punishment Older child to protect themselves from being hit Immersion burns		Circumferential linear marks on neck, wrists, ankles Circular/oval bruises on chest, upper arms, ear pinna Oral injuries: Frenulum tear, mouth lacerations Bruises/burns on buttocks, thighs, genitalia Bruises on volar surface of forearms Stocking/glove distributions
Severity	Extensive More severe Multiple, various ages, various stages of healing Various locations Bilateral, symmetric	Mild First degree burn, superficial Few, isolated Nonprotected areas Unilateral (accidental fall generally does not injure both sides of body)	Severe 2nd or 3rd degree burn Bilateral orbital fractures/contusions

Burns	No splash marks
	  Uniform
	  Regular
	  Circumferential
	  Predominately 2nd or 3rd degree
	  Clear, sharply demarcated edges
		Splash marks
		Variable
		No severe
		Predominately 1st degree
		Indistinct irregular edges
			Accidental injury: Spill, cup of hot liquid, decreasing severity and splash marks from initial site of contact

unable to accurately interpret genital findings,[96] which is why some child abuse experts recommend the use of providers specially trained and experienced in completing child sexual abuse examinations and reviewing evidence of abuse.[69]

It is desirable to perform pediatric sexual abuse evaluations in a pleasant, nonthreatening environment using resources or facilities designed for this type of examination. Most sexual abuse examinations are not emergent and may be scheduled at a later, more convenient time, with some exceptions: evidence of injury or bleeding, an assault within the past 72 hours in which the transfer of

biological material is thought to have occurred and older children who have complaints of pain.[69] Evaluation under anesthesia should be considered in order to minimize the emotional trauma of the examination. Documentation via photography or video colposcopy should be done.

Studies indicate that there is a very low yield on forensic evidence testing in pediatric sexual abuse cases. In one study of pediatric sexual abuse victims that compared urgently seen (<72 hours) versus nonurgently seen children younger than 13 years of age, a positive forensic finding was obtained in only 9% of urgently seen children.[95] Positive examination findings were found in

Patterns of Nonaccidental Bruises

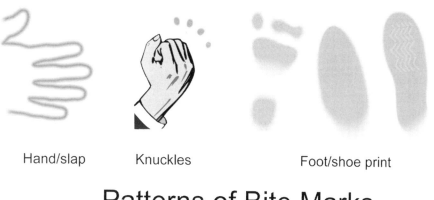

Hand/slap   Knuckles   Foot/shoe print

Patterns of Bite Marks

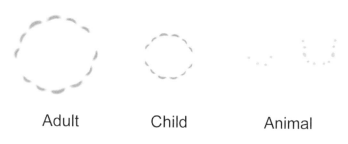

Adult   Child   Animal

DNA Analysis

Bruise Patterns - Household Items

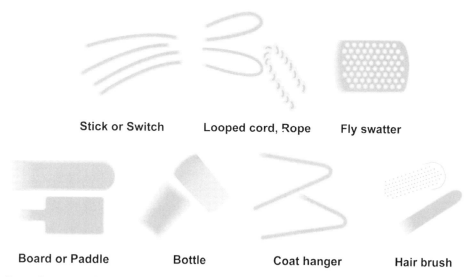

Stick or Switch   **Looped cord, Rope**   **Fly swatter**

Board or Paddle   **Bottle**   **Coat hanger**   **Hair brush**

Figure 24.I.4 A and B. Patterns of nonaccidental bruises. (Modified from *Nelson Textbook of Pediatrics*, 18th ed. 2007:174, 176.)

13.2% of urgently seen children and 3.8% of nonurgently seen children.[94] There was no recovery of semen in children seen more than 24 hours after the initial incidence.[94] A key finding was that in young children, semen was recovered only from clothing or body linen and not from body sites. Semen or sperm were recovered from body sites only in children older than age 10 or on clothing or objects.[95]

A thorough, well-documented history is essential when working with an alleged sexual abuse victim because this

Patterns of Nonaccidental Burns

Immersion burns

Kitchen items

Knife   Forks   Spoon   Pot/pan   Hot plate

Household items

Iron   Curling iron   Light bulb   Barbecue grill   Automobile   Cigarette
                                                                               cigarette lighter

Figure 24.I.5. Patterns of nonaccidental burns. Modified from *Nelson Textbook of Pediatrics*, 18th ed. 2007:174, 176.)

history frequently provides the sole or primary diagnostic evidence. A thorough physical examination includes a complete physical examination and notation of any anogenital abnormalities, although a speculum examination is not indicated and is inappropriate in prepubertal children. If intravaginal trauma is suspected, evaluation under anesthesia in the operating room is indicated.

Magnification aids in the detection of micro-trauma and mild changes in the hymen that can be missed by the naked eye.[70] A handheld magnifier or otoscope, which is usually readily available in an ED, can be used. Colposcopes, which allow for both magnification and photography, can be used to collect forensic evidence. Toluidine blue, a dye that is preferentially taken up by exposed endothelial cells, is used to aid in detecting minor injuries.[70] If the assault is acute, then forensic specimens for detection of the perpetrator's DNA and for sperm is warranted.

The evaluation of pediatric sexual abuse victims for sexually transmitted diseases (STDs) is complicated, particularly in infants and very young children. This is why many clinicians consult with pediatric sexual abuse experts for both evaluation and treatment.[47] Numerous variables need to be considered when evaluating a pediatric patient

for possible STDs, including the nature of the abuse, the disease prevalence in the community and the patient's symptoms.[69,70]

Herpes simplex viruses and human papillomaviruses are no longer automatically considered STDs; however, syphilis, gonorrhea and chlamydia are still considered STDs and, if it is an acute assault, prophylactic treatment is recommended. Whether to give prophylaxis against human immunodeficiency virus is dependent on variables such as disease prevalence in the community, and, generally, a consult with the local infectious disease expert is obtained before beginning such therapy. In addition to treating the child for the usual STDs, if the child is not immunized and the perpetrator has an acute hepatitis B infection, hepatitis B immune globulin (HBIG) plus the first dose of a series of three doses of the hepatitis B vaccine (HBV) is indicated.[70] Ideally, a protocol for post-exposure prophylaxis is developed with the input of local infectious disease and child abuse specialists.

Although an initial medical evaluation may be indicated in the ED to begin treatment of the abused infant or child and to determine his or her safe disposition, a more detailed or definitive forensic evaluation by a child abuse specialist and follow-up with their pediatrician or primary care provider is indicated. [47,69,70]

UNEXPLAINED INFANT DEATH

Sudden infant death syndrome (SIDS), also referred to as *crib death,* is the sudden unexplained death of an infant younger than 1 year of age. Some cases of SIDS have been attributed to infant abuse, neglect or homicide.[97] A previous study found a high incidence (85% or 33/39 infants) of child abuse in the form of attempted suffocation in hospitalized infants with an apparent life-threatening event (ALTE) discovered by covert video surveillance.[98] In 30% of the infants, the referring physician had no clue that the ALTE may be secondary to abuse.[98]

It is difficult to distinguish between infant nonaccidental asphyxiation and SIDS.[97,99–102] Infanticide may account for up to 5% of deaths attributed to SIDS, according to some estimates. An American Academy of Pediatrics (AAP) policy statement lists the following as parameters suggestive of nonaccidental asphyxiation: occurrence in an infant older than or equal to 6 months of age, blood in the infant's mouth or nose, simultaneous or near simultaneous death of twins and unexplained or unexpected death of a sibling.[102] Recommendations from the AAP include prompt death scene investigation to include interviews of household members, examination of the dead infant at the ED by a child abuse specialist and collation of patient history from records and health care providers.[102]

CHILD DEATH REVIEW TEAMS

Most suspicious child deaths occur in very young children; half the fatal child abuse victims are infants younger than 1 year of age.[103] Child Death Review Teams promote a multidisciplinary approach to the investigation of an unexplained infant death which incorporates medical history, record review, autopsy and death scene investigation, while protecting the child and family's rights.[102]

PITFALLS

- Failure to recognize that child maltreatment is common and occurs in all socioeconomic, racial, ethnic and cultural groups. Child maltreatment can be differentiated into neglect, physical abuse, sexual abuse, emotional abuse, and Munchausen's syndrome.
- Failure to recognize that nonaccidental head trauma, is the number one case of traumatic death and serious head injury in infants. Approximately one third of cases of shaken baby syndrome are misdiagnosed in the ED.
- Failure to include child maltreatment in the form of suffocation, in the differential diagnosis of SIDS and ALTE.

REFERENCES

1. Gaudiosi JA. Reports. *Child Maltreatment 2005.* U.S. Department of Health and Human Services, Children's Bureau. Washington, DC: U.S. Government Printing Office; 2007:5.
2. Child Welfare Information Gateway. *Child Abuse and Neglect Fatalities: Statistics and Interventions.* U.S. Department of Health and Human Services, Children's Bureau. Washington, DC: U.S. Government Printing Office; 2006:2.
3. Alexander RC. Statistics of child abuse. In: Jones G, Levitt CJ; American Academy of Pediatrics Section on Child Abuse and Neglect, eds. *A Guide to References and Resources in Child Abuse and Neglect,* 2nd ed. Chicago, IL: American Academy of Pediatrics; 1998:81–182.
4. National Center for Child Abuse and Neglect. *National Study of the Incidence and Severity of Child Abuses and Neglect.* Washington, DC: U.S. Department of Health and Human Services; 1988. Publication OHDS 81-30329.
5. Herman-Giddens ME, Brown G, Verbies S, et al. Under-ascertainment of child abuse mortality in the United States. *JAMA.* 1999;282(5):463–467.
6. Crume TL, DiGuiseppti CD, Byers T, et al. Under ascertainment of child maltreatment fatalities by death certificates, 1990–1998. *Pediatrics.* 2002;110:e18.
7. Wang CT, Daro D. *Current Trends in Child Abuse Reporting and Fatalities: The Results of the 1996 Annual Fifty-State Survey.* Chicago, IL: National Committee to Prevent Child Abuse; 1997.
8. Keshavarz R, Kawashima R, Low C. Child abuse and neglect presentations to a pediatric emergency department. *J Emerg Med.* 2002;4:341–345.
9. Overpeck MD, Brenner RA, Trumble AC, et al. Risk factors for infant homicide in the United States. *N Engl J Med.* 1998;339:1211–1216.
10. Advisory Board on Child Abuse and Neglect. *A Nation's Shame. Fatal Child Abuse and Neglect in the United States.* Washington, DC: Department of Health and Human Services; 1995. Report No. 5.
11. Marshall WN, Puls T, Davidson C. New child abuse spectrum in an age of increased awareness. *Am J Dis Child.* 1988;142:664–667.
12. Green FC. Child abuse and neglect. A priority problem for the private physician. *Pediatr Clin North Am.* 1975;22(2):329–339.
13. Ventura SJ, Peters KD, Martin JA, et al. Births and deaths: United States, 1996. *Mon Vital Stat Rep.* 1997;46(1 Suppl 2):1–40.
14. Malinosky-Rummel R, Hansen DJ. Long-term consequences of childhood physical abuse. *Psychol Bull.* 1993;114:68–79.
15. Wisdom CS. Post-traumatic stress disorder in abused and neglected children grown up. *Am J Psychiatry.* 1999;156:1223–1229.
16. Worley KB. Psychological impact of child maltreatment. In: Jones G, Levitt CJ; American Academy of Pediatrics Section on Child Abuse and Neglect, eds. *A Guide to References and Resources in Child Abuse and Neglect,* 2nd ed. Chicago, IL: American Academy of Pediatrics; 1998:122–127.
17. Felitti VJ, Anda RF, Nordenberg D, et al. Relationship of childhood abuse and household dysfunction to many of

the leading causes of death in adults: the adverse child-hood experience (ACE) study. *Am J Prev Med.* 1998;14:245–258.

18. Dube SR, Anda RF, Felitti VJ, et al. Childhood abuse, household dysfunctions and the risk of attempted suicide throughout the lifespan: findings from the adverse child-hood experiences study. *JAMA.* 2001;286:3089–3096.

19. King WK, Kiesel EL, Simon HK. Child abuse fatalities. Are we missing opportunities for intervention? *Pediatr Emerg Care.* 2006;22(4):211–214.

20. Loder RT, Bookout C. Fracture patterns in battered children. *J Orthop Trauma.* 1991;5:428–433.

21. Rosenberg LA, Wissow LS. Effects of maltreatment on the child. In: Wissow LS. *Child Advocacy for the Clinician: An Approach to Child Abuse and Neglect.* Baltimore, MD: Williams & Wilkins; 1990:12.

22. Ellaway BA, Payne EH, Rolfe K, et al. Are abused babies protected from further abuse? *Arch Dis Child.* 2004;89:845–846.

23. Mace SE. Child abuse. In: Weinstock M, Longstreth R, eds. *Bounce Backs.* Columbus, OH: Anadem Publishing; 2006:439–451.

24. Mace SE. Child physical abuse: a state of the art approach. *Pediatr Emerg Med Pract.* 2004;1(2):1–20.

25. Mace SE. Child maltreatment: physical abuse of the child and infant. *Crit Decisions Emerg Med.* 2006;21(2):14–21.

26. Baren JM, Mace SE, Hendry PL. Children's mental health emergencies, part 3: special situations: child maltreatment, violence, and response to disasters. *Pediatr Emerg Care.* 2008.

27. Rosenberg NM, Meyers S, Shackleton N. Prediction of child abuse in an ambulatory setting. *Pediatrics.* 1982;70(6):879–882.

28. Kelleher K, Chaffin M, Hollenberg J, et al. Alcohol and drug disorders among physically abusive and neglectful parents in a community-based sample. *Am J Public Health.* 1994;84(10):1586–1590.

29. Murphy JM, Jellinek M, Quinn D, et al. Substance abuse and serious child mistreatment: prevalence, risk, and outcome in a court sample. *Child Abuse Negl.* 1991;15(3):197–211.

30. Ross SM. Risk of physical abuse to children of spouse abusing parents. *Child Abuse Negl.* 1996;20(7):589–598.

31. O'Keefe M. Predictors of child abuse in maritally violent families. *J Interpersonal Violence.* 1995;10:3–25.

32. Robin M. Innocent victims. The connection between animal abuse and violence toward humans. *Minn Med.* 1999;82(8):42–44.

33. Cadzow SP, Armstrong KL, Fraser JA. Stressed parents with infants: reassessing physical abuse risk factors. *Child Abuse Negl.* 1999;23(9):845–853.

34. Schlosser P, Pierpont J, Poertner J. Active surveillance of child abuse fatalities. *Child Abuse Negl.* 1992;16:3–10.

35. Starling SP, Holden JR, Jenny C. Abusive head trauma: the relationship of perpetrators to their victims. *Pediatrics.* 1995;95(2):259–262.

36. National Clearinghouse on Child Abuse and Neglect Information. Reports from the States to the National Child Abuse and Neglect Data System (NCANDS). http://child.cornell.edu. Accessed on May 22, 2008.

37. Schutzman S. Injury – head. In: Fleisher GR, Ludwig S, Henretig FM, et al, eds. *Textbook of Pediatric Emergency Medicine.* Philadelphia, PA: Lippincott Williams &Wilkins; 2006:373–381.

38. Gerber P, Coffman K. Non-accidental head trauma in infants. *Childs Nerv Syst.* 2007;23:499–507.

39. Duhaime AC, Alario AJ, Lewander WJ, et al. Head injury in very young children: mechanisms, injury types, and oph-thalmologic findings in 100 hospitalized patients younger than 2 years of age. *Pediatrics.* 1992;90(2 Pt 1):179–185.

40. Keenan HT, Runyan DK, Marshall SW, et al. A population-based study of inflicted traumatic brain injury in young children. *JAMA.* 2003;290:621–626.

41. Billmire ME, Myers PA. Serious head injury in infants: accident or abuse? *Pediatrics.* 1985;75(2):340–342.

42. Starling S, Holden JR, Jenny C. Abusive head trauma: the relationship of perpetrators to their victims. *Pediatrics.* 1995;95(2):259–262.

43. Caffey J. Multiple fractures of the long bones in infants suffering from chronic subdural hematoma. *AJR.* 1946;56:163–173.

44. Caffey J. On the theory and practice of shaking infants. Its potential residual effects of permanent brain damage and mental retardation. *Am J Dis Child.* 1972;124:161–169.

45. Duhaime AC, Christian CW, Rorke LB, et al. Nonaccidental head injury in infants – the "shaken baby syndrome." *N Engl J Med.* 1998;338:1822–1829.

46. Duhaime AC, Gennarelli TA, Thibault LE, et al. The shaken baby syndrome. A clinical, pathological, and biomechanical study. *J Neurosurg.* 1987;66(3):409–415.

47. Newton AW, Vadeven AM. Update on child maltreatment. *Curr Opin Pediatr.* 2007;19:223–229.

48. Atwal GS, Rutty GN, Carter N, et al. Bruising in non-accidental head injured children: a retrospective study of the prevalence, distribution, and pathological associations in 24 cases. *Forensic Sci Int.* 1998;96:215–230.

49. Eisenbrey AB. Retinal hemorrhage in the battered child. *Childs Brain.* 1979;5:40–44.

50. Zimmerman RA, Bilaniuk LT, Bruce D, et al. Computed tomography of craniocerebral injury in the abused child. *Radiology.* 1979;130:687–690.

51. Sinal SH, Ball MR. Head trauma due to child abuse: serial computerized tomography in diagnosis and management. *South Med J.* 1987;80:1505–1512.

52. Gilliland MG, Luckenbach MW, Chenier TC. Systemic and ocular findings in 169 prospectively studied child deaths: retinal hemorrhages usually mean child abuse. *Forensic Sci Int.* 1994;68:117–132.

53. Ewing-Cobbs L, Kramer L, Prasad M, et al. Neuroimaging, physical, and developmental findings after inflicted and noninflicted traumatic brain injury in young children. *Pediatrics.* 1998;102:300–307.

54. Jenny C, Hymel KP, Ritzen A, et al. Analysis of missed cases of abusive head trauma. *JAMA.* 1999;281:621–626.

55. Kivlin JD, Simons KB, Lazoritz S, et al. Shaken baby syndrome. *Ophthalmology.* 2000;107:1246–1254.

56. Hughes LA, May K, Talbot JF, et al. Incidence, distribution, and duration of birth related retinal hemorrhages: a prospective study. *J AAPOS.* 2006;10:102–106.

57. Hymel KP, Abshire TC, Luckey DW, et al. Coagulopathy in pediatric abusive head trauma. *Pediatrics.* 1997;99:371–375.

58. Aryan HE, Ghosheh FR, Jandial R, et al. Retinal hemorrhage and pediatric brain injury: etiology and review of the literature. *J Clin Neurosci.* 2005;12:624–631.

59. Morad Y, Kim YM, Armstrong DC, et al. Correlation between retinal abnormalities and intracranial abnormalities in the shaken baby syndrome. *Am J Ophthalmol.* 2002;134:354–359.

60. Schloff S, Mullaney PB, Armstrong DC, et al. Retinal findings in children with intracranial hemorrhage. *Ophthalmology.* 2002;109:1472–1476.

61. Wygnanski-Jaffe T, Levin AV, Shafiq A, et al. Postmortem orbital findings in shaken baby syndrome. *Am J Ophthalmol.* 2006;142:233–240.

62. Quintana EC. Nonophthalmologist accuracy in diagnosing retinal hemorrhages in the shaken baby syndrome. *Ann Emerg Med.* 2004;43(6):796–797.

63. Sinal SH, Ball MR. Head trauma due to child abuse: serial computerized tomography in diagnosis and management. *South Med J.* 1987;80:1505–1512.

64. Case ME, Graham MA, Handy TC, et al. Position paper on fatal abusive head injuries in infants and young children. *Am J Forensic Med Pathol.* 2001;22:112–122.

65. Diagnostic imaging of child abuse. *Pediatrics.* 2000;105(6): 1345–1348.

66. Huyer D. Abdominal injuries in child abuse. *The APSAC Advisor.* 1994;7:5–7, 24.

67. O'Neill JA Jr, Meacham WF, Griffin JP, et al. Patterns of injury in the battered child syndrome. *J Trauma.* 1973;13:332–339.

68. Ledbetter DJ, Hatch EI Jr, Fedlman KW, et al. Diagnostic and surgical implications of child abuse. *Arch Surg.* 1998;9:1101–1105.

69. Hudson M, Kaplan R. Clinical response to child abuse. *Pediatr Clin North Am.* 2006;53:27–39.

70. Berkowitz CD. Child maltreatment. In: Marx JA, Hockberger RS, Walls RM, et al, eds. *Rosen's Emergency Medicine Concepts and Clinical Practice,* 6th ed. Philadelphia: Mosby Elsevier; 2006:968–976.

71. Thomas SA, Rosenfield NS, Leventhal JM, et al. Longbone fractures in young children: distinguishing accidental injuries from child abuse. *Pediatrics.* 1991;88(3):471–476.

72. Blakemore LC, Loder RT, Hensinger RN. Role of intentional abuse in children 1 to 5 years old with isolated femoral shaft fractures. *J Pediatr Orthop.* 1996;16(5):585–588.

73. McClelland CQ, Heiple KG. Fractures in the first year of life. A diagnostic dilemma. *Am J Dis Child.* 1982;136(1):26–29.

74. Merten DF, Radkowski MA, Leonidas JC. The abused child: a radiological reappraisal. *Radiology.* 1983;146(2):377–381.

75. Leventhal J, Thomas S, Rosenfield N, et al. Fractures in young children: distinguishing child abuse from unintentional injuries. *Am J Dis Child.* 1993;147:87–92.

76. Kleinman PK, Marks SC Jr. A regional approach to classic metaphyseal lesions in abused infants: the distal tibia. *Am J Roentgenol.* 1996;166:1207–1212.

77. Kleinman PK, Marks SC Jr. A regional approach to classic metaphyseal lesion in abuse infants: the proximal tibia. *Am J Roentgenol.* 1996;166:421–426.

78. Kleinman PK, Marks SC Jr, Nimkin K, et al. Rib fractures in 31 abused infants: postmortem radiologic-histopathologic study. *Radiology.* 1996;200:807–810.

79. Kleinman PK, Marks SC Jr, Richmond JM, et al. Inflicted skeletal injury: a postmortem radiologic-histopathologic study in 31 infants. *Am J Roentgenol.* 1005;165:647–650.

80. Kleinman PK, Marks SC. Vertebral body fractures in child abuse: radiologic-histopathologic correlates. *Invest Radiol.* 1992;27:715–722.

81. Thomas SA, Rosenfield NS, Leventhal JM, et al. Longbone fractures in young children: distinguishing accidental injuries from child abuse. *Pediatrics.* 1991;88:471–476.

82. Hettler J, Greenes DS. Can the initial history predict whether a child with a head injury has been abused? *Pediatrics.* 2003;111(3):602–607.

83. Warrington SA, Wright CM for the ALPSAC Study Team. Accidents and resulting injuries in premobile infants: data from the ALPSAC study. *Arch Dis Child.* 2001;85:104–107.

84. Hennrikus WL, Shaw BA, Gerardi JA. Injuries when children reportedly fall from a bed or couch. *Clin Orthop.* 2003;407:148–151.

85. Lyons RJ, Oates RK. Falling out of bed: a relatively benign occurrence. *Pediatrics.* 1993;92:125–127.

86. Spevak MR, Kleinman PK, Belanger PL, et al. Cardiopulmonary resuscitation and rib fractures in infants: a postmortem radiologic-pathologic study. *JAMA.* 1994;272(8):617–618.

87. Feldman KW, Brewer DK. Child abuse, cardiopulmonary resuscitation, and rib fractures. *Pediatrics.* 1984;73(3):339–342.

88. Betz P, Liebhardt E. Rib fractures in children-resuscitation or child abuse? *Int J Legal Med.* 1994;106:215–218.

89. Anilkumar A, Fender LJ, Broderick NJ, et al. The role of the follow-up chest radiograph in suspected non-accidental injury. *Pediatr Radiol.* 2006;36:216–218.

90. Smith FW, Gilday DL, Ash JM, et al. Unsuspected costovertebral fractures demonstrated by bone scanning in the child abuse syndrome. *Pediatr Radiol.* 1980;10:103–106.

91. Berenson AB, Chacko MR, Wiemann CM, et al. A casecontrol study of anatomic changes resulting from sexual abuse. *Am J Obstet Gynecol.* 2000;182:820–834.

92. Heger A, Ticson L, Belasquez O, et al. Children referred for possible sexual abuse: medical findings in 2384 children. *Child Abuse Negl.* 2002;26:645–659.

93. Christian CW, Lavelle JM, DeJong AR, et al. Forensic findings in prepubertal victims of sexual assault. *Pediatrics.* 2000;106:100–104.

94. Young KL, Jones JG, Worthington T, et al. Forensic laboratory evidence in sexually abused children and adolescents. *Arch Pediatr Adolesc Med.* 2006;160:585–588.

95. Palusci VJ, Cox EO, Shatz EM, et al. Urgent medical assessment after child sexual abuse. *Child Abuse Negl.* 2006;30:367–380.

96. Makoroff KL, Brauley JL, Brandner AM, et al. Genital examinations for alleged sexual abuse of prepubertal girls: findings by pediatric emergency medicine physicians compared with child abuse trained physicians. *Child Abuse Negl.* 2002;26:1235–1242.

97. Meadow R. Suffocation, recurrent apnea, and sudden infant death. *J Pediatr.* 1990;117:351–357.

98. Southall DP, Plunkett MCB, Banks MW, et al. Covert video recordings of life-threatening child abuse: lessons for child protection. *Pediatrics.* 1997;100:735–760.

99. Reece RM. Fatal child abuse and sudden infant death syndrome: a critical diagnostic decision. *Pediatrics.* 1993;91: 423–429.

100. American Academy of Pediatrics. Committee on Child Abuse and Neglect. Addendum: Distinguishing sudden infant death syndrome from child abuse fatalities. *Pediatrics.* 2001;108(3):812.

101. American Academy of Pediatrics. Committee on Child Abuse and Neglect. American Academy of Pediatrics. Distinguishing sudden infant death syndrome from child abuse fatalities. *Pediatrics.* 2001;107(2):437–441.

102. Kairys SW, Alexander RC, Block RW, et al. American Academy of Pediatrics. Committee on Child Abuse and Neglect and Committee on Community Health Services. Investigation and review of unexpected infant and child deaths. *Pediatrics.* 1999;104(5 Pt 1):1158–1160.

103. Durfee MJ, Gellert GA, Tilton-Durfee D. Origins and clinical relevance of child death review teams. *JAMA.* 1992;267:3172–3175.

SECTION II. MINOR HEAD INJURY

Sharon E. Mace

INTRODUCTION

Injury is the number one cause of death and disability in children and infants.[1] More than 10 million children in the United States, or about 1 out of every 6 children, are treated annually in the emergency department (ED) for injuries, and more than 10,000 children die each year from serious injury.[1]

Head trauma is one of the most common injuries of children and infants.[2,3] On an annual basis, pediatric head trauma accounts for approximately 650,000 ED visits, 250,000 hospital admissions, 550,000 hospital days and hospital care costs greater than $1 billion per year.[4,5]

Head or traumatic brain injury (TBI) is the most common cause of pediatric morbidity and mortality in developed countries.[6,7] Each year in the United States, about 3000 children and infants die from TBI.[6] More than 5 million Americans live with disabilities secondary to TBI.[8,9] There are also various non–health care costs. These costs include psychosocial problems for the child such as learning disabilities and school problems; sleep disturbances, memory problems, mood changes and persistent

Table 24.II.1. Differences between the brain of the child or infant and the adult

- The infant's brain doubles in size in the first 6 months of life (an infant's weight also doubles in the first 6 months and triples in the first 12 months).
- At 2 years of age, the child's brain size is 80% of the adult brain size.
- At birth, there is incomplete neuronal synapse formation, arborization, myelinization.
- Neuronal plasticity occurs after birth.
- The subarachnoid space is relatively smaller in the child and infant than in the adult.
- Subarachnoid space offers less protection to the brain (because of less buoyancy).
- Head momentum (from trauma) is more likely to result in parenchymal structural damage in the child than in the adult.
- The normal cerebral blood flow in a child increases proportionately to almost twice that of the adult by age 5, then decreases.

This is partly responsible for the child's severe susceptibility to cerebral hypoxia.

- The infant's/young child's thinner skull affords less protection for the brain than the older child's or adult's thicker skull.
- There is a greater (per unit) cerebral oxygen and glucose requirement in the infant and child than in the adult.

headache; and parent or caregiver loss of productivity, loss of wages, loss of time from job or school, and anxiety.[9]

About 80% of all head injuries are considered minor.[10] There is much discussion and controversy regarding the appropriate evaluation and management of patients with minor head injuries, especially infants.[11–14]

DIFFERENCES BETWEEN THE BRAIN OF THE CHILD OR INFANT AND THE BRAIN OF THE ADULT

There are many anatomic and physiologic differences between the brain of a child or infant and that of the adult. These differences account, in part, for the higher frequency of brain injuries from blunt trauma in the pediatric patient as well as for the child's marked susceptibility to cerebral hypoxia[1,15] (Table 24.II.1).

There are also numerous differences between the child or infant and the adult in terms of injury mechanisms[1,10,15] (Table 24.II.2). Evaluation of the infant or child differs from evaluation of the adult and can be more difficult, especially in nonverbal children, for many reasons including inability to report symptoms, limited behavioral responses and frequent lack of symptoms with

Table 24.II.2. Differences in injury mechanisms between the child or infant and the adult

- The infant or child with a head injury is more likely to have other injuries (↑ likelihood of multiple trauma).
- The infant or child has a smaller body mass, thus, any trauma has a greater force per unit body area.
- This more "concentrated" energy is transmitted to a body with closer proximity of multiple organs, less fat and less connective tissue.
- This leads to a higher frequency of multiple organ injuries (multiple trauma) than in the adult.
- The child and infant's head is proportionately much larger than the adult's, resulting in a higher frequency of blunt brain injuries.
- There is a greater body surface area to body volume in the child than in the adult with a greater heat loss and the early development of hypothermia.
- The outcome in a child <3 years of age is worse than a similar injury in an older child.
- Children have an increased susceptibility to secondary brain injury caused by hypovolemia, hypoxia, seizures or hyperthermia.
- In adults and older children, hypotension is almost never due to head injury.
- Infants can become hypotensive from blood loss into the subdural or epidural space or scalp because of the infant's smaller blood volume (~80 cc/kg blood volume in infants).
- The infant's open fontanel and mobile cranial sutures may allow for expansion of an intracranial mass lesion with clinical signs masked until late when rapid decompensation may occur
- An infant with bulging fontanelles or diastatic cranial sutures should be treated as having a serious intracranial injury even if there are few or no clinical signs of a mass lesion such as an altered mental status or coma
- With Traumatic Brain Injury (TBI), children and infants have fewer focal mass lesions than adults
- Children and infants have a greater incidence of diffuse intracerebral injuries or diffuse axonal injuries than adults
- Increased intracranial pressure from cerebral edema is more common in children and infants than adults
- The Glasgow Coma Scale (GCS) is modified for pediatric patients (Table 24.II.3)
- The child/infant may compensate early on when hemorrhage occurs then precipitously deteriorate so resuscitate early and with adequate fluid and consult trauma surgeon or neurosurgeon early

Table 24.II.3. Glasgow coma scale

	Standard glasgow coma scale	Pediatric glasgow coma scale
Eye Opening (E)	Spontaneous 4 To speech 3 To pain 2 None 1	Spontaneous 4 To speech 3 To pain 2 None 1
Best Verbal Response (V)	Oriented 5 Confused 4 Inappropriate words 3 Incomprehensible sounds 2 None 1	Coos, Babbles 5 Irritable, cries 4 Cries to pain 3 Moans to pain 2 None 1
Best Motor Response (M)	Follows commands 6 Localizes pain 5 Withdraws to pain 4 Flexion to pain 3 Extension to pain 2 None 1	Normal spontaneous movement 6 Withdraws to touch 5 Withdraws to pain 4 Abnormal Flexion 3 Abnormal extension 2 None 1

skull, because they have a proportionately greater cerebral blood flow (with corresponding greater cerebral oxygen and glucose requirements), and because they have increased susceptibility to decreased cerebral blood flow and cerebral hypoxia.[1,10,15] Children younger than 3 years of age who experience severe brain injury have a worse outcome than older children or adults with a similar injury.[1,10,15]

DEFINITION OF MINOR HEAD INJURY

Various criteria have been used to define minor head trauma. Traditionally, *minor head injury* (MHI) was defined by a Glasgow Coma Scale (GCS) rating of 13 to 15 and no focal neurologic deficits.[2] Advanced Trauma Life Support (ATLS) defines *mild brain injury* as a GCS of 14 or 15, *moderate brain injury* as a GCS of 9 to 13 and *severe brain injury* as a GCS less than or equal to 8[10] (Table 24.II.3). In other literature, *minor head trauma* is defined as a GCS of 13 to 15,[16] or 15 alone,[17,18] versus 14 or 15[19.] The American Academy of Pediatrics, in a recent guideline, defined children with *MHI* as "those who have normal mental status at the initial examination, who have no abnormal or focal findings on neurologic examination, and who have no physical evidence of skull fracture."[20]

There are several confounding factors affecting the definition of MHI. Within the category of MHI patients, there

intracranial injury (ICI). Infants and children are also at greater risk for abuse, which makes evaluation difficult. It has been stated that "up to one half of infants with ICI have no symptoms of brain injury"[6] (see Section I. Child Abuse in Infancy).

Children and especially infants have a greater incidence of head and multiple trauma because their brains are less protected in the smaller subarachnoid space by a thinner are significant differences among patients with a GCS of 13 or 14 versus 15 with a greater incidence of ICI and a higher likelihood of needing neurosurgical intervention (NSI) as the GCS decreases. [21] A patient with a GCS of 13 has a greater likelihood of having a significant brain injury, having a more severe TBI and needing NSI than a patient with a higher GCS of 14 or 15.[21] This is further complicated by the imprecision of the GCS; patients with the same GCS (e.g., GCS 15) may have very different ICIs and prognoses. Clinical decision rules or algorithms may further subdivide MHI patients into different categories based on whether the GCS is 13 or 14 or 15. Thus, risk stratification of MHI patients, based on clinical variables, is made difficult because, although some patients with the same GCS rating of 15 may have a normal mental status, others may have abnormal behavior, lethargy or even a localized or focal motor and/or sensory deficit. Diagnostic algorithms, in order to risk-stratify MHI patients, are often dependent on nonspecific clinical variables, such as loss of consciousness (LOC), vomiting, headache and post-traumatic amnesia.[11–14,22] Furthermore, such clinical variables often have very different definitions.

EVALUATION OF MINOR HEAD INJURY

Clinical signs and symptoms in children and especially in infants can be subtle and nonspecific compared with adults; therefore, the age of the patient also is a factor with most pediatric clinical decision rules differentiating between infants and older children. There has been no uniform agreement about which clinical variables are the best predictors of ICI and need for NSI, especially in infants.[11–14,22]

In general, the consensus from the various studies has been that a patient with MHI and a GCS of 13 or 14 needs neuroimaging.[13,22] A patient with MHI and a GCS of 15 who is symptomatic with LOC or post-traumatic amnesia should be strongly considered for neuroimaging.[13] When dealing with a patient with a GCS of 15 who is asymptomatic, the physician may reserve neuroimaging for selected high-risk cases such as those with focal neurological findings, clinical evidence of a skull fracture, an abnormal mental status or a coagulopathy.[13]

Because there are concerns about the long-term consequences of radiation causing an increased cancer risk, the occasional need for sedation in order to obtain neuroimaging, and the increased health care costs, several alternatives to neuroimaging have been suggested.

Observation, preferably in an observation or short-stay unit, is more cost-effective than an inpatient admission, thus it is a viable alternative.[23–25] Sending the patient home to be observed by reliable family or friends or, in the case of an infant or child, by the parents or caregivers, has also been suggested. There are, however, several pitfalls to this approach, especially in infants. There is the possibility that the injury may be due to parental or caregiver abuse or neglect. Next, what is a "reliable" caregiver? Studies indicate that the assessment of the caregiver's reliability shows wide variability among health care professionals not to mention the other qualifications for discharge such as ability to return to the ED (e.g., available transportation and reasonably short travel time).[26]

INTRACRANIAL INJURIES IN NEUROLOGICALLY NORMAL CHILDREN

Of greater concern is the fact that signs and symptoms in patients with ICI, especially infants, may be subtle or nonexistent.[2,6,22] Furthermore, there is a low but not zero incidence of ICI and need for NSI in MHI patients. Thus, ICI with need for NSI can occur in pediatric patients who are alert and have no neurologic deficits.[2,6,22] Pediatric patients younger than 2 years of age who are neurologically intact following blunt head trauma are at an even greater risk for ICI and need for NSI.[6,22] Reasons for the increased risk and a correspondingly lower threshold for obtaining neuroimaging in this vulnerable age group (<2 years old) include the following: more difficult to evaluate, greater risk of both skull fractures and ICIs (based on pathophysiology and vulnerability to child abuse), increased likelihood of being asymptomatic (up to 50% of infants with ICIs are asymptomatic)[6] and a greater risk for inflicted injury.[6,22] Occult ICI is noted most often in the youngest infants,[27,28] with 27% of infants younger than 6 months of age and 15% of infants 6 months to 1 year of age being asymptomatic versus none of the infants older than 1 year of age being asymptomatic in one study.[28]

NEUROIMAGING OF PATIENTS WITH MINOR HEAD INJURY

Skull Radiographs

In the past, skull radiographs were used to screen for skull fractures in order to identify patients at risk for ICI.[2,13,14] Numerous studies have documented that the risk of ICI is increased in the presence of a skull fracture.[3,15,27–36] In adults, the presence of a skull fracture and an impaired LOC carries up to a 25% risk of an intracranial hematoma.[29] Similar results were noted in pediatric patients.[30] The presence of a skull fracture is one of the strongest predictors of ICI, especially in pediatric patients younger than 2 years old. In one study, skull x-rays were ordered in pediatric patients (mean age 7 years, range 2 months – 16 years) who were admitted with a head injury (N = 846) or had a skull fracture and were not admitted (N = 37). Skull fractures were seen on 19% (162/870) of the skull radiographs of whom 65% had a CT scan of the head. Of the 106 CT scans done in children with a skull fracture, 13% (14/106) had an ICI.[37] This report found a 65% sensitivity and 83% negative predictive value of skull x-rays for ICI.[37] In another report, skull fractures were found in 95% of patients with occult ICI.[28] Studies indicate that 15% to 30% of linear skull fractures,[27,38–42] 30% of closed depressed skull fractures[43] and 21% of basilar skull fractures are associated with ICI.[44] However, the absence of a skull fracture does not rule out ICI.

Conversely, reports have found that 40% to 100% of cases of ICI have an associated skull fracture.[27,35,36,39,40,45–47] The relative risk for ICI is increased from 4- to 20-fold,[6,32,35,36] even up to 100-fold[15] in the presence of a skull fracture. Therefore, if a skull fracture is found on a plain skull x-ray, then a CT scan of the brain is indicated.[2,6,10,14]

In infants, skull fractures can have significant complications.[14,15,48,49] Unlike adults and older children, skull fractures in infants have the potential to develop leptomeningeal and porencephalic cysts.[48] Such cysts can occur when tissue becomes interposed between the *diastatic* (or separated) skull fracture segments. These cysts can increase in size and create a mass effect on the brain with resultant neurological symptoms and complications. Growing skull fractures that can enlarge over time generally occur in infants or young children with diastatic fractures and can present months to years after the initial injury.[14,15,48,49]

Another complication that can occur with a basilar skull fracture is a dural tear causing a leak of cerebrospinal fluid (CSF).[6,10,15] The patient with a CSF leak has a risk of meningitis until the dural tear is surgically repaired or heals. Depressed skull fractures, especially with a greater than or equal to 1-cm depression, usually require surgical repair to prevent a mass effect on the brain and for cosmetic repair of the skull deformity.[15] There is also a

high incidence of child abuse in infants with skull fractures (see Section I. Child Abuse in Infancy).

For all these reasons, it is important to diagnose a skull fracture, especially in infants and young children, which is a second indication (in addition to detecting ICI) for neuroimaging in infants and young children with MHI.

The incidence of skull fractures in pediatric head injury outpatients presenting for evaluation ranges from 2% to 20%,[36,37,46,49,50] with a higher incidence in infants and younger children (especially ages <1–2 years) in whom there is also a high frequency of child abuse.[36,37,46,49,50]

Skull fractures can be diagnosed by skull radiography (94%–99% sensitivity for linear depressed fractures),[22,27,36,41,51] although one report found only 64% sensitivity.[46] The advantage of skull radiography is that it is readily available, does not require procedural sedation with its inherent risk and has less radiation than CT scanning, which may not detect some skull fractures.[27,36,41,51]

The main drawback to skull radiography is that it yields no information about ICI so that it has been largely supplanted by CT scanning.[2,13,14,15] However, there may still be some utility for skull radiographs in an era where CT scanning is widely available.[6,14,15,52] These indications include skull radiographs are part of the x-ray panel for child abuse (see Section I. Child Abuse in Infancy), can be used to follow diastatic skull fractures and, if CT is not available, can provide screening information especially in asymptomatic infants younger than 1 year of age with scalp hematomas or contusions because these infants have a higher incidence of skull fractures and the possibility of nonaccidental trauma exists.[6,14,15,52]

Head CT Scans

There is a wide variation in the CT neuroimaging of pediatric MHI patients. The overall CT scan rate was 15%, with a range from 6% to 26% for children younger than or equal to 16 years of age with MHI (no definition of MHI was given) in one retrospective chart review.[53] The percentage of abnormal CTs compared with all CT scans ranged from 11.1% to 50% among the participating hospitals.[53] The incidence of ICI in all MHI patients detected by brain CT scan was 5%, but this incidence also varied substantially from 1% to 9% and the need for NSI was 0.2%. A recent report from the pediatric emergency care applied research network (PECARN), which enrolled 35,140 children younger than 18 years with blunt head trauma at 25

EDs, also found a wide variability in CT neuroimaging for children with minor head trauma.[54] Head CTs were obtained in about one third of MHI patients (36.8%), with a site-specific range from 9.7% to 71.1%.[54] Positive head CTs were obtained in 11.2%, of which 30% were isolated skull fractures.[54]

Magnetic Resonance Imaging

Magnetic resonance imaging (MRI) may be more sensitive than CT scanning for the detection of small intracranial hematomas, brainstem and cortical parenchymal injuries and diffuse axonal injuries (DAIs), but MRI may be less sensitive than CT scanning for the detection of isolated subarachnoid hemorrhages.[55–57] MRI is generally more difficult to obtain, especially in an acutely head injured pediatric patient, and is more expensive, whereas CT scanning is readily available. Furthermore, there has been no demonstrable significant clinical advantage of MRI over CT scanning for the acutely injured trauma patient.[58,59]

Risks Associated With Neuroimaging: Head CT Scans

Head CT scanning can detect ICIs and skull fractures, which we do not want to miss; therefore, why not CT scan all pediatric patients with MHIs? The answer is twofold: the risk of ICI in patients with MHI is low and the need for NSI is even lower, and there are risks associated with CT scanning. Although the risk for ICI in MHI patients is low, it is not zero, and there are reports of patients (both adults and children) who "talk and die," indicating that sudden severe deterioration and even death can occur after a lucid (or "normal") period.[2,25,32,60–62]

Obtaining a CT scan involves the transport of the child or infant away from the ED, increased ED length of stay, exposure to ionizing radiation with its associated long-term risk of the development of malignancy, frequent need for procedural sedation with its associated risk and increased health care costs. In order to obtain the CT scan, especially in infants and young children, procedural sedation with its own inherent risks may be necessary. CT scans take time and personnel to obtain, which can impact patient flow in a busy ED. There is also an issue of cost. With the cost of an individual CT scan at $500 to $800, the total annual cost for obtaining CT scans of the brain in all ED patients with MHIs is estimated at $135 to $216 million annually.[63]

Perhaps more importantly are the long-term risks secondary to the radiation needed for neuroimaging. There is also a concern for the risks of radiation, especially in young children and infants, because cancer risk is cumulative over time and children and infants have a longer post imaging lifetime in which a radiation-related cancer may manifest. Image quality is improved with higher radiation doses, and infants and young children receive a higher radiation dose than older children and adults for the same CT setting. It has been estimated that the cranial CT radiation from our current generation CT scanners may cause one lethal malignancy for every 2000 imaged infants and for every 5000 imaged children.[64,65] Children and infants receiving radiation therapy are at risk for long-term cognitive disorders and endocrine dysfunction.[66] Whether there are long-term side effects from the diagnostic radiation needed for an isolated cranial CT in a pediatric patient considering the smaller one-time radiation dose, is unknown.

CLINICAL VARIABLES USED IN THE EVALUATION OF MINOR HEAD INJURY

There is a dilemma associated with the neuroimaging of MHI patients. How do we detect all clinically significant ICI and the need for NSI and not miss the patient with MHI who "talks and dies" while decreasing unnecessary neuroimaging studies, which have an associated cost and some risk to the individual patient?

Multiple individual clinical variables have been associated with an increased incidence of ICI and need for NSI and thus have been suggested as indications for cranial CT scanning in MHI patients. No single variable has 100% sensitivity or specificity; therefore, various algorithms have been devised in an attempt to ascertain which MHI patients need neuroimaging.

What are the current clinical recommendations and what is the consensus? CT scan neuroimaging should be obtained in patients with the following variables[10,13,31,67–69]:

1. Focal neurologic findings
2. GCS of 13 or 14
3. Skull fracture
4. History of a bleeding diathesis, which includes patients on anticoagulants (there is an estimated

10-fold increase in the likelihood of an intracranial hematoma after MHI[69])

5. Major mechanism of injury

Once these five variables are excluded, consensus ends and controversy begins.

The risk for ICI with MHI varies depending on the definition of MHI and the patient's age. Studies indicate that the risk of ICI is inversely related to the GCS. The incidence of ICI in a prospective study of pediatric patients with blunt head trauma was as follows: 33% with GCS 13, 11% for GCS 14 and 5% for GCS 15.[70] Two studies in adults confirmed this finding with an incidence of abnormal cranial CT of 37% for GCS 13, 24% for GCS 14 and 13% for GCS 15 in one study,[71] and 20.5% for GCS 13, 13.6% for GCS 14, 5.5% for GCS 15 with NSI in 1.3% (GCS 13), 0.9% for GCS 14 and 0.4% for GCS 15.[72] Overall, pediatric patients with a GCS of 13 or 14 have an incidence of ICI from 14% to 33% with up to 12% requiring NSI.[39,40,46,73] Based on these reports, the recommendation has been to obtain a cranial CT scan in MHI patients with a GCS of 13 or 14. With a GCS of 15 in pediatric blunt head trauma patients, the incidence of ICI was 4% to 12% with a 0% to 7% incidence of NSI.

The controversy over "to CT scan or not to CT scan" exists for the patient with a GCS of 15 (who does not have focal neurologic findings or a skull fracture, does not have a bleeding dialysis, does not have a major mechanism of injury and has a normal mental status). In one prospective study, 28% of the patients with ICI had a GCS of 15.[46] Other variables that have been considered to determine whether a CT scan is warranted include scalp abnormalities, LOC, post-traumatic amnesia (in older children and adults), vomiting, headache, seizures, irritability and age.

Scalp Abnormalities Such as Hematomas

Scalp abnormalities (e.g., scalp hematomas), especially in infants, have been suggested as a predictor of ICI. Children, especially infants, with scalp abnormalities have a significantly higher incidence of ICI. There is a strong association of ICI with scalp hematoma in most studies. According to one report, 98% of infants with skull fractures had evidence of scalp trauma.[41] Similar results were noted in another study in which 96% of infants with isolated skull fractures had local findings (either swelling or

palpable fracture).[51] Scalp hematomas were predictive of skull fractures in infants younger than 1 year of age but were not predictive of ICI according to one study.[36] Soft-tissue swelling (detected on CT scan) was found in all cases of acute skull fracture in another report.[71] The conclusion is that presence of a scalp hematoma in an infant suggests a high likelihood of skull fracture or ICI.[18,24,27,36,37,42] One caveat needs to be mentioned. If the patient is seen immediately post trauma, then the swelling or hematoma may not have had time to develop; therefore, parents of young infants should be advised to seek medical care if these signs develop later.

Loss of Consciousness

LOC occurs in 5% to 30.6% of pediatric MHI patients (compared with 61.3% of adult MHI patients).[72] Most studies have noted that LOC is a significant predictor of ICI,[30,36,39,46,53,73–75] although a few studies found otherwise.[40,68,76] The definition of LOC (e.g., momentary or a "few seconds" versus longer than 20–30 seconds or 1 minute) and whether it is associated with other clinical variables (e.g., amnesia or vomiting) or isolated may be a factor.[77,78] The duration of LOC may be a variable. One study found that LOC was associated with ICI if the LOC lasted longer than 20 seconds. A meta-analysis of variables that predict significant ICI in MHI patients found that LOC was significantly associated with ICI as well as focal neurology, GCS lower than 15, skull fracture and seizure; whereas headache and vomiting were not associated with ICI.[79] Several clinical decision rules have included LOC as a variable and noted that LOC was a positive predictor of ICI.[72,80] An expert panel felt that a child or infant younger than 2 years old with LOC (per caretakers) longer than 1 minute should undergo CT neuroimaging.[31]

Seizures

The incidence of post-traumatic seizures with MHI is up to 8% in pediatric patients[18,40,72,75,80] and 23% in adults.[72] Post-traumatic or impact seizures have been significantly associated with an increased likelihood of ICI in children[75,80,81] and adults,[72,82] with some exceptions.[27,40,42] Again, the expert consensus is that a child younger than 2 years of age with a post-traumatic seizure should have a head CT.[31]

Post-traumatic Amnesia

Obviously, this clinical variable is not used for clinical decision rules in infants and young children who are unable to verbalize their symptoms. The incidence of post-traumatic amnesia longer than 30 minutes in adults status post MHI with a GCS of 13 to 15 was 28.8%.[72] Some studies have evaluated LOC and amnesia as a single clinical variable.[74,77] In the reports that have looked at amnesia as an independent variable, persistent post-traumatic amnesia (≥ 4 hours, 2–4 hours) or persistent antegrade amnesia was found to be a significant predictor of ICI.[72]

Vomiting

Any vomiting, which has been reported as high as 21% to 30.6% in pediatric patients[80,83] versus 10.8% in adults[72] with MHI, has been noted to have poor sensitivity and specificity.[27,36,40,42,81] However, persistent vomiting may be an important clinical sign.[14,72] Some clinicians suggest that a patient vomiting five or more times per hour should be considered at high risk for ICI with a cranial CT scan recommended, whereas three to four episodes of vomiting place the patient at intermediate risk and, with any potential indicators of brain injury, this intermediate risk patient warrants a head CT or observation.[14] Some reports have linked post-traumatic vomiting in children with a personal or family predisposition to vomit.[7]

What constitutes a limited period or repeated vomiting varies and is not well-defined. Pediatric patients may have a greater tendency to vomit after blunt head trauma than adults, in whom any vomiting has been used as a predictor of ICI in clinical decision rules.[72] However, repeated or persistent vomiting (versus no vomiting or a single episode of emesis) in children or infants has been shown to be a significant predictor of ICI.[75] Again, the consensus of experts is that progressive or worsening vomiting is an indication for CT in the infant or child younger than 2 years old with MHI.[31]

Other Clinical Variables

Headache has been noted in up to 21% of children with MHI.[80] Headache does not have a high sensitivity and specificity, although prolonged or worsening headache is significantly associated with ICI in both pediatric[75] and adult[83] patients.

In infants, two other variables place the infant in a high-risk group for ICI: *irritability* (defined as not easily consoled) and *bulging fontanel* (suggestive of increased intracranial pressure). If either of these clinical variables is present following MHI, a CT scan is indicated.[31]

HETEROGENICITY OF STUDIES AND RESULTS

There are many reasons for variable results among studies. What definition of MHI is being used? Which clinical variables are included and how are they defined? For example, is vomiting one episode or more than one episode or persistent defined by length of time or a combination of duration and number of episodes? What is the patient population (e.g., inclusion and exclusion criteria)? Is it a GCS of 15 and LOC, emesis, and headache; just GCS of 15 plus LOC alone; or just GCS of 15? With the outcome, how is ICI defined? Do they include just mass lesions or any ICI? Are skull fractures without associated underlying brain injury included? What is meant by the need for treatment or NSI? Is it operative neurosurgical procedures only or is it medical management, such as medications, supportive therapy with IV fluids or observation or both? Is it a retrospective case series in which some data (e.g., headache or vomiting) may not be documented or a prospective study? Is there a small number of patients from one center or a large multicenter study? Finally, what is the patient population: all ages, adults, children, infants, newborns, younger than 1 year, younger than 2 years, younger than 5 years, and so on?

CONCLUSION: CLINICAL INDICATORS OF INTRACRANIAL INJURY

Although the presence of certain clinical variables increases the relative risk of an ICI, no one clinical finding, either alone or in combination, has adequate sensitivity and specificity to detect all clinically significant ICIs. These clinical parameters include focal neurological findings, skull fracture, GCS lower than 15 (e.g., MHI with GCS 13 or 14), *prolonged LOC* (usually defined as >20–30 seconds or 1 minute), persistent vomiting (generally two or more episodes of emesis), prolonged or persistent headache, seizure and persistent post-traumatic amnesia. Two additional parameters – bulging fontanel and irritability – place infants at high risk for ICI and are indications for a head CT scan.

CLINICAL DECISION RULES FOR MINOR HEAD INJURY

Because no one (or two) clinical parameters can predict all ICIs in patients with MHIs, various algorithms have been proposed. One of the first large clinical decision rules created regarding MHI was the New Orleans criteria.[84] This ED study included 1429 (first phase 520, second phase 909) adults and children (>3 years old) with a normal GCS of 15 and a normal neurologic examination. A positive head CT scan was significantly associated with seven findings: headache, vomiting, age older than 60 years, intoxication (drug or alcohol), short-term memory deficits, physical evidence of trauma above the clavicles, and seizure.

The National Emergency X-Radiography Utilization Study II (NEXUS II) is a prospective, observational, multicenter study of all ED patients (of all ages) with blunt head trauma (GCS 13–15) who underwent cranial CT imaging. They identified eight criteria that were independently and highly associated with ICI in the 13,728 enrolled patients: evidence of skull fracture, scalp hematoma, neurologic deficit, altered level of alertness, abnormal behavior, coagulopathy, persistent vomiting, and age 65 years or higher.[85]

The Canadian CT Head Rule (CCHR) study included 3121 adults (GCS 13–15) with MHI in 10 Canadian EDs.[63] The authors derived a CT head rule with five high-risk factors: failure to reach GCS of 15 within 2 hours, suspected open skull fracture, any sign of basal skull fracture, vomiting 2 or more episodes and age 65 years or higher; and two medium risk factors: amnesia before impact more than 30 minutes and dangerous mechanism of injury.[86]

The CT in Head Injury Patients (CHIP) study from the Netherlands enrolled 3181 adult (≥16 years) ED patients (GCS 13–15) and found 7.6% ICI and 0.5% need for NSI.[72] They used 10 major criteria and 8 minor criteria. A head CT was indicated in the presence of 1 major or at least 2 minor criteria.[72] The major criteria were pedestrian/cyclist versus vehicle, ejected from vehicle, vomiting, post-traumatic amnesia longer than or equal to 4 hours, clinical signs of skull fracture, GCS lower than 15, GCS deterioration of 2 or more points (1 hour after presentation), anticoagulant use, post-traumatic seizure, and age 60 years or higher. Minor criteria were fall from any elevation, persistent retrograde amnesia, contusion of skull,

neurologic deficits, LOC, GCS deterioration of 1 point (1 hour after presentation), and age 40 to 60 years.[72]

A meta-analysis of 22,420 children (16 reports) analyzed variables that predict significant ICI in children younger than 18 years old with MHI; this meta-analysis found a statistically significant correlation with skull fracture, focal neurology, LOC and abnormal GCS.[79] Headache, vomiting and seizures were not predictive.[79] The authors conducted a similar meta-analysis in adults (83,636 patients, 35 reports) and found eight history factors and six examination findings that significantly increased the risk of ICI.[83] The history parameters were severe headache, nausea, vomiting, LOC, amnesia, seizure, age (>60 years) and male gender.[83] The examination variables were skull fracture, GCS lower than 15, focal neurology, basilar skull fracture, other significant trauma and alcohol intake.[83]

The University of California–Davis rule was derived from a prospective observational study of 2043 children (age <18 years, GCS 13–15).[70] They found 7.7% ICIs and an acute intervention rate of 5.1%. The acute intervention rate may be higher than other studies at least partly because of their definition of intervention, which included neurosurgical procedure, antiepileptic therapy longer than 1 week, 2 or more hospitalization days and neurological deficit until discharge. They identified five statistically significant factors: abnormal mental status, clinical signs of skull fracture, history of vomiting, scalp hematoma (if age <2 years) and headache. Presence of any of these five parameters predicted ICI on CT (97 of 98 children)(99%; 95% CI 94% to 100%) and those needing acute intervention (105 of 105 children)(100%, 95% CI 97% to 100%).[70]

Using the pediatric subset (1666 patients age <18 years, GCS 13–15) of NEXUS II, which identified eight variables in their decision instrument, an ICI of 8.3% was noted. The pediatric tool had only seven parameters because the variable age older than 65 years was deleted.[86] The seven variables used in their decision rule were significant skull fracture, altered level of alertness, neurological deficit, persistent vomiting, scalp hematoma, abnormal behavior and coagulopathy. The pediatric decision instrument had 98.6% sensitivity, 99.1% negative predictive value and 15.1% specificity.[63]

A prospective multicenter cohort study in Italy evaluated 3806 children (age <16 years) and found 27.8% ICI, and an NSI rate of 0.2%.[75] This higher ICI than most studies is likely due to broader inclusion criteria. The statistically significant variables that predicted ICI were LOC, prolonged headache, persistent drowsiness, abnormal mental status, focal neurological signs and signs of basilar or nonfrontal skull fracture, and their sensitivity for ICI was 100%.[75]

The Children's Head Injury Algorithm for the Prediction of Important Clinical Events (CHALICE) study from England analyzed 40 clinical variables for 22,772 children; only 3% of these children received a CT scan of whom 281 children had CT scan abnormalities, 137 had a neurosurgical operation and 15 died.[80] The CHALICE rule has a 98% sensitivity and an 87% specificity. A CT scan was indicated if *any* of the following criteria are present: LOC longer than 5 minutes duration, amnesia (antegrade or retrograde) (>5 minutes duration), abnormal drowsiness, three or more vomits, suspicion of nonaccidental injury and seizure in a patient with no history of epilepsy; GCS lower than 14 or GCS less than 15 if younger than 1 year old, suspicion of penetrating or depressed skull injury or tense fontanel, signs of a basal skull fracture, positive focal neurology and presence of bruise, swelling or laceration larger than 5 cm if younger than 1 year old; high-speed road traffic accident (pedestrian, cyclist or occupant), fall of greater than 3 meters in height or a high-speed injury from a projectile or an object.[80]

The Canadian Assessment of Tomography for Childhood Head Injury (CATCH), which enrolled 3781 children in a prospective multicenter cohort study, used 28 variables and a 14-day telephone follow-up.[87] CATCH excluded patients with known penetrating or depressed skull fracture, focal neurological deficit, referred patients with CT scan, known CSF shunt, severe neurological delay and known or suspected child abuse. Their inclusion criteria were LOC, amnesia, disorientation, at least two vomiting episodes or irritability (≤2 years old), GCS 13 to 15 and age younger than 16 years. The ICI on CT scan was 4.5%, and 0.7% received NSI (neurosurgery, intubation, intracranial pressure monitor and/or anticonvulsants). High-risk factors were GCS lower than 15, suspected open skull fracture, worsening headache and irritability. Medium-risk factors were scalp hematoma, signs of basilar skull fracture and dangerous mechanism of injury. Preliminary results (abstract only reported so far) using only the four high-risk factors yielded a sensitivity equal to 100% and specificity of 70.4% for NSI with only 29.6% of children needing CT. With only medium-risk

factors, the clinical decision rule is 98.3% sensitive and 50.1% specific for ICI with 49.9% needing CT.[87]

The largest pediatric study of MHI so far is from PECARN.[54] This study excluded patients with trivial trauma and included patients with a GCS 14 to 15 and age younger than 18 years with blunt head trauma. The incidence of ICI was 5% with neurosurgery performed on 0.14%. There were 42,495 enrolled, of whom 33,873 were used to derive the decision rules and 8622 to validate the rules. Preliminary analysis (abstract only reported so far) suggests that altered mental status, signs of skull fracture, any emesis, severe mechanism of injury and a few other clinical variables increase the risk for ICI. Clinical decision rules will be validated for two separate groups: those younger than 2 years old and those 2 years of age or older.[54]

CONCLUSION: CLINICAL DECISION RULES

The different clinical decision rules use similar clinical parameters in varying combinations. Most algorithms have included both adults and children. Clinical decision rules that deal with just pediatric patients are limited in number and there are even fewer studies analyzing only infants and very young children. So far there have been no validated clinical decision rules evaluating only infants and very young children (age <2 years), which is the age group that is the most difficult to evaluate. However, with the anticipated publication of the large multicenter prospective studies, such as PECARN and CATCH, and validation of the proposed clinical decision rules, we should have some guidance in the management of the infant or child with MHI in the near future.

LONG-TERM PSYCHOSOCIAL OUTCOMES OF MINOR HEAD INJURY

Severe head injuries are known to cause significant disabilities in adults as well as children.[9,88] There is also evidence that MHI may not be as benign as previously thought.[1,9,15,88] Impairments in the activities of daily living (ADLs), cognition and behavior following mild TBI have been reported.[9] Long-term psychosocial problems can occur,[9] particularly when the head injury occurs during the preschool years.[89] Increased hyperactivity or inattention and conduct disorder were more prevalent especially if the MHI occurred before age 5 years.[89]

BIOMARKERS OF BRAIN INJURY

Central nervous system (CNS) trauma produces injury via *primary* (the initial direct injury) and *secondary* mechanisms (hypoxia and hypoperfusion of the brain causing further injury).[10] Neuropeptides found in CNS neurons are released extracellularly after injury. These endogenous opioid peptides released in response to original trauma are postulated to have a role in the secondary or *indirect* CNS injury. Substances that antagonize the physiologic effects of these endogenous neuropeptides, specifically opiate antagonists and thyrotropin-releasing hormone, have improved the neurologic and cerebrovascular status (as well as the cardiovascular and metabolic status) following TBI in experimental studies.[90]

Neuronal and glial cell protein levels are elevated in acute head injured patients; therefore, several biomarkers have been studied to assess their ability to correlate with the presence of and severity of TBI. The enzyme ubiquitin C-terminal hydrolase (UCH-L1) measured in the CSF was increased significantly in severe TBI patients and correlated with GCS scores.[91] Whether the results of this study prove to be valid in children and infants and in patients with mild TBI not just in severe TBI needs to be determined.

A study of β-endorphin levels in the CSF following TBI noted significantly higher β-endorphin levels in head injured patients compared to the control non–head injury group.[90] Unfortunately, the β-endorphin levels did not correlate with GCS scores.[90] Alpha-spectrin is elevated with severe TBI.[92] N-acetylaspartate has also been studied as a biomarker.[93] After excluding older patients in whom the N-acetylaspartate may be low for reasons secondary to aging, a trend toward significance was found.[92] High levels of serum S-100-β levels have been noted in patients with intracranial pathology.[94–97]

Unfortunately, these biomarker studies measured levels in the CSF not the serum,[90–97] which limits their usefulness in the acute setting in the ED. A study that did measure serum levels of the tau protein in patients with blunt head trauma found no significant difference between patients with ICI versus patients with only a linear skull fracture.[98]

Preliminary data suggest that the use of biomarkers to detect acute brain injury has a promising future. However, several questions need to be answered. In terms of practicality, does the biomarker measured in serum reflect CSF levels and head injury severity? Does the biomarker correlate with GCS, thereby helping to distinguish between mild head injury and moderate or severe head injury? Does the biomarker correlate with the diagnosis and prognosis? Are there age-related or other factors affecting the validity of the biomarkers such as decreased levels in the very young (due to lesser brain mass) or conversely decreased levels in the geriatric patient secondary to the atrophy from the aging process?

USE OF ULTRASOUND IN PEDIATRIC PATIENTS WITH HEAD TRAUMA

Ultrasound has been used in patients with head trauma.[99–102] In infants with an open fontanel, major intracranial bleeding can be diagnosed.[99] Ultrasound has also been recommended as a tool to assess the condition of the dura in patients with a diastatic skull fracture.[99] A third use of ultrasound is to evaluate cerebral perfusion, which can be estimated by measuring the velocity of blood passing through the circle of Willis. If severe cerebral edema is present, perfusion in the major branches of the circle of Willis is decreased. Ultrasound has also been used to diagnose traumatic dissection of the common carotid. Patients with abnormal cerebral blood flow evaluated by ultrasound following an acute closed head injury were divided into three groups:

1. Global hyperemia
2. Vasospasm
3. Early cerebral circulatory arrest

The global hyperemic patients had the best outcome.[101] This suggests that global hyperemia represents a recovery phase of impaired cerebral hemodynamics.[101]

The major drawback to the use of ultrasound in head trauma patients is its limited applicability.[99] Currently, ultrasound can be used to evaluate the brain only if the following are true:

1. There is an open fontanel, thus it is only available in young infants.
2. There are skull fractures with dural tears located in a position accessible to ultrasound (some fractures are located in positions inaccessible to ultrasound, e.g., orbital roof fractures).
3. There are extracranial carotid dissections, with the intracranial segment of the common carotid being inaccessible to ultrasound.

Other drawbacks to ultrasound use with head trauma patients are that there is the limited experience with the use of ultrasound in patients with TBI, and the effectiveness of ultrasound is highly operator-dependent.[99]

PITFALLS

- Failure to recognize that signs and symptoms in infants with ICI may be subtle or nonexistent
- Failure to recognize that occult ICI is noted most often in the youngest infants (27% of infants <6 months may be asymptomatic). Patients, especially infants, with ICI may have a normal GCS and a normal examination
- Failure to realize that no one clinical variable can predict all ICI in all MHI patients, although numerous variables are associated with an increased risk of ICI
- Failure to recognize that infants with scalp hematomas have a significantly higher incidence of ICI

REFERENCES

1. Head trauma. In: American College of Surgeons. *Advanced Trauma Life Support Program for Doctors*, 7th ed. Chicago, IL: American College of Surgeons; 2004:151–175.
2. Quayle KS. Minor head injury in the pediatric patient. *Pediatr Clin North Am.* 1999;46(6):1189–1199.
3. Homer CJ, Kleinman L. Technical report: minor head injury in children. *Pediatrics.* 1999;104(6):e78.
4. National Center for Injury Prevention and Control. *Traumatic Brain Injury in the United States: Assessing Outcomes in Children.* Atlanta, GA: Centers for Disease Control and Prevention; 2002.
5. Centers for Disease Control and Prevention. *2000 National Hospital Ambulatory Medical Care Survey, Emergency Department File 2002* [on CD-ROM]. Hyattsville, MD: National Center for Health Statistics; 2002. Vital Health Series 13, No. 33.
6. Schutzman SA. Injury – head. In: Fleisher GR, Ludwig S, Henretig F, et al, eds. *Textbook of Pediatric Emergency Medicine*, 5th ed. Philadelphia, PA: Lippincott Williams & Wilkins; 2006:373–381.
7. DaDalt L, Andreola B, Facchin P, et al. Characteristics of children with vomiting after minor head trauma: a case-control study. *J Pediatr.* 2007;150:274–278.
8. Thurman D, Alverson C, Dunn K, et al. Traumatic brain injury in the United States: a public health perspective. *J Head Trauma Rehabilitation.* 1999;14(6):602–615.
9. Facts about concussion and brain injury and where to get help. *CDC Injury Center.* www.cdc.gov/ncipc/tbi. Accessed on October 29, 2007.
10. Pediatric head trauma. In: *Advanced Trauma Life Support Program for Doctors*, 7th ed. Chicago, IL: American College of Surgeons; 2004:243–261.
11. Kupperman N. Intracranial injury in minor head trauma. *Arch Dis Child.* 2004;89:593–594.
12. Greenes DS. Decision-making in pediatric minor head trauma. *Ann Emerg Med.* 2003;42:515–518.
13. Savitsky EA and Votey SR. Current controversies in the management of minor pediatric head injuries. *Am J Emerg Med.* 2000;18:96–101.
14. Thiessen ML, Woolridge DP. Pediatric minor closed head injury. *Pediatr Clin North Am.* 2006;53:1–26.
15. Francel PC, Honeycutt J. Mild brain injury in children, including growing skull fractures and growing fractures. In: Winn HR, ed. *Youmans Neurological Surgery*, 5th ed. Philadelphia, PA: Saunders; 2004:3461–3472.
16. Gedeit R. Head injury. *Pediatr Rev.* 2001;22:118–123.
17. Miller JD, Murray LS, Teasdale GM. Development of a traumatic intracranial hematoma after a "minor" head injury. *Neurosurgery.* 1990;27:669–673.
18. Davis RL, Mullen N, Makela M, et al. Cranial computed tomography scans in children after minimal head injury with loss of consciousness. *Ann Emerg Med.* 1994;24:640–645.
19. Tepas J, DiScala C, Ramenofsky ML, et al. Mortality and head injury: the pediatric perspective. *J Pediatr Surg.* 1990;25:92–95.
20. Committee on Quality Improvement, American Academy of Pediatrics. The management of minor closed head injury in children. *Pediatrics.* 1999;104:1407–1415.
21. Fuchs S, Lewis RJ. Tools for the measurement of outcome after minor head injury in children: summary from the ambulatory pediatric association/EMSC outcomes research conference. *Acad Emerg Med.* 2003;10:368–375.
22. Schutzman SA, Greenes DS. Pediatric minor head trauma. *Ann Emerg Med.* 2001;37(1):65–74.
23. Ochoa-Gomez J, Villar-Arias A, Echeverria-Echarri L, et al. Attendance of patients with a minor head injury in an emergency department observation ward. *Eur J Emerg Med.* 2000;7:267–270.
24. Mace SE. Pediatric observation medicine. *Emerg Med Clin North Am.* 2001;9(1):239–254.
25. Aitken ME, Herrerias CT, Davis R, et al. Minor head injury in children. Current management practices of pediatricians, emergency physicians, and family physicians. *Arch Pediatr Adolesc Med.* 1998;152:1176–1180.
26. Sobo EJ, Kurtin P. Variation in physicians' definitions of the competent parent and other barriers to guideline adherence: the case of pediatric minor head injury management. *Soc Sci Med.* 2003;56:2479–2491.
27. Greenes DS, Schutzman SA. Clinical indicators of intracranial injury in head-injured infants. *Pediatrics.* 1999;104:861–867.
28. Greenes DS, Schutzman SA. Occult intracranial injury in infants. *Ann Emerg Med.* 1998;32:680–686.
29. Mendelow AD, Teasdale G, Jennett B, et al. Risks of intracranial haematoma in head injured adults. *BMJ.* 1983;287:1173–1176.
30. Teasdale GM, Murray G, Anderson E, et al. Risks of acute traumatic intracranial haematoma in children and adults: implications for managing head injuries. *BMJ.* 1990;300:363–367.
31. Schutzman SA, Barnes P, Duhaime AC, et al. Evaluation and management of children younger than two years old with apparently minor head trauma. Proposed guidelines. *Pediatrics.* 2001;107:983–993.

32. Dacey RG Jr, Alves WM, Rimel RW, et al. Neurosurgical complications after apparently minor head injury. Assessment of risk in a series of 610 patients. *J Neurosurg.* 1986;65:203–210.

33. Bonadio WA, Smith DS, Hillman S. Clinical indicators of intracranial lesion on computed tomographic scan in children with parietal skull fracture. *Am J Dis Child.* 1989;143:194–196.

34. Chan KH, Yue CP, Mann KS. The risk of intracranial complications in pediatric head injury. Results of multivariate analysis. *Child Nerv Syst.* 1990;6:27–29.

35. Godano U, Serracchioli A, Servadei F, et al. Intracranial lesions or surfical interest in minor head injuries in paediatric patients. *Childs Nerv Syst.* 1992;8:136–138.

36. Quayle KS, Jaffe DM, Kupperman N, et al. Diagnostic testing for acute head injury in children: when are head computed tomography and skull radiographs indicated? *Pediatrics.* 1997;99(5):E11.

37. Lloyd DA, Carty H, Patterson M, et al. Predictive value of skull radial intracranial injury in children with blunt head injury. *Lancet.* 1997;349(9055):821–824.

38. Duhaime AC, Alario AJ, Lewander WJ, et al. Head injury in very young children: mechanisms, injury types, and ophthalmologic findings in 100 hospitalized patients younger than 2 years of age. *Pediatrics.* 1992;90:179–185.

39. Hahn YS, McLone DG. Risk factors in the outcome of children with minor head injury. *Pediatr Neurosurg.* 1993;19:135–142.

40. Schunk JE, Rodgerson JD, Woodward GA. The utility of head computer tomographic scanning in pediatric patients with normal neurologic examination in the emergency department. *Pediatr Emerg Care.* 1996;12:160–165.

41. Shane SA, Fuchs SM. Skull fractures in infants and predictors of associated intracranial injury. *Pediatr Emerg Care.* 1997;13:198–203.

42. Gruskin KD, Schutzman SA. Head trauma in children younger than 2 years: are there predictors for complications? *Arch Pediatr Adolesc Med.* 1999;153:15–20.

43. Ersahin Y, Mutluer S, Mirzai H, et al. Pediatric depressed skull fractures: analysis of 530 cases. *Childs Nerv Syst.* 1996;12:323–331.

44. Kadish HA, Schunk JE. Pediatric basilar skull fracture: do children with normal neurologic findings and no intracranial injury require hospitalization? *Ann Emerg Med.* 1995;26:37–41.

45. Schutzman SA, Barnes PD, Mantello M, et al. Epidural hematomas in children. *Ann Emerg Med.* 1993;22:535–541.

46. Dietrich AM, Bowman MJ, Ginn-Pease ME, et al. Pediatric head injuries: can clinical factors reliably predict an abnormality on computed tomography? *Ann Emerg Med.* 1993;22:1535–1540.

47. Shugeman RP, Paez A, Grossman DC, et al. Epidural hemorrhage: is it abuse? *Pediatrics.* 1996;97:664–668.

48. Gupta SK, Reddy NM, Khosla VK, et al. Growing skull fractures: a clinical study of 41 patients. *Acta Neurochir.* 1997;139:928–932.

49. Harwood-Nash CE, Hendrick EB, Hendrick EB, et al. The significance of skull fractures in children. A study of 1187 patients. *Radiology.* 1971;101:151–156.

50. Boulis ZF, Dick R, Barnes NR. Head injuries in children – aetiology, symptoms, physical findings and x-ray wastage. *Br J Radiol.* 1978;51:851–854.

51. Greenes DS, Schutzman SA. Infants with isolated skull fracture: what are their clinical characteristics, and do they require hospitalization? *Ann Emerg Med.* 1997;30:253–259.

52. Diagnostic imaging of child abuse. *Pediatrics.* 2000; 105(6):1345–1348.

53. Klassen TP, Reed MH, Stiell IG, et al. Variation of utilization of computed tomography scanning for the investigation of minor head trauma in children: a Canadian experience. *Acad Emerg Med.* 2000;7:739–744.

54. Kuppermann N, Holmes JF, Dayan PS, et al. Blunt head trauma in the Pediatric Emergency Applied Research Network (PECARN). *Acad Emerg Med.* 2007;(5s1):S94–95.

55. Snow RB, Zimmerman RD, Gandy SE, et al. Comparison of magnetic resonance imaging and computed tomography in the evaluation of head injury. *Neurosurgery.* 1986;18:45–52.

56. Kelley AB, Zimmerman RD, et al. Head trauma: comparison of MR and CT experience in 100 patients. *AJNR.* 1988;9:699–708.

57. Doezema D, King JN, Tandeberg D, et al. Magnetic resonance imaging in minor head injury. *Ann Emerg Med.* 1991;20:1281–1285.

58. Pitts L. The role of neuroimaging in minor head injury. *Ann Emerg Med.* 1991;20:1286–1388.

59. Levin HS, Amparo E, Eisenberg HM, et al. Magnetic resonance imaging and computerized tomography in relation to the neurobehavioral sequelae of mild and moderate head injuries. *J Neurosurg.* 1987;66:706–713.

60. Snoek JW, Minderhoud JM, Wilmink JT. Delayed deterioration following mild head injury in children. *Brain.* 1984;107:15–36.

61. Humphreys RP, Hendrick EB, Hoffman HJ. The head-injured child who "talks and dies": a report of 4 cases. *Childs Nerv Syst.* 1990;6:139–142.

62. Bruce DA. Delayed deterioration of consciousness after trivial head injury in childhood. *BMJ.* 1984;289:715–716.

63. Stiell IG, Wells GA, Vandemheen K, et al. The Canadian CT rule for patients with minor head injury. *Lancet.* 2001;357:1391–1396.

64. Brenner D, Elliston C, Hall E, et al. Estimated risks of radiation-induced fatal cancer from pediatric CT. *AJR.* 2001;176:289–296.

65. Brenner DJ. Estimating cancer risks from pediatric CT: going from the qualitative to the quantitative. *Pediatr Radiol.* 2002;32:228–233.

66. Duffner PK. Long-term effects of radiation therapy on cognitive and endocrine function in children with leukemia and brain tumors. *Neurologist.* 2004;10(6):293–310.

67. Schynoll W, Overton D, Krome R, et al. A prospective study to identify high-yield criteria associated with acute intracranial computed tomography findings in head injured patients. *Am J Emerg Med.* 1993;11:321–326.

68. Simon B, Letourneau P, Vitorino E, et al. Pediatric minor head trauma: indications for computed tomographic scanning revisited. *J Trauma Injury.* 2001;51:231–238.

69. Saab M, Gray A, Hodgkinson E, et al. Warfarin and the apparent minor head injury. *J Accid Emerg Med.* 1996;13:208–209.

70. Palchak MJ, Holmes JF, Vance CW, et al. A decision rule for identifying children at low risk for brain injuries after blunt head trauma. *Ann Emerg Med.* 2003;42:492–506.

71. Stein SC, Ross S. Mild head injury: a plea for routine early CT scanning. *J Trauma.* 1992;33:11–13.

72. Smits M, Dippel DWJ, Steyerberg EW, et al. Predicting intracranial traumatic findings on computed tomography in patients with minor head injury: the CHIP prediction rule. *Ann Intern Med.* 2007;146:397–405.

73. Rivara F, Tanaguchi D, Parish RA, et al. Poor prediction of positive computed tomographic scans by clinical criteria in symptomatic head trauma. *Pediatrics.* 1987;80:579–584.

74. Halley MK, Silva PD, Foley J, et al. Loss of consciousness: when to perform computed tomography. *Pediatr Crit Care Med.* 2004;5:230–233.

75. Da Dalt L, Marchi AG, Laudizi L, Crichuitti G, et al. Predictors of intracranial injuries in children after blunt head trauma. *Eur J Pediatr.* 2006;165(3):142–148.

76. Miller EC, Derlet RW, Kinser D. Minor head trauma: is computed tomography always necessary? *Ann Emerg Med.* 1996;27(3):290–294.

77. Palchak MJ, Holmes JF, Vance CW, et al. Does an isolated history of loss of consciousness or amnesia predict brain injuries in children after blunt head trauma? *Pediatrics.* 2004;113:e507–e513.

78. Kupperman N, Palchak MJ, Holmes JF. Loss of consciousness and/or amnesia after blunt head trauma in children. *Pediatr Crit Care Med.* 2005;6(1):93–94.

79. Dunning J, Batchelor J, Stratford-Smith P, et al. A meta-analysis of variables that predict significant intracranial injury in minor head trauma. *Arch Dis Child.* 2004;89:653–659.

80. Dunning J, Daly JP, Lomas JP, et al. Derivation of the children's head injury algorithm for the prediction of important clinical events decision rule for head injury in children. *Arch Dis Child.* 2006;91:885–891.

81. Ramundo M, McKnight T, Kempf J, et al. Clinical predictors of computed tomographic abnormalities following pediatric traumatic brain injury. *Pediatr Emerg Care.* 1995;11:27–30.

82. Zubovic C, Fogarty E, Shamdasani S, et al. Minor head injuries in children. *Ir Med J.* 2006;99(4):121–123.

83. Dunning J, Stratford-Smith P, Lecky F, et al. A meta-analysis of clinical correlates that predict significant intracranial injury in adults with minor head trauma. *J Neurotrauma.* 2004;21(7):877–885.

84. Haydel MJ, Preston CA, Mills TJ, et al. Indications for computed tomography in patients with minor head injury. *N Engl J Med.* 2000;343:100–105.

85. Mower WR, Hoffman JR, Herbert M, et al. Developing a decision instrument to guide computed tomographic imaging of blunt head injury patients. *J Trauma Injury.* 2005;59:954–959.

86. Oman JA, Cooper RJ, Holmes JF, et al. Performance of a decision rule to predict need for computed tomography among children with blunt head trauma. *Pediatrics.* 2006;117(2):e238–246.

87. Osmond MH, Klassen TP, Stiell IG, et al. The CATCH rule: a clinical decision rule for the use of computed tomography of the head in children with minor head injury. *Acad Emerg Med.* 2006;13(5s1):S11.

88. Doppenberg EMR, Ward JD. Pediatric head injury. In: Winn HR, ed. *Youmans Neurological Surgery,* 5th ed. Philadelphia, PA: Saunders; 2004:3473–3480.

89. McKinlay A, Kalrymple-Alford JC, Horwood LJ, et al. Long-term psychosocial outcomes after mild head injury in early childhood. *J Neurol Neurosurg Psychiatry.* 2002;73:281–288.

90. Paşaoğlu H, Karakucuk EI, Kurtşoy A, Paşaoğlu A. Endogenous neuropeptides in patients with acute traumatic head injury, I: cerebrospinal fluid β-endorphin levels are increased within 24 hours following the trauma. *Neuropeptides.* 1996;30(1):47–51.

91. Papa L, Hayes R, Robertson C, et al. Levels UCH-L1 in human CSF and severity of injury following severe traumatic brain injury. *Acad Emerg Med.* 2007;(5S1):S60.

92. Pineda JA, Lewis SB, Valadka AB, et al. Clinical significance of alpha II-spectrin breakdown products in cerebrospinal fluid after severe traumatic brain injury. *J Neurotrauma.* 2007;24(2):354–366.

93. Castillo M. Whole-brain *N*-acetylaspartate: a marker of the severity of mild head trauma. *AJNR.* 2007;28(5):914–915.

94. Ingebrigtsen T, Waterloo K, Jaconsen LA, et al. Traumatic brain damage in minor head injury: relation of serum S-100 protein measurements to magnetic resonance imaging and neurobehavioral outcome. *Neurosurgery.* 1999;45:468–476.

95. Woertgen C, Rothoerl RD, Metz C, et al. Comparison of clinical, radiologic, and serum marker as prognostic factors after severe head injury. *J Trauma.* 1999;47:1126–1130.

96. Woertgen C, Rothoerl RD, Metz C, et al. Comparison of clinical, radiologic, and serum marker as prognostic factors after severe head injury. *J Trauma.* 1999;47:1126–1130.

97. Ingebrigtsen T, Rominer B, Marup-Jensen S, et al. The clinical value of serum S-100 protein measurements in minor head injury: a Scandinavian multicentre study. *Brain Injury.* 2000;14:1047–1055.

98. Kavalci C, Pekdemir M, Durukan P, et al. The value of serum tau protein for the diagnosis of intracranial injury in minor head trauma. *AJEM.* 2007;25:391–395.

99. Décarie JC, Mercier C. The role of ultrasonography in imaging of paediatric head trauma. *Childs Nerv Syst.* 1999;15:740–742.

100. Mandera M, Larysz D, Wojtacha M. Changes in cerebral hemodynamics assessed by transcranial Doppler ultrasonography in children after head injury. *Childs Nerv Syst.* 2002;18:124–128.

101. Lee EJ, Chio CC, Chang CH, et al. Prognostic significance of altered cerebral blood flow velocity in acute head trauma. *J Formos Med Assoc.* 1997;96:5–12.

102. Tsung JW, Blaivas M, Cooper A, et al. A rapid noninvasive method of detecting elevated intracranial pressure using bedside ocular ultrasound: application to 3 cases of head trauma in the pediatric emergency department. *Pediatr Emerg Care.* 2005;21(2):94–98.

SECTION III. ORTHOPEDIC INJURIES

Jamie G. Lien and Ghazala Q. Sharieff

INTRODUCTION

Children present with different types of injuries than are commonly seen in adults due to unique aspects of the structure and physiology of their musculoskeletal system. This chapter section discusses musculoskeletal injuries that are unique to the pediatric population.

Bones in children are significantly more porous and pliable than those of adults, resulting in decreased stiffness and a greater tendency toward fracture. Children also have open growth plates, which are weaker than ligamentous attachments. As a result, fractures occur more frequently than sprains, dislocations and strains in children. The most common terms used in pediatric orthopedics are listed in Table 24.III.1.

Physical Examination

In an infant with a suspected orthopedic injury, a thorough physical examination guided by an accurate detailed history is necessary to avoid overlooking any findings. Understanding the mechanism of injury and force involved provides information about the possible location and severity of injury. A caregiver-provided history that is inconsistent with physical exam findings or a significant delay in seeking medical treatment may indicate intentional trauma.

On physical examination, start by observing the infant's behavior, looking for signs of pain such as guarding of an extremity, refusal to bear weight or persistent crying. The infant should be fully unclothed to facilitate visual inspection for areas of swelling, deformity, ecchymosis, abrasion, laceration or puncture. Palpation and manipulation of

Table 24.III.1. Definitions in pediatric orthopedics

- *Physis:* The cartilaginous growth plate that appears lucent on radiographs
- *Epiphysis:* A secondary ossification center at the end of a long bone that is separated by the physis from the remainder of the bone
- *Apophysis:* A secondary ossification center at the insertion of tendon onto bone
- *Diaphysis:* The shaft of a long cortical bone
- *Metaphysis:* The widened portion of the end of a bone adjacent to the physis

areas of suspected injury, which may cause increased discomfort, should be performed after completing the rest of the exam. The soft tissues and joints immediately proximal and distal to the affected site should be examined. In addition, it is important to perform a comparison examination of the contralateral side. Any extremity with a suspected orthopedic injury should be assessed specifically for neurovascular compromise.

Patients with orthopedic injuries should not be allowed to consume any food or drink until evaluation and treatment are completed, in the event that procedural sedation is needed. Appropriate pain management should be provided as soon as possible in all patients, including splinting and analgesics (see Chapter 3).

Radiographic Examination

When performing plain radiographs of children's bones, at least two views of the injured site that are perpendicular to one another should be obtained. Additional views may be helpful when initial radiographs show no abnormality but clinical suspicion for fracture is high. In addition, radiographs of the joints above and below the injury should be performed. Comparison views of the contralateral side can help discern normal growing anatomy from abnormal findings. Specific abnormalities such as fat pad signs in the elbow can help identify subtle fractures.

Interpreting radiographs of pediatric bones can be complicated by the appearance of epiphyseal centers at different ages. Normal growth centers may be mistaken for fracture fragments, highlighting the value of comparison views of the uninjured extremity. Figure 24.III.1 identifies the appearance of common ossification centers in the elbow.

Appearance of Ossification Centers (CRITOE)

Capitellum 1 to 8 months
Radial head 3 to 5 years
Internal (medial) epicondyle 5 to 7 years
Trochlea 7 to 9 years
Olecranon 8 to 11 years
External (lateral) epicondyle 11 to 14 years

FRACTURES UNIQUE TO CHILDREN

The anatomic and physiologic differences between the musculoskeletal systems of children and adults result

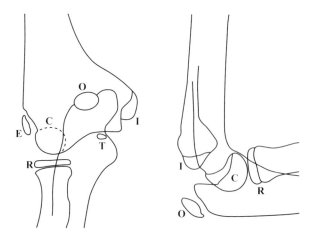

Figure 24.III.1. Ossification centers of the elbow. C = **C**api-tellum; R = **R**adial head; I = **I**nternal (medial) epicondyle; T = **T**rochlea; O = **O**lecranon; E = **E**xternal (lateral) epicondyle

in types of fractures unique to the pediatric population. These include physeal fractures, greenstick fractures, bowing fractures, torus fractures and metaphyseal fractures.

Physeal Fractures

The Salter-Harris classification is the most widely used system for describing physeal fractures (Figure 24.III.2). This is a radiological classification and is not anatomic, nor is it related to the mechanism or severity of injury. Increasing Salter-Harris classification type correlates with a worse prognosis for growth disturbance.

A *Salter-Harris type I fracture* is through the physis without extension proximally or distally. These fractures account for 6% of all physeal fractures; they may be displaced or nondisplaced. A nondisplaced type I fracture may not be obvious on x-ray acutely; therefore, clinical suspicion is the key to making the diagnosis. Patients typically present with circumferential tenderness along the physeal area. Prognosis is generally good, as long as near-anatomic alignment is achieved.

A *Salter-Harris type II fracture* extends through the physis and continues into the metaphysis. These fractures account for 75% of all physeal fractures. Undisplaced type II fractures generally do not cause growth disturbances.

A *Salter-Harris type III fracture* extends through the physis and continues into the epiphysis. These fractures account for approximately 8% of all physeal fractures and

usually occur in children who are older with a partially closed physis.

A *Salter-Harris type IV fracture* extends through the physis and into both the metaphysis and the epiphysis disrupting the intraarticular surface. These fractures account for 10% of physeal fractures. Types III and IV fractures need accurate reduction as partial or complete growth arrest may occur if correct positioning is not obtained.

A *Salter-Harris type V fracture* is a crush injury of the physis, resulting from axial compression, and is the most serious type of physeal fracture. Fortunately, type V fractures account for only 1% of physeal fractures. Type V fractures may not be clearly visible at the time of injury and are often diagnosed in retrospect when growth arrest is noted. Comparison views of the contralateral limb may be helpful in making the diagnosis acutely.

Greenstick Fractures

A *greenstick fracture* is incomplete and describes a fracture through only the tension side of a bone undergoing a deforming stress. The periosteum in pediatric bone is particularly thick and remains intact on the concave side of greenstick fractures. These fractures are typically angulated and may require conversion to a complete fracture in order to correct the deformity.

Bowing Fractures

Bowing fractures occur when the bone undergoes plastic deformation after an injury and does not recoil back to its original position (Figure 24.III.3). The fibula and ulna are most commonly involved. If there is a fracture of the adjacent bone, bowing can inhibit reduction of the fractured bone. Remodeling does not occur readily in bowing fractures, and thus anatomic reduction of a bowing deformity is necessary to prevent persistent deformation.

Torus Fractures

Torus, or *buckle*, *fractures* involve a failure of cortical bone with a compressive mechanism (Figure 24.III.4). These fractures occur over the metaphyseal region, particularly in the distal radius. Torus fractures are very common and stable, and they heal readily when immobilized. Complications are quite rare.

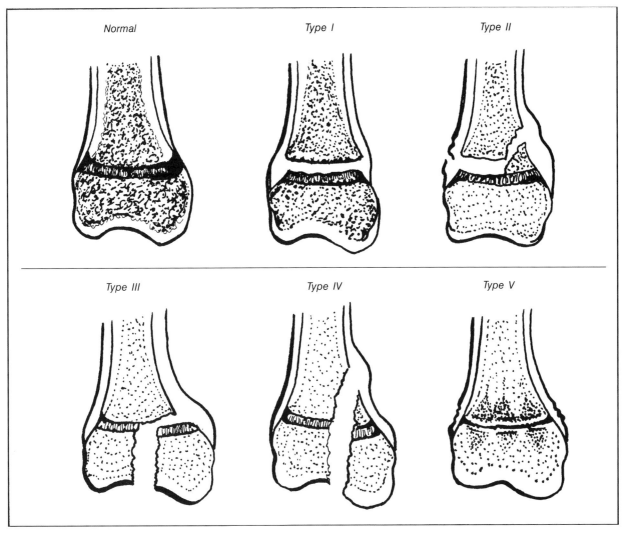

Figure 24.III.2. Salter-Harris classification. (Used with permission from Sharieff G. Pediatrics. In: Simon B, Sherman S, Koenisgsknecht, eds. *Emergency Orthopedics,* 5th ed. New York, NY: McGraw-Hill; 2007:91–118.)

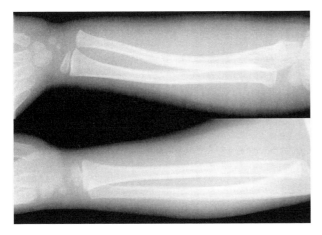

Figure 24.III.3. AP and lateral views of a bowing fracture of the ulna. (Courtesy of Loren Yamamoto, MD, Kapiolani Medical Center for Women and Children, University of Hawaii, John A. Burns School of Medicine.)

Metaphyseal Fractures

Also called *bucket handle* or *corner fractures, metaphyseal fractures* are planar fractures through the most immature part of growing bone and occur most frequently in the distal femur (Figure 24.III.5). Metaphyseal fractures in children who are not yet walking are highly suspicious for traumatic abuse. These fractures may be associated with minimal periosteal reaction and heal quickly (10 days to several weeks); therefore, they may be easily overlooked on radiograph.

NECK INJURIES

The level of cervical spine injury varies with age due to the effect of the relatively large head and ligamentous laxity in

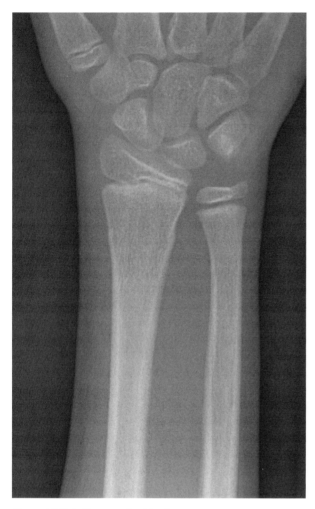

Figure 24.III.4. Torus, or buckle, fracture.

children. Therefore, when injury occurs in young children, high torques and shear forces are typically applied to the C1 to C3 region.[1] The incidence of neurologic deficit associated with cervical spine fractures or dislocations is 20% in children younger than 8 years of age and approximately 40% in children 8 to 16 years of age.[2]

In any patient with potential cervical spine or spinal cord injury, immobilization of the cervical spine in the neutral position is desired. Because of the relatively larger head compared to the torso in children younger than 8 years, and particularly under 4 years, supine placement on a flat surface results in a position of forced flexion, and it is recommended that either the torso be elevated or an occipital recess be created to achieve a more neutral position.[3]

Anteroposterior (AP) and lateral cervical spine radiographs are indicated in children who have experienced trauma and cannot communicate due to age or head injury or have a neurological deficit, neck pain or a painful distracting injury.[4]

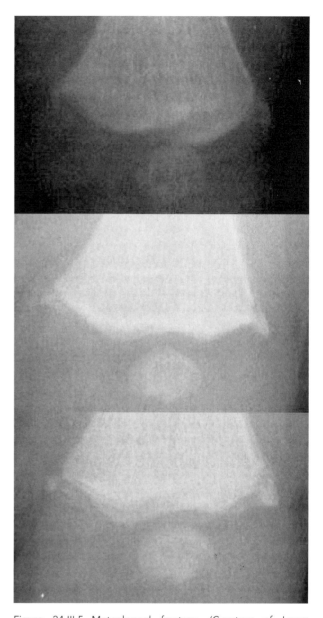

Figure 24.III.5. Metaphyseal fracture. (Courtesy of Loren Yamamoto, MD, Kapiolani Medical Center for Women and Children, University of Hawaii, John A. Burns School of Medicine.)

Pseudosubluxation

The extreme laxity of the cervical ligaments can increase the vertebral override of adjacent vertebrae in 46% of children younger than 8 years old.[1] This finding, known as *pseudosubluxation*, is most commonly found at the C2 to C3 level (Figure 24.III.6). To distinguish pseudosubluxation from true subluxation, Swischuk defined the *posterior cervical line* (Figure 24.III.7). This line is drawn by connecting the anterior aspects of the spinous processes of C1 and C3. If the anterior aspect of the spinous process of C2 misses this line by 2 mm or more, a true subluxation

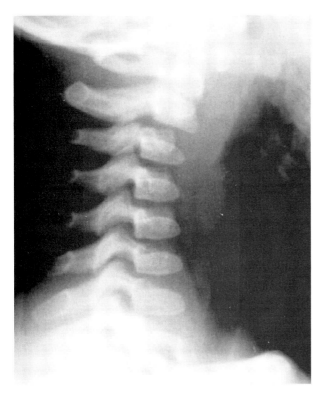

Figure 24.III.6. Pseudosubluxation of C2 on C3. (Courtesy of Loren Yamamoto, MD, Kapiolani Medical Center for Women and Children, University of Hawaii, John A. Burns School of Medicine.)

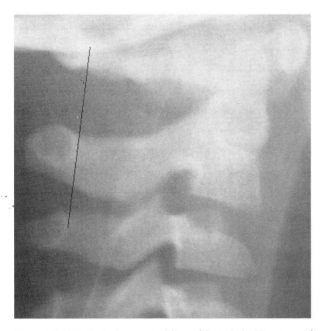

Figure 24.III.7. Posterior cervical line of Swischuk. (Courtesy of Loren Yamamoto, MD, Kapiolani Medical Center for Women and Children, University of Hawaii, John A. Burns School of Medicine.)

or a hangman's fracture of the neural arches of C2 should be suspected.

Spinal Cord Injury Without Radiographic Abnormality

In addition to vertebral injuries visible on plain radiographs, children may also suffer spinal cord injury without radiographic abnormality (SCIWORA). In children, the vertebral column is more elastic and flexible than the spinal cord. Therefore, a distraction injury may cause cord traction or ischemia without anatomic defects. Mechanisms that may result in SCIWORA include spinal cord traction, spinal cord concussion, vertebral artery spasm, hyperextension with inward bulging of the interlaminar ligaments and flexion compression of the cord.

The incidence of SCIWORA ranges from 18% to 38%, with most cases occurring in children younger than 8 years of age.[5] The upper cervical spine is involved in up to 80% of cases.[6] Most cases of SCIWORA present with some type of neurologic symptom, most commonly paresthesias and partial cord syndromes. However, delayed onset of neurologic deficit and complete cord transection can occur. Patients with suspected spinal cord injuries should be treated with a loading dose of methylprednisolone 30 mg/kg over 15 minutes, followed by a maintenance infusion of 5.4 mg/kg/hour for either 24 hours (if initiated <3 hours after injury) or 48 hours (if initiated 3–8 hours after injury).[7]

UPPER EXTREMITY INJURIES

Clavicle Fractures

The clavicle is the bone most commonly injured during delivery. Although there is a higher incidence of clavicle fractures following deliveries that require oxytocin, instrumental extraction, maneuvers for dystocia and prolonged second stage labor, clavicle fractures can occur during both vaginal deliveries and Cesarean sections. Clavicle fractures in neonates are typically greenstick fractures. These neonates may present with decreased or absent movement in the arm of the affected side, tenderness with manipulation, deformity and discoloration at the fracture site, and crepitus along the clavicle. In older children, clavicle fractures usually result from falls or direct blows and most commonly involve the middle one third of the clavicle. The majority of these fractures can be managed without orthopedic referral. Fractures of the clavicle can be treated with an arm sling, which is more comfortable than a figure-of-eight splint. Clavicle fractures in infants older than newborn should raise suspicion for nonaccidental trauma.

Elbow

The elbow is a common site for fractures in children. The typical history is a fall on an outstretched arm with hyperextension at the elbow and resultant injury to the distal humerus.

Radiographic evaluation of a child's elbow is made more complicated because of the six ossification centers around the elbow, which appear at different ages, earlier in girls than boys (see Figure 24.III.2). Consider obtaining comparison views of the opposite elbow if there is any question about a possible fracture.

Supracondylar Fractures

Supracondylar fractures are generally extra-articular, account for 50% to 70% of all elbow fractures and are most commonly seen in children between the ages of 3 and 11 years. The most common mechanism encountered is a fall on the outstretched arm with the elbow in extension.

Distal humeral fractures are associated frequently with neurovascular complications, even in the absence of displacement. The most commonly injured structures are the median nerve and the brachial artery. The physician must initially document the presence and strength of the radial, ulnar and brachial pulses. The presence of a pulse, however, does not exclude a significant arterial injury. The physician must also examine and document the motor and sensory components of the radial, ulnar and median nerves.

Routine imaging of a pediatric elbow with suspected injury must include AP and lateral projections with comparison to the uninjured extremity. Oblique views may also be helpful. Subtle changes, such as an abnormal anterior humeral line, an abnormal radiocapitellar line or the presence of a posterior fat pad, may be the only radiographic clues to the presence of a fracture. The *anterior humeral line* is a line drawn on a lateral radiograph along the anterior surface of the humerus through the elbow. Normally, this line transects the middle third of

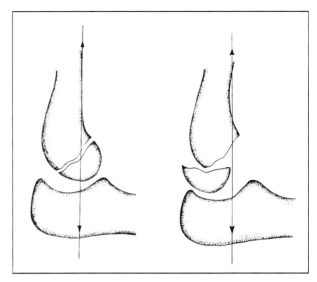

Figure 24.III.8. Anterior humeral line. (Used with permission from Sharieff G. Pediatrics. In Simon B, Sherman S, Koenisgsknecht, eds. *Emergency Orthopedics*, 5th ed. New York, NY: McGraw-Hill; 2007:91–118.)

the capitellum. With a supracondylar extension fracture, this line either transects the anterior third of the capitellum or passes entirely anterior to it (Figure 24.III.8). The *radiocapitellar line* is a line drawn through the radial neck and should pass through the capitellum (Figure 24.III.9). The two fat pads overlying the joint capsule along the distal humerus are displaced when there is fluid in the joint space, and these fat pads indicate occult fracture if no other abnormalities are seen. The *anterior fat pad* is

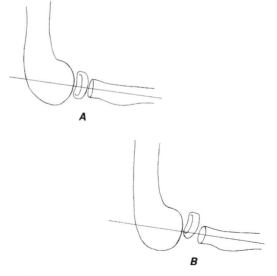

A

B

Figure 24.III.9. Radiocapitellar line. (Used with permission from Sharieff G. Pediatrics. In Simon B, Sherman S, Koenisgsknecht, eds. *Emergency Orthopedics*, 5th ed. New York, NY: McGraw-Hill; 2007:91–118.)

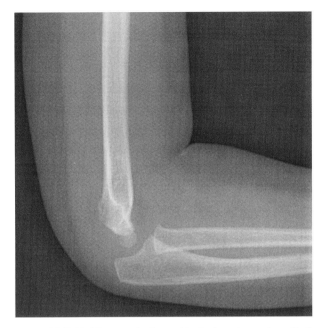

Figure 24.III.10. The anterior fat pad is displaced, creating a "sail sign." The posterior fat pad is also visible.

normally visible on a lateral radiograph, but when displaced it can create a *sail sign* (Figure 24.III.10). A visible *posterior fat pad* is always pathologic and raises the index of suspicion for a fracture (Figure 24.III.11).

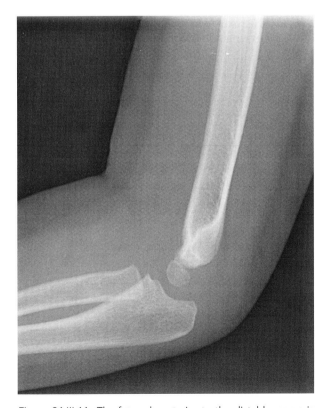

Figure 24.III.11. The fat pad posterior to the distal humerus is visible, indicating joint effusion and the presence of a fracture.

Nondisplaced supracondylar fractures are treated with cast immobilization. All displaced fractures require emergent consultation with an experienced orthopedic surgeon and admission for neurovascular monitoring.

Radial Head Subluxation (Nursemaid's Elbow)

Radial head subluxation (nursemaid's elbow) is a common orthopedic injury occurring in early childhood. The peak incidence is in the toddler years; however, the condition does occur in the first year of life and has been described as late as age 6 years.[8] The annular ligament provides support for the radial head, maintaining the head in its normal relationship with the humerus and the ulna. In children, there is little structural support between the radius and the humerus. With sudden traction of the hand or the forearm such as occurs when a parent pulls a child up by the arm to prevent a fall, the annular ligament is pulled over the radial head and is interposed between the radius and the capitellum[9] (Figure 24.III.12).

Children with radial head subluxation present because they are unable to use the affected arm, and they are noted to hold the arm at their side with the forearm in a pronated position. It is important to note that patients with radial head subluxation do not have swelling, warmth or ecchymosis about the elbow, and they have normal radiographs. Radiographs should be performed prior to reduction attempts in cases in which aspects of the history (e.g., witnessed direct trauma to the upper extremity) and examination findings (e.g., swelling, bruising or warmth over the joint) suggest that infection or fracture are more likely than radial head subluxation. Patients who present with a history and exam findings

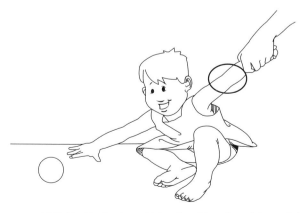

Figure 24.III.12. Mechanism of injury in subluxation of the radial head (nursemaid's elbow).

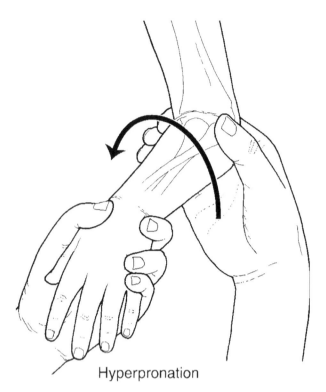

Figure 24.III.13. Hyperpronation technique for radial head sub-luxation reduction. (Used with permission from Sharieff G. Pediatrics. In: Simon B, Sherman S, Koenisgsknecht, eds. *Emergency Orthopedics*, 5th ed. New York, NY: McGraw-Hill; 2007:91–118.)

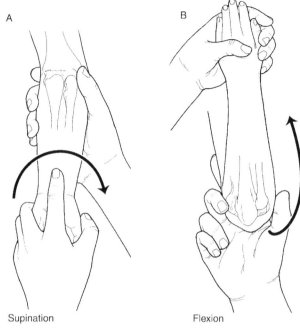

Figure 24.III.14. Supination/flexion technique for radial head subluxation reduction. (Used with permission from Sharieff G. Pediatrics. In: Simon B, Sherman S, Koenisgsknecht, eds. *Emergency Orthopedics*, 5th ed. New York, NY: McGraw-Hill; 2007: 91–118.)

consistent with radial head subluxation need not undergo radiography prior to reduction attempts. If radiographs of a subluxed radial head are obtained, they appear normal.

There are two different methods commonly used to reduce a nursemaid's elbow. Prospective studies comparing the two methods reveal that the hyperpronation technique has a higher initial success rate (95%) than the supination/flexion technique (77%).[10,11]

The *hyperpronation* method involves the examiner cradling the child's elbow with one hand (with thumb or forefingers overlying the radial head) while the examiner's other hand is used to hyperpronate the child's forearm by holding and turning the child's hand into a hyperpronated position. With successful reduction, a "click" is felt about the child's elbow by the examiner (Figure 24.III.13).

The *supination/flexion* technique involves the examiner cradling the child's elbow with one hand (again with thumb or forefingers over the radial head) and supinating the patient's hand completely. The examiner then fully flexes the child's elbow by bringing the supinated hand up

toward the shoulder. With successful reduction, a "click" is felt near the elbow (Figure 24.III.14).

Regardless of which reduction technique is used, the child typically begins to use the arm normally within 15 minutes. A failed reduction attempt should be followed by a second attempt using either the same or alternate technique. This second attempt often meets with success. If the reduction is unsuccessful after two or three attempts, radiographs of the upper extremity should be obtained to help exclude fracture or other pathology as the cause of the child's symptoms.

The child with a successfully reduced nursemaid's elbow does not need specific follow-up with the primary care provider unless symptoms (pain or disuse of the arm) return. Parents and caregivers should be cautioned about refraining from any activity that involves pulling on the child's arm as the condition recurs in about 25% of children who have experienced at least one episode.[12]

The patient who does not respond to attempts at reduction of presumed radial head subluxation requires close primary care follow-up and possibly orthopedic consultation.

HIP INJURIES

Developmental Dysplasia of the Hip

Developmental dysplasia of the hip (DDH) is an intra-articular displacement of the femoral head from its normal position within the acetabulum. DDH occurs more often in girls than in boys. The displacement of the femoral head leads to an interruption in the normal development of the joint occurring before or shortly after birth.[13] At birth, the acetabular fossa is shallow with the superior portion of the acetabulum poorly developed, offering little resistance to the upward movement of the head by muscle pull or weight-bearing. This can lead to a condition called *congenital subluxation of the femoral head,* in which the femoral head is displaced laterally and proximally and articulates with the outer portion of the acetabulum. In complete dislocation of the hip, the femoral head is located completely outside the acetabulum and rests against the lateral wall of the ilium. Later, a false acetabulum forms with a capsule interposed between the femoral head and the ilium.

In the normal infant, one sees folds in the groin, below the buttocks and along the thigh, which are symmetrical. In an infant with subluxation or dislocation of the hip, these folds are asymmetrical. When the examiner places the infant on the table, the pelvis and the limb on the affected side are pulled proximally by muscle action. This proximal displacement of the limb causes apparent shortening of the limb.

The Barlow and Ortolani tests should be performed as a routine part of every examination on all infants younger than 1 year of age, including patients seen in the emergency department. The *Barlow provocative test* is performed with the newborn positioned supine and the hips flexed to 90 degrees. The leg is then gently adducted while posteriorly directed pressure is placed on the knee. A palpable clunk or sensation of movement is felt as the femoral head exits the acetabulum posteriorly in an abnormal hip. In the *Ortolani click test*, the hip is flexed 90 degrees and the thigh is abducted. In the normal infant, the lateral aspect of both thighs nearly touch the table. In subluxation or dislocation, abduction is restricted and the involved hip is unable to be abducted as far as the normal one, producing an audible or palpable click as the femoral head slips over the acetabular rim. These maneuvers are performed one hip at a time.

Repeat examination of the infant is mandatory until the child starts walking because the lack of symptoms, including pain, and the subtle physical findings make early diagnosis difficult. Early treatment can prevent life-long complications. Patients with late-presenting DDH will typically present with a painless limp. There is usually a history of a delay in walking with the age of onset being between 14 and 15 months of age, instead of 12 months of age. The affected lower leg may be shortened, and the patient develops a positive Trendelenburg test. If the hip dysplasia is bilateral, the toddler may walk with a waddle. If untreated, these patients have persistent limp, external rotation and adduction deformity and limitation of internal rotation and abduction.

A radiograph of the pelvis after the infant is 4 months of age helps to confirm the diagnosis. Ultrasound may be effective for early diagnosis of this disorder in infants younger than 4 to 6 months of age.[14] However, the use of screening ultrasounds without risk factors (e.g., breech position in utero and family history) is not recommended. Close physical examination and referral to orthopedics for suspected cases is appropriate.[15] Early treatment involves use of a Pavlik harness, which maintains the hips in controlled flexion and abduction, preventing dislocation and allowing the acetabulum to develop normally.

Transient Synovitis

Transient synovitis is the most common cause of acute hip pain in children between 3 and 10 years of age. Typically, these children present with hip pain of 1 to 3 days' duration, accompanied by a limp or a refusal to bear weight. The extremity is held in flexion, adduction and internal rotation while the child resists all attempts at passive motion resulting from muscle spasm. The temperature is usually normal to slightly elevated and is rarely high. This condition has an uncertain etiology, and it is diagnosed through a process of exclusion. Patients often report a preceding viral or bacterial infection. The disorder is usually unilateral, although it can be bilateral.

Septic arthritis must first be ruled out because femoral head destruction and degenerative arthritis will result if septic arthritis is not treated promptly. In a recent study, a univariate analysis showed significant differences in body temperature, serum white blood cell (WBC) count, erythrocyte sedimentation rate (ESR) and C-reactive protein (CRP) levels between patients with septic arthritis and those with transient synovitis. Plain radiographs showed a displacement or blurring of periarticular fat pads in patients with acute septic arthritis, and multivariate regression analysis revealed that a fever, ESR greater than 20 mm/hour, CRP greater than 1 mg/dL, WBC higher than 11,000/mL and an increased hip joint space of greater than 2 mm were independent predictors of acute septic arthritis.[16] However, if any doubt exists as to the etiology of the pain, aspiration of the hip joint and culture of the synovial fluid are mandatory. The treatment for transient synovitis is rest and anti-inflammatory medication with close follow-up.[17]

Septic Arthritis and Osteomyelitis

Septic arthritis and osteomyelitis are not uncommon in children. The pathologic origin is hematogenous seeding, local invasion from contiguous infection or direct inoculation of the bone, either surgically or after trauma.

The presentation of septic arthritis usually consists of a fever, which may be low-grade, and *pseudoparalysis*, a refusal of the child to use a limb. Gentle passive motion, however, is usually allowed. Presenting symptoms in neonates may be as vague as increased irritability, fever or poor feeding.

Children with osteomyelitis have fever and tenderness to palpation particularly over the metaphysis. The femur and tibia are by far the most common bones affected. When the hip and shoulder are involved in osteomyelitis, the pus can track under the periosteum of the metaphysis into the adjacent joint and thus the patient may have findings of both osteomyelitis and septic arthritis.

The most common organisms involved in newborns with septic arthritis include staphylococci, *Haemophilus influenza* and gram-negative bacilli. In infants and children, *Staphylococcus aureus* is the most common major organism, as *H. influenza* disease has markedly decreased due to universal vaccination.

S. aureus is the pathogen in most cases of hematogenous osteomyelitis, with group A beta-hemolytic streptococci a distant second. *H. influenza* type B occurs more often in neonates and patients who are not immunized. Patients with sickle cell disease are also at risk for salmonella osteomyelitis.

The diagnosis of septic arthritis can be made when a child presents with a fever and elevations in the WBC count, CRP and ESR. Approximately 70% of patients

with an ESR of more than 30 mm/hour have arthralgia or arthritis of infectious or inflammatory origin. Those with an ESR of 40 mm/hour or more have bacterial infections as the cause of their refusal to walk.[18]

The diagnosis of osteomyelitis can be made by the presence of any two of the following diagnostic criteria:

- Purulence of the bone
- Positive bone or blood culture
- Localized erythema, edema or both
- Positive imaging study on radiography, scintigraphy or magnetic resonance imaging

Cultures taken from bone result in a yield of 80%. Blood cultures should be drawn on all patients suspected of having osteomyelitis, as these cultures are positive in up to 50% of patients.

Plain films are generally normal as it takes 7 to 10 days for radiographic changes to appear in either osteomyelitis or septic arthritis.[19] Soft tissue, however, may show changes earlier. The younger the child, the more likely one is to see widening of the joint space. Abnormal subluxation of the hip with widening of the joint space is the most common x-ray finding. Because plain radiographs are usually not helpful early in the course of this disease, negative films should be followed by skeletal scintigraphy. Scintigraphically guided aspiration of the hip evacuates pus, decreases damage to articular surfaces, differentiates joint sepsis from other effusions and helps direct antibiotic therapy. Computed tomography scans are not useful in establishing a diagnosis of acute musculoskeletal sepsis.[20]

In treating children with osteomyelitis and septic arthritis, oxacillin or cefazolin should be used. Clindamycin or vancomycin should be used in cases of suspected or confirmed methicillin-resistant *Staphylococcus aureus*.[21]

LOWER EXTREMITY INJURIES

Toddler's Fracture

A *toddler's fracture* is a nondisplaced spiral or oblique fracture of the lower third of the tibial shaft. This fracture occurs in patients between the ages of 9 months and 3 years and results from torsion of the lower leg (Figure 24.III.15). A fibula fracture is not present. Often, the parents do not recall any trauma, and the only complaint is an acute onset of difficulty walking or resistance to weight-bearing.

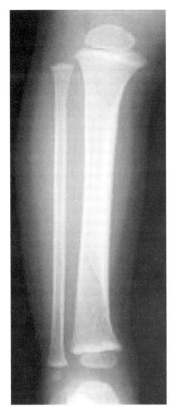

Figure 24.III.15. Toddler's fracture of the distal tibia.

Physical exam often fails to reveal swelling but may show increased warmth and pain with palpation of the lower third of the tibia.

AP and lateral films may appear normal; if clinical suspicion for a fracture is high, oblique views may confirm the diagnosis. Subperiosteal bone formation is seen on films obtained 2 to 3 weeks after injury, confirming the presence of a fracture which may not be visible on initial radiographs.

The treatment of radiographically confirmed toddler's fractures consists of a below-knee walking cast for approximately 3 weeks. The treatment of a presumed toddler's fracture, in which no fracture is visualized on the initial radiograph, is somewhat controversial. Some advocate splinting for comfort and repeating radiographs in 10 days, whereas others recommend casting all children with a history of acute injury, inability to walk or limp, no constitutional signs and negative radiographs in order to avoid a delay in treatment.[22]

OSTEOGENESIS IMPERFECTA

Osteogenesis imperfecta (OI) is a rare disorder of congenital bone fragility, caused by mutations in the genes that code for type I procollagen, an important structural component of many tissues. The severity of the disease ranges from mild to severe, with the most affected forms associated with death in the perinatal period. There are also many syndromes that resemble OI, which are associated with distinct clinical or histologic features. Most cases of OI are due to new mutations, although some patients have a family history of the disorder.

Patients with OI present with repeated fractures after minor trauma, often beginning in the childhood period. The most severe cases have in utero fractures. Patients have high pain tolerance, and their fractures may remain undetected. Most patients have normal bone healing. Blue sclera, easy bruising, progressive deafness, poor exercise tolerance and reduced muscle strength are other possible associated findings.

Diagnosis of OI is confirmed by skin biopsy. Management of fractures should involve an orthopedic surgeon, and long-term management of patients with OI requires a multidisciplinary approach.

PITFALLS

- Failure to obtain radiographs of a joint above and a joint below the area of pain
- Failure to suspect child abuse in patients with metaphyseal bucket handle or corner fractures
- Failure to suspect fracture in patients with soft tissue swelling of the elbow and performing reduction attempts for nursemaid's elbow
- Failure to perform the Barlow and Ortolani tests in all non-ambulatory infants
- Failure to suspect septic joint or osteomyelitis in patients with fever and decreased range of limb motion

REFERENCES

1. Baker C, Kadish H, Schunk JE. Evaluation of pediatric cervical spine injuries. *Am J Emerg Med.* 1999;17(3):230–234.
2. Apple JS, Kirks DR, Merten DF, et al. Cervical spine fractures and dislocations in children. *Pediatr Radiol.* 1987;17(1):45–49.
3. Nypayer M, Treloar D. Neutral cervical spine positioning in children. *Ann Emerg Med.* 1994;23:208–211.
4. Management of pediatric cervical spine and spinal cord injuries. *Neurosurgery.* 2002;50(3 Suppl):S85–99.
5. Proctor MR. Spinal cord injury. *Crit Care Med.* 2002;30(11 Suppl):S489–S499.
6. Kokoska ER, Keller MS, Rallo MC, et al. Characteristics of pediatric cervical spine injuries. *J Pediatr Surg.* 2001;36(1)100–105.

7. Bracken MB, Shepard MJ, Holford TR, et al. Administration of methylprednisolone for 24 or 48 hours or tirilazad mesylate for 48 hours in the treatment of acute spinal cord injury. Results of the Third National Acute Spinal Cord Injury Randomized Controlled Trial. National Acute Spinal Cord Injury Study. *JAMA.* 1997;277(20):1597–1604.

8. Schutzman SA, Teach S. Upper-extremity impairment in young children. *Ann Emerg Med.* 1995;26(4):474–479.

9. Bretland PM. Pulled elbow in childhood. *Br J Radiol.* 1994;67(804):1176–1185.

10. Macias CG, Bothner J, Wiebe R. A comparison of supination/flexion to hyperpronation in the reduction of radial head subluxations. *Pediatrics.* 1998;102(1):e10.

11. McDonald J, Whitelaw C, Goldsmith LJ. Radial head subluxation: comparing two methods of reduction. *Acad Emerg Med.* 1999;6(7):715–718.

12. Teach SJ, Schutzman SA. Prospective study of recurrent radial head subluxation. *Arch Pediatr Adolesc Med.* 1996;150(2):164–166.

13. Aronsson DD, Goldberg MJ, Kling TF Jr, et al. Developmental dysplasia of the hip. *Pediatrics.* 1994;94(2 Pt 1):201–208.

14. Roovers EA, Boere-Boonekamp MM, Castelein RM, et al. Effectiveness of ultrasound screening for developmental dysplasia of the hip. *Arch Dis Child Fetal Neonatal Ed.* 2005;90(1):F25–F30.

15. Clinical practice guideline: early detection of developmental dysplasia of the hip. Committee on Quality Improvement, Subcommittee on Developmental Dysplasia of the Hip. American Academy of Pediatrics. *Pediatrics.* 2000;105(4 Pt 1):896–905.

16. Jung ST, Rowe SM, Moon ES, et al. Significance of laboratory and radiologic findings for differentiating between septic arthritis and transient synovitis of the hip. *J Pediatr Orthop.* 2003;23(3):368–372.

17. Kermond S, Fink M, Graham K, et al. A randomized clinical trial: should the child with transient synovitis of the hip be treated with nonsteroidal anti-inflammatory drugs? *Ann Emerg Med.* 2002;40(3):294–299.

18. Lawrence LL. The limping child. *Emerg Med Clin North Am.* 1998;16(4):911–929, viii.

19. Barkin RM, Barkin SZ, Barkin AZ. The limping child. *J Emerg Med.* 2000;18(3):331–339.

20. Connolly LP, Connolly SA. Skeletal scintigraphy in the multimodality assessment of young children with acute skeletal symptoms. *Clin Nucl Med.* 2003;28(9):746–754.

21. Bradley J, Nelson J. *Nelson's Pocket Book of Pediatric Antimicrobial Therapy*, 16th ed. Buenos Aires, Argentina: Alliance for World Wide Editing; 2006:31.

22. Halsey MF, Finzel KC, Carrion WV, et al. Toddler's fracture: presumptive diagnosis and treatment. *J Pediatr Orthop.* 2001;21(2):152–156.

Pediatric Formulas

Maureen McCollough and Ghazala Q. Sharieff

Endotracheal Intubation

a. Tube size

   (16 + age in years)/4 or 4 + (age in years/4) for uncuffed tube
   3 + (age in years/4) for cuffed ETT

b. ETT placement: 10 + age in years (centimeters at the lips)
   1 kg newborn: 7
   2 kg newborn: 8
   3 kg newborn: 9
   4 kg newborn: 10
   or 3 × ETT size

Resuscitation Endotracheal Tube Sizing

   ETT size based on uncuffed formula
   2 × ETT size = NG/OG/Foley size
   3 × ETT size = ETT position at the lips
   4 × ETT size = Chest tube size

Rough Estimate of Weight in Kilograms

a. (2 × age in years) + 8
b. 1 year old weighs 10 kg; takes size 4.0 ETT
   5 year old weighs 20 kg; takes size 5.0 ETT
   10 year old weighs 30 kg; takes size 6.0 ETT

Systolic Blood Pressure Parameters

a. Preferred formula: (2 × **age in years**) + **90**
   This is the 50th percentile
b. Newborn systolic blood pressure: 60 mm Hg

Initial Fluid Bolus

a. Newborn: 10cc/kg NS or LR
b. Child: 20cc/kg NS or LR
   10cc/kg of PRBCs or FFP

ETT, endotracheal tube; FFP, fresh frozen plasma; LR, lactated Ringer's solution; NG, nasogastric; NS, normal saline; OG, orogastric; PRBC, packed red blood cell.

APPENDIX 2

Immunizations

Marla J. Friedman

Table A2.1. Childhood immunization schedule – United States, 2008

	Birth	1 mo	2 mos	4 mos	6 mos	12 mos	15 mos	18 mos	24 mos	4–6 yrs	11–12 yrs	15–18 yrs
Hepatitis B	HepB											
		|_____HepB_____|			|_____HepB 3_____|			|_____catch-up series_____|				
DTaP			DTaP	DTaP	DTaP		|__DTaP__|			DTaP	Tdap	|__catch-up series__|
HiB			HiB	HiB	HiB*	|__HiB__|						
Polio			IPV	IPV	|_____IPV_____|					IPV	|_____catch-up series_____|	
MMR						|__MMR__|				MMR	|_____catch-up series_____|	
Varicella						|_Varicella_|				Varicella	|_____catch-up series_____|	
Pneumococcal			PCV	PCV	PCV	|___PCV___|			|_____high-risk groups[†]_____|			
Influenza					|_____Influenza (Annually)_____|							
Rotavirus			Rota	Rota	Rota							
Hepatitis A						|_Hep A (2 doses)_|			|_____high-risk groups[‡]_____|			
Meningococcal									|___MPSV4[¶]___|	MCV4	|__catch-up series__|	
HPV											HPV	|__catch-up series__|

* Not required if vaccine containing PRP-OMP (Comvax, PedvaxHIB) given at 2 and 4 months.

[†] High-risk groups: sickle cell disease, HIV, asplenia, diabetes, heart/pulmonary disease.

[‡] High-risk groups: chronic liver disease, clotting disorders, travel to developing countries, illicit drug use, homosexual adolescent males.

[¶] Children 2–10 years of age with anatomic/functional asplenia, terminal complement deficiencies, travel to or residence in areas of epidemic meningococcal disease.

DTaP, diphtheria, tetanus, acellular pertussis; HiB: *Haemophilus influenza* type B; HPV: human papillomavirus; MMR, measles, mumps, rubella; Tdap, tetanus and diphtheria toxoids, acellular pertussis.

Adapted from recommendations of the Advisory Committee on Immunization Practices (www.cdc.gov/vaccines/recs/acip), the American Academy of Pediatrics (www.aap.org), and the American Academy of Family Physicians (www.aafp.org).

Table A2.2. Combination vaccines

	Approved use	Notes
Pediarix (DTaP, IPV, hepatitis B)	Only for 3-dose primary series at 2, 4, 6 mos; ages 6 wks–6 yrs	Do not use for booster doses
MMRV (ProQuad) (measles, mumps, rubella, varicella)	12 mos–12 yrs	2 doses ≥3 mos apart
Comvax (HiB, hepatitis B)	6 wks–15 mos; for children born to HBsAg negative mothers	If given at 2 and 4 mo, no dose needed at 6 mo
TriHIBit (DTaP, HiB)	Only as a booster dose after other HiB vaccine; age ≥12 mo	Cannot be used for primary series
Twinrix (hepatitis A, hepatitis B)	Age ≥18 yrs	3 doses within 4 wks (0, 7, 21–30 days); booster dose at 12 months

DTaP, diphtheria, tetanus, acellular pertussis; HBsAg, hepatitis B surface antigen; HiB, *Haemophilus influenza* type B; IPV, inactivated poliovirus.

Table A2.3. Factors that are not contraindications to immunization

Mild local reaction (soreness, redness, swelling) to previous vaccination
Fever after previous vaccine dose
Mild acute illness with or without fever
Current antimicrobial therapy
Prematurity (infants should receive same dosage and schedule as full-term infants)
Recent exposure to infectious disease
Unimmunized household contact
Immunocompromised or pregnant household contact
HIV infection (unless low CD4+ counts)

Table A2.4. Children at risk for invasive pneumococcal infections

High risk
　Sickle cell disease and/or asplenia
　Immunodeficiency
　Chronic renal, cardiac or pulmonary disease
　Diabetes
　Cochlear implants
Moderate risk
　Children 24–35 months of age
　Children 36–59 months of age in out-of-home daycare
　African American or American Indian children aged 36–59 months
　Low socioeconomic status
　Homelessness
　Chronic exposure to tobacco smoke
　History of recurrent otitis media or tympanostomy tubes

Pediatric Procedures

Maureen McCollough and Ghazala Q. Sharieff

PEDIATRIC FOREIGN BODY REMOVAL

Ear
- Round objects: Use loop curettes
- Insects: Use Alligator forceps
- Don't forget to check other ear!

Nose
- Occlude nonobstructed nostril and have parent blow gently but quickly into child's mouth. Warn parent this might result in snot on parent's cheek.
- Occlude nonobstructed nostril and blow into child's mouth gently but quickly with a bag-valve-mask.
- Insert 6-French Foley catheter past the obstruction, gently inflate and pull out foreign body.

Esophagus
- Acute coin ingestions that are above the thoracic inlet should be removed. However, if the coin was ingested prior to emergency department (ED) arrival and the patient is asymptomatic, a radiograph may be obtained to check for downward movement of the coin.
- A coin in the mid-esophagus or distal esophagus can be observed for 24 hours. If the coin has not moved into the stomach, it should be removed.
- All button batteries in the esophagus should be removed.

NEEDLE THORACOSTOMY AND PERCUTANEOUS CHEST TUBES

Diagnosis
- Children requiring positive-pressure ventilation in the ED are at high risk for pneumothoraces or tension pneumothoraces.
- Remember mnemonic for sudden deterioration of an intubated patient:
  - D – Dislodgement – check endotracheal tube (ETT) placement
  - O – Obstruction – suction ETT
  - P – Tension pneumothorax – diagnosis of exclusion
  - E – Equipment failure – check tubing, O_2 source, ventilator
- *Tension pneumothorax:* Sudden desaturation, hypotension and bradycardia. There also may be decreased breath sounds, shift of PMI, decreased chest rise, hyperresonance or tympany of the chest.
- In young infants, it may be possible to transilluminate chest wall.
- If there is a true tension pneumothorax, do not wait for an x-ray.

Needle Thoracostomy
- Prepare skin with povidone-iodine.
- Connect 3-way stopcock between 18- or 20-gauge Angiocath and syringe; open stopcock to the Angiocath
- Insert Angiocath at a 45-degree angle to the skin, directed cephalad, in the 4th or 5th intercostal space, just over top of ribs, below breast tissue, in the anterior axillary line.
- Withdraw on the syringe as you are inserting the Angiocath until you get a rush of air.
- As the angiocatheter enters the pleural space, decrease the angle to 15 degrees above the chest wall and slide the catheter in while removing the needle stylet.
- Withdraw the needle stylet from the catheter and reattach the catheter to the stopcock and continue withdrawing air, then close the stopcock to the child and depress the syringe to evacuate the air in it.

- Alternatively, you can use a butterfly needle, inserted at a 90-degree angle to the skin in the 2nd or 3rd intercostal space, midclavicular line, attached to stopcock and syringe as described earlier.

Percutaneous Chest Tubes

Rough rule for chest tube size $= 4 \times$ ETT size.

- This procedure is similar to percutaneous central line placement using guidewire and dilators.
- Chest tube should be placed in the 4th or 5th intercostal space.
- Measure the chest tube length necessary, from the area of skin insertion to the mid-clavicle area.
- Using a finder needle to enter the pleural air space. A few milliliters of normal saline in the syringe will help to identify air as bubbles will appear. Once the pleural space is entered, remove the syringe and insert the guidewire into the pleural space through the finder needle.
- Remove the finder needle; nick the skin with the blade going directly on top of the guidewire.
- Place the first dilator over the guidewire and insert it into the chest.
- Remove the first dilator and proceed, in order, with subsequently larger and larger dilators.
- After the last dilator has been used and removed, the tract that has been created should be large enough to accommodate the chest tube chosen.
- Place chest tube over the guidewire and remove the guidewire.
- Observe for humidity or bubbling in chest tube to verify intrapleural location.
- Connect the chest tube to the drainage system without putting tension on tube.
- Secure chest tube to skin with a pursestring suture.

Complications

- Misdiagnosis with resultant unnecessary chest tube placement
- Lung laceration or perforation, puncture of liver, damage to breast tissue, chylothorax
- Horner's syndrome due to nerve damage or phrenic nerve injury
- Misplacement of tube: into subcutaneous tissue, with last side-hole outside of pleural space, or with tip of chest tube across the mediastinum

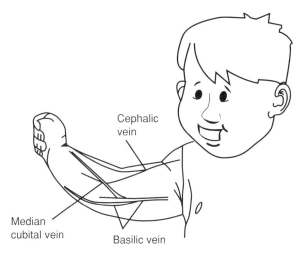

Figure A3.1.

- Infection
- Subcutaneous emphysema

VASCULAR ACCESS

Peripheral Access

- Effective for blood samples or administration of fluid or medications
- External jugular has low risk of pneumothorax or injury to carotid and is relatively safe in a child with a coagulopathy.
- Preferred sites (Figures A3.1 and A3.2)
  Antecubital

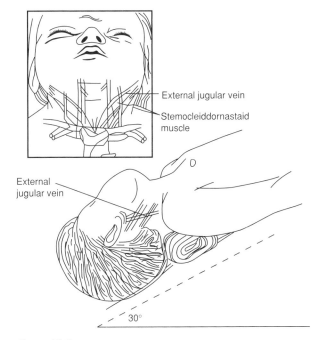

Figure A3.2.

Dorsum of hand

Basilic/cephalic vein

Saphenous vein

Scalp veins

External jugular

- 22- or 24-gauge catheters are the ones used primarily in children.

Saphenous Vein Cutdown

- The location is 1–2 cm anterior to medial malleolus.
- Externally rotate the leg.
- Make a 2-cm transverse incision over the medial malleolus.
- Perform a blunt dissection parallel to the vein.
- Tie-off the distal end of the vein.
- Loosely wrap a tie around the proximal ends of the vein.
- Make an incision in the upper one third of the vein; advance the catheter into the vein.
- Secure the catheter with the proximal tie already in place

Cutdown Complications

- Bleeding
- Phlebitis or infection
- Nerve damage

CENTRAL VENOUS ACCESS*

Femoral Vein

- This is a dirty area for central vein access but it is the easiest of the central veins to find in small kids.
- Remember, NERVE – ARTERY – VEIN from lateral to medial (Figure A3.3).
- If a line is drawn between the anterior superior iliac spine and symphysis pubis, the femoral artery runs directly across at the midpoint, and medial to that is the vein
- When accessing the femoral vein using the needle that advances the guidewire, try finding the vein *without a syringe on the needle;* when the needle advances into the vein, blood will fill the hub of the needle; at this point, insert the guidewire and advance it into the vein.

Subclavian Vein – Tips for Access

- Higher risk of pneumothorax
- Place the child in the Trendelenburg position and place a small rolled towel under the thoracic area to open it up.

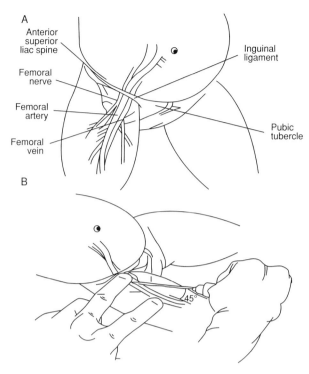

Figure A3.3.

- Use a tuberculin syringe instead of a large syringe to find the vessel; a larger syringe may collapse the vein and make it possible to miss the flash.

Internal Jugular Vein

- Landmarks may be difficult to find in small children; remember that the vein tends to lie lateral to the artery.
- Risk of puncturing carotid artery
- Contraindicated if the child has a coagulopathy

* as with all vascular access, ultrasound can improve the practitioner's ability to find and cannulate the vessel

Complications

- Pneumothorax
- Bleeding and hematoma secondary to laceration of the vessel
- Arterial puncture
- Air or catheter embolism
- Infection
- Hemothorax

INTRAOSSEOUS LINE*

- Reserved for situations in which a child in severe shock has failed 3 attempts at intravenous (IV) access or 90 seconds have elapsed in the attempt.

- Use this vascular access route as FIRST-LINE approach for pediatric CARDIAC ARRESTS (nearly impossible to achieve peripheral access in a young child in full arrest).

* Pediatric Advanced Life Support recommendation is to use intraosseous (IO) lines as needed in all pediatric age groups.

Absolute Contraindications*
- Previous attempt in that bone
- Ipsilateral fracture

* In both of these situations, any fluid or medication given will flow out of the bone marrow area and into the surrounding subcutaneous tissue.

Relative Contraindications
- Osteogenesis imperfecta
- Local infection

Preferred Sites
- Proximal aspect of tibia
- Distal aspect of tibia on malleoli
- Distal aspect of femur

Equipment
- IO needle or bone marrow needle
- 10-cc syringe
- Saline flush

- 3-way stopcock
- T-connector IV tubing

Procedure
- Clean the area with povidone-iodine solution
- Proximal tibia landmarks: 2 fingerbreadths distal to the tibial tuberosity, on the flat part of the tibia (medially)
- Insert the IO needle perpendicular to the bone using twisting back-and-forth motion with gentle pressure.
- If possible, during insertion, angle the needle away from the epiphyseal growth plate.
- Placement is verified by lack of resistance, needle standing erect in bone without support, aspiration of bone marrow and free flow of fluids (Figure A3.4).
- New devices are available such as the EZ-IO and the BIG (bone injection gun).

Complications
- Complications are very rare with IO lines; the rate of infection is higher for peripheral IV access compared to IO line placements.
- Osteomyelitis <1% or other infections
- Extravasation of fluid, cellulitis, fractures, epiphyseal cartilage
- Fat embolism
- Compartment syndrome
- Skin necrosis

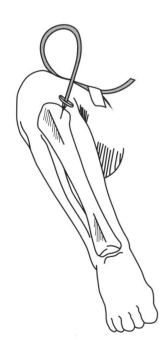

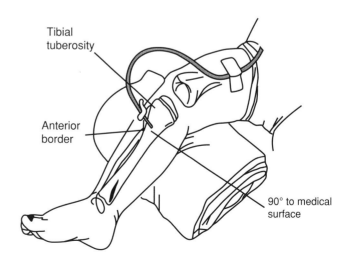

Figure A3.4.

UMBILICAL VEIN CATHETERIZATION

- The umbilical vein remains patent for at least 1 week after birth; it is used to provide access in newborns or young neonates who require emergent vascular access after peripheral attempts have been unsuccessful.

Equipment
- Antiseptic solution and sterile gauze pads
- Sterile drapes
- Umbilical tape or 3-0 silk suture on a straight needle
- Small hemostat
- Sterile scalpel
- 3.5- or 5-French umbilical catheter (can also use 5-French feeding tubes)
- 3-way stopcock
- 10-cc syringe
- Saline flush

Procedure
- Place the newborn supine and restrain extremities as necessary.
- Place newborn on a cardiac monitor and pulse oximeter; also monitor newborn's temperature; use warming bed or lamps, if possible.
- Attach a 5-French umbilical catheter (or feeding tube) to the 3-way stopcock and syringe filled with saline.
- Flush the catheter with saline.
- Clean the umbilical stump and abdomen from xyphoid to pubic symphysis.
- Loosely tie umbilical tape or silk suture around the base of the umbilical stump.
- Cut the cord 1–2 cm from the abdominal wall.
- Identify the vessels (the umbilical vein is a single, thin walled, large diameter lumen, usually located at the 12-

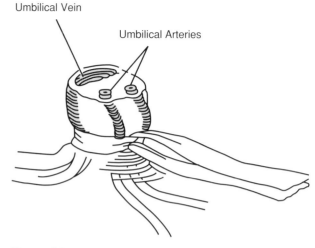

Umbilical Vein

Umbilical Arteries

Figure A3.5.

o'clock position; the arteries are paired and have thicker walls with a smaller diameter lumen.
- The cut end of the cord resembles "Oh no, Mr. Bill" from *Saturday Night Live* (Figure A3.5).
- Gently remove any clot from the umbilical vein.
- Insert the catheter until there is a free return of blood.
- Confirm catheter placement with an abdominal x-ray. The catheter should not curve into the right upper quadrant; it might be entering hepatic portal circulation. The x-ray should show placement at or above the diaphragm.

Complications
- Infection
- Embolization or thrombosis
- Vessel perforation
- Hemorrhage
- Ischemia of extremities or intra-abdominal organs

Other Environmental Emergencies*

Ghazala Q. Sharieff

*Adopted from Sharieff G, Joseph M, Wylie T. Pediatric Quick Glance. McGraw-Hill 2005.

PATHOPHYSIOLOGY

- 300 injuries/100 fatalities per year in the United States.
- 2/3 of lightning strike survivors have permanent sequelae.
- The fetus is at higher risk of injury than the mother due to the 200-fold less resistance of fetal skin and also because the hyperemic pregnant uterus and amniotic fluid also conduct electricity well.
- Extent of injury is determined by:
  - **Tissue resistance**
    1. ↑ Resistance generates greater heat and resultant thermal injury
    2. (**Highest**) Resistance bone> fat > tendon > skin > muscle > vessels > blood > nerves (**lowest**)
  - **Intensity of current**
    1. Skin with lower resistance (i.e. thin, high H_2O content, newborn) allows for deeper tissue damage
    2. Pregnancy: (fetal death) alternating current (AC) > lightning > direct current (DC)
  - **Pathway of current flow**- contact to "ground"
    1. **Hand to hand** (↑ mortality due to transection of the spinal cord from C4-C8)
    2. **Hand to foot** (causes dysrhythmias)
    3. **Foot to foot**-mortality is < 5%
  - **Types of current**
    1. **AC:** Causes tetany, "lock on" phenomenon
       a. Commercial high voltage
       b. Household low voltage
    2. **DC:** Massive energy, but brief contact resulting in a single strong contraction
       a. Lightning (direct strike, side, stride potential, flash over phenomenon)
       b. Defibrillation

DEFINITIONS

- **Direct strike:** most serious type, major current flow is through the victim's body.
- **Side Flash:** Lightning passes from the primary strike area through the air to a nearby victim.
- **Stride potential:** current hits the ground, enters one leg of the victim and exits through the other leg. Mortality rate of 30% in patients with leg burns due to stride potential.
- **Flash over phenomenon:** lightning energy flows outside the body of the victim usually via wet clothes. Pathognomonic featherlike skin burns may be present.

CLINICAL MANIFESTATIONS

- Cardiac
  - Primary cause of death (dysrhythmias, myocardial damage, secondary to respiratory arrest)
  - AC current results in ventricular fibrillation
  - DC current results in asystole
  - Lightning is direct current (asystole)
- Pulmonary
  - Respiratory center paralysis or forced tetanic contractions of respiratory muscles
  - Aspiration, acute respiratory distress syndrome (ARDS), pulmonary edema
  - Duration of apnea appears to be the critical factor in patient survival, so aggressive management in the clinically dead is indicated.
- Central Nervous System
  - Most frequently involved system
  - Immediate effects are loss of consciousness, paralysis, visual disturbances, amnesia, intracranial hematoma, Horner's syndrome
  - Later complications include: paraplegia, brachial plexus injury, syndrome of inappropriate secretion

of antidiuretic hormone (SIADH), diabetes insipidus (DI), hearing loss, neuropathy, seizures
- Renal
  - ↑ Injuries with high voltage electrical injury
  - Hypoxic renal injury is a direct effect of current on tissue
  - Myoglobinuria (most common- especially with "lock on" tetany)
- Oral
  - "Child bites cord" or "sucks on live cord"
  - Intense heat causes coagulation necrosis and liquefaction- lesions are painless because the nerves are destroyed.
  - Lip commissure burn/eschar complication "delayed bleeding of labial artery" 5–14 days later
  - Long term effects: microstomia, speech problems, adhesions, abnormal dentition/arch formation
- Ocular
  - Cataracts, optic neuritis/neuropathy, extraocular muscle paralysis
- Fractures/ compartment syndrome

MANAGEMENT

- Prehospital
  - Extrication, removal from source, cut wires with wooden cutters
  - Cervical spine immobilization
- Hospital
  - IV- NS or LR 20cc/kg bolus. Titrate to urine output > 1 cc/kg/hr
  - Intubate for intracranial injuries
  - Minimal fluid resuscitation for lightning injuries due to CNS effects
  - CBC, chemistry panel, urinalysis, myoglobin, creatine phosphokinase (CPK), electrocardiogram (ECG), x-rays as needed
  - Myoglobinuria: keep urine pH > 7.45, lasix (1 mg/kg), mannitol (0.5 mg/kg)
  - Aggressive respiratory management even if patient seems "dead"
  - Cardiac arrest from lightning injury have higher survival rates
  - Dysrhythmias- ACLS/ PALS protocol
  - Fasciotomy may be needed for compartment syndrome

- Admit all children (except those with minor burns and those who are asymptomatic after a minor household injury)
- Admit all lightning injuries
- Tetanus booster

HEAT INDUCED ILLNESSES

OVERVIEW
- Neonates and infants < 2 years lack good thermoregulatory control, have greater surface area:mass ratio, and have a high metabolic rate.
- Older children differ from adults in that they do not sweat as much, have greater surface area:mass ratio; do not instinctively replace losses or limit exertion in extreme heat.
- Teenagers exercise in the heat and athletes push themselves to their limits, may not adequately replace losses, especially over consecutive days of exertion.
- Chronic diseases such as cystic fibrosis (CF), quadriplegia, and anhidrosis may ↓ ability to sweat.
- Drugs causing heat production include amphetamines and cocaine; phencyclidine (PCP) and D-lysergic acid diethylamide (LSD) ↓ sweating, as do antihistamines, phenothiazines, anticholinergics, diuretics, β-blockers & alcohol.

PATHOPHYSIOLOGY
- **Endogenous** heat production due to physical activity, thyroid activity, epinephrine, and fever (pyrogens stimulate prostaglandins, resetting the hypothalamus).
- **Exogenous** heat is environmental.
- **Usual core temperature** is 37° C +/− 0.6 (98.6° F +/−1)
- **Heat illness**
  - Results when heat cannot be dissipated by:
    1. Conduction
    2. Convection
    3. Radiation (usually 60% of losses)
    4. Evaporation (25%)
- **Hypothalamus**
  - Controls heat by:
    1. Dilation of cutaneous blood vessels by inhibition of sympathetic stimulators in the posterior hypothalamus (maximal at 40° C)
    2. Stimulation of sweating via sympathetic stimulation

3. Inhibition of heat production by stopping shivering, which causes ↓ release of thyrotropin releasing hormone
- **Temperature > 40° C**
  - Causes splanchnic vasoconstriction resulting in:
    1. Nausea, vomiting, diarrhea
    2. ↓ Urine output, ↑ liver enzymes, blood urea nitrogen (BUN), creatinine
    3. Hypocalcemia, hyper/hypokalemia
    4. Changes in blood sugar level
  - Acute renal failure commonly occurs in severe heatstroke, rhabdomyolysis being a major contributing factor.
  - Persistent temperature > 42° C causes CNS disturbances (disorientation, seizures, coma) with cellular injury possible.
  - Death occurs due to circulatory or respiratory collapse, disseminated intravascular coagulation (DIC), electrolyte imbalance, or cerebral edema.

TYPES OF HEAT ILLNESSES

- Prickly heat
  - (Miliaria) acute inflammatory skin eruption with sweat gland blockage caused by heat and humidity. Rash is maculopapular with erythema and vesicles.
  - **Treat** by wearing light loose clothing and maintaining a cool environment; avoid talcs and powders.
- Heat edema
  - Dependent swelling of hands and feet with sudden changes in temperature. Self-limited and resolves spontaneously probably caused by aldosterone production.
  - **Treat** by being in a cool environment
- Heat syncope
  - Seen during early heat acclimation, associated with postural hypotension and dehydration, worsened by prolonged standing or vigorous activity.
  - **Treat** by removing from heat, supine position, oral rehydration, rest.
- Heat cramps
  - Occur in active muscle groups with spasms during or after activity, sometimes with ↑ body temperature. Etiology thought to be salt depletion and drinking hypotonic fluids.
  - **Treat** by removing from heat, oral (one teaspoon of salt in 500cc water) or IV rehydration depending on severity of dehydration.

- Heat exhaustion
  - Temperature is < 40° C and mental status is **normal**
  - **Two types:**
    1. **Water-depletion** with quick onset after high temperatures and insufficient fluids.
    2. **Salt-depletion** with onset over several days in people rehydrating with inadequate salt; more in unacclimatized people whose sweat contains more salt.
  - **Laboratory studies:** ↑ hematocrit (HCT), ↑ BUN, ↓ glucose, hypernatremia or hyponatremia
  - **Caused by:**
    1. High temperatures
    2. Excessive sweating
    3. Inadequate water and salt replenishment
  - **Symptoms:** headache, nausea, vomiting, lethargy, irritability, thirst, anorexia
  - May be a precursor to heat stroke
  - **Treat** with removal from heat, fluid replacement (oral if mild, IV if severe), rest.
- Heatstroke
  - Medical emergency with temperature > 40.6° C (105° F), neurologic dysfunction and often anhidrosis.
  - Loss of thermostatic control with uncontrolled rise in temperature causing:
    1. Cellular injury (edema, vacuolization, hemorrhage) including rhabdomyolysis
    2. Renal failure
    3. Hepatocellular necrosis
    4. Myocardial damage
    5. Cerebral edema.
  - **Classic** – nonexertional, infants/elderly, develops over days during a heat wave
  - **Exertional** – develops rapidly in young, vigorously exercising individuals who are unacclimatized to a hot environment
  - Laboratory studies: show electrolyte disturbances, evidence of liver and renal injury
  - Disseminated intravascular coagulation (DIC) may develop
  - For each degree > 37° C, adjustments need to be made for (pH ↓ 0.015, PCO_2 ↑4.4, PO_2 ↑ 7.2)
  - **Treat** by airway stabilization, remove clothing, ice packs to axillae, groin and neck; spray with water and fan until temperature is < 39° C; IV rehydration with normal saline 20 cc/kg, consider central venous monitoring if considering further fluids

ACCIDENTAL HYPOTHERMIA AND FROSTBITE

HYPOTHERMIA

- **Definition**- Core body temperature ≤35° C (95° F).
- **Moderate Hypothermia**-Core temperature = 30–32° C (86–89° F).
- **Profound Hypothermia**- Core temperature < 28° C (82° F).
- **Afterdrop**- Continued ↓ in core temperature; even after the patient is removed from the cold stress.
- **Aftershock**- State of depletion of intravascular volume that occurs with rewarming.
- **Complications of hypothermia:**
  - Gastrointestinal (GI) bleeding
  - Acute renal failure
  - Pancreatitis
  - Deep vein thrombosis (DVT)
  - Disseminated intravascular coagulation
  - Pulmonary edema
  - Dysrhythmias
- **Factors that influence thermoregulatory balance in infant and children:**
  - Large surface area/body weight ratio
  - Minimal subcutaneous fat
  - Thin skin with ↑ permeability
  - Delayed shivering and inefficient ability to generate heat
  - Immature or inappropriate behavioral response to environment
  - Infants and young children have specialized body cells called "brown fat cell"- allows for a tripling of heat production by infants- mostly found in neck and shoulder region
- **Mechanisms of heat loss**
  - **Radiation**-65% of heat loss
  - **Conduction**-transfer of heat from one object to another
  - **Convection**-heat flow from one object to a moving object
  - **Evaporation**-heat transfer as matter changes form
- **Signs and Symptoms of Hypothermia**
  - 35° C (95° F): Maximal shivering and slurred speech
  - 32° C (89° F): Altered level of consciousness (ALOC), dilated, but reactive pupils, shivering stops
  - 30° C (86° F): Resuscitation drugs may be inactive, ↓ respiratory rate
  - 28° C (82° F): Bradycardia refractory to atropine, Osborne, (J) waves; pupils nonreactive

- 25° C (79° F): Fixed and dilated pupils, maximum risk of ventricular fibrillation (V. Fib), areflexia
- 20° C (68° F): Cardiac systole common
- **Poor Prognostic Indicators:**
  - Core temperature <15° C (59° F)
  - Potassium >10 mEq/l
  - Fibrinogen < 50
  - Exposure > 24 hours
  - Absence of cardiac rhythm
- **Management**
  - **Prehospital**
    1. Avoid rewarming of frozen limbs until cardiovascular and metabolic problems are under control.
    2. No first-line resuscitation drugs if core temperature < 30° C
    3. Volume re-expansion is a key aspect to therapy for hypothermic patients- administration of IV saline before rewarming reduced mortality rate from 75% to 17%.
  - **Hospital**
    1. Primary consideration- return to normothermia
    2. Use pre-warmed normal saline (NS); thoracic, peritoneal, gastric cavity lavage with heated IV fluids
- **Resuscitation attempts**
  - V. Fib- try 1 J/kg, then initiate resuscitation drugs when core temperature is > 30° C
  - No need for intubation prophylaxis
  - Atrial arrhythmias more common and usually respond to rewarming
  - Use NS **not** lactated ringers (LR), since cold liver does not metabolize lactate
  - Rewarm frozen extremities after core temperature is 32–34° C (89–93° F), then use 40° C water immersion
  - Antibiotics recommended in patients with moderate to severe hypothermia
  - Rewarm patient to 30° C (86° F) prior to declaring the patient dead; prefer 32° C (89° F) if possible, "no one is dead, until they are warm and dead."
  - Laboratory studies: potassium, glucose (may be ↑), prothrombin time (PT)/partial thromboplastin time (PTT), fibrinogen, CBC, electrolytes, ABG
  - Classic ECG finding is the Osborne wave, seen at 30°

FROSTBITE

- Associated with tissue freezing and vascular disruption, caused by significant environmental cold stress associated with ↓ in blood flow to the involved skin and body area.

- **Superficial Frostbite**- involves skin and immediate underlying layers of subcutaneous tissue; no pain or sensation before rewarming. Usually have blister formation.
- **Deeper Frostbite**- involves skin, subcutaneous tissues and deeper structures- muscles, tendons, nerves, bones. No pain while frozen or even during rewarming process- usually no blister formation.
- Treatment:
  - Rewarm for 20-30 minutes for superficial and up to 1 hour for deep. Do not rewarm if there is a chance that additional freezing injury may occur.
  - Give IV pain medications prior to rewarming.
  - Use water that is 38–43° C for immersion therapy.
  - Td booster
  - Delayed amputation until tissue demarcation lines are determined.

HIGH ALTITUDE ILLNESS AND DYSBARISM

ACUTE MOUNTAIN SICKNESS (AMS)

- Most common type of altitude sickness.
- Highest incidence in 1–20 year old group.
- Onset: 6–24 hours after ascent and lasts up to 4 days.
- Starts at 8,000 feet, most people affected at 10,000 feet.
- Predisposing factors: rapid ascent, exercise, pre-existing lung disease or infection, previous episode of high altitude sickness.
- Physical Examination findings: ataxia, tachycardia, oliguria, and localized rales in 25–35%.
- **Symptoms**: nausea, vomiting, fatigue, headache (HA), irritability, shortness of breath (SOB).
- **Treatment**: usually self-limited, high carbohydrate diet, rest, hydration, no alcohol (ETOH) or smoking.
- **Prevention**: when climbing between 10–14,000 feet, take one day to ascend each 1,000 feet. Take 2 days for each 1000 feet above 14,000 feet.
  - Diamox- 5–10 mg/kg/24hours BID (adults 250 mg BID); start medications 24 hours before climb and continue for 2–3 days after reaching altitude
  - Decadron- 4 mg PO q 6 hours starting 48 hours before climb
  - Combination of the two agents

HIGH ALTITUDE PULMONARY EDEMA (HAPE)

- Symptoms: fatigue, nonproductive cough with dyspnea on exertion (DOE)→ productive cough with pink, frothy sputum, fever, confusion.
- Occurs 24–96 hours after arrival at altitude.
- Affects 10% of people above 14,500 feet.
- Predisposing factors: more common in kids (38%) and young adults, rapid ascent, exercise.
- **Laboratory studies**: ABG- respiratory alkalosis; urinalysis-proteinuria and high specific gravity; CBC hemoconcentration
- **Radiology/cardiac studies**: chest x-ray- diffuse patchy infiltrates; ECG -RV strain
- **Treatment:** Descent- as little as 1–2,000 feet can improve pulmonary status, rest, O_2, end expiratory positive pressure (EPAP) via Down mask- works via alveolar recruitment and can ↑ hemoglobin (HGB) O_2 saturation by 10%. Diuretics, digoxin, theophylline, steroids are not effective.
- **Prevention**: nifedipine may prevent HAPE and can also be used acutely. Other measures to prevent HAPE include the prophylactic use of acetazolamide or dexamethasone.

HIGH ALTITUDE CEREBRAL EDEMA (HACE)

- Most severe form of acute mountain sickness. Hypoxia → cerebral vasodilatation.
- Symptoms: severe headache, ataxia, hallucinations, lethargy, coma, death.
- Rare below 12,000 feet.
- Onset 2–3 days after ascent.
- **Diagnosis**: Head computed tomography (CT) reveals slit-like ventricles.
- **Treatment**: Rapid descent, O_2, elevate head of bed (HOB), intubate using vecuronium, pentothal, lidocaine. Decadron 4 mg q 6 hours. Diamox not helpful.

HIGH ALTITUDE RETINAL HEMORRHAGES
- Painless
- 50% of climbers above 16,000 feet and 100% above 21,000 feet.
- **Symptoms:** ↓ visual acuity (VA) may imply macular involvement, retinal hemorrhages. May be a warning sign of HACE.
- **Treatment:** Descent if there are visual changes.
- **Prevention:** 2–4 day stay at 5–7,000 feet for ultimate ascent to 8–14,000 feet, for ascent to 14–22,000 feet

additional 2–4 day stay at 10–12,000 feet. For > 14,000 feet, only ascend 1,000 feet per day with rest every other day.

AIR TRAVEL

- **Do not fly if:**
  - Unstable congestive heart failure (CHF)
  - Cyanotic heart disease
  - Acute pneumonia with borderline O$_2$ saturations at sea level
  - Pneumothorax or recent thoracic surgery ≤ 3 weeks
  - Abdominal or eye surgery ≤ 2 weeks
  - Newborns < 24 hours of age
  - Scuba diving ≤ 24 hours of flight
- **Relative contraindications:**
  - Sickle cell disease (SCD) or SC-Thalassemia – 20% will have vasoocclusive crisis at cabin pressures of 5,000 feet.
  - Anemia with Hgb < 7gm/dl
  - Acute otitis media (AOM) or sinusitis
  - Patients with cardiopulmonary disease can fly if sea level Pao$_2$ is 67 mmHg.

ANIMAL AND HUMAN BITES

OVERVIEW

- Boys are bitten by dogs twice as often as girls.
- The most common dog involved in bites is the German shepherd.
- The pit bull is implicated in over 70% of dog bite fatalities.
- Up to 60% of dog bites in children involve the head and neck region.
- Less than 5% of dog bites become infected.
- Cat bites and scratches cause less tissue damage than dog bites but are infected more often than dog bites. Girls are involved more often than boys.
- Deep tissue penetration can occur with cat bites due to their sharp teeth. Tendon sheaths of the hand or finger joints may be involved.
- For human bites, measure the distance between the center of the canine teeth (3rd tooth on each side of the lateral incisor). If the distance is > 3cm, the biter has permanent teeth.
- Intracranial involvement can occur with animal bites to the head particularly in infants.

- Wound infections are more common on the extremities. Puncture wounds account for up to 40% of infected wounds.
- The most common flora involved in dog and cat bite infections are *Pasteurella multocida* (most common) and *Staphylococcus aureus* with signs of infection developing within 72 hours of the injury.
- *Pasteurella* infections are more virulent and symptoms occur within 12–24 hours of the bite, while *S. aureus* infections occur later.
- Cat scratch disease occurs 3–50 days after a scratch and is accompanied by regional lymphadenopathy.
- The human mouth has many organisms including *Eikenella corrodens,* Streptococci, anaerobes and *S. aureus.*
- Human mouth bites of the hand often involve puncture of the joint space or extensor tendon of the hand by an incisor and are accompanied by high rates of infection.

MANAGEMENT

- Radiographs should be obtained if there is a deep wound or puncture of a joint space is suspected. Skull films should be considered in children with significant wounds on the scalp.
- Most bites should be left open; however, for cosmetic reasons bites on the face are often sutured after copious irrigation and within 6 hours of the bite. Deep puncture wounds especially from cats should not be closed.
- Td should be updated and the wound should be copiously irrigated using a high-pressure system.
- Bites involving the periorbital area should be referred to ophthalmology. Up to 40% of cat wounds close to the eye involve a corneal abrasion
- Prophylactic antibiotics are typically given for: hand wounds, deep puncture wounds, wounds that have sutures placed, and wounds in immunocompromised patients. Copious irrigation is essential.
- *Pasteurella* is penicillin-resistant and therefore treatment requires either a combination of penicillin and cephalexin or augmentin (amoxicillin/clavulanate). Trimethoprim/sulfa can also be used to cover for *Pasteurella* in patients with penicillin allergies.
- Patients with wounds that are not responding to outpatient management, or those who appear toxic on initial evaluation should be admitted and treated with IV antibiotics (nafcillin and penicillin).

VENOMOUS ANIMAL BITES AND STINGS

Type	Description	Clinical presentation	Management	Other

Crotalidae (Pit vipers)
 	
Rattlesnakes
    Copperheads
    Moccasins
	• Vertical elliptical pupils
	• Triangular head
	• Pit between eye & nostril
	• Venom = peptides + enzymes
		Local:
		• Tissue damage to vascular endothelial cells
		• Progressive edema and subcutaneous hemorrhage at bite site
		• RBC hemolysis and muscle cell necrosis
		Systemic:
		• ↓ Fibrinogen
		• ↓ Platelets
		• ↑ FSP*
		• DIC*
		Severe envenomation:
		• Hypotension
		• Acute renal failure
		• Pulmonary edema
		• Serum sickness
			• No tourniquet
			• Mark level of edema
			• Transport to nearest medical facility
			Labs:
			• CBC* + differential
			• Coagulation studies
			• FSP*
			• Fibrinogen
			• CK* (if severe)
			• Observe 6-8 hrs if asymptomatic
			• If envenomation confirmed; give antivenom
				• Copperhead is least toxic
				• If skin test +, dilute vials
				• H1 & H2 blockers
				• If anaphylactic shock:
				- Fluids
				- Colloids
				• Td updated
				• Snakes hibernate in winter (90% bites occur between April & October)
				• 40% nonaccidental (snake-handlers)

Elapidae (Coral Snakes)	• Round pupils • Yellow/red rings "Red on yellow, kill a fellow."	Neurotoxin: • Cranial nerve palsies • Mild bite site swelling	• Antivenom not always required • Antivenom is always required for any confirmed bite regardless of presence or lack of presence of symptoms • Supportive care: i.e.: (ETT)*; volume	• Found in Arizona & Southern gulf states
Latrodectus Black widow spider	• Black with red hour glass • 2 small fang marks • Venom: releases ACH*	• HA*, nausea/vomiting • Severe muscle cramps-paralysis • Systemic HTN* Upper extremity bite • Can cause respiratory distress Lower extremity bite • Abdominal pain/rigidity	• No labs indicated • Supportive care: - Valium - Analgesics • Antivenin if: - Severe cramps - HTN - Children < 6 years of age	• Severe in kids due to higher dose of venom relative to body size
Loxosceles reclusa Brown Recluse	• Brown with violin shaped mark • Usually painless bite • Venom: (Sphingomyelinase D): - Damages endothelium - RBC* hemolysis - Activates platelet thrombosis	• Causes local infarction/necrosis	Mild: • Resolves 5–7days Treatment: Corticosteroid Cream Severe: • Systemic-nausea, vomiting, fever, chills, muscle tissue Necrosis • DIC (rare) • Treatment: Dapsone debridement, plastic surgery repair	HBO* is experimental

(continued)

(continued)

Type	Description	Clinical presentation	Management	Other
Scorpions (Centruroides) Sculptured scorpion is only species dangerous to humans All other ones harmless	• Venom: releases ACH & norepinephrine • Lives in southwestern US & Mexico	• Cardiotoxic • Marked local hyperesthesia	Mild: • Cold compresses • Local injection of anesthetic • Monitor for several hours Severe: • ↑ HR* • CNS* stimulation – convulsions-Treatment: barbiturates • Muscle twitching & incoordination can cause respiratory compromise • HTN-Treatment: Hydralazine, Nifedipine	• No narcotics, may worsen dysrhythmias • Antivenom experimental in Arizona
Triatoma Kissing bug Texas bedbug	• Feed on vertebrate blood • Black- 2.5cm length long probosas	• Symptoms range from itching to severe anaphylaxis	• Cool compress • Corticosteroid cream (oral if moderate symptoms are present) • Oral antihistamines	• Sensitization increases with subsequent bites
Centipedes	• Cytolytic venom: - Phosphatase - Histamine - Serotonin	• Superficial necrosis • Nausea • Dizziness	• Symptomatic Care • Tetanus prophylaxis	• Venom not toxic, but can cause rhabdomyolysis & acute renal failure
Millipedes	• No venom apparatus	• Toxin causes contact dermatitis • "Mahogany discoloration" • Blepharospasm, conjunctivitis, periorbital edema, corneal ulceration may develop	• Copious irrigation; Treat as 2nd degree Chemical burn • Refer eye injury to ophthalmologist	
Coelenterata Jellyfish Anemones Corals	• Venom apparatus composed of nematocysts • Venom: proteins, histamines, catecholamines, heat stable	Mild: • Local reaction • Burning • Paresthesias-may progress to necrosis/ulceration Severe: • CNS- HA, vertigo, seizure, coma, paralysis	• Bathe in salt water (fresh activates!) • Vinegar inactivates nematocysts • Scrape off with razor/ knife • Treatment: topical corticosteroids, analgesics • Td update	• Cardiac dysrhythmias, respiratory failure (rare) • No antivenom for North American jellyfish, Portuguese man-of-war or sea-anemones
Echinodermata Starfish Sea urchin	• Spines may have venom	Local: • Burning pain • Rapid swelling • Redness • Pain Systemic: • Weakness • Syncope • Facial muscle paralysis • Respiratory failure	• X-ray: localize spine • Removal technique-controversial (Cautious of multiple small spines with invisible sheath) • Treatment-may need antibiotics if infection develops	• Must remove spines as they cause a foreign body reaction & infection • If spine penetrates joint-removal in operating room is necessary

Type	Description	Clinical presentation	Management	Other
Stingrays	• Venomous organ is on dorsal tail • Punctures feet • Venom: contains serotonin, PDE*, nucleotides	Local: • Barb pieces imbedded • Pain • Edema • Hemorrhage Systemic: • Muscle cramps • Nausea/Vomiting • Weakness • ↑ HR • ↓ BP*	• Copious irrigation • Hot water immersion-inactivates venom • Foreign body removal • Debridement • Supportive care	• Death (rare)
Scorpaenidae Sculpin Lionfish Stonefish	• Coastal waters (CA, FL, HI) • Venomous spine: heat labile protein-cardiotoxic	Local: • Ischemic & cyanotic (immediately) • Edema • Paresthesias • Necrosis Systemic: • GI* • CNS • CV*	• Copious irrigation • Hot water immersion-inactivates venom • Foreign body removal • Debridement • Supportive care	• Antivenom for stone fish

RBC = Red blood cell; FSP = Fibrin split products; DIC = Disseminated intravascular coagulation; CK = creatine kinase; ETT = Endotracheal tube; ACH = Acetycholine; HA = Headache; HTN = Hypertension; HBO = Hyperbaric O_2; PDE = phosphodiesterase; HR = Heart Rate; BP = Blood pressure; GI = Gastrointestinal; CNS = Central Nervous System; CV = Cardiovascular; CBC = Complete Blood Count

INHALATIONAL INJURIES

• **Types of Inhalants:**
   • Categorized by Gases, Smokes, Volatiles and Vapors
   • The most common agents that are abused are: glues, adhesives, nail polish removers, paints, gasoline, deodorants.
• **Stages of Pulmonary Injury after Smoke Inhalation:**
   • Respiratory insufficiency and bronchospasm at 1–12 hours after exposure
   • Pulmonary edema at 6–72 hours after exposure
   • Bronchopneumonia at >60 hours after exposure
• **Specific Inhalation Injuries:**
   • **Smoke**
      1. Thermal and toxic gases including carbon monoxide (CO) and cyanide.
      2. Most house fires occur at night between December and March.
      3. Mortality ranges from 45–78%.
      4. Toxicity is affected by heat (as low as 150° C may cause injury), particulate matter, and toxic gases (most common is CO)
      5. The upper and lower airways may be affected, resulting in respiratory failure, asphyxiation, and systemic poisoning.
      6. Evaluation should include an ABG with co-oximetry to check the carboxyhemoglobin level. The initial chest x-ray is an insensitive indicator of smoke injury.
      7. Management is supportive with humidified O_2, suctioning, and early airway support.
   • **Carbon Monoxide**
      1. An odorless, tasteless, and colorless gas
      2. Toxicity is associated with smoke injuries, heating equipment, and automobile exhaust.
      3. CO binds hemoglobin 230–270 times stronger than O_2 and children may have symptoms of syncope or altered mental status from levels as low as 18–24%.
      4. Although the child may have cyanosis or paleness, the classic presentation is the cherry-red color of the skin and mucous membranes.
      5. Retinal hemorrhages are occasionally seen with this poisoning. Immediate death may occur at levels of 70–80%.

6. Long-term complications involve neuropsychiatric problems.

7. Must measure with co-oximetry

8. Comparisons of levels with symptoms are not reliable in children.

9. The Pao$_2$ may be normal despite cyanosis in a patient.

10. **Management:**

   a. Delivery of 100% O$_2$, which ↓ the half-life of carboxyhemoglobin from 4–6 hours to 46–60 min

   b. Alternatively, a hyperbaric oxygen (HBO_chamber) reduces the half-life to 20–30 min; if available HBO should be used for symptomatic patients, pregnant patients, levels >25–30% or symptoms that fail to resolve with 100% O$_2$.

- **Hydrocarbon Aspiration**

1. Most hydrocarbons are derivatives of petroleum, but common childhood ingestions include kerosene and gasoline products that are left in nonsecure containers.

2. Toxicity is primarily dependent on the viscosity:

   a. The lower the viscosity, the higher risk of aspiration

   b. Mineral oil has a low viscosity

   c. Mineral seal oil and kerosene have moderate viscosity

   d. Gasoline and naptha have high viscosity.

   e. Patients with low viscosity hydrocarbon ingestion should not undergo gastric emptying due to the higher risk of aspiration

3. Side effects include:

   a. Aspiration pneumonitis (most common)

   b. CNS effects, dysrhythmias, and cardiomyopathy

   c. An ABG will demonstrate a normal Paco$_2$ with significant hypoxemia.

   d. CBC may demonstrate a leukocytosis with a left shift ≤ 1 hour of ingestion.

4. Management

   a. Supportive with O$_2$ and cutaneous decontamination

   b. All children with ingestion and suspicion of aspiration should be admitted for observation.

- **CHAMP mnemonic for hydrocarbons that should undergo GI decontamination:**

1. C-camphor containing compounds

2. H-halogenated hydrocarbons

3. A-aromatic hydrocarbons such as benzene

4. M-heavy metals such as lead, cadmium and selenium

5. P-pesticide-containing hydrocarbons

- **Chlorine Gas**

1. A yellow-green gas that destroys the mucous membranes on contact.

2. Diagnostic findings include:

   a. Lacrimation

   b. Rhinorrhea

   c. Conjunctival irritation

   d. Cough

   e. Sore throat

   f. Laryngeal edema

3. Onset may occur within minutes of the exposure

4. **Management** is supportive and decontamination

- **Solvent abuse**

1. Patients present with:

   a. Euphoria

   b. Headache

   c. Nausea/vomiting

   d. Slurred speech and ataxia (drunk appearance).

2. **Management** includes O$_2$, skin decontamination, and screening for methemoglobinemia

- **Ammonia**

1. Alkaline, colorless, and lighter than air

2. Most home products are 5–10% aqueous ammonia solutions and side effects are mostly local irritation and superficial mucosal membrane burns.

3. Ammonia causes a liquefactive necrosis and therefore high concentrations can result in airway irritation (upper airway edema, bronchospasm), chemical burns of the eyes, and partial or full-thickness skin burns.

4. Management

   a. Supportive with humidified O$_2$ or emergent intubation for severe cases.

   b. Some ENT physicians recommend steroids for the laryngeal edema.

   c. Skin and eye irrigation should be performed and an ophthalmologist should be consulted for eye burns.

RADIATION EXPOSURE

- Children are more vulnerable to radiation due to larger quantity of rapidly dividing cells.

- Types of radiation:
  - Nonionizing:
    1. Solar rays, microwaves, radio waves
    2. Can be harmful
    3. Do not cause radiation sickness or radioactive contamination
  - Ionizing:
    1. Nuclear weapons/reactors, x-ray machines
    2. Penetrating or nonpenetrating
    3. Damage by exposing DNA to free radicals

- Nausea, vomiting, malaise, depression of white cells/platelets
- Absolute lymphocyte count 48 hours after exposure to whole body irradiation is the best estimator of ultimate prognosis:
  1. If count >1200, prognosis good
  2. If count = 300–1200, prognosis fair
  3. If count <300, prognosis poor
- Complications
  - ↑Incidence of cancer (leukemia, thyroid, breast, head/neck), cataracts

Types	Characteristics	Examples	Effects of radiation
Alpha	• + Charge • Limited to epidermis • Not harmful • Travel few centimeters	• Plutonium • Uranium • Radium	• Generally not harmful
Beta	• Electrons • Travel few meters • Cause burns	• Tritium • C14 • Phosphorus	• Generally not harmful
Gamma	• Penetrate deeply • Main cause of radiation syndrome	• X-rays	• 75–125 rads-minimum dose that produces nausea/vomiting in 20% • 125–200 rads-lymphocyte depression of 50% by 48 hours • 240–340 rads-lymphocyte depression of >75% by 48 hours • 500 + rads- GI complications, death and bleeding • 5,000 + rads-CNS, GI, and CV involvement with death by 24–72 hours
Neutrons	• No electrical charge • Penetrate deep layers	• Nuclear reactors • Accelerators • Weapons	

- Clinical effects on CNS, GI, genetic, hematopoetic depend on:
  - Type and amount of radiation exposure
  - Length of exposure
  - Distance from radiation source
  - Type of shielding
  - Continuous versus intermittent exposure
- Definitions
  - Irradiation:
    1. Exposure to a source of radiation
    2. Does not cause patient to be overreactive
  - Contamination
    1. Deposition of radioactive material in or on the body
    2. Alpha, beta, and neutron effects
- Diagnostic Findings
  - The earlier the onset of symptoms, the greater the amount and length of exposure.

- ↓Life span
- Genetic mutations
- Management
  - Airway, breathing, circulation (ABCs)
  - Minimize internal contamination
  - Minimize spread of unsealed radioisotope contamination
  - Evaluate and treat acute radiation syndrome
  - Enter emergency room by separate door
  - Cover patient with sheet
  - Closed ventilation to room
  - Wear protective gear
  - Maximum exposure allowed per contact: 5 rems
- Contamination
  - External Contamination
    1. Removing clothing results in 70–90% decrease in radiation

2. Wash patient with warm water and soap, shampoo hair
3. Irrigate eyes, trim nails
4. Treat open wounds first

- **Internal Contamination**
  1. Gastric lavage or emesis followed by antacids
  2. Use of cathartics recommended
  3. Remove inhaled contaminants with bronchopulmonary lavage
  4. Chelation ethylene diamine tetraacetic acid (EDTA), diethylenetriamine pentaacetic acid (DTPA)
     a. Aluminum phosphate gel-star, BaSO4 or MgSO4 is used for S++Ra
     b. Prussian blue for cesium, rubidium and thallium
     c. Potassium iodide for radioactive iodide
     d. EDTA and penicillamine for radioactive lead
     e. DTPA for trasuranic metals

- **Disposition**
  - **Survival probable**
    1. No symptoms or mild symptoms that subside in few hours
    2. Exposure <200 rads
    3. Normal initial leukocyte count
  - **Survival possible**
    1. Exposure to 200–800 rads
    2. Nausea and vomiting brief 24–48 hours
    3. Asymptomatic after nausea/vomiting
    4. Later, thrombocytopenia, granulocytopenia, lymphopenia
    5. Admit for fluid and electrolyte monitoring
  - **Survival improbable**
    1. Exposure ≥ 800 rads
    2. Rapid onset of fulminant nausea/vomiting/diarrhea
    3. Dismal prognosis
    4. Death within 2–10 days

- **Basis for estimating exposure dose and prognosis**
  1. Type of exposing radiation (alpha, beta, gamma, neutron)
  2. Duration of exposure
  3. Distance between exposing agent and victim and amount of exposing agent present
  4. History of exposure
  5. Rapidity of onset of symptoms
  6. Type of symptoms
  7. Initial leukocyte count

INDEX